Electrophysical Agents

Electrophysical Agents

Evidence-Based Practice

THIRTEENTH EDITION

Edited by

Tim Watson, PhD, BSc, FCSP
Professor of Physiotherapy, Department of Allied Health Professions, Midwifery and Social Work University of Hertfordshire, Hatfield, UK

Ethne L. Nussbaum, PhD, MEd, BScPT
Adjunct Clinical Professor, Physical Therapy, Western University, London, Ontario
Adjunct Professor, Physical Therapy, University of Toronto, Ontario, Canada

ELSEVIER Edinburgh London New York Oxford Philadelphia St. Louis Sydney 2021

First edition 1948 as Clayton's Electrotherapy and Actinotherapy
Eighth edition 1981 as Clayton's Electrotherapy
Eleventh edition 2002 as Electrotherapy: Evidence-Based Practice
Twelfth edition 2008
Thirteenth edition 2021 as Electrophysical Agents: Evidence-Based Practice

---

Notices

ISBN: 978-0-7020-5151-7

Content Strategist: Poppy Garraway
Senior Content Development Specialist: Helen Leng
Publishing Services Manager: Shereen Jameel
Project Manager: Aparna Venkatachalam
Design: Margaret Reid
Illustration Manager: Muthukumaran Thangaraj
Marketing Manager: Ed Major

Printed in Great Britain

Last digit is the print number: 9 8 7 6 5 4 3

Working together to grow libraries in developing countries

www.elsevier.com • www.bookaid.org

CONTENTS

PREFACE

"If you can't explain it simply, you do not understand it well enough."

Albert Einstein

The new edition of this time-honoured text has been substantially revised. In the first instance, the title of the text is changed to reflect a global move away from the term 'Electrotherapy' to the more inclusive 'Electrophysical Agents'. Whilst the former term was historically taken to include all modalities utilized by therapists, agents such as ultrasound, laser (photobiomodulation), shockwave, vibration-based therapy, and many others, do not strictly fit under this label. The phrase Electrophysical Agents (some use Electrophysical Modalities) is technically more accurate and reflects a more inclusive range of agents including those that do not deliver electrical energy to the tissues.

The chapters which have been added to this revised edition reflect the widening scope of practice with these agents in the therapeutic environment. Existing chapters have been thoroughly revised to reflect the significant volume of evidence that has been published since the previous edition.

The structure of each of the modality chapters now follows a common format which will assist the reader searching for information. Following a brief introduction, any specific physical principles not covered in Chapter 2 are outlined. The biophysical effects are detailed, followed by a review of the therapeutic uses and then clinical application issues. The clinical evidence is critically reviewed, followed by a succinct summary and a full reference list for the papers cited. The weighting of the material is structured such that evaluation of the clinical evidence remains the most substantial section – thus reflecting the title of the text. Much as clinical application issues are addressed, this is not intended to be a 'how to do it' text – it is intended to take an objective and critical view of the available evidence and provide an informed guide to underpin practice, fully referenced for the reader.

Evidence-based practice (EBP) continues to dominate clinical practice across all health-related professions. The philosophy of the editors, and indeed, the chapter authors, is that this is a central tenet to modern practice. Whilst healthcare professionals' understanding of EBP has increased, there are numerous professional groups who are developing their use of these agents but whose exposure to them during their education may be limited. This text is aimed at multiple professions. Whilst historically, the use of these agents was dominated by the physiotherapy/physical therapy profession, this is no longer the case. The term 'therapist' is widely employed in this edition to reflect this shift.

Original research with EPAs is flourishing and there are substantially more systematic reviews and meta-analyses available to the clinician, student and researcher than there were 10 years ago. This is reflective of the research-led developments in our professional fields. There remain numerous gaps in our knowledge, and the editors and authors have striven to reflect not only the increased volume and quality of evidence, but to recognize where knowledge gaps persist. There is no attempt to 'paper over the cracks' or to imply that everything that needs to be known is now known.

Given the proliferation of pre-programmed, menu driven devices, it may be considered unnecessary to work through a text such as this. It is our view that the application of Electrophysical Agents as a component of a therapy programme should be based on a sound clinical decision-making process, tailored to the individual patient, taking into account their specific presentation and individual needs. There is no automatic programme or machine-driven menu system which can perform such a task. The knowledge, skill and clinical ability of the practitioner remains paramount. The material in this text aims to facilitate sound clinical decision making and thus improve patient care.

The widely cited quotation which leads the preface is not to be taken lightly. Most of us who are involved in education fully appreciate what Einstein meant. We have all sat through lectures and presentations by the most eminent in their field, only to walk away more confused than when we took our seat. Making a topic understandable – and thus, simply explained – does not mean that the authors of this material are being simplistic. Quite the reverse in fact. They are fully conversant with the complexities of their material. They are, however, making strenuous effort to make this material understandable and therefore useful to the student, the clinician, the researcher and the academic. This is no mean feat, and they are to be congratulated for their efforts.

The uptake and popularity of Electrophysical Agents varies between countries, between professional groups and across various clinical specialities. Whichever country, whichever profession and whichever clinical speciality you consider yourself part of, the evidence is the evidence, and this text aims to make it available to you in an accessible format. We trust that it might be of benefit to you and your patients.

Tim Watson and Ethne Nussbaum
September 2019

ACKNOWLEDGEMENTS

As with any multi author text of this size and complexity, there are a myriad of people who have made significant effort and whose efforts need to be acknowledged, and we would like to thank the following.

The authors and contributors of the chapters, without whom, the whole venture could not have been achieved. They have made strenuous efforts to critically review the evidence in their topic area, summarise that material and explain the complexities. They have accepted the suggestions that we made from the Editorial team with generosity of spirit and have been committed to our philosophy from the start of the project.

At Elsevier, there have been many individuals who have assisted greatly in getting the publication into its final form, but in particular, we are very grateful to Helen Leng and Poppy Garraway who have supported and assisted the planning process and facilitated production. Aparna Venkatachalam, Project Manager, has provided tenacious and detailed production support and we are immensely grateful for her attention to detail.

Our spouses, Hazel and John, who have endured prolonged Skype / WhatsApp conference calls, late nights and prolonged keyboard activity.

Colleagues in the EPA community – academics, researchers, clinicians – whose names may not appear later in the text, but whose willingness to participate in debate, discussion and deliberation is very much appreciated.

There are, no doubt, many others who could be mentioned, and we apologise if your being omitted by name causes offence – none is intended.

The students, post grads and PhDs, researchers, colleagues and patients who have, over the years asked questions which have (maybe unbeknown to them) prompted me to go away and find out something more, something new or set up another research programme.

Paul Standing and Jimmy Guest (Mr Guest to almost all of us!), both of West Middlesex Physiotherapy, and both sadly, no longer with us, were instrumental in my passion for the subject and tolerated my early inane questions and repeated abstract discussions. Professor John Mellerio at University of Westminster who woke up the researcher in me and encouraged a style of thinking that I value to this day.

-Tim-

I credit the physiotherapy faculty at Witwatersrand University, South Africa, for teaching me that practice decisions regarding electrophysical agents depended on the connectedness between patient's issues and the relevant anatomy, physiology and physical science. To a meaningful extent we practiced evidence based patient care long before such an approach assumed the aura of an obligation. Years later, in Toronto, Canada, despite as a new immigrant having no expectations of creating a professional niche for myself, I experienced ideal opportunities to practice alongside skilled evidence-based practitioners, to study further, conduct research and teach. The support, encouragement and challenges provided by my Canadian colleagues, clinical and academic, have carried me to this point. I thank them all.

-Ethne-

LIST OF CONTRIBUTORS

The editors would like to acknowledge and offer grateful thanks for the input of all previous editions' contributors, without whom this new edition would not have been possible.

Maryam M. Al-Mandeel, PhD
Assistant Professor
Physical Therapy
Kuwait University
Kuwait

Joseph Anthony, PhD, BPhty (Hons)
Associate Dean
Health Professions
Faculty of Medicine
Clinical Professor
Physical Therapy
The University of British Columbia
Vancouver, Canada

G. David Baxter, TD, BSc(Hons), DPhil, MBA, FCSP
Centre for Health
Activity and Rehabilitation Research
University of Otago
Dunedin, New Zealand

Chris Bleakley, BSc, PhD
Associate Professor
Physical Therapy
High Point University
North Carolina, USA

Sally Durham, MCSP
Clinical Specialist
Physiotherapist
Gait Laboratory
Queen Mary's Hospital
London, UK

Cliff Eaton, BSc(Hons), MSc
Clinical Specialist
Recovery Science
DJO Global
Guildford, UK

Jorge Fuentes C, MSc, PhD
Adjunct Professor
Department of Physical Therapy
Catholic University of Maule, Talca, Chile
Adjunct Assistant Professor
Rehab Med Faculty
University of Alberta
Edmonton, Canada

Gail ter Haar, MA, MSc, PhD, DSc
Professor
Division of Radiotherapy and Imaging
The Institute of Cancer Research
London, UK

Mark I. Johnson, PhD, BSc, PGCertHE
Professor
Centre for Pain Research
School of Clinical and Applied Sciences
Leeds Beckett University
Leeds, UK

Luther Kloth, BS, PT, MS, FAPTA, FACCWS
Professor Emeritus
Physical Therapy
Marquette University
Milwaukee
Wisconsin, USA

Binoy Kumaran, MSc, PgDip, FHEA, PhD
Research Fellow
Physiotherapy
Department of Allied Health Professions
Midwifery and Social Work
University of Hertfordshire
Hatfield, UK

Freddy Man Hin Lam, PhD, BScPT
Postdoctoral Fellow
Department of Medicine and Therapeutics
Faculty of Medicine
The Chinese University of Hong Kong
Hong Kong

John Leddy, BSc Physiotherapy
Sonographer
MSK Service
Circle MSK
Bedford, UK

Michael C. Lescallette, DPT, ECS, R.NCS.T#630
Senior Faculty
Education
The American Academy of Clinical Electrodiagnosis
Indiana, Pennsylvania, USA;
Drayer Physical Therapy Institute
Harrisburg, Pennsylvania

Mark Maybury, MSc Neuromusculoskeletal Health Care, BSc(Hons) Sports Science, BSc (Hons) Physiotherapy, PgD Biomechanics, PgD Medical Ultrasound (MSK)
NIHR Biomedial Research Centre Birmingham
Research Physiotherapist/MSK Sonographer
Rheumatology Research Group
Inflammation Research Facility
University of Birmingham Research Laboratories
University Hospitals Birmingham
Queen Elizabeth Hospital
Birmingham, UK

Ethne L. Nussbaum, PhD, MEd, BScPT
Adjunct Clinical Professor
Physical Therapy
Western University
London, Ontario;
Adjunct Professor
Physical Therapy
University of Toronto
Ontario, Canada

Marco Pang, BScPT, PhD
Professor
Department of Rehabilitation Sciences
Hong Kong Polytechnic University
Kowloon, Hong Kong

Anna Polak, PT, PhD
Associate Professor
Institute of Physioterapy and Health Sciences
The Jerzy Kukuczka Academy of Physical Education
Katowice, Poland;
Rehabilitation Center "Technomex"
Gliwice, Poland

Oscar Ronzio, PT, DHSc
Associate Professor
Department of Physical Therapy
Universidad Nacional Arturo Jauretche
Florencio Varela, Buenos Aires, Argentina
Head of Physical Therapy program
Universidad Maimónides
Ciudad Autónoma de Buenos Aires, Argentina

David M. Selkowitz, PT, PhD, DPT, OCS, DAAPM
Associate Professor
Department of Physical Therapy
MGH Institute of Health Professions
Boston, Massachusetts, USA

Kathleen A. Sluka, PT, PhD, FAPTA
Professor
Physical Therapy and Rehabilitation Science
Pain Research Program
University of Iowa
Iowa City
Iowa, USA

Sarah Taylor, MSc Clinical Sciences (Clinical Engineering), MEng Medical Engineering
Senior Clinical Scientist
Gait Laboratory
Queen Mary's Hospital
London, UK

Tim Watson, PhD, BSc, FCSP
Professor of Physiotherapy
Department of Allied Health Professions
Midwifery and Social Work
University of Hertfordshire
Hatfield, UK

Introduction to Scientific Concepts

Introduction and General Concepts

Tim Watson, Ethne L. Nussbaum

INTRODUCTION

Electrophysical agents (EPAs) have a long-established place in patient care; the first edition of *Clayton's Electrotherapy and Actinotherapy* was published in the UK in 1948 and an interesting historical review can be found in Kahn (1994). The most popular modalities used in current practice are in many respects quite dissimilar to those of 60 or more years ago though of course they are based on the same principles. Even in the last 10 years there has been a noticeable change in emphasis and delivery methods. The most striking change over time, however, is likely in the approach to their use: nowadays they are seen as an adjunct to treatment embedded within a comprehensive programme, rather than as a stand-alone solution to a clinical problem. There are instances where EPAs can be rightly considered to be the focus of the treatment, but this is arguably the exception rather than the rule.

Given that many of the EPAs that have been used in the past have waned in popularity, and that every year new machines and new 'treatments' come to the marketplace, it can be difficult for the therapist to know whether a 'new' treatment is in fact new, or just a revamped version of an existing intervention. New interventions and manipulation of existing treatments are often driven by a demand from patients and from manufacturers. Research is another driving force for change in practice; however, it is widely recognized that there are challenges when it comes to translating research into practice. To claim that all current EPA practice is 'evidence-based' would be naive, although there is room for debate as to what actually constitutes evidence-based practice. Some of these issues will be explored in this introductory chapter.

The evidence base for the implementation of EPAs is substantial, and many of the modalities have been exposed to rigorous evaluation. Some of the research can appear daunting, and a substantial proportion is not published in the therapy journals per se, which can make access more problematic, but the evidence is there. Searching for and evaluating the evidence is an integral part of evidence-based practice. This text attempts to present the evidence without bias. Readers will note that both positive and negative findings are reported. Parameters of application are based, to the extent possible, on research rather than on favourite approaches of the individual authors.

The most highly valued research is considered to be systematic reviews (SRs) with meta-analysis and review of reviews. However, in the field of EPAs, adopting the conclusions of authors of SRs might direct practitioners away from potentially beneficial treatments for some patients. EPAs can be applied with a bewildering array of parameters, particularly of energy dose. Therapies such as laser, ultrasound, shortwave and ultraviolet (UV) can be delivered at a level that changes cellular activity, involving enzymes and proteins that are substrates for healing, and generally stimulate cell metabolism. At a different level of delivery, the same modalities can kill bacteria, inhibit scar tissue and heat tissue to the point of modifying protein structure for the purpose of increasing tissue length. Modalities such as transcutaneous electrical nerve stimulation (TENS), Neuromuscular Electrical Stimulation, Interferential Current, and other types besides, can be delivered with a bewildering array of settings. The 'right' dosage is not necessarily the same for different stages of a patient's recovery – acute, subacute and chronic conditions present with different tissue problems, and therefore different treatment goals and, accordingly, different dosages when using EPAs to address the problems.

How does this relate to SRs? Unfortunately, there are too many meta-analyses involving the pooling of data among studies involving patient conditions, where there is no attempt to evaluate suitability of the treatment approach: for example, investigating ultrasound effectiveness on chronic shoulder stiffness, and including among other studies that use thermal ultrasound, a study that applies pulsed low dose ultrasound to an area about 200 cm^2 around the shoulder. Pooling a mix of data, as in this instance, is bound to lead to a conclusion that ultrasound is ineffective for shoulder injuries. And bias creeps into SRs simply by selecting inclusion and exclusion criteria that determine the outcome – it has been noted that authors who have performed SRs as well as their own research study in that field usually reach a conclusion in keeping with their own results. So should a clinician disregard SRs? Not at all; but it is unproductive to read SR abstracts only. Clinicians should evaluate details of every included study. Just because it is the conclusion of an SR does not mean that it is good enough evidence to underpin practice.

Not all Randomized Controlled Trial are well designed – some practitioners assume that if published, the research is good and the conclusion is to be believed. Sometimes papers get to press (i.e. into the journal) despite peer review. A study (Ainsworth et al 2007) considering the value of using ultrasound therapy as a component of shoulder pain treatment inadvertently makes this point. The randomized controlled trial was multicentred, double blind and placebo controlled. Patients were randomly allocated to receive manual therapy plus ultrasound or manual therapy with placebo ultrasound. All patients were provided with an exercise schedule and advice. The conclusion was that the addition of ultrasound did not significantly improve patient outcomes. It is only when one looks at the detail (rather than the abstract) that some of the issues begin to emerge: performing multicentre trials is an excellent way to achieve reasonable patient numbers – but the ultrasound 'dose' was determined by the individual therapists delivering the treatment. This is a reflection of a 'real world' situation – pragmatic trial – BUT the doses varied tremendously, as did the decision whether to use ultrasound or not. Eighty-eight percent of the treatment sessions used ultrasound (not 100% as one might expect; moreover, dose information was not available for about 25% of ultrasound treatments). The power output range was from 0.2–1.0 Wcm^{-2} (the strongest dose was therefore five times stronger than the weakest dose) and

at different frequencies (both 1 and 3 MHz), with differing treatment times (230% difference between the shortest and the longest treatments) and pulse regimens. The conclusions therefore are based on a (relatively) homogenous patient group but a heterogeneous intervention. In fairness, this study does not convincingly demonstrate a lack of benefit of ultrasound for this patient group.

In research, the treatment protocol is sometimes inappropriate to the condition at hand and yet the study is well powered and appears in an influential journal. For example, the VenUS III study, involving 337 patients, examined the effect of ultrasound on chronic venous ulcer healing and reported finding no benefit (Watson 2011). The outcome is not surprising given that treatment was applied once weekly for 12 weeks. The treatment frequency was likely totally inadequate to produce any effects. When treatment protocols stray far from usual practice (from clinical guidelines, expert opinion, RCTs, etc.) clinicians should be guarded with regard to weighing up the new evidence.

For those who wish to undertake their own evaluation of the literature, the chapters in this text are extensively referenced. In fact, the ideal would be for all readers to go back to the original papers and check them out. Some will do so – but rightly or wrongly, the majority will not. Many will accept that somebody has trawled through the material, evaluated it, ranked it, and presented it in a digestible format. Interestingly, for those who do explore the reference material, differences in interpretation will inevitably occur. The more people that access and read the original material, the more widespread the knowledge and the stronger the drive to change practice. EPAs are effective when used appropriately; used inappropriately, they may achieve nothing. If they are omitted from a therapist's practice, a patient may not in fact be receiving the best 'evidence-based' treatment. EPAs are not appropriate for all patients or necessary for the effective management of all clinical presentations. They have a place in the package of care alongside exercise, manual therapy, acupuncture and a wide range of other interventions. Their selection needs to be founded on the best evidence, and that is what this text aims to facilitate. Unfortunately, there remain substantial areas of EPA therapy where there is not a full range of research – so if we continue to deliver these therapies, are we delivering practice that is not evidence-based? Sackett suggests that it is not only RCTs that count:

"Evidence-based medicine is not restricted to randomised trials and meta-analyses. It involves tracking down the best external evidence with which to answer our clinical questions…and if no randomised trial has been carried out for our patient's predicament, we follow the trail to the next best external evidence and work from there."

By best available external clinical evidence we mean clinically relevant research, often from the basic sciences of medicine, but especially from patient centred clinical research.

Sackett et al 1996

From the published and experiential evidence, it appears that EPAs can be clinically effective and need not be written off as something that is 'old fashioned' and that no longer deserves a place in the therapeutic tool kit. That it can be applied in a clinically effective manner is evidenced in the chapters that follow. That it can also be delivered in an ineffectual manner is something that will be recognized by practitioners from many disciplines. The evidence would suggest that when the appropriate modality is applied at the 'right' dose for the presenting problem, it can make a significant contribution to the improvement and well-being of the patient. The fact that it does not work in all cases is not surprising at all. This would be a common feature of any therapy – whether manual therapy, exercise or drug therapy. There are patients who fail to respond to therapy A, but do very well with therapy B. The reasons for these individual differences are poorly understood, but certainly add to the richness of clinical experience. If therapy was simply a matter of applying the right recipe to the patient presenting with a given problem, clinical practice would lose a deal of its attractiveness. For any therapeutic intervention to be effective there is the need for a clear assessment, a rationalization of the problem(s), and the construction of a proposed treatment plan that matches the needs of the individual taking into account their holistic circumstances, not just their presenting signs and symptoms. The applied intervention is that which is deemed to be most likely to be effective. This is no guarantee that there will be 100% success, but the best odds for a beneficial outcome. The thinking therapist then re-evaluates the outcomes as the treatment progresses, modifying the treatment package in the light of these results.

One of the problems with the research applicable to EPAs, as well as in other fields, is that the research tends to be somewhat reductionist in approach. A clinical trial that evaluates, for example, the effect of ultrasound for patients with a tear of the medial collateral ligament of the knee, aims to construct a methodology that readily identifies the contribution that ultrasound makes to the clinical outcome. By keeping all other treatment parameters 'constant' – the advice, exercise, manual therapy, environment, number of treatment and treatment intervals – the real effect of the ultrasound therapy can be evaluated.

The clinical reality is that it is the *package* of care that is clinically effective, rather than any one individual component of it. If a patient has received several forms of intervention (e.g. electrotherapy, manual therapy and exercise coupled with appropriate advice and education) and comes back for the next session with an improvement, it is extraordinarily difficult to know which elements of the treatment package were responsible for the change. It could be that all were necessary in that particular combination; it could be that one could have been safely omitted and the equivalent outcome would have been achieved.

When making a clinical decision, practitioners will put together the package that in their opinion is most likely to be effective for that patient. Some patients will not take advice well, others will almost certainly not undertake the exercises that are suggested, and others might have a strong aversion to the idea of electrical stimulation. The effective package is the one that matches the patient's presentation and the treatment context. Some patients might be treated several times a week whereas others can only be seen once every 2 or 3 weeks on a 'check-up' basis. Package tailoring is an essential skill for any therapist.

The current stage of research in EPAs is still at the point where the building blocks of these packages are being evaluated. We might know, in absolute terms, the effect of this particular treatment, at this particular dose on a specific problem in a controlled research environment. We might not know what happens when the same therapy is used in a different combination – there are almost too many variables to evaluate at the current time.

The research evidence suggests that EPAs can be effective as an element of treatment. Further work is needed to evaluate the combinations – or treatment packages – that are most effective. Practitioners will have, from their own experience, ideas about combinations that are more or less effective. This is the source of the richness of therapeutic experience and until substantially more work has been completed – both in the laboratory and in clinical practice, using reductionist, holistic and pragmatic methodologies – the full story is unlikely to emerge.

The intention of this publication is to provide a review of the background, evidence and clinical applicability of various modalities. The authors of each chapter are writing because they know their subject and, although there might be gaps in the knowledge that deserve to be filled, there is sufficient evidence out there from which clinical decision making can be enhanced and further developments achieved.

CURRENT CONCEPTS IN ELECTROPHYSICAL AGENTS

There has been a progressive shift over recent years away from the term 'electrotherapy' towards a more encompassing term 'electrophysical agents'. There are several reasons for this, but to a great extent, it relates to the fact that 'electrotherapy' in the strictest sense relates to the delivery of electrical energy and therefore interventions such as therapeutic ultrasound, laser therapy and shockwave therapy would be excluded from this grouping. Classification of EPAs is not straightforward because no matter which classification one uses, there is no one correct way to divide and categorize the modalities. One could, for example, use a thermal/non-thermal division, but reading the literature on thermal versus non-thermal versus microthermal treatments will soon demonstrate that this is an almost certainly flawed proposition. One could attempt to categorize by type of applied energy: light (e.g. laser, ultraviolet) versus electrical stimulation (e.g. TENS, interferential) versus the high-frequency radiations (shortwave, microwave). Therapeutic ultrasound would have to sit in a category of its own, and diagnostic ultrasound would seemingly not belong anywhere because ultrasound images inside the body are captured in real-time as a result of reflection of high-frequency ultrasound waves off the body structures. This division could also be challenged in that, for example, the effects of continuous shortwave are similar but clinically different from those of pulsed shortwave. The fundamental energy might be the same but the mode of delivery makes a substantial difference to the treatment outcome.

Furthermore, there is an issue with the inclusion of 'new' therapies into the classification. Magnetic therapy is a swiftly developing field although, one would suggest, still in its clinical infancy. Should it have a category of its own or should it incorporate with shortwave that also employs an electromagnetic field

The modalities covered in this text include those that are in common clinical use, and have been divided where feasible into sections that reflect the type of energy employed, for example, the thermal energies are grouped as are various forms of electrical stimulation. The grouping of non-thermal and microthermal EPAs (laser, ultrasound, etc.) does not imply a common energy type or mode of action, but rather their individuality.

MODELS OF ELECTROPHYSICAL AGENTS

All EPAs – whether in current use, abandoned from the past or yet to be 'invented' – actually follow a very straightforward model that is presented in subsequent section. It is sufficiently robust to explain current practice, yet sufficiently flexible to incorporate future developments. It has been refined over the years and will almost certainly be subject to further refinement in the future.

In principle, the model identifies that the delivery of energy from a machine or device is the starting point of the intervention (Fig. 1.1). The energy entry to the tissues results in a change in one or more physiological events.

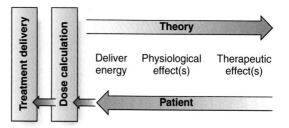

Fig. 1.1 A simple model of electro therapy.

Some are very specific whereas others are multifaceted. The capacity of the energy to influence physiological events is key to the ensuing processes and will be reflected throughout this publication. The physiological shift that results from the energy delivery is used in practice to generate what is commonly referred to as a therapeutic effect.

This is a fairly classical learning sequence for many therapists. One learns what the energy is, where it goes, what it does when it gets there and what the outcome might be. One has to learn the material somehow, and this is possibly as good a way as any.

The clinical application of the model is best achieved by what appears to be a reversal of this process. Start with the patient and their problems, which are identified from the clinical assessment. Once the problems are known, the treatment priorities can be established and the rationale for the treatment determined. Knowing what it is that is intended to be achieved generates the target for the intervention. Moving one step back through the model, the question then arises: 'If that is the intended outcome or therapeutic effect, which physiological process(es) need to be stimulated, modified or affected in order for the outcome to be achieved?' Once the physiological changes are established, one further step back through the model will enable the determination of the most appropriate modality that can be used to achieve this effect, based on the best available evidence. If, for example, the patient presents with a chronic hamstring muscle tear, with pain, disturbed movement patterns and functional difficulty, the clinician and patient together should then decide what needs to be changed, stimulated or activated to get a clinically beneficial outcome. Once this is decided, it is a matter of deciding from the evidence whether any particular modality would be a critical factor in achieving the desired outcome, or at least would accelerate the achievement of these results. It might be that EPAs have no role in the management of this particular patient.

The effects of EPAs appear to be modality dependent. The primary decision that has to be made is critical, in that some modalities have a limited subset of effects that are fundamentally different from another modality. They are not necessarily interchangeable, although they might be.

Having identified the modality that is best able to achieve the effects required, the next clinical stage is to make a 'dose' selection. Not only is it critical to apply the right modality, but it needs to be applied at the appropriate 'dose' for maximal benefit to be achieved. There is a substantial and growing body of evidence that the same modality can be applied at different doses and the results will not be the same. An obvious example might be laser therapy. Applied at a low dose, laser has effects that are harnessed by therapists when treating a variety of open wounds and musculo-skeletal tissue problems. Applied at a higher dose, the same light energy is used by the surgeon as a means to ablate or vaporize tissue. The energy might be the same, but the dose is different and the outcome is easily distinguished.

One might argue that this is an extreme example, which in some ways it is, but the point is that the effects of the therapy are both modality and dose dependent. There are 'therapeutic windows' when using modalities (as there are in almost all therapeutic interventions) and, to achieve the 'best' outcome, it is essential to get as close to this window as one possibly can. The theory of these windows will be briefly explored in the next section.

This fundamental model could be applied to many interventions: drug therapy, manual therapy, exercise therapy, etc. In this respect, therefore, EPAs are similar to other interventions in the treatment realm. It is a tool that, when applied at the right time, at the right dose and for the right reason, has the capacity to be beneficial. Applied inappropriately, it is not at all surprising that it has the capacity to achieve nothing. The skilful practitioner uses the available evidence combined with experience to make the best possible decision taking into account the psycho-social and holistic components of the problem – it is not a simple reductionist solution.

ELECTROTHERAPEUTIC WINDOWS

Windows of opportunity are topical in many areas of medical practice and are not a new phenomenon at all. It has long been recognized that the 'amount' of a treatment is a critical parameter. This is no less true for EPAs than for other interventions. Literally hundreds of research papers illustrate that the same modality applied in the same circumstances, but at a different 'dose', will produce a different outcome. The illustrations used in this section are deliberately taken from cell, animal and clinical research studies to illustrate the breadth of the principle. Furthermore, the examples used are not intended to criticize the researchers reporting these results. Knowing where the window 'is not' is possibly as important as knowing where it is.

Given the research evidence, there appear to be several aspects to this issue. Using a very straightforward model, there is substantial evidence, for example, that there is an *amplitude window* or *strength window*. An energy delivered at a particular amplitude has a beneficial effect, whereas the same energy at a lower amplitude might have no demonstrable effect. The laser example above is a simple extension of this case – one level will produce a distinct cellular response whereas a higher dose can be considered to be destructive. (Karu 1987) demonstrated and reported these principles related to laser energy. The concept is included in the laser review by Tumilty et al (2010) and the research reported by Vinck et al (2003).

There are many examples of amplitude windows in the electrotherapeutic-related literature, and in some instances, the researchers have not set out to evaluate window effects but have none the less demonstrated their existence. Papers by Larsen et al (2005) measuring ultrasound parameter manipulation in tendon healing, Aaron et al (1999) investigating electromagnetic field strengths, Goldman et al (1996) considering the effects of electrical stimulation in chronic wound healing, Zhang et al (2014) and Speed (2014) relating to shockwave use, Rubin et al (1989) investigating electromagnetic field strength and osteoporosis and Cramp et al (2002) comparing different forms of TENS and its influence on local blood flow all provide evidence in this field. Hughes et al (2013) and Johnson (2014) provide supporting evidence relating to frequency based evidence pertaining to TENS clinical use. A summary of the evidence is considered in Watson and Goh (2015) – relating the principle to the oft cited 'Goldilocks principle'.

Along similar lines, *frequency windows* are also apparent. A modality applied at a specific frequency (pulsing regimen) might have a measurable benefit, whereas the same modality applied using a different pulsing profile might not appear to achieve equivalent results.

Electrical stimulation frequency windows have been proposed and there is clinical and laboratory evidence to suggest that there are frequency-dependent responses in clinical practice. TENS applied at different frequencies appears to produce different outcomes in an equivalent patient population. Studies by Han et al (1991), Kararmaz et al (2004) and Sluka et al (2005) are among the many that have demonstrated frequency-dependent effects of TENS. Several authors have appeared to demonstrate that frequency parameters are possibly less critical, especially in clinical practice, and Chapters 15 and 18, on TENS and interferential therapy, include useful discussion on these issues. Frequency windows are not confined to TENS treatments and there are examples from other areas, including electromagnetic fields (Blackman et al 1988), ultrasound (Schafer et al 2005), laser (Nussbaum 2002) and interferential (Noble et al 2000).

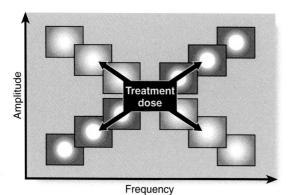

Fig. 1.2 Basic windows of opportunity.

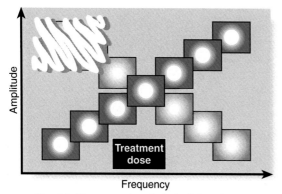

Fig. 1.3 Treatment dose 'missing' the window.

A simple therapeutic windows model is illustrated in Fig. 1.2, using amplitude and frequency as the critical parameters. The figure shows that the 'ideal' treatment dose would be that combination of modality amplitude and frequency contained in the central effective zone. It can be suggested (from the evidence) that if the right amplitude and the right frequency are applied at the same time, then the maximally beneficial effect will be achieved. Unfortunately, there are clearly more ways to get this combination 'wrong' than 'right'. A modality applied at a less than ideal dose will not achieve best results. Again, this does not mean that the modality is ineffective, but more likely, that the ideal window has been missed. The same principle can be applied across many, if not all areas of therapy.

In Fig. 1.3, the most effective treatment window (black box, lower central) has clearly been missed by the delivered treatment (upper left) and hence whatever the effect of the therapy, it will fail to be maximally effective.

The situation is complicated by the apparent capacity of the windows to 'move' with the patient's condition. The position of the therapeutic window in the acute scenario appears to be different from the window position for the patient with a chronic version of the same problem. A treatment dose that might be very effective for an acute problem may fail to be beneficial with a chronic presentation.

In Fig. 1.4, the effective 'acute window' shown in the left-hand picture is in a different position to the most effective 'chronic window' shown in the right-hand picture. A consideration of a dose-response curve is illustrated in Fig. 1.5.

Given the rapidly increasing complexity seen in this simple two-parameter model (amplitude and frequency) with two levels of condition (acute and chronic), it is easy to see how difficult clinical reality might be. As the volume of published work continues to increase, new results can be included in the existing framework, and this helps to identify where the windows are (positive research outcomes) and where they are not (negative outcomes). If this methodology is pursued, it is interesting to note how the effective treatments cluster when plotted, adding weight to the therapeutic windows theory.

Assuming that there are likely to be more than two variables to the real-world model, some complex further work needs to be invoked. There is almost certainly an energy- or time-based window (e.g. Hill et al 2002) and then another factor based on treatment frequency (number of sessions a week or treatment intervals). Work continues in our own, and other, research units to identify the more and less critical parameters for each modality across a range of clinical presentations.

One research style that has proved to be helpful in this context is to test a treatment on non-injured subjects in the laboratory using a variety of doses, and then to take the same protocol out into the clinical environment and repeat the testing procedure with real patients with particular clinical problems. Preliminary results indicate that there are distinct differences between the responses on 'normal' and 'injured' tissues at equivalent doses and further work is essential to maximize our understanding of these behaviours. Research that demonstrates significant effect in a laboratory study might, or might not, transfer directly to the clinical environment. Work with pulsed shortwave therapy (Al Mandil & Watson 2006) clearly demonstrated a different magnitude of physiological effect when the same 'treatment' was delivered to asymptomatic subjects in the laboratory and real patients in a clinical setting: the physiological changes were similar, but of a different magnitude.

CLINICAL DECISION MAKING USING ELECTROPHYSICAL AGENTS

When it comes to making a decision with regard to EPAs as a component of treatment (and taking into account the issues discussed in previous sections', the first determination

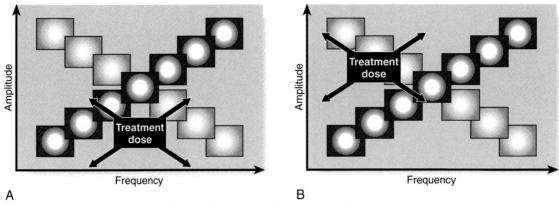

Fig. 1.4 Moving acute (A) and chronic (B) windows.

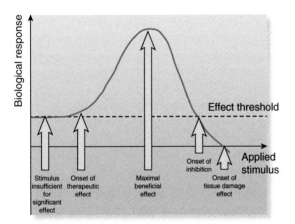

Fig. 1.5 A general dose-response curve which can be applied to all electrophysical agents (EPAs).

needs to be which modality to use; the secondary decision, although still of importance, is that of dosage.

This having been said, it is important to remember that in clinical practice an EPA is a component of a whole treatment programme. Modalities may well have been overused in the past; currently, however, their incorporation into practice is more evidence-based and selective, and hence should be more effective.

The detailed chapters in this text examine the evidence base for each of the included modalities and, within that evidence, the areas where the modality has the capacity to be effective and those where there is insufficient evidence at the present time. A commonly cited phrase that is important in this context relates to the difference between a *lack of evidence* as opposed to an *evidence of lack*; in other words, there are many areas of practice, including several areas involving EPAs, where there is a substantial lack of evidence – it is simply not there – whereas in other areas

there is evidence that demonstrates a lack of effect. In the former circumstance, the clinician might have to make a clinical decision based on experience and expert opinion in the absence of published research. In the latter circumstances, the clinician who takes account of the available evidence would refrain from adopting that particular clinical approach in favour of another.

If it were a matter of learning a set of rules or guidelines, the use of EPAs in practice might appear to be somewhat simpler but, in reality, there are no rule sets that would govern every possible clinical scenario, and therefore clinical decision making remains an art with a scientific bias, or a science with an integrated art, depending on which philosophy you follow. Whichever one of these it is, the employment of EPAs into current clinical practice cannot be reduced to a simple rule set. The evidence will continue to close the gaps, although, inevitably, by closing down one gap, another will become apparent, and hence further research will be needed.

The individual chapters in this text aim to identify the key issues about each modality, examine the evidence for their effects and relate this to clinical practice. None of the chapters aims to provide clinical recipes, but will enable practitioners to evaluate the available evidence in order to facilitate their clinical decision making.

CONCLUSION

Incorporation of EPA modalities into clinical management can result in significant benefit for the patient. Used unwisely, it is at best an inefficient use of resources and at worst, can easily have effects that are neither wanted nor beneficial. Critical thinking, an understanding of the capacity of the various modalities to influence the tissues combined with other critically appraised aspects of practice, such as manual therapy and exercise therapy, can result in gains for the patient. Patients who are routinely denied EPA modalities because the clinician does not believe them to be effective would seem, based on the evidence presented in this text, to be denied potential benefit.

REFERENCES

Aaron, R. K., Ciombor, D. M., Keeping, H., et al. (1999). Power frequency fields promote cell differentiation coincident with an increase in transforming growth factor-beta(1) expression. *Bioelectromagnetics, 20*(7), 453–458.

Al-Mandeel, M., & Watson, T. (2006). An evaluative audit of patient records in electrotherapy with specific reference to pulsed short wave therapy (PSWT). *International Journal of Rehabilitation Research, 13*(9), 414–419.

Blackman, C. F., Benane, S. G., Elliott, D. J., et al. (1988). Influence of electromagnetic fields on the efflux of calcium ions from brain tissue in vitro: a three-model analysis consistent with the frequency response up to 510 Hz. *Bioelectromagnetics, 9*(3), 215–227.

Cramp, F. L., McCullough, G. R., Lowe, A. S., et al. (2002). Transcutaneous electric nerve stimulation: The effect of intensity on local and distal cutaneous blood flow and skin temperature in healthy subjects. *Archives of Physical Medicine and Rehabilitation, 83*(1), 5–9.

Goldman, R., & Pollack, S. (1996). Electric fields and proliferation in a chronic wound model. *Bioelectromagnetics, 17*(6), 450–457.

Han, J. S., Chen, X. H., Sun, S. L., et al. (1991). "Effect of low- and high-frequency TENS on Met-enkephalin-Arg-Phe and dynorphin A immunoreactivity in human lumbar CSF." *Pain, 47*(3), 295–298.

Hill, J., Lewis, M., Mills, P., et al. (2002). Pulsed short-wave diathermy effects on human fibroblast proliferation. *Archives of Physical Medicine and Rehabilitation, 83*(6), 832–836.

Hughes, N., Bennett, M. I., & Johnson, M. I. (2013). An investigation into the magnitude of the current window and perception of transcutaneous electrical nerve stimulation (TENS) sensation at various frequencies and body sites in healthy human participants. *Clinical Journal of Pain, 29*(2), 146–53.

Johnson, M, I. (2014). *Transcutaneous Electrical Nerve Stimulation (TENS): Research to support clinical practice.* Oxford University Press.

Kahn, J. (1994). Principles and Practice of Electrotherapy, Churchill Livingstone.

Kararmaz, A.S, .Kaya, H.Karaman and S. Turhanoglu2004). "Effect of the frequency of transcutaneous electrical nerve stimulation on analgesia during extracorporeal shock wave lithotripsy." *Urol Res, 32*(6), 411–415.

Karu, T. I. (1987). Photobiological fundamentals of low power laser therapy. *IEEE Journal of Quantum Electronics, 23*(10), 1703–1717.

Larsen, A., Kristensen, G., Thorlacius-Ussing, O., et al. (2005). The influence of ultrasound on the mechanical properties of healing tendons in rabbits. *Acta Orthopaedica, 76*(2), 225–230.

Noble, J. G., Henderson, G., Cramp, A. F., et al. (2000). The effect of interferential therapy upon cutaneous blood flow in humans. *Clinical Physiology, 20*(1), 2–7.

Nussbaum, E. L., Lilge, L., & Mazzulli, T. (2002). Effects of 630-, 660-, 810-, and 905-nm laser irradiation delivering radiant exposure of 1–50 J/cm^2 on three species of bacteria in vitro. *Journal of Clinical Laser Medicine & Surgery, 20*(6), 325–333.

Rubin, C. T., McLeod, K. J., Lanyon, L. E., et al. (1989). Prevention of osteoporosis by pulsed electromagnetic fields. *Journal of Bone and Joint Surgery, 71*(3), 411–417.

Sackett, D. L., Rosenberg, W. M., Gray, J. A., Haynes, R. B., & Richardson, W. S. (1996). Evidence based medicine: What it is and what it isn't. *British Medical Journal, 312*(7023), 71–72.

Schafer, S., Kliner, S., Klinghammer, L., et al. (2005). Influence of ultrasound operating parameters on ultrasound-induced thrombolysis in vitro. *Ultrasound in Medicine & Biology, 31*(6), 841–847.

Sluka, K. A., Vance, C. G., Lisi, T. L., et al. (2005). High-frequency, but not low-frequency, transcutaneous electrical nerve stimulation reduces aspartate and glutamate release in the spinal cord dorsal horn. *Journal of Neurochemistry, 95*(6), 1794–1801.

Speed, C. (2014). A systematic review of shockwave therapies in soft tissue conditions: Focusing on the evidence. *British Journal of Sports Medicine, 48*(21), 1538–1542.

Tumilty, S., Munn, J., McDonough, S., Hurley, D. A., Basford, J. R., & Baxter, G. D. (2010). Low level laser treatment of tendinopathy: A systematic review with meta-analysis. *Photomedicine and Laser Surgery, 28*(1), 3–16.

Vinck, E. M,. Cagnie, B. J., Cornelissen, M. J., et al. (2003). Increased fibroblast proliferation induced by light emitting diode and low power laser irradiation. *Lasers in Medical Science, 18*(2), 95–99.

Watson, J. M., Kang'ombe, A. R., Soares, M. O., et al. (2011). Use of weekly low dose high frequency ultrasound for hard to heal venous leg ulcers: The VenUS III randomised controlled trial. *British Medical Journal, 342*, d1092.

Watson, T., Goh, A. C. (2015). *Dose dependency with electro physical agents: both the Arndt Schulz law and the Goldilocks principle provide an explanatory model.* World Confederation Physical Therapy Congress 2015, Singapore, Physiotherapy.

Zhang, X., Yan, X., Wang, C., Tang, T., & Chai, Y. (2014). The dose-effect relationship in extracorporeal shock wave therapy: The optimal parameter for extracorporeal shock wave therapy. *IEEE Journal of Quantum Electronics, 186*(1), 484–492.

Biophysical and Physiological Constructs

Physical Principles of Sound, Electricity and Magnetism

Gail ter Haar

INTRODUCTION

Electrophysical agents are used by physiotherapists to treat a wide variety of conditions. These agents include both electromagnetic and sound waves, in addition to muscle- and nerve-stimulating currents. In part, these techniques are used to induce tissue heating. This chapter contains, in simple terms, an introduction to the effects of heat on tissue and the basic physics necessary for the understanding of the remainder of the book.

For centuries, early philosophers speculated on the nature of heat and cold. Opinions were divided as to whether heat was a substance or an effect of the motion of particles, but in the eighteenth century, physicists and physical chemists came to the conclusion that what gave our senses the impression of heat or cold was the speed of motion of the constituent molecules within the body or object. An accurate investigation of the relationship between the work done in driving an apparatus designed to churn water, and the heat developed while doing so, was undertaken by Dr JP Joule of Manchester in 1840. He showed quite clearly that the amount of heat produced by friction depended on the amount of work done. Subsequently, his work also contributed to the theory of the correlation of forces and, in 1847, he stated the law of the conservation of energy (the basis of the first law of thermodynamics).

It became the accepted view that heat can be regarded as a form of energy that is interchangeable with other forms, such as electrical or mechanical energy. The theory supposed that, when a body is heated, the rise in temperature is due to the increased energy of motion of molecules in that body. The theory went further and explained the transmission of radiant energy from one body to another, as from the sun to an individual on earth. Evidence was found in favour of the supposition that light is an electromagnetic wave, and exactly the same evidence was adduced with regard to radiant energy. Apart from the fact that radiant heat waves (e.g. infrared radiations) have a longer wavelength than light waves, their physical characteristics are the same. It was therefore suggested that the molecules of a hot body are in a state of rapid vibration, or are the centre of rapid periodic disturbances, producing electromagnetic waves, and that these waves travel between the hot body and the receiving body, causing a similar motion in its molecules. The sensation of heat may thus be excited in an organism by waves of radiant heat energy that emanate from a hot object, just as the sense of sight is excited by waves of light that arise from a luminous object.

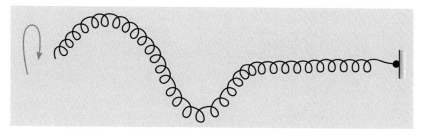

Transverse wave

Fig. 2.1 If a spring that is attached at one end is flicked up and down, a transverse wave is produced.

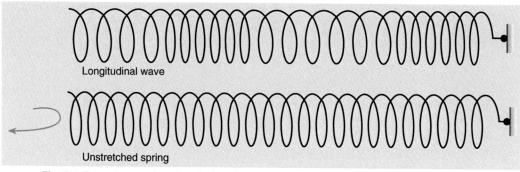

Longitudinal wave

Unstretched spring

Fig. 2.2 Extending a spring along its length and letting it go again produces a longitudinal wave.

An understanding of wave motion is central to getting to grips with the physics of any form of therapy that uses either electrical or mechanical energy. Therefore, a general description of wave motion here precedes more detailed treatment of electricity and magnetism, and of ultrasound.

WAVE MOTION

Wave motion transfers energy from one place to another. Think of a cork floating in a pond into which a stone is dropped. Ripples move out from where the stone enters the water and some of the stone's energy is transferred to the pond's edge. The cork bobs up and down but does not move within the pond.

An easy way to demonstrate wave motion is to use a Slinky spring toy. Two types of wave exist: *transverse waves*, which can be mimicked by raising and lowering one end of the spring rapidly, as shown in Fig. 2.1, and *longitudinal waves*, which can be demonstrated by extending the spring along its length and then letting it go (Fig. 2.2). Water waves, the motion of a violin string and electromagnetic waves – as used in short-wave diathermy, infrared and interferential current therapy – are examples of transverse waves. Sound, as used in ultrasound therapy, propagates in soft tissues mainly as longitudinal waves.

It is much more difficult to picture a longitudinal wave than a transverse wave. If the spring with the wave travelling down it (Fig. 2.2) is compared with an unstretched spring, some regions can be seen where the coils are closer together, and other regions where the coils are further apart. The part of the spring where the coils are closely spaced is called a region of *compression*, and the region where they are separated more widely is the *rarefaction* region.

Waves on the sea are generally described in terms of peaks and troughs. The movement up to a wave crest, down to a trough, and back up to the crest again is known as a *cycle of oscillation*. A cork floating in the sea bobs up and down as the waves go past. The difference in height of the cork between a crest and a trough is twice the *amplitude*. Perhaps a simpler way of visualizing the amplitude is as the difference in water height above the seabed between a flat, calm sea and the crest of the wave. The number of wave crests passing the cork in a second is the wave *frequency* (f). Frequency is measured in *Hertz* (Hz), where 1 Hz is 1 cycle/second. The time that elapses between two adjacent wave crests passing the cork is the

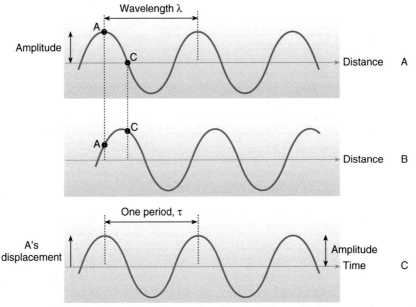

Fig. 2.3 Parts (A) and (B) show the position of two points A and C in the path of a wave as it passes through. The displacements shown are frozen at two different times, between which the wave has moved on a fraction of a wavelength. (C) shows the displacement of the point during two cycles.

period (τ) of the oscillation. This has units of time: if each cycle takes τ seconds, there must be $1/\tau$ cycles in each second. The number of cycles that occur in a second has already been defined as the frequency, and so can be written as follows:

$$f = 1/\tau \qquad [1]$$

$$\tau = 1/f \qquad [2]$$

The distance between two adjacent wave crests is the *wavelength* (λ).

Fig. 2.3A and B shows a wave frozen at two moments, a short time apart. It can be seen that the different points on the wave have changed position relative to the central line but have not moved in space. In fact, if you tracked the motion of point A over several periods, the movement up and down would look like the picture shown in Fig. 2.3C. The speed at which the wave crests move is known as the wave *speed*. As the wave moves a wavelength (λ) in one cycle, and as one cycle takes a time equal to the period τ, then the wave speed (c) is given by the equation:

$$c = \lambda/\tau \qquad [3]$$

It is known that $1/\tau$ is the same as the frequency f, and so:

$$c = f\lambda \qquad [4]$$

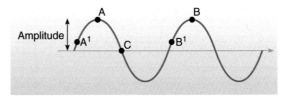

Fig. 2.4 Points A and B, and also A^1 and B^1, are always in the same relative position in the wave. They are in phase. Points A and C are out of phase.

In Fig. 2.4, points A and B on the wave (or, equally, A^1 and B^1) are moving in the same way and will reach the crest (or trough) together. These points are said to be in *phase* with each other. The movement from A to B (or A^1 to B^1) represents one cycle of the wave motion. A and C, however, are not in phase: C is a quarter of a cycle ahead of A and they are said to have a *phase difference* (ϕ) of a quarter cycle. Phase is usually expressed as an angle, where a complete cycle is 2π radians (or 360°). A quarter cycle therefore represents a phase difference of $\pi/2$ radians (90°). This is illustrated in Fig. 2.5.

Reflection and Refraction of Waves

When waves travelling through a medium arrive at the surface between two media, some of the energy is reflected back into the first medium and some is transmitted through

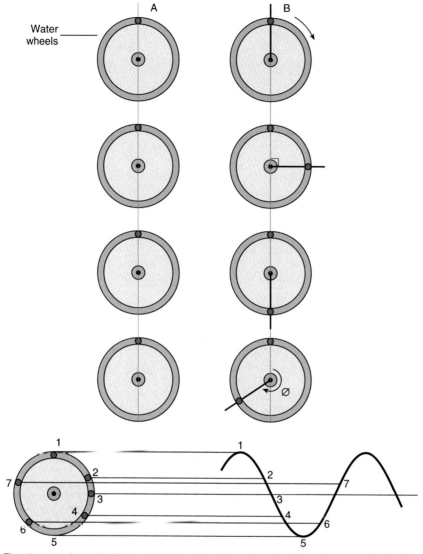

Fig. 2.5 The phase angle can be likened to the turning of a water wheel. Imagine two wheels, A and B, both with a mark on their rim. A does not move but B turns and, as it does, the rim mark executes the circles, each complete turn representing one *cycle*. The angle through which the mark turns in one cycle is 360° (2π radians). Thus, for example, compared with A, when the mark on B's rim has moved around a quarter of a turn (cycle), the angle between the two marks is a quarter of 360° (90° or π/2 radians); after half a turn, the angle between the two marks is 180° or π radians. This angle between the two marks is analogous to the *phase difference*. As B rotates, the height of the mark above the wheel's hub varies. If the wheel turns at a constant speed, then the mark's height traces out a *sine wave* when plotted against time.

into the second medium. The proportion of the total energy that is reflected is determined by the properties of the two media involved. Fig. 2.6 shows what happens when waves are reflected by a flat (plane) surface. An imaginary line drawn perpendicular to the surface is called the *normal*. The *law of reflection* states that the angle between the incident (incoming) wave and the normal is always equal to the angle between the reflected wave and the normal. If the incident wave is at normal incidence (perpendicular to the surface), the wave is reflected back along its path.

The waves that are transmitted into the second medium may also undergo *refraction*. This is the bending of light

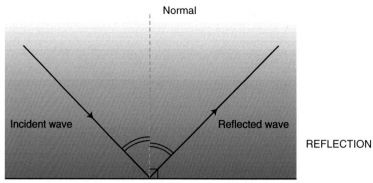

Normal

Incident wave   Reflected wave

REFLECTION

Fig. 2.6 The law of reflection states that the angle of incidence equals the angle of reflection.

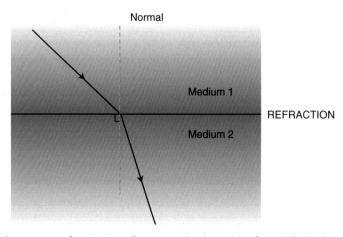

Normal

Medium 1

REFRACTION

Medium 2

Fig. 2.7 When a beam passes from one medium to another it can be refracted (i.e. it changes its direction).

towards the normal when it travels from one medium into one in which the wave speed is lower, or away from the normal when the wave speed in the second medium is higher (Fig. 2.7). For example, light bends towards the normal as it enters water from air since it travels more slowly in water than in air, and so a swimming pool may appear shallower than it really is.

As has been discussed earlier, waves carry energy. There are conditions, however, in which the transport of energy can be stopped, and the energy can be localized. This happens in a *standing (stationary) wave*. A standing wave is produced when an incident wave meets a returning reflected wave with the same amplitude. When the two waves meet, the total amplitude is the sum of the two individual amplitudes. Thus, as can be seen in Fig. 2.8A, if the trough of one wave coincides with the crest of the other, the two waves cancel each other out. If, however, the crest of one meets the crest of the other, the wave motion is reinforced (Fig. 2.8B) and the total amplitude doubles. In

the reinforced standing wave there are points that always have zero amplitude; these are called *nodes*. Similarly, there are points that always have the greatest amplitude, and these are called *antinodes*. Nodes and antinodes are shown in Fig. 2.8B. The distance between adjacent nodes, or adjacent antinodes, is one-half of the wavelength ($\lambda/2$).

Polarization

When flicking the Slinky spring up and down to produce a transverse wave, one has an infinite number of choices as to the direction in which to move it, so long as the motion is at right angles to the line of the spring. If the spring is always moved in a fixed direction, the wave is said to be *polarized* – the waves are in that plane only. However, if the waves (or directions in which the spring is moved) are in a number of different directions, the waves are *unpolarized*. It is possible to polarize the waves by passing them through a filter that allows through only waves that are in one plane. This can be visualized by envisaging a piece of

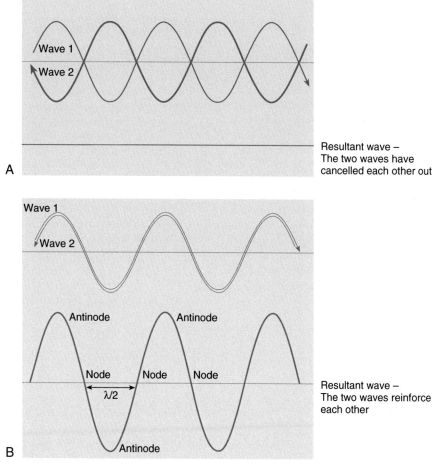

Fig. 2.8 A standing wave is formed when two waves of equal amplitude travelling in opposite directions meet. (A) The two waves cancel each other out; (B) the two waves add to reinforce each other.

card with a long narrow slit in it. This will allow the waves formed in the plane of the slit to go through, but no others – the card therefore acts as a polarizing filter.

ELECTRICITY AND MAGNETISM

Everyone is familiar with effects of electrical charges, even if they are not aware of their causes. The 'static' experienced when brushing newly washed hair, or undressing, and the electrical discharge obvious in lightning are examples of the effects of charges.

Electricity

Matter is made up of atoms, an atom being the smallest particle of an element that can be identified as being from that element. The atom consists of a positively charged central nucleus (made up of positively charged *protons*

and uncharged *neutrons*), with negatively charged particles (*electrons*) orbiting around it, resembling a miniature solar system. An atom contains as many protons as there are electrons, and so has no net charge. If this balance is destroyed, the atom has a non-zero net charge and is called an *ion*. If an electron is removed from the atom it becomes a *positive ion*, and if an electron is added the atom becomes a *negative ion*.

Two particles of opposite charge attract each other, and two particles of the same charge repel each other (push each other away). Hence, an electron and a proton are attracted to each other, whereas two electrons repel each other.

The unit of charge is a *coulomb* (C). An electron has a charge of 1.6×10^{-19} C, so it takes a very large number (6.2×10^{18}) of electrons to make up one coulomb.

The force between two particles of charge q_1 and q_2 is proportional to the product of q_1 and q_2 ($q_1 \times q_2$), and inversely proportional to the distance between them (d)

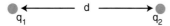

Fig. 2.9 Two particles of charge q_1 and q_2 a distance of d apart experience a force between them that is proportional to $q_1 q_2/d^2$.

squared (Fig. 2.9). Thus, the force is proportional to $q_1 q_2/d^2$. The constant of proportionality (i.e. the invariant number) necessary to allow one to calculate the force between two charges is $1/4\pi\varepsilon$, where ε is the *permittivity* of the medium containing the two charges:

$$F = q_1 q_2/4\pi\varepsilon d^2 \qquad [5]$$

If one of the charges is negative, then the force is attractive. If the particles are in a vacuum, the permittivity used is ε_0; this is known as the *permittivity of free space*. For a medium other than a vacuum, the permittivity is often quoted as a multiple of ε_0, where the multiplying factor, κ, is known as the *relative permittivity* or *dielectric constant*. So:

$$\varepsilon = \kappa\varepsilon_0, \text{ or} \qquad [6a]$$

$$\kappa = \varepsilon/\varepsilon_0 \qquad [6b]$$

Electric Fields

An *electric field* exists around any charged particle. If a smaller charge that is free to move is placed in the field, the paths it will move along are called *lines of force* (or *field lines*). Examples of fields and their patterns are shown in Fig. 2.10.

The *electric field strength*, E, is defined as the force per unit charge on a particle placed in the field. A little thought shows that $E = F/q$, where F is the force and q is the particle's charge. The units used to describe E are newtons/coulomb (N/C).

If E is the same throughout a field, it is said to be uniform. In this case, the field lines are parallel to each other as shown in Fig. 2.10D. If a charged particle is moved in this field, work is done on it, unless it moves perpendicular to the field lines. This is somewhat analogous to moving a ball around on earth. If the ball is always kept at the same height, and moved horizontally, its potential energy remains constant. If the ball is raised or lowered, its potential energy is changed. The ball has no potential energy when it lies on the ground. In a non-uniform field where the lines are not parallel, moving a charged particle always results in a change of potential energy. The *electric potential*, V, is defined as the potential energy per unit charge of a positively charged particle placed at that point. Electric potential is measured in units of *volts*. As the position at which the electric potential energy is zero is taken as

infinity, another way of thinking of the electrical potential at a point is as the work done in moving the charge to that point from infinity. In practice it is easier to compare the electrical potential at two points in the field than to consider infinity. The difference in the work required to move a charge from infinity to a point, A, and that required to move it to another point, B, is called the *potential difference* (p.d.) between the two points; this is also measured in *volts*. The p.d. is best thought of as a kind of pressure difference. Between the two points there will be a gradient in potential (just as there is a pressure gradient between the top and bottom of a waterfall). This gradient is described in units of volts/metre. In a uniform field between parallel plates with potential difference V, and separation d, the potential gradient is given by V/d. If a particle of charge q is moved from one plate to another, the work done is qV. Work is force × distance, and so the force, F, is given by:

$$F = qV/d \qquad [7]$$

As the electric field strength, E, is given by:

$$E = F/q \qquad [8]$$

it follows that:

$$E = V/d \qquad [9]$$

Remember that V/d is the potential gradient. From equation [9] we can see that the electric field strength can be increased by bringing the two plates closer together. Although the derivation is more complicated, the electric field strength at any point in a non-uniform field can also be shown to be the same as the potential gradient at that point.

Any electric circuit needs a supply of power to drive the electrons around the conductors. A power source has one positive and one negative terminal, with the electrons originating from its negative terminal. Electrical energy can be produced within the source by a number of means. Dynamos convert mechanical energy into electrical energy, solar cells convert the sun's energy into electrical energy, and batteries convert chemical energy into electrical energy. The force acting on the electrons is called the *electromotive force* (e.m.f.). This is defined as the electrical energy produced per unit charge inside the source. The unit in which e.m.f. is measured is the volt, because 1 volt is 1 joule/coulomb.

Electric Current

An *electric current* is the flow of electric charge. In some materials (e.g. metals) where the atoms are bound into a lattice structure, the charge is carried by electrons. In materials in which the atoms are free to move, the charge is carried by ions. A liquid in which the ions are the charge carriers is called an *electrolyte*. An *insulator* is a material that has no free charge carriers, and so is unable to carry an electric current.

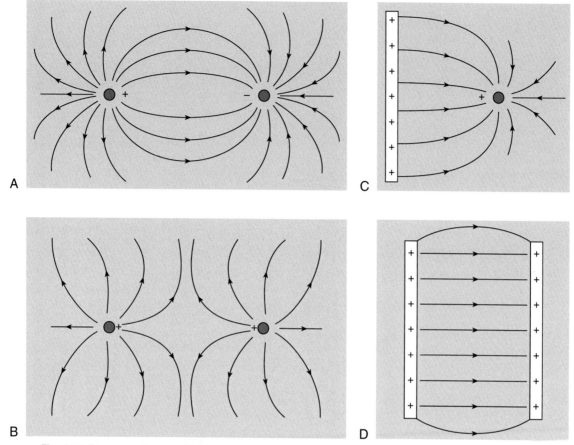

Fig. 2.10 Examples of electric fields near charged particles and plates: (A) field between two particles of equal and opposite charges; (B) field between two positively charged particles; (C) field between a charged particle and an oppositely charged plate; (D) field between two oppositely charged plates.

Current is measured using an ammeter, and the unit in which it is given is the *ampere* (A). An ampere represents 1 coulomb of charge flowing through a point in 1 second.

There are two types of electric current. A *direct current* (DC) is one in which the flow of electrons is in one direction only, and an *alternating current* (AC) is one in which the current flows first one way and then another. In considering electric circuits, it is easiest to think first of direct currents. A later section points to the differences between AC and DC circuits.

Resistance and Ohm's Law

The flow of electric charge through a conductor is analogous to the flow of water through pipes. If water is pumped round the system, narrow pipes put up more resistance to flow than wide ones. Electrical conductors also put up a *resistance* to the flow of charge. As the charged particles move through a conductor they collide with other charge carriers and with the resident atoms; the constituents of the conductor thus impede the current flow.

Georg Ohm was able to demonstrate that the current flowing in a circuit is proportional to the potential difference across it. His law (*Ohm's law*), formally stated, is:

The current flowing through a metallic conductor is proportional to the potential difference that exists across it, provided that all physical conditions remain constant.

So, $I \propto V$; this can also be written as $V \propto I$, where the constant of proportionality is the *resistance*, R. The equation resulting from Ohm's law is therefore:

$$V = IR \qquad [10]$$

R is measured in ohms (Ω). The ohm is defined as the resistance of a body such that a 1-volt potential difference across the body results in a current of 1 ampere through it.

The resistance of a piece of wire increases with its length, and decreases as its cross-sectional area increases. A property, the *resistivity*, is defined. This is a property of the material only, and not of the material's shape. The resistance R of a piece of wire with resistivity ρ, length L and area A is given by:

$$R = \rho L / A \qquad [11]$$

When electrons flow through a conductor, they collide with the atoms in the conductor material and impart energy to those atoms. This leads to heating of the conductor. The unit used for measuring energy is the *joule*. It has been seen earlier (see equation [7]) that the potential difference measured in volts is the work done in moving a unit charge between two points. So it follows from this that since the potential difference is the work done per unit charge:

$$volt = joule/coulomb \qquad [12a]$$

and so:

$$joule = volt \; coulomb \qquad [12b]$$

The unit of power measurement is the *watt*. Power is the rate of doing work, so a watt is a joule/second. It follows from the equation above that:

$$1 \; watt = 1 \; joule/second \qquad [13a]$$
$$joule = 1 \; volt \; coulomb/second \qquad [13b]$$

From the definition given it is known that a coulomb/second is an ampere. So, therefore:

$$1 \; watt = 1 \; volt \bullet ampere \qquad [14]$$

In other words, the electrical power developed in a circuit is given by:

$$Power = VI \qquad [15]$$

where V is in volts, I is in amperes, and the power is in watts.

From Ohm's law, substitutions can be made into this equation to express power in terms of different combinations of V, I and R. So:

$$W = VI \qquad [16a]$$

$$W = I^2 R \qquad [16b]$$

$$W = V^2/R \qquad [16c]$$

are equivalent equations, where W is in watts, V is in volts and R is in ohms.

Capacitance

Any passive device capable of storing electric charge is called a *capacitor*. This is the electrical equivalent of a compressed spring, which stores energy until it is allowed to expand. A capacitor stores charge until it can release it by becoming part of a completed electrical circuit. If you apply an electric potential, V, between two plates of a capacitor, one plate becomes positively charged and the other becomes charged with an equal but opposite negative charge. If an insulating material, known as a *dielectric*, is placed between the plates, the capacity to store charge is increased. The *relative permittivity*, or *dielectric constant* mentioned earlier, has another definition: it is also the ratio of the charge that can be stored between two plates with a dielectric material between them, to that which can be stored without the dielectric.

A capacitor is drawn in a circuit diagram as a pair of vertical parallel lines. Its *capacitance*, C, is defined as the charge (Q) stored per unit potential difference across its plates.

$$C = Q/V \qquad [17]$$

As Q is measured in coulombs, and V is measured in volts, the unit for capacitance is the coulomb/volt, known as the *farad*. Commonly, the capacitance of a capacitor found in an electric circuit is a few micro- (10^{-6}) or pico- (10^{-12}) Farads.

A capacitor is *charged* by applying a potential difference across its plates. It is *discharged* (i.e. the charge is allowed to flow away from the plates) by providing an electrical connection between the plates.

Electric Circuits

The symbols used to denote different components used in electrical circuits are shown in Fig. 2.11. Two electrical components are said to be in *series* if they carry the same current. The potential difference across a series of components is the sum of the potential differences across each one. The components are in *parallel* if they have the same potential difference across them. The current is then the sum of the currents flowing through them.

Resistors in series. If several resistors are joined in series with each other, the same current flows through them all, since electrons cannot be lost on the way through. From Ohm's law, the potential, V_i across each resistance in Fig. 2.12A, is given by:

$$V_i = IR_i \qquad [18]$$

If the total potential across the whole string is V, then:

$$V = V_1 + V_2 + V_3 + ... + V_i \qquad [19]$$

So:

$$V = IR_1 + IR_2 + IR_3 + ... + IR_i$$
$$= I[R_1 + R_2 + R_3 + ... + R_i] \qquad [20]$$

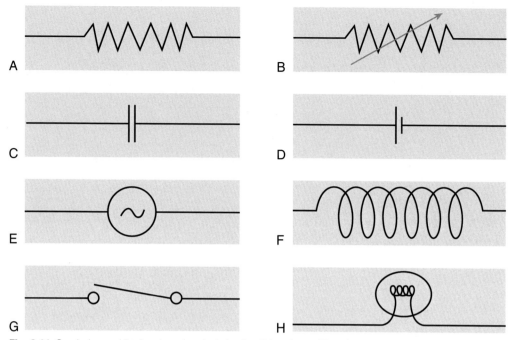

Fig. 2.11 Symbols used in drawing electrical circuits: (A) resistor; (B) variable resistor; (C) capacitor; (D) DC source; (E) AC source; (F) inductance; (G) switch; (H) bulb.

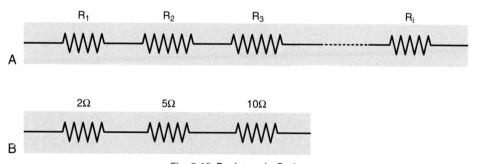

Fig. 2.12 Resistors in Series

Thus the single resistance needed to have the same effect as the string of resistors, R_{total}, is the sum of all the resistances:

$$R_{total} = R_1 + R_2 + R_3 + \ldots + R_i \qquad [21]$$

For example, in the string shown in Fig. 2.12B, the total resistance, R_{total}, is $2 + 5 + 10\Omega = 17\Omega$.

Resistors in parallel. Resistors can also be wired up in parallel, as shown in Fig. 2.13A. The electron flow splits up at A, electrons taking different routes to B where they join up again. The total flow of current through all resistors, I, is the same as the sum of the currents through each resistor:

$$I = I_1 + I_2 + I_3 + \ldots + I_i \qquad [22]$$

The potential difference across each resistor is identical. Using Ohm's law in the above equation, we can write:

$$I = V/R_1 + V/R_2 + V/R_3 + \cdots + V/R_i$$
$$= V[1/R_1 + 1/R_2 + 1/R_3 + \cdots + 1/R_i] \qquad [23]$$

Therefore the single resistance that could replace these parallel resistors has a value:

$$1/R_{total} = 1/R_1 + 1/R_2 + 1/R_3 + \cdots + 1/R_i \qquad [24]$$

For example, if three resistors of 2, 5 and 10 Ω are in parallel, as shown in Fig. 1.13B, the equivalent resistor to

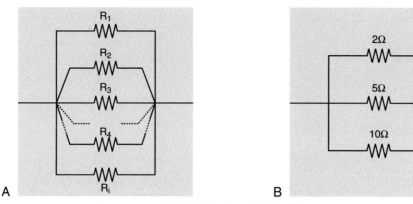

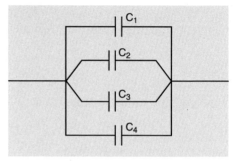

A   B

Fig. 2.13 Resistors in Parallel

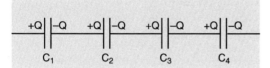

Fig. 2.14 Capacitors in Series

Fig. 2.15 Capacitors in Parallel

replace these is $1/(\frac{1}{2} + \{\frac{1}{5}\} + \{1/10\})$, which is $1/(0.5 + 0.2 + 0.1) = 1/0.8 = 1.25\ \Omega$.

Capacitors in series. A voltage applied across four capacitors in series induces charges of $+Q$ and $-Q$ on the plates of each (Fig. 2.14). Using equation [17] we know that:

$$1/C = V/Q$$

The potential difference across the series row is the sum of the potentials across each capacitor, and so the single capacitance, C, equivalent to the four capacitors C_1, C_2, C_3 and C_4 is given by:

$$1/C = [V_1 + V_2 + V_3 + V_4]/Q \qquad [25]$$

$$= V_1/Q + V_2/Q + V_3/Q + V_4/Q$$

$$= 1/C_1 + 1/C_2 + 1/C_3 + 1/C_4 \qquad [26]$$

If the capacitances are 2, 1, 5 and 10 μF, then $C = 0.56$ μF.

Capacitors in parallel. If capacitors are connected in parallel (Fig. 2.15), the total charge developed on them is the sum of the charges on each of them. The current is never negative. The potential difference is the same across all the capacitors.

The effective capacitance of all the capacitors put together is given by the expression:

$$C = Q/V$$

where:

$$Q = Q_1 + Q_2 + Q_3 + Q_4$$

and so:

$$C = Q_1/V + Q_2/V + Q_3/V + Q_4/V \qquad [27]$$

$$= C_1 + C_2 + C_3 + C_4 \qquad [28]$$

If the capacitances are 1, 2, 5 and 10μF, then C is 18μF.

Direct and Alternating Current

As discussed earlier, two types of electric current exist: direct current (DC) and alternating current (AC). The most common type of alternating current has a sinusoidal waveform, such as that found in the electricity mains. For sinusoidal AC, the relationships between frequency and period, etc., defined in the first section hold true. The variation of current can be described by the relationship:

$$I = I_0 \sin [2\pi ft] \qquad [29]$$

and, similarly, the voltage is described by:

$$V = V_0 \sin [2\pi ft] \qquad [30]$$

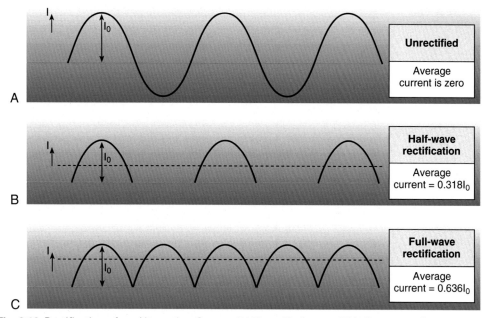

Fig. 2.16 Rectification of an Alternating Current (A) Unrectified wave; (B) half-wave rectification; (C) full-wave rectification.

where $\sin[2\pi ft]$ is the expression that tells you that the wave form is a sine wave of frequency f, and I_0 and V_0 are the maximum values of current and voltage (the amplitude of the oscillation). Clearly, the average current over one cycle in Fig. 2.16A is zero – the current is positive as much as it is negative – and the same applies to the voltage.

In some instances, an alternating current may be *rectified*, as shown in Fig. 2.16B and C. Here, the average current is clearly not zero. For *half-wave rectification*, the average current is $0.318I_0$, and for *full-wave rectification* the average current is $0.636I_0$.

If an alternating current flows through a resistor the average current is zero, but the heating effect is not. On each pass through the resistor, the electrons heat it slightly, whatever the direction of flow. Clearly, despite the zero net current, some energy is expended in the circuit, and an *effective current* is defined to account for this. The effective current (also known as the *root mean square (RMS) current*, I_{RMS}), is the value of the constant current that if allowed to flow for the same length of time would expend the same amount of electrical energy for a fixed voltage as the alternating current. An *effective voltage* (*root mean square (RMS) voltage*, V_{RMS}) is defined in a similar way as the constant voltage that, if present for the same length of time, would expend the same amount

of electrical energy for a fixed voltage as the alternating voltage.

From equation [16] the power, W, in DC circuits is given by:

$$W = VI$$

where W is in watts, V is in volts, and I is in amperes. Similarly, in an AC circuit:

$$W = V_{RMS} I_{RMS} \qquad [31]$$

Ohm's law can be used if the effective currents and voltages are used. Thus the power may also be written:

$$W = I_{eff}^2 R \qquad [32]$$

or

$$W = V_{eff}^2 / R \qquad [33]$$

It can be shown that $I_{eff} = I_0/\sqrt{2} = 0.707I_0$ and that $V_{eff} = V_0/\sqrt{2} = 0.707V_0$.

Capacitors allow alternating currents to flow. The resistance across capacitor plates is known as the *impedance* (Z). This is defined as the ratio of the amplitudes of the voltage and current in the same way as resistance is given by V/R for direct current. It can be shown that:

$$Z = 1/\omega C \qquad [34]$$

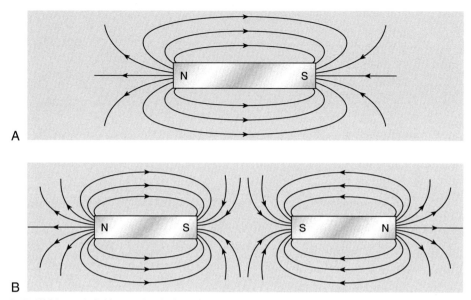

Fig. 2.17 (A) Magnetic field around a single permanent bar magnet; (B) magnetic field around two bar magnets.

where C is the capacitance and ω (the *angular frequency*) = $2\pi f$.

Magnetism

Those who have used a compass know that the needle swings around to point North–South. The compass is a permanent bar magnet that aligns itself with the earth's magnetic field.

There are two magnetic poles: the North pole and the South pole. In many ways, the two poles of a magnet act in the same way as opposite electric charges. Like magnetic poles repel each other, and unlike poles attract. There is a force between two magnets a distance d apart from each other, and the equation describing this force is very similar to that in equation [5]:

$$F = m_1 m_2 / 4\pi\mu d^{2\mu} \qquad [35]$$

Here, μ is the *permeability* of the medium, μ_0 (the permeability of free space) is used when the magnets lie in a vacuum. The strength of a magnet, m, is measured in units of *webers* (Wb). The unit of permeability is the *henry/metre* (H/m). *Relative permeability*, μ_r, is defined by the relationship:

$$\mu_r = \mu / \mu_0 \qquad [36]$$

A *magnetic field* exists at a point if a small magnet put there experiences a force. It will line up along the *magnetic field lines*. The fields around some permanent magnets are shown in Fig. 2.17.

The number of magnetic lines of force passing through an area, A, is known as the *magnetic flux* (N). The magnetic flux going through a unit area that is aligned perpendicular to the field is the *magnetic flux density* (B). Magnetic flux density is measured in units of *teslas* (T); 1 tesla = 1 Wb/m².

Electromagnetism

Wires carrying an electric current produce magnetic fields around them. The magnetic field around a long straight wire forms a series of concentric circles with the wire at their centre. A solenoid (i.e. a coil of wire) creates a field somewhat similar to that produced by a permanent bar magnet, the main difference being that there is a uniform field inside it. This uniformity of field is used to advantage in short-wave diathermy applications. Fig. 2.18 illustrates these fields.

The electromagnetic spectrum. Light is a form of electromagnetic radiation. It can be split up into its different component parts using a prism, with each colour of the 'rainbow' having a different wavelength. Electromagnetic waves are electrical and magnetic fields that travel together through space without the need for a carrier medium (Fig. 2.19). They travel at a speed of 3×10^8 m/s in a vacuum. There is a whole spectrum of such waves of which light is only a small part. Other radiations in the electromagnetic spectrum include radio waves, microwaves and x-rays; the spectrum is shown in Fig. 2.20. The behaviour of electromagnetic radiation can be usefully described, not only in terms of wave motion, but also in terms of 'particles'. It can be thought of as discrete 'packets' of energy and momentum, sometimes referred to as *quanta*. The energy in joules

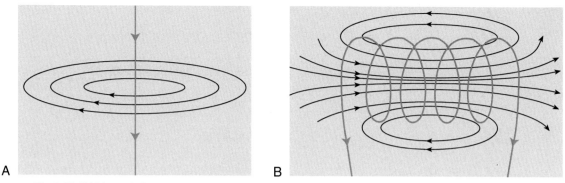

A   B

Fig. 2.18 (A) Magnetic field around a long straight wire carrying an electric current; (B) magnetic field around a coil carrying an electric current.

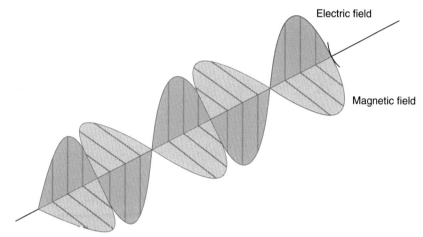

Electric field

Magnetic field

Fig. 2.19 An electromagnetic wave; the electric and magnetic fields travel together.

of a quantum of radiation is determined by its frequency, v, and is given by the equation:

$$E = hv \qquad [37]$$

where h is *Planck's constant* ($h = 6.62 \times 10^{-34}$J). It is more usual to quote electromagnetic energies in *electron-volts* (eV); $1\text{eV} = 1.6 \times 10^{-13}$J. It can be seen from Fig. 2.20 that energies at the long-wavelength end of the spectrum are very small. It is generally thought that energies in excess of 30 eV are required to ionize atoms, and so this allows the spectrum to be classified into two bands: those of 'ionizing' and 'non-ionizing' radiation.

The wavelength of the radiation determines the size of objects with which it will interact. A wave with a wavelength of 100 m (a radio wave) will not 'see' something of the size of an atom and will pass by undisturbed. However, a wave with a wavelength of 10^{-12}m (a gamma ray) will interact with the atomic nucleus, with which it is a comparable size. Infrared radiation has a wavelength comparable to the size of atoms or molecules and so can interact with them, imparting kinetic energy (heat).

Electromagnetic induction. The dynamo on a bicycle wheel that is used to power the bicycle's lights makes use of electromagnetic induction. Electromagnetic induction is in many ways the reverse of electromagnetism. When a magnet and a conducting wire move relative to one another, a current is induced in the wire. In the bicycle wheel, a magnet is made to rotate near a fixed coil of wire that forms part of a circuit that includes the lamp bulb. Current is induced in the wire and the lamp is lit.

The electrons in the wire approaching (or being approached by) a magnetic field experience a force as they enter the field. All of the electrons are displaced towards one end of the wire, and so that end becomes negatively charged. Conversely, the other end takes up a positive charge. An electromotive force is therefore induced between the two ends, and, if the circuit is completed, a current will flow. If the wire is coiled, the

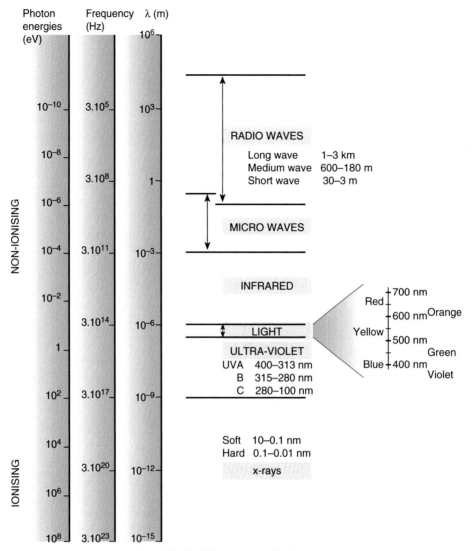

Fig. 2.20 The Electromagnetic Spectrum

induced current is increased. A coil of conducting wire used in this way is called an *inductor*. The e.m.f. induced in the conductor equals the rate of change of flux linkage – this is *Faraday's law* of electromagnetic induction. The direction of the induced current is always such that it opposes the change that caused it: *Lenz's law*. In this sense, inductors act as resistances in circuits; they are often used to block changing voltages while allowing steady (DC) voltages through.

An inductor (L) and capacitor (C) are sometimes used in series or in parallel to produce *LC-tuned* circuits (Fig. 2.21). It can be shown that these circuits have a resonant frequency, *f*, such that series LC-tuned circuits offer a very low impedance to waves of that frequency, but an extremely high impedance to everything else, whereas parallel LC-tuned circuits offer a very high resistance to waves of frequency *f* and allow other frequencies through. They therefore act as filters. The resonant frequency is given by the equation:

$$f = 1/2\pi \sqrt{(LC)}$$

[38]

Mutual Induction

A changing magnetic field from a current-carrying conductor can induce an e.m.f. and current in a second conductor nearby. This current will vary, and in its turn can produce its own varying magnetic field that induces an e.m.f. and current in the first conductor. Each conductor therefore induces a current in the other (Fig. 2.22). This is called *mutual inductance*. The mutual inductance is 1 henry if 1 volt is induced in one conductor by a current change of 1 ampere per second in the other. An AC transformer makes use of mutual inductance.

Self-inductance

When a current is switched on in a coil, the growing current in the coil causes a change in magnetic flux in the coil. This, in turn, causes an e.m.f. that opposes the e.m.f. of the battery. This is called a *back e.m.f.* This effect is increased if there is a soft iron core in the coil.

A conductor has a self-inductance of 1 henry if a back e.m.f. of 1 volt is induced by a changing current of 1 ampere/second.

MECHANICAL WAVES

The most important mechanical wave used in physiotherapy is ultrasound. Sound waves differ from electromagnetic waves in one major way: the waves are a form of *mechanical energy* and, as such, cannot propagate through a vacuum.

This is because energy passes through the medium by the movement of molecules, which transfer their momentum to their near neighbours in the direction of the wave. Sound is produced by a moving surface; this may be a diaphragm in a loudspeaker, for example, or a transducer front face in medical ultrasound. As the surface moves forward, it *compresses* the molecules immediately in front. These molecules in turn push forward against their neighbours in an attempt to restore their former arrangement, and these in turn push their neighbours. The compression therefore moves away from its source. If the surface now moves in the opposite direction, the density of the molecules is reduced next to it (a region of *rarefaction* is created), and so molecules move in to fill the space. This in turn leaves a low-density region which is immediately filled by more molecules, and so the rarefaction moves away from the source (Fig. 2.23). This type of wave is called a *longitudinal* wave because the displacement of the molecules is along the direction in which the wave moves.

Ultrasound

The velocity of sound in air is 330 m/s. The human ear can hear frequencies up to about 18,000 Hz (18 kHz). The wavelength of audible sound (calculated using equation [4]) where the ear is most sensitive (about 1.6 kHz) is about 20 cm. At ultrasonic frequencies (above 18 kHz), the wavelength becomes so short that the sound does not travel far through air. (At 1.5 MHz, the wavelength is about 0.2 mm.) However,

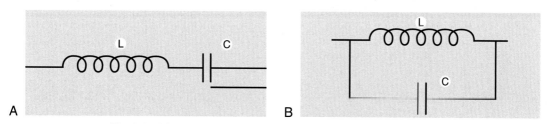

A   B

Fig. 2.21 LC-tuned Circuits (A) Series LC circuit; (B) parallel LC circuit.

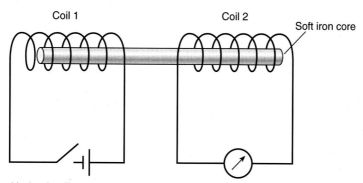

Fig. 2.22 Mutual Induction The changing magnetic field in one coil can induce a current in a second coil. The magnetic field thus created will create a current in the first coil. A soft iron core enhances this effect.

ultrasound will travel through water, a medium for which the sound velocity is 1500 m/s. At 1.5 MHz the wavelength in water is 1 mm. This fact is used in medicine since most body tissues are comprised mainly of water, and the millimetre wavelengths at the low megahertz frequencies used (0.75–10 MHz) are comparable with the size of the tissue structures with which interaction is required.

Ultrasound is generated from a *transducer*, i.e. a device that transforms one form of energy into another. The transducer most commonly used in ultrasound changes electrical energy into mechanical energy using the *piezo-electric effect*. A piezoelectric crystal has the property that if a voltage is applied across it, it will change its thickness, and alternatively if the crystal thickness is changed then a voltage develops across the crystal (this is the *inverse*

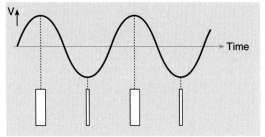

Fig. 2.23 **The Piezoelectric Effect** The crystal gets fatter and thinner, depending on the polarity of the voltage.

piezoelectric effect). Thus, if an oscillating voltage is applied across the crystal it will alternately get thicker and thinner than its resting thickness, following the polarity of the voltage (see Fig. 2.23). As the front face of the transducer moves backwards and forwards, regions of compression and rarefaction move out from it, forming an ultrasonic wave. The piezoelectric material most commonly used for physiotherapy transducers is lead zirconate titanate.

The voltage across the ultrasound transducer may either be applied continuously over the whole treatment time (*continuous wave*, CW), or may be applied in bursts – on for a time, off for a time, and so on; this is known as *pulsed mode*. The wave trains for a continuous wave and for pulsed mode are shown in Fig. 2.24.

In the pulsed mode, the pulsing regimen may be described in one of three ways (Fig. 2.24B):

1. *x* seconds on; *y* seconds off
2. *m*:*s*, where *m* represents the 'mark' and *s* represents the 'space', where the ratio represents that of the on time to the off time; this is called the *mark:space ratio*. So, if the on time is twice the off time, *m*:*s* is 2:1. To discover the true pulsing regimen, it is also necessary to know the pulse length
3. The *duty cycle*: this is the pulse length as a percentage of the total on and off time, so it is given by $x/(x+y) \times 100\%$.

Take, for example, a common pulsing regimen as shown in Fig. 2.25. This may be described as 2 ms on: 8 ms off, as 1:4 mark:space ratio, pulse length 2 ms, or as a

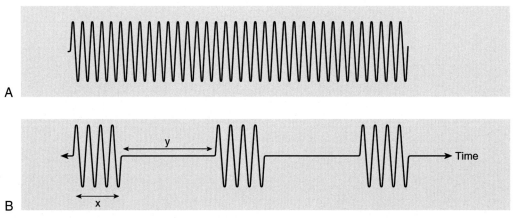

Fig. 2.24 (A) Continuous wave ultrasound; (B) pulsed ultrasound. In this example, the sound is on for *x* seconds and off for *y* seconds.

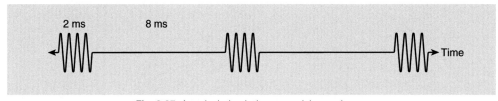

Fig. 2.25 A typical physiotherapy pulsing regimen.

TABLE 2.1 Extent of Near Field for Different Ultrasound Transducers		
Frequency (MHz)	r (cm)	r^2/λ (cm)
0.75	0.5	1.25
	1.0	5
	1.5	11.25
1.0	0.5	0.6
	1.0	6.7
	1.5	15
1.5	0.5	2.5
	1.0	10
	1.5	22.5
3.0	0.5	5
	1.0	20
	1.5	45

λ, Ultrasonic wavelength; r, transducer radius.

20% ($\{2/10\}\times100\%$) duty cycle. It is worth noting that, at 1 MHz, a pulse of length 2 ms contains 2000 cycles.

Intensity

The energy in an ultrasound wave is characterized by *intensity*. This is the energy crossing a unit area perpendicular to the wave in unit time; the units used are *watts/m²*. However, for clinical applications, the square metre is an inappropriately large area in terms of regions of the human body to be treated, and so the unit used in medical ultrasound is watts/cm² ($1 \text{ W/m}^2 = 10^4 \text{ W cm}^{-2}$).

Several types of intensity are used to describe ultrasound exposures. The field from a flat circular piezoelectric disc is complex. Near the transducer there are many peaks and troughs, but as the beam moves further from the transducer the field pattern becomes more uniform. The region near the transducer is known as the *near field* or *Fresnel zone*; the region beyond that is called the *far field* or *Fraunhoffer zone*. The boundary between the two zones is at a distance given by r^2/λ where r is the transducer radius and λ is the wavelength of the ultrasound. This is the position of the peak of intensity on the beam axis that is furthest from the transducer. Physiotherapy ultrasound commonly operates at 0.75, 1.0, 1.5 or 3 MHz. The extent of the near field is shown in Table 2.1 for a number of frequencies and transducer sizes. This demonstrates that most physiotherapy ultrasound exposures are carried out in the near field, which has many peaks of intensity. It also indicates that a number of intensities need to be identified.

The transverse field profiles shown in Fig. 2.26 illustrate the problem. Both profiles have the same peak intensity, I_0, but the levels are rather different if they are averaged over the whole beam. Peak levels are the most significant parameter if the beam is held stationary over one tissue volume for a long time, but if the transducer is kept in continuous motion the average value becomes more important since this is more representative of what the tissue will experience. In a continuous wave field, therefore, two intensities are defined, the *spatial peak intensity* (I_{SP}) and the *spatial average intensity* (I_{SA}).

Things become more complicated in a pulsed field. Here, the analogy is of a boy standing up to his ankles in the sea. As the waves come in, the water rises up his legs, and drops again as the wave moves past, only to come up again on the next wave. There is a high-water mark on the boy's legs, representing the highest point reached by the wave while he was standing there (the *temporal peak*) and there is an average water level experienced during the paddle (the *temporal average*). In the same way, a *temporal peak intensity* and a *temporal average intensity* can be identified as the highest intensity experienced at a point in tissue over a period of time, and the average intensity experienced at that point over a time, where the averaging is done over both on-times and off-times. If these temporal intensities are measured at the point in tissue where the spatial peak intensity is found, then a *spatial peak temporal peak intensity* (I_{SPTP}) and a *spatial peak temporal average intensity* (I_{SPTA}) can be determined. If these temporal intensities are combined with spatial averaging, the *spatial average temporal average* (I_{SATA}) and *spatial average temporal peak intensities* (I_{SATP}) can also be defined. These are demonstrated in Figs 2.27 and 2.28.

For example, take a beam with $I_{SP} = 3$ W cm^{-2} and $I_{SA} = 2$ W cm^{-2} while the sound is on, pulsed 2 ms on, 8 ms off. Whatever the temporal peak, the temporal average will be 20% of this since the sound is on for only a fifth of the time. Thus, $I_{SPTP} = 3$ W cm^{-2}, $I_{SPTA} = 0.6$ W cm^{-2}, $I_{SATP} = 2$ W cm^{-2}, $I_{SATA} = 0.4$ W cm^{-2}.

The ultrasound field can also be described in terms of the pressures involved. It can be seen from Fig. 2.29 that the pressure oscillates around the ambient level in the medium through which it passes. The field can therefore also be characterized in terms of *pressure amplitude* (usually the *peak positive pressure amplitude*, p_1, and the *peak negative pressure amplitude*, p_2) found anywhere in the field.

Intensity and pressure are related in a plane wave by the expression:

$$I = p^2/2\rho c \qquad [39]$$

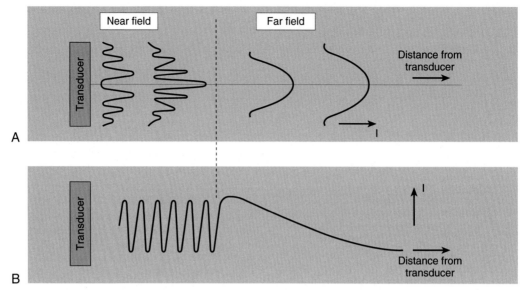

Fig. 2.26 (A) Transverse intensity distributions at different distances from the transducer; (B) intensity distribution on axis.

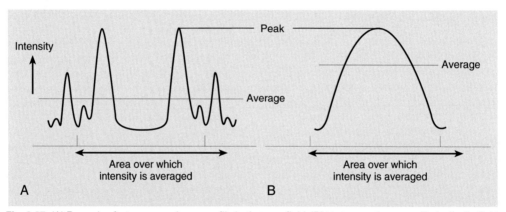

Fig. 2.27 (A) Example of a transverse beam profile in the near field; (B) transverse beam profile in the far field. This has the same peak intensity as the profile in (A).

where ϱ is the density and c is the speed of sound in the medium.

Ultrasound interacts with tissue in several ways. The two mechanisms thought to be most important are heat and cavitation. Cavitation is the activity of bubbles in an ultrasonic field. The oscillating pressure can cause bubbles to grow and to oscillate. An oscillating bubble causes the liquids around it to stream, and considerable shear stresses may occur. In some instances they may become *resonant*, in which case they start to oscillate unstably and may undergo violent collapse, causing tissue damage in their vicinity. When the amount of tissue heating is being considered, spatially averaged intensities are the most relevant parameters. However, when cavitation is considered, it is the peak negative pressure that is the most relevant parameter.

Calibration

Ultrasound fields can be calibrated using a number of methods, depending on the information required. The pressure distribution can be mapped using a pressure-sensitive polyvinylidene difluoride (PVDF) membrane hydrophone, which makes use of the inverse piezoelectric effect. Field plotting is a lengthy and detailed process usually undertaken by manufacturers or medical physics departments. It is always advisable to have transducers calibrated in this way before

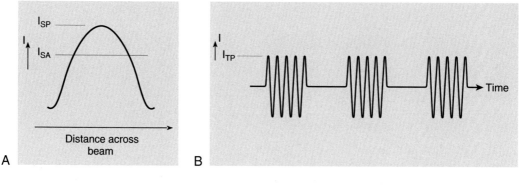

A

B

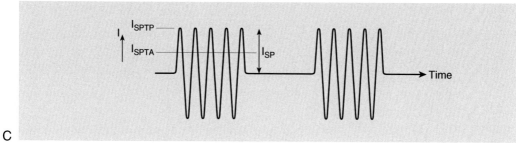

C

Fig. 2.28 **The Different Types of Intensity** I_{SA}, Spatial average; I_{SP}, spatial peak; I_{SPTA}, spatial peak temporal average; I_{SPTP}, spatial peak temporal peak; I_{TP}, temporal peak.

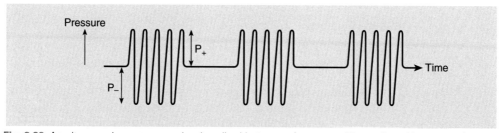

Fig. 2.29 An ultrasound exposure can be described in terms of pressure. The peak positive pressure amplitude, P_1, and the peak negative pressure amplitude, P_2, are shown.

use, and again when a fault is suspected; it provides an easy way of identifying damaged crystals. The calibration method of choice within a physiotherapy department should be a radiation pressure balance. When ultrasound hits a target in water, it exerts a force on the target (radiation pressure) and tries to move it. If this is suitably counterbalanced, the radiation force can be calculated. This device averages over the target area, and allows a rapid assessment of reproducibility of output from day to day. This is an important check that should be incorporated into any treatment routine.

Reflection of Ultrasound Waves

Tissue offers resistance to the passage of ultrasound. This resistance is called the *acoustic impedance, Z*, and may be calculated from the expression:

$$Z = \rho c \qquad [40]$$

where ρ is the density and c is the velocity of sound. The unit in which Z is reported is the *rayl*.

The amount of sound reflected from a plane surface between two materials of impedance Z_1 and Z_2 is $(Z_2 - Z_1)/(Z_2 + Z_1)$, and the amount of sound transmitted is $2Z_2/(Z_2 + Z_1)$. Water has an impedance of 1.5×10^6 rayl, fat has an impedance of 1.4×10^6 rayl, muscle of 1.7×10^6 rayl and bone of 7×10^6 rayl.

Attenuation

As ultrasound passes through tissue, some of the energy is reflected by the structures in its path (*scattering*), and some of the energy is absorbed by the medium itself, leading to local heating (*absorption*). Attenuation (the loss of energy from the beam) is due to these two mechanisms, with absorption accounting for 60–80% of the

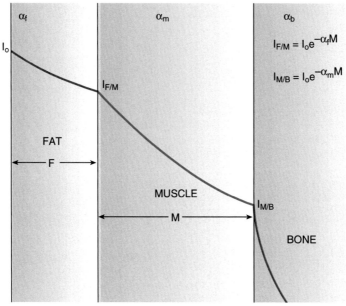

Fig. 2.30 Ultrasound energy is attenuated exponentially as it travels through tissue. Bone attenuates most strongly.

energy loss. If the intensity incident on tissue is I_0, and the intensity after travelling through x cm of tissue of attenuation coefficient α, is I, these are related by the expression:

$$I = I_0 e^{2 - \alpha x} \qquad [41]$$

The way in which the intensity drops as it goes through tissue is shown in Fig. 2.30; this is known as *exponential decay*.

Attenuation coefficient values are often quoted in dB/cm/MHz or nepers/cm/MHz (1 dB/cm = 4.34 nepers/cm). The decibel (dB) represents a ratio of intensity levels such that the intensity level quoted in decibels is $10 \log_{10} [I_0/I]$. It can be shown that when the intensity level is 3 dB the ratio of intensities is 2. The attenuation coefficient is quoted as a function of frequency, as they are approximately linearly related.

Table 2.2 shows relative attenuation coefficients for different biological tissues. Also shown are half-value thicknesses. This is the thickness of tissue needed to reduce the intensity by a factor of 2. It can be seen that bone and lung attenuate the sound very rapidly and very little energy gets into them. They are therefore not suited to physiotherapy ultrasound treatments. In fact, care should be taken when treating over such regions because the lost energy goes into heating the tissue locally. It can also be seen that the half-thickness layer decreases with increasing frequency and so, where deep treatments are required, low frequencies should be used.

Coupling Agents

It can be seen from Table 2.2 that megahertz-frequency sound does not travel through air. Therefore, when a patient is being treated, it is essential for an effective treatment that no air comes between the transducer and the skin. There are a number of methods by which ultrasound is applied. The most common method is to use a 'contact' application, where a thin layer of oil or gel is applied to the skin prior to treatment. The requirement for the coupling medium is that it has a similar acoustic impedance to skin. Mineral oils and water-based gels are most commonly used. Awkward geometries can most readily be treated in a water bath, with both the limb to be treated and the transducer being immersed.

HEAT AND TEMPERATURE

The fact that when various forms of energy are converted into heat there is always a constant ratio between the amount of energy that is lost and the amount of heat produced suggests that in all these processes, energy is neither created nor destroyed. This principle is a partial expression of the *first law of thermodynamics*: 'in all processes occurring in an isolated system, the energy of the system remains constant'. Electrical, chemical, magnetic and other forms of energy can be converted into heat energy with 100% efficiency, but it is not possible to achieve the reverse and transform all heat energy stored in the microstructure of matter to some other energy form. Again, if one form of energy is

TABLE 2.2	Tissue Ultrasound Attenuation Coefficients and Half-value Layers		
Tissue	Attenuation (dB/cm/MHz)	Half-value layer at 1 MHz	Half-value layer at 3 MHz
Blood	0.2	15 cm	5 cm
Fat	0.6	5 cm	1.6 cm
Liver	1.0	3 cm	1 cm
Muscle	1.3–3.3	1–2 cm	3–6 mm
Bone	20	1.5 mm	0.5 mm
Lung	41	0.7 mm	0.2 mm
Air	342 (1 MHz)	0.02 mm	
Water	0.002	1500 cm	500 cm

converted to another (e.g. chemical to mechanical) the process is not 100% efficient and some of the energy is always converted to heat. The tendency to randomize molecular motion into heat energy eventually suggests that heat is a primordial component in the structure of matter.

The concepts of *heat* and *temperature* are rigorously differentiated in physics and the distinction needs to be similarly maintained in the theory of electrotherapy. Supposing that the same quantity of heat (Q) is distributed over a large or a small volume of the same material, the larger volume will have a lower temperature (T_1) than the smaller volume (T_2). Thus, while the quantity of heat is a form of energy, the temperature of an object is a measure of the *average kinetic energy* of the constituent molecules. Because it is related to the 'average' movement of molecules, the concept of temperature can be applied only to bodies consisting of a large number of molecules.

The only term for temperature that allows consistent expression of all states of matter, solid, liquid and gas in accord with the laws of thermodynamics is the thermodynamic temperature, the base unit of which is the *kelvin* (K). In this system, introduced by Lord Kelvin in 1848, the linear scale starts at the absolute zero of temperature (0 K). The thermodynamic Celsius scale is subdivided into the same intervals as the Kelvin scale but has a zero point displaced by 273.15. The Celsius scale is divided into 100 unit intervals between two fixed points: the condensing point of steam (100°C = 373.15 K) and the melting point of ice (0°C = 273.15 K). Absolute zero on the Celsius scale is −273.15°C. The *Fahrenheit* (F) scale does not conform to the International System (SI) of units but continues to be used in many regions of the world particularly for meteorological data; 0°C is 32°F, 100°C is 212°F, so 1° on the Celsius scale is equivalent to 1.8° on the Fahrenheit scale.

Heat Units

Energy, work and the *amount of heat* are physical quantities with the same dimensions and ideally should be measured by a common unit. Traditional units such as the calorie are deeply rooted in technical as well as in dietary usage, but in accordance with SI strategy, the calorie is a 'noncoherent' unit. To conform with the SI, a quantity of heat should be expressed in *joules* (J). Heat exchanges are usually described in terms of *power* (energy per unit time), for example joules per second (watt or W). The watt is probably more familiar in everyday use as a measure of power consumption of electrical appliances, for instance in kilowatt hours (kWh), which is actually energy per unit time × time.

The amount of heat energy required to raise a unit mass of material by 1°C is known as the *specific heat* of the material. The specific heat of water is 4.185 J/g per °C. Far less heat is needed to raise the temperature of a gas (e.g. the specific heat of air is 1.01 J/g per °C). The human body comprises approximately 60% water and not surprisingly has a relatively high specific heat (3.56 J/g per °C). The specific heats of skin, muscle, fat and bone are respectively 3.77, 3.75, 2.3 and 1.59 J/g per °C. It is thus readily calculated that if the mean body temperature of a 65-kg person is increased by 1°C over a period of 1 hour then an extra 231 kJ of heat has been stored in the body.

Physical Effects of Heat

When heat is added to matter, a number of physical phenomena result from increasing the kinetic energy of its microstructure. These can be summarized as follows:
1. Temperature rise: the average kinetic energy of constituent molecules increases.
2. Expansion of the material: increased kinetic energy produces a greater vibration of molecules, which move further apart and expand the material. Gases will expand more than liquids, and liquids more than solids. If, for example, a gas is enclosed so that expansion cannot take place, a rise in gas pressure will occur instead.

3. Change in physical state: changing a substance from one physical state (phase) to another requires a specific amount of heat energy (i.e. latent heat). For example, the latent heat of fusion is the energy required for, or released by, 1 g ice at 0°C to convert it to 1 g water at 0°C (336 joules), and the latent heat of vaporization is the energy needed to convert 1 g water at 100°C to 1 g steam at 100°C (2268 joules).

4. Acceleration of chemical reactions: van't Hoff's law states that 'any chemical reaction capable of being accelerated, is accelerated by a rise in temperature; the ratio of the reaction rate constants for a reaction occurring at two temperatures 10°C apart is the Q_{10} of the reaction'.

5. Production of an electrical potential difference: if the junction of two dissimilar metals (e.g. copper and antimony) is heated, an e.m.f. (electromotive force or electrical potential difference) is produced between their free ends (the Seebeck or thermocouple effect). Conversely, an e.m.f. applied to the junction of two metals can cause a rise in temperature at the junction (Peltier effect).

6. Production of electromagnetic waves: when energy is added to an atom (e.g. by heating) an electron may move out into a higher-energy electron shell. When the electron returns to its normal level, energy is released as a pulse of electromagnetic energy (a photon).

7. Thermionic emission: heating of some materials (e.g. tungsten) may cause such molecular agitation that some electrons leave their atoms and may break free of the metal. This leaves a positive charge which tends to attract electrons back. A point is reached where the rate of loss of electrons equals the rate of return, and a cloud of electrons then exists as a space charge around the metal. This process is known as thermionic emission.

8. Reduction in viscosity of fluids: dynamic viscosity is the property of a fluid (liquid or gas) of offering resistance (internal friction) to the non-accelerated displacement of two adjacent layers. The molecules in a viscous fluid are quite strongly attracted to one another. Heating increases the kinetic movement of these molecules, reducing their cohesive mutual attraction and making the fluid less viscous.

Heat Transfer

The laws of thermodynamics govern processes involving the movement of heat energy from one point to another. Mention has previously been made of the first law, which deals with the conservation and interchange of different forms of energy. The second law of thermodynamics states that 'heat cannot by itself, i.e. without performance of work by some external agency, pass from a colder to a warmer body'. These general laws establish the principles that govern heat exchanges (gain or loss) within the body and between the body and its environment. In electrotherapy we are concerned with the transfer of heat energy between the external environment and the body surface, and between the component tissues and fluids of the body itself as well as with the therapeutic effects of heat.

Conduction

Conduction is the mechanism of energy exchange between regions of different temperature, from hotter to colder regions, which is accomplished by direct molecular collision. The energy thus transferred causes an increased vibration of molecules, which is transmitted to adjacent molecules. A simple example of this process is the metal bar heated at one end which, by heat conduction, eventually becomes hot at its other end. The application of a cold pack to the skin surface induces skin cooling by heat conduction from the warm skin, and vice versa for a hot pack. The rate of heat transfer depends on the difference in temperature between the regions in contact, the surface area of contact at the boundary and the thermal conductivity of the materials in contact. Thermal conductivity is a specific property of the material itself; for example, metals are better conductors than wood, water a better conductor than air.

Convection

Convection is the heat transfer mechanism that occurs in a fluid due to gross movements of molecules within the mass of fluid. If a part of a fluid is heated, the kinetic energy of the molecules in that part is increased, the molecules move further apart and the fluid becomes less dense. In consequence, the heated fluid rises and displaces the more dense fluid above, which in turn descends to take its place. The immediate process of energy transfer from one fluid particle to another remains one of conduction, but the energy is transported from one point in space to another primarily by convective displacement of the fluid itself. Pure conduction is rarely observed in a fluid, owing to the ease with which even small temperature differences initiate free convection currents.

Thermal Radiation

Heat may be transmitted by electromagnetic radiation emission from the surface of a body whose surface temperature is above absolute zero. The heating of certain atoms causes an electron to move to a higher-energy electron shell; as it returns to its normal shell, the energy is released as a pulse of electromagnetic energy. This radiation occurs primarily in the infrared band, with wavelengths of about 10^{25}cm to 10^{22}cm (0.1–100 mm, or 10^3–10^6Å). A thermal radiation incident upon a surface can be:

1. reflected back from that surface
2. transmitted through it
3. absorbed.

In many everyday circumstances, objects are radiating and absorbing the same amount of infrared energy, thus maintaining a constant temperature. The amount of radiation from an object is proportional to the fourth power of the temperature (in kelvins). The rate of emission from a surface also depends on the nature of the surface, being greatest for a black body. A perfect black body absorbs all the radiation, whereas other surfaces absorb some and reflect the remainder.

Evaporation

Thermal energy is required to transform a liquid into vapour; the rate at which this proceeds is determined by the rate at which the vapour diffuses away from the surface. The rate depends on the power supplied and the vapour pressure of the air above the liquid. Evaporation follows laws very similar to those governing convection. When water vaporises from the body surface (e.g. during sweating) the latent heat required is extracted from the surface tissue, thereby cooling it. The converse process, condensation, entails latent heat gain at the surface as vapour is changed into liquid.

Body Heat Transfer

In thermoregulation, heat is exchanged by conductive, convective, radiative and evaporative transfer processes between the body surface and the environment so that the body's core temperature remains constant, and equilibrium is maintained between internal (metabolic) heat production and heat loss (or gain) from the skin's surface.

Heat transfer within tissues takes place primarily by conduction and convection. The temperature distribution will depend on the amount of energy converted into heat at a given tissue depth and the thermal properties of the tissue (e.g. specific heat, thermal conductivity). Physiological factors are important in determining tissue temperature: for example, when a raised tissue temperature produces increased local blood flow, cooler blood reperfusing the heated tissue will selectively tend to cool the tissue by conduction. The technique of application of a treatment modality will also clearly modify the tissue temperature through variations in time and intensity, etc. When deep treatment is applied (e.g. short-wave diathermy, microwave, or ultrasound) conversion of the energy into heat occurs as it penetrates into the tissues.

In thermotherapy, the important properties concerned with heat conduction in tissues are thermal conductivity, tissue density and specific heat. Convection involves these properties also but, in addition, fluid viscosity becomes important. Understanding of the interaction of electromagnetic waves within biological media requires knowledge of the dielectric properties of tissues with different water contents.

3

Physiological Principles

Tim Watson, Kathleen A. Sluka

THE NEUROBIOLOGY OF PAIN AND ANALGESIA

INTRODUCTION

Pain is a complex experience unique to each individual. Pain can occur as a result of damage or potential damage to tissue innervated by nociceptors, or can occur in the absence of tissue damage. The impact of pain spreads beyond the perception of pain and can affect a person's social and emotional states. For example, there is a significant impact on participation in recreational activities and activities of daily living for those with acute and chronic pain (Foundation 2006). Pain is the number one reason a person seeks medical attention; chronic pain affects one third of the population, and 20% of individuals report moderate to severe pain (Committee on Advancing Pain Research 2011; Gaskin & Richard 2012; Johannes et al 2010).

The International Association for the Study of Pain (IASP) has defined pain as an unpleasant sensory and emotional experience associated with actual or potential tissue damage or defined in terms of such damage. Melzack and Casey (1968) propose three dimensions of pain (Fig. 3.1). The sensory-discriminative component conveys the intensity, location, quality and duration of pain; the motivational-affective component conveys the unpleasantness of pain; and the cognitive-evaluative component puts pain in context of current and past experiences. The IASP has defined three mechanistic terms to describe different types of pain. The first is nociceptive pain, which is pain that arises from actual or potential tissue damage to non-neuronal tissue and is due to activation of nociceptors. The second is neuropathic pain and is the result of a lesion or disease of the somatosensory nervous system. The third is nociplastic pain and is defined as pain that arises from altered nociception despite no clear evidence of actual or potential tissue damage causing activation of nociceptors or disease or lesion of the somatosensory system.

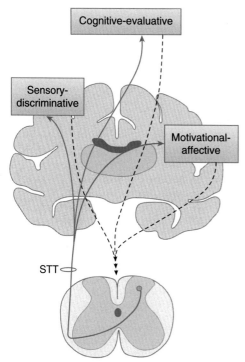

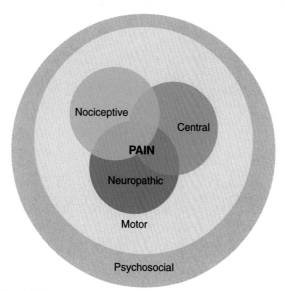

Fig. 3.1 The Three Dimensions of Pain The sensory-discriminative dimension is concerned with the intensity, duration, location and quality of pain. The motivational-affective dimension of pain is concerned with the unpleasantness and emotional components of pain. The cognitive-evaluative dimension of pain can modulate the experience in light of past experiences and current context. *STT*, spinothalamic tract.

Fig. 3.2 A conceptual model as an expansion of the biopsychosocial model of pain to include potential mechanisms that include nociceptive, central (nociplastic) or neuropathic contributors. The model also includes psychosocial and motor systems that can be influenced by and that can influence the pain experience.

A number of theories and models have been proposed to explain pain and provide treatment. These have been reviewed elsewhere (Sluka 2016). This chapter will use a biopsychosocial model of pain that takes into account the three biological mechanistic terms provided by the IASP, described above, with psychological, social and motor systems (Chimenti et al 2018; Sluka 2016) (Fig. 3.2). We will describe the underlying neurobiology of nociceptive transmission and perception of pain, the biology of analgesic systems and how non-pharmacological treatments can impact these systems.

PERIPHERAL NERVOUS SYSTEM

The peripheral nervous system plays a major role in the generation and maintenance of both acute and chronic pain. Nociceptors are sensory receptors that innervate peripheral tissues, and they consist of free nerve endings. A nociceptor responds to noxious stimuli, defined as damaging or potentially damaging stimuli. Once activated, they convey information to the central nervous system through thinly myelinated Aδ and unmyelinated C-fibres. The cell bodies of these primary afferent fibres are located in the dorsal root ganglia (DRG), which have a unique pseudounipolar structure. The axons have two branches, with one going to the peripheral tissues and one to the central nervous system (Fig. 3.3). Each tissue type, e.g. muscle or skin, has a unique set of noxious stimuli that will activate nociceptors. For example, cutaneous nociceptors are activated by cutting the skin, while visceral nociceptors respond to distension but not cutting the visceral tissue. Additionally, nearly all tissues contain silent, or mechanically insensitive, nociceptors. These nociceptors, which comprise about a third of the population, do not respond to mechanical stimuli in normal uninjured tissues; however, after tissue injury, they begin to fire in response to mechanical stimuli (Gebhart 1996; Neugebauer & Schaible 1988; Schmidt et al 1995). Thus, nociceptors innervate nearly every tissue in the body and provide unique information about noxious stimuli from peripheral tissues to the central nervous system (Fig. 3.3).

Peripheral sensitization The sensitivity of nociceptors is modifiable and can increase or decrease its response to noxious stimuli. Sensitization is a term used to describe the increased responsiveness of nociceptive neurons to their normal input. This is a normal response to injury and could result in increased response to noxious stimuli, decreased

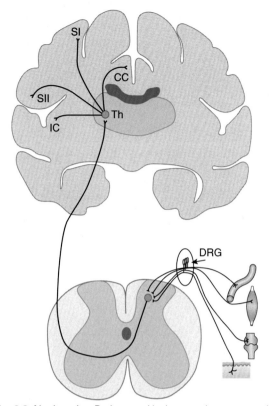

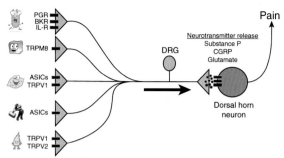

Fig. 3.4 The Diversity of Stimuli and Receptors that are Found on Nociceptors Chemical stimulators associated with inflammation can activate prostaglandin (*PG*), bradykinin (*BK*) and interleukin (*IL*) receptors; cold activates TRPM8 receptors; decreases in pH (protons) can activate TRPV1 and acid sensing ion channels (*ASICs*); mechanical stimuli are hypothesized to activate ASICs; and heat stimuli activate TRPV1 and TRPV2 receptors. These signals are transmitted to the dorsal horn of the spinal cord where primary afferents release excitatory neurotransmitters to activate dorsal horn neurons that send signals to higher brain centres to result in the perception of pain. *CGRP*, Calcitonin gene-related peptide; *DRG*, dorsal root ganglia; *TRP*, transient receptor potential channel.

Fig. 3.3 Nociceptive Pathways. Nociceptors innervate multiple types of tissue and send input to the spinal cord sending signals through the spinothalamic tract and to the cortex. Multiple sites are involved in nociceptive processing including the somatosensory cortices (*SI* and *SII*), and the insular (*IC*) and cingulate (*CC*) cortices. *DRG*, Dorsal root ganglia; *Th*, thalamus.

threshold to noxious stimuli, and/or increased spontaneous firing of the neuron. For example, recording the activity of peripheral nerves after the induction of joint inflammation, Schaible and Schmidt (1985, 1988) show increases in responsiveness to joint movement in nociceptors innervating the joint. This enhanced activity has been shown in numerous animal models after tissue injury that results in nerve damage or inflammation. Thus, tissue injury results in a general increase in the activity of nociceptors, including an increased firing of silent nociceptors, which increases the input to the central nervous system. This increased activity in nociceptors after tissue injury explains the hyperalgesia and localized pain that normally occurs after tissue injury (Ringkamp et al 2013).

Chemical mediators Noxious mechanical, thermal and chemical stimuli can activate and sensitize nociceptors through unique receptors located on nociceptors (Fig. 3.4). A number of neurotransmitters, receptors and ion channels located within or on the peripheral terminals of primary afferent fibres are capable of producing pain and inflammation (Fig. 3.5).

Neuropeptides. Neuropeptides, such as substance P and calcitonin gene-related peptide (CGRP) are contained in small diameter afferents (group III and IV), and can be released from peripheral terminals of primary afferent fibres, a process termed neurogenic inflammation. Neuropeptides released from primary afferent fibres in the periphery produce an inflammatory response (Brain & Williams 1985; Levine et al 1985; Sousa-Valente & Brain 2018; White & Helme 1985; Yaksh 1988), indicating that sensory neurons are involved in the generation of inflammation. Indeed, substance P and CGRP are increased in the inflamed knee joint in both animal models and human subjects with arthritis (Appelgren et al 1991; Larsson et al 1989; Mapp et al 1990; Pereira da Silva & Carmo-Fonseca 1990). Conversely, chemical or surgical elimination of primary afferent fibres reduces the inflammatory response (Colpaert et al 1983; Lam & Ferrell 1989, 1991; Sluka et al 1994). This neurogenic component of inflammation also involves the CNS through the generation of action potentials in the spinal cord that transmit to the periphery, termed dorsal root reflex. This dorsal root reflex releases neuropeptides from the peripheral terminal to enhance the inflammatory response (Rees et al 1994, 1995; Sluka & Westlund 1993; Sluka et al 1995).

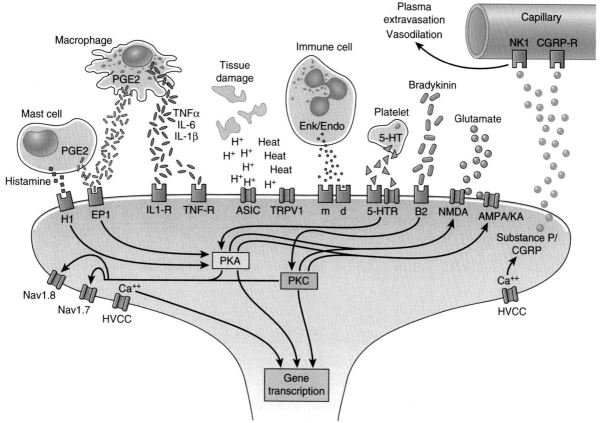

Fig. 3.5 The Multitude of Receptors and Stimuli that Activate Receptors on Nociceptors Release of a variety of chemicals from non-neuronal cells may act directly or indirectly to sensitize nociceptors. Release of substance P, calcitonin gene-related peptide (CGRP), or glutamate from nociceptors can further enhance the inflammatory response by acting on non-neuronal cells and capillaries to cause plasma extravasation and inflammation. Intracellular signalling pathways can be activated by receptors and can subsequently turn on gene transcription or phosphorylate receptors to enhance or reduce their activity

Glutamate. This excitatory neurotransmitter in the nervous system is found in primary afferent fibres, and its receptors are found on peripheral terminals of nociceptors (Carlton et al 1995; Svensson et al 2003b; Westlund et al 1992). Injection of glutamate peripherally produces hyperalgesia in human and animals, and sensitizes primary afferent fibres (Cairns et al 2003; Du et al 2001; Jackson et al 1995; Lawand et al 1997; O'Neill et al 2007; Svensson et al 2003b). Glutamate is increased in synovium after joint inflammation (Lawand et al 2000; McNearney et al 2000), and in muscle in those with temporomandibular disorder or myofascial pain (Gerdle et al 2014; Shah et al 2005). In both humans and animals, blockade of glutamate receptors peripherally reduces pain and hyperalgesia (Cairns et al 2006; Castrillon et al 2007).

Ion Channels. There are both ligand-gated and voltage-gated ion channels that are found on nociceptors and

contribute to the generation of nociception and pain. Acid sensing ion channels (ASICs) are activated by protons and lactate, which increase after tissue injury or fatigue, and play a significant role in musculoskeletal pain conditions (Abdelhamid & Sluka 2015; Sluka & Gregory 2015). Transient receptor potential channels (TRP) are activated by thermal stimuli with TRPV1 showing a significant role in heat nociception and TRPM8 showing a significant role in cold pain. Further inflammatory mediators can sensitize both the ASICs and TRPV1 to enhance the response to noxious stimuli (Abdelhamid & Sluka 2015; Ringkamp et al 2013; Sluka & Gregory 2015).

Further, voltage-gated ion channels that are important in neurotransmission and action potential propagation, such as sodium or calcium, can be upregulated by tissue injury, and make the nociceptor more excitable. $Na_v1.7$

and Na$_v$1.8 play critical roles in nociception (Black et al 2004; Cummins et al 2007; Dib-Hajj et al 2007; Drenth & Waxman 2007) with a change in sodium channel composition after peripheral neuropathy resulting in physiological changes that contribute to hyperexcitability of DRG neurons (Gold et al 2003). Mutations in the genes encoding for Na$_v$1.7 result in the painful syndrome erythromelalgia and the paroxysmal extreme pain disorder, or a complete loss of functional Na$_v$1.7 resulting in insensitivity to pain (Black et al 2004; Dib-Hajj et al 2005; Dib-Hajj et al 2007; Drenth & Waxman 2007; Gold et al 2003).

Inflammatory mediators. It is well established that the immune system, and factors released from immune cells (e.g. cytokines and chemokines), play a critical role in the generation of both acute and chronic pain (Fig. 3.5). Evidence for mast cells, neutrophils, macrophages, dendritic cells and T-cells show their involvement in a variety of pain conditions (Dawes et al 2013), and for macrophages in the analgesia by non-pharmacological treatments like acupuncture and exercise (da Silva et al 2015; Leung et al 2016). Substances released by immune cells include serotonin, bradykinin, prostaglandins, cytokines and chemokines. During inflammation, cytokines are released by infiltrating macrophages at the site of injury, and these pro-inflammatory cytokines (e.g. IL-1β, IL-6, TNFα) sensitize nociceptors and produce mechanical and thermal hyperalgesia in animals and humans (Cunha et al 1992; Feldmann et al 1995; Ferreira et al 1988; Kaneko et al 2000; Kaneyama et al 2002; McNearney et al 2004; Ozaktay et al 2002; Watkins et al 1994; Watkins et al 1995). As stated above, these inflammatory mediators can sensitize the ASIC and TRPV1 channels to make them more responsive to acidic, mechanical and thermal stimuli. Together these data can increase input to the central nervous system to result ultimately in the perception of pain.

Nerve growth factor. NGF is a neurotrophic factor that is produced by muscle and during tissue injury (Amano et al 1991; Hayashi et al 2011; Wu et al 2009) and activates and sensitizes nociceptors through its TrkA (high affinity) receptors (Hoheisel et al 2007; Murase et al 2010; Snider & McMahon 1998). Injection of NGF in humans and animals produces long-lasting hyperalgesia and results in an upregulation of proteins involved in pain transmission, including substance P, TRPV1 and Nav1.8, and alters N-methyl-D-aspartate (NMDA) glutamate receptor sensitivity (Basbaum et al 2009; Ji et al 2002; Svensson et al 2003a; Wong et al 2014) which enhances nociceptor excitability.

Consequences of nociceptor activation. Activation of nociceptors can result in multiple and complex outputs. Nociceptors send signals to the central nervous system that activate neurons in the nociceptive pathways, ultimately sending a signal to the cortex that it interprets as pain. It is important, however, to recognize that activation of nociceptors, or the nociceptive pathways, does not always result in pain. Nociceptive signalling and pain are under significant cortical and subcortical modulation. In addition to pain as an outcome for activation of nociceptors, there can be alterations in motor output often recognized as limb guarding, muscle spasm or reduced activity. The effects on the motor system are complex and varied (Chimenti et al 2018; Sluka 2016). Activation of nociceptors can also modulate the autonomic nervous system. For example, in animal models of chronic pain and in individuals with fibromyalgia there is decreased heart rate variability, decreased baroreceptor sensitivity and increased blood pressure variability (Kulshreshtha & Deepak 2013; Sabharwal et al 2016). Lastly, there are alterations in mood and affect by activation of nociceptors, including increased depression, anxiety, fear of movement and pain catastrophizing (Eccleston et al 2014; Flor 2014; Sluka & Clauw 2016). Thus, nociceptor activation clearly results in alterations in sensory, motor, autonomic and psychological factors.

CENTRAL NERVOUS SYSTEM

Nociceptive pathways. The nociceptive pathways in the central nervous system are complex and involve multiple anatomical pathways and nuclei at cortical and subcortical sites (Sluka 2016). Initial input from nociceptors reaches the central nervous system at the level of the spinal cord dorsal horn. From the spinal cord, nociceptive information is transmitted to supraspinal structures through the spinothalamic tract, which is subsequently relayed to cortical sites for perception of pain. The spinomesencephalic and spinoreticular pathways serve to integrate nociceptive information with areas involved in descending inhibition, facilitation and autonomic responses associated in the brainstem with pain.

The spinothalamic tract transmits information to neurons in the ventroposterior lateral (VPL) nucleus and medial thalamic nuclei. From here the VPL projects to the somatosensory cortex (SI and SII) and this pathway is thought to be involved in the sensory-discriminative component of pain (i.e. location, duration, quality and intensity) (Hofbauer et al 2001; Rainville et al 1997). The ascending projections from the medial thalamic nuclei are more diffuse and include areas such as the anterior cingulate and insular cortices, which are thought to be the basis for the motivational-affective component of pain (i.e. unpleasantness) (Hofbauer et al 2001; Rainville et al 1997) (Fig. 3.6).

The central nervous system balances excitatory and inhibitory activity across the nociceptive sites and pathways.

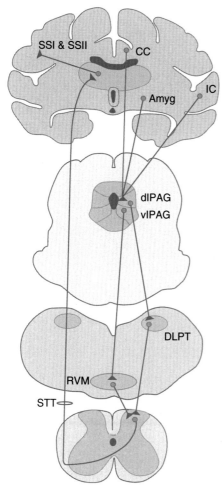

Fig. 3.6 The ascending spinothalamic tract (STT) and the descending inhibitory and excitatory pathways involved in nociception. *Amyg*, Amygdala; *CC*, cingulate cortex; *dlPAG*, dorsolateral PAG; *DLPT*, dorsolateral pontine nuclei; *IC*, insular cortex; *PAG*, periaqueductal grey; *RVM*, rostral ventromedial medulla; *SI, SII*, somatosensory cortex I, II; *vlPAG*, ventrolateral PAG.

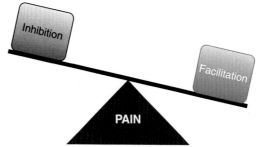

Fig. 3.7 The altered balance between central nervous system processing of inhibitory and excitatory signals that can result in pain.

Conceptually, an increase in excitatory activity and/or a decrease in inhibitory activity results in the perception of pain. Goals of treatment are to rebalance the nervous system by reducing activity at sites involved in facilitating nociception and pain and increasing activity at sites involved in inhibiting nociception and pain (Fig. 3.7).

Spinal cord. Neurons in the dorsal horn of the spinal cord are classified as high threshold, wide dynamic range and low threshold. High threshold neurons respond only to noxious stimulation; low threshold neurons respond only to innocuous stimuli; and wide dynamic range neurons respond to both noxious and innocuous stimuli.

Transmission of nociceptive information through the dorsal horn occurs through high threshold and wide dynamic range neurons.

Brainstem sites. Neurons in the medulla, pons and midbrain can modulate pain, and play a role in the facilitation as well as inhibition of nociceptive information. In the medulla the rostral ventromedial medulla is a key nucleus in nociception (Burgess et al 2002; Coutinho et al 1998; Terayama et al 2000; Tillu et al 2008; Urban et al 1999; Vera-Portocarrero et al 2006). In the pons, the locus coeruleus, and subcoeruleus and parabrachial nuclei are key players in nociception. In the midbrain, the periaqueductal grey is involved in nociception. More rostrally, the periaqueductal grey (PAG), pontine nuclei, amygdala and anterior cingulate cortex (ACC) also play a role in descending facilitation (Calejesan et al 2000; DeSantana & Sluka 2008; Holden et al 1999; Neugebauer & Li 2003). The PAG sends input to the rostral ventral medial medulla (RVM) and the pontine tegmentum, which subsequently send input to the spinal cord to modulate nociception.

Cortical sites. Cortical processing of pain in humans involves multiple brain sites that convey and process different aspects of the pain experience. Brain imaging studies have shown several areas that are routinely activated by painful stimuli including the somatosensory cortices (SI and SII), anterior cingulate cortex and anterior insular cortex (Coghill et al 1994; Hofbauer et al 2001; Rainville et al 1997). Additional cortical sites implicated in processing painful information include: amygdala, which is involved in fear and emotion; hippocampus, which is involved in learning and memory; prefrontal cortex, which is involved in planning complex behaviours, personality, and decision making; and motor cortex, which is involved in function and movement.

Glial cells and pain. Glial cells in the central nervous system, particularly the spinal cord, play a critical role in processing of nociceptive information (for review see Watkins et al 2001; Watkins & Maier 2002). Glia express receptors for

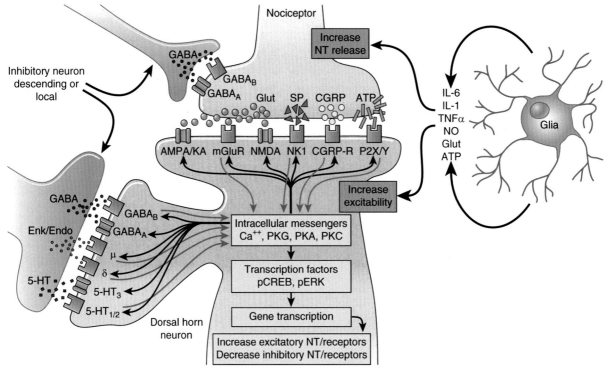

Fig. 3.8 A neuron in the dorsal horn receiving input from nociceptors, descending inhibitory signals (*green*) or glial cells. Neurotransmitters released from nociceptors activate receptors on dorsal horn neurons to enhance excitability. This can result in increased activation of intracellular signalling pathways that phosphorylate transcription factors to result in gene transcription. Glial cells release neuroactive substances that can increase release of neurotransmitters from nociceptors and enhance excitability of dorsal horn neurons. Descending inhibitory neurons can synapse pre-synaptically to modulate nociceptor activity or post-synaptically to modulate dorsal horn neuron activity. *AMPA/KA*, Non-NMDA glutamate receptors; *ATP*, adenosine triphosphate; *CGRP*, calcitonin gene-related peptide; *GABA*, gamma-amino-butyric acid; *Glut*, glutamate; *IL-1*, interleukin-1; *IL-6*, interleukin-6; *mGluR*, metabotropic glutamate receptors; *NK1*, neurokinin-1 receptor; *NMDA*, N-methyl-D-aspartate; *NO*, nitric oxide; *NT*, neurotransmitter; *PKA*, protein kinase A; *PKC*, protein kinase C; *PKG*, protein kinase G; *SP*, substance P; *TNFa*, tumour necrosis factor alpha.

many neurotransmitters, including glutamate receptors, and are involved in the clearance of neurotransmitters from the synaptic cleft. Activation of astrocytes and microglia occur in a number of pain models including neuropathic and inflammatory (Fu et al 1999; Garrison et al 1991; Sweitzer et al 1999), and release substances that sensitize neurons (Fig. 3.8).

Central sensitization Central sensitization, as defined by the IASP, is an increased responsiveness of nociceptive neurons in the central nervous system to their normal or sub-threshold afferent input. Following tissue injury, there is sensitization of neurons in the nociceptive systems, including the spinal cord. Central sensitization is manifested as an increase in receptive field size, increased responsiveness to innocuous or noxious stimuli, and/or decreased threshold to innocuous or noxious stimuli (Hoheisel et al 1993; Nahin

et al 1989; Palecek et al 1992; Schaible et al 1987). Central sensitization is thought to underlie secondary hyperalgesia, referred pain and pain that persists beyond normal tissue healing time clinically. Unique to central neurons is an increased responsiveness to innocuous stimuli after tissue injury, which is thought to be the basis of allodynia, a painful response to innocuous stimuli. It should be pointed out, however, that central sensitization is a phenomenon attributed to neurons, and as such cannot be directly measured in human subjects. For this reason, the IASP has used the term nociplastic pain to refer to human subjects that present with pain without observable tissue damage.

Sensitization of nociceptive neurons can be maintained by input from sensitized nociceptors. In this case, the goal of therapy is to reduce the input from peripherally sensitized nociceptors, which will decrease sensitization of dorsal horn neurons and the consequent pain. However, central sensitization can be initiated by input from sensitized nociceptors and can persist in the absence of nociceptive input. For example, central sensitization and contralateral hyperalgesia in a variety of animal models continues after application of local anaesthetics to the site of injury or deafferentation of the limb (Coderre & Melzack 1985,1987; Sluka et al 2001; Woolf & Wall 1986). If the central sensitization predominates and remains after peripheral injury, treatments should be focused on central mechanisms to reduce central sensitization.

Neurotransmitters and Mediators

There are a number of neurotransmitters, receptors and intracellular signalling molecules that have been identified to play a role in nociception throughout the central nervous system. It is beyond the scope of this review to describe them all; we refer the reader to other sources (Willis & Coggeshall 2004). Therefore, we will describe a few of the well-characterized systems to provide a general overview to the reader. We have also provided information on molecules that have been modified by non-pharmacological approaches to manage pain.

Neuropeptides. The neuropeptides, substance P and calcitonin gene-related peptide (CGRP), are located in the central terminals of primary afferent fibres in the dorsal horn and transmit nociceptive information to spinal cord dorsal horn neurons (Millan 1999). Substance P activates the neurokinin 1 (NK1) receptor to produce nociceptive-like behaviours (Wilcox 1988), activate and sensitize dorsal horn neurons (Radhakrishnan & Henry 1991) and enhance NMDA glutamate receptor function (Dougherty & Willis 1991). In contrast, blockade of NK1 receptors or loss of NK1-containing neurons in the spinal cord reduces hyperalgesia and sensitization of dorsal horn neurons (Fleetwood-Walker et al 1990; Neugebauer et al 1995; Radhakrishnan & Henry 1995; Sluka et al 1997; Suzuki et al 2002; Yashpal et al 1993). Similarly, CGRP antagonists reduce sensitization of dorsal horn neurons (Neugebauer et al 1996), and CGRP enhances the effects of substance P in the spinal cord (Schaible et al 1992; Woolf & Wiesenfeld Hallin 1986).

Glutamate. Glutamate mediates excitatory synaptic transmission between primary afferent nociceptors and dorsal horn neurons (Schneider & Perl 1985, 1988), and plays a role in supraspinal nociceptive sites in the brainstem and cortex (Kolber et al 2010; Radhakrishnan & Sluka 2009). Glutamate exerts its actions through ionotropic and metabotropic receptors. At the spinal and brainstem level the N-methyl-D-aspartate (NMDA) glutamate receptors, calcium channels with a voltage dependent Mg^{++} block, are implicated in synaptic plasticity associated with nociceptive transmission (Coderre et al 1993; Coderre et al 1997). Spinal or supraspinal application of NMDA glutamate receptor antagonists, or modulation of NMDA receptor subunits, decreases hyperalgesia in a variety of animal models of pain (Calcutt & Chaplan 1997; Chapman & Dickenson 1995; Coderre & Melzack 1992; da Silva et al 2010a; da Silva et al 2010b; Dougherty et al 1992; Mao et al 1992; Neugebauer et al 1993; Ren et al 1992; Skyba et al 2002; Sluka and Westlund 1993; Sluka et al 2012). In the amygdala, blockade of the metabotropic glutamate receptor 5 reverses hyperalgesia in a variety of pain models (Crock et al 2012; Kolber et al 2010).

Intracellular messengers. Neurotransmitters activate complex intracellular signalling pathways to modulate other neurotransmitter systems, receptor function and gene expression. Ionotropic receptor activation increases calcium influx to activate intracellular pathways, while G-protein coupled receptors (GPCRs) directly activate intracellular pathways. These signalling pathways would include protein kinases that phosphorylate receptors, cellular proteins, or transcription factors (Fig. 3.8). Phosphorylation of intracellular receptor proteins, by a variety of protein kinases, can enhance or reduce the activity of the channel, alter the transport of receptors to the cell membrane and increase gene transcription. For excitatory neurotransmitters, there is enhanced phosphorylation of receptors that increases channel excitability, enhances transport to the synapse and increases production of receptors (Guan et al 2003; Sluka et al 2013; Sluka 2016). For inhibitory neurotransmitters, phosphorylation reduces effectiveness of the receptors Lin et al., 1996. Thus, phosphorylation and intracellular signalling enhance excitability and reduce inhibition of central nociceptive systems ultimately resulting in more excitability.

Endogenous Inhibition

The body has the capacity to inhibit and modulate nociceptive neurons peripherally and centrally. Centrally, the PAG, the rostral ventral medial medulla (RVM) and the lateral pontine tegmentum (Fig. 3.6) are key nuclei involved in inhibition. Stimulation, either electrically or chemically, of the PAG, RVM or lateral pontine tegmentum produces analgesia and reduces dorsal horn activity and sensitization (Gebhart et al 1983; Heinricher 1997; Jones & Gebhart 1987; Liebeskind et al 1973; Reynolds 1969; Tsuruoka & Willis 1996; Zhao & Duggan 1988). Anatomically, the PAG sends projections to the RVM and the lateral pontine tegmentum, but not directly to the spinal cord (Cameron et al 1995). The RVM and lateral pontine tegmentum then project to the spinal cord and modulate dorsal horn neuron activity and ultimately nociceptive information. It is generally thought that there is a balance between facilitation and inhibition from these descending modulatory pathways (Fig. 3.7) so that in conditions with pain there is an increase in facilitation and a decrease in inhibition.

Conditioned pain modulation (CPM) is an inhibitory mechanism used in human subjects to test central inhibition capability. It is analogous to diffuse noxious inhibitory controls (DNIC) in animals. CPM can predict the development of chronic pain after surgery and is reduced in most chronic pain conditions (Correa et al 2015; Daenen et al 2013; Dailey et al 2013; Normand et al 2011; Peters et al 1992; Sandrini et al 2006; Yarnitsky et al 2008). The dorsal reticular nucleus of the medulla, not the PAG or RVM, is a key nucleus in the DNIC response (Bouhassira et al 1993; De Resende et al 2011).

There are several key neurotransmitters involved in inhibition including gamma-amino-butyric acid (GABA), endogenous opioids, serotonin and noradrenaline. These neurotransmitters are generally found in central inhibitory sites and can be altered by tissue damage and pain. The endogenous inhibitory neurotransmitters outlined below have been shown to mediate analgesia by a variety of non-pharmacological treatments.

Endogenous opioids Endogenous opioids are located in peripheral tissues, immune cells and central nervous system pain modulation sites. Opioid analgesia has been extensively studied in endogenous pain control mechanisms. After peripheral inflammation, in both animals and human subjects, there is an upregulation of opioid receptors on the peripheral terminals of primary afferent fibres. Local immune cells all contain opioid peptides, and the amount of endogenous opioid peptides in these cells increases in inflamed tissues (Machelska & Stein 2006; Stein 1995; Stein et al 1990).

In the central nervous system, endogenous opioids are located in key pain inhibition nuclei, including the PAG, RVM and spinal cord. Enkephalins, endomorphins and dynorphins and their receptors μ, δ and κ are located in neurons in the brain and dorsal horn in areas known to be involved in analgesia, such as the PAG, RVM and dorsal horn of the spinal cord (Fields et al 2006; Millan 2002). Activation of opioid receptors with selective agonists, systemically or locally in the PAG, RVM, or spinal cord, produces analgesia and reduces hyperalgesia in a number of pain models, including inflammatory pain, acid-induced muscle pain and neuropathic pain (Fields et al 2006; Millan 2002; Yaksh 2006).

GABA Gamma-amino-butyric acid (GABA) is an inhibitory neurotransmitter located in neuronal cell bodies throughout the nervous system, including in pain-inhibitory pathways. It exerts its actions through activation of the ionotropic receptor, $GABA_A$, and the metabotropic receptor, $GABA_B$. There is an upregulation of GABA following peripheral inflammation and a decrease in GABA following peripheral neuropathy (Baba et al 2003; Castro-Lopes et al 1992), and activation of GABAergic receptors in the spinal cord produces analgesia (Baba et al 2003; Castro-Lopes et al 1992; Hammond Drower 1984). One potential mechanism that may contribute to hyperalgesia is a reduction in GABAergic inhibition. For example, STT cells show a reduced responsiveness to GABA agonists after induction of inflammation with capsaicin (Lin et al 1996).

Serotonin Serotonin is a neurotransmitter that is found in the RVM in neurons that send projections to the spinal cord (Basbaum & Fields 1984). Application of serotonin to the spinal cord can decrease activity of dorsal horn neurons and produces analgesia (Carruba et al 1992; Deakin & Dostrovsky 1978), and increases in serotonin in the RVM produce analgesia (Barbaro et al 1985; Brodie & Proudfit 1986). Serotonin concentrations are modulated by the serotonin transporter (SERT), and increases in SERT in chronic pain models are associated with hyperalgesia (Brito et al 2017). In the spinal cord, multiple serotonin receptors are present and have been extensively reviewed (Millan, 2002). The role of individual serotonin receptors and receptor subtypes in nociceptive transmission is controversial because 5-HT receptors have been implicated in both facilitation and inhibition of nociception, including non-pharmacological treatments for pain.

Norepinephrine Norepinephrine (i.e. noradrenaline) terminals in the spinal cord arise primarily from the DLPT (Clark & Proudfit 1991; Millan 2002). Spinally, norepinephrine inhibits nociceptive stimuli through activation of α_2-adrenergic receptors (Goldin et al 1997; Kuraishi et al 1985; Proudfit 1988). On the other hand, activation of spinal dorsal horn α_1-adrenergic receptors mediates descending facilitation of nociception (Nuseir & Proudfit, 2000). Thus, norepinephrine is involved in descending facilitatory and inhibitory nociceptive signalling depending on receptor activation.

PRINCIPLES OF CHRONIC PAIN

Chronic pain is associated with increased central excitability and reduced central inhibition. These changes in central pathways can occur in response to continued peripheral drive as a result of nociceptor sensitization, or can be independent of nociceptor input and maintained by central sensitization (Fig. 3.9A). Most commonly, patients present with a combination of peripheral and central factors driving their chronic pain. Further, chronic pain conditions with increased central excitability can result in peripheral manifestations such as increased autonomic activity, increased

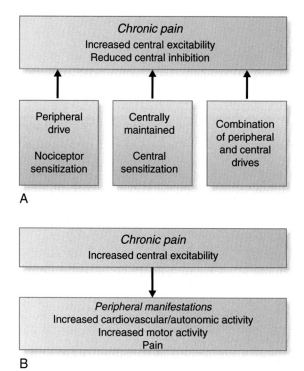

A

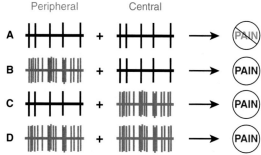

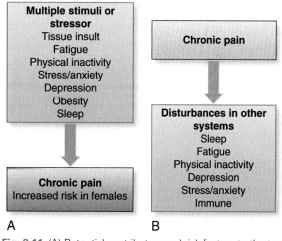

Fig. 3.10 How Underlying Peripheral and Central Sensitization Can Lead to Pain (A) Shows that under normal conditions the nervous system does not feel pain. (B) Shows a condition with primarily peripheral sensitization. Enhanced nociceptor activity activates unsensitized central neurons to result in pain. (C) Shows the condition with primarily central sensitization. Normal input from a nociceptor will activate sensitized neurons in the central nervous system to result in pain. (D) Shows the condition with both peripheral and central sensitization. Sensitized nociceptors activate sensitized central nervous system neurons and result in pain.

Fig. 3.9 (A) The increased central excitability and the reduced central inhibition that occurs with chronic pain can be driven by nociceptor sensitization, can be maintained by central sensitization independent of nociceptor activity or can be a combination of both peripheral and central sensitization. (B) Illustration showing that increased excitability in chronic pain can drive changes peripherally including autonomic activity, motor activity and result in pain without a nociceptor input.

Fig. 3.11 (A) Potential contributors and risk factors to the transition from acute to chronic pain and (B) the potential consequences of chronic pain.

motor activity and pain and hyperalgesia in peripheral tissues (Fig. 3.9B). Fig. 3.10 illustrates each of these conditions showing that peripheral sensitization, central sensitization or a combination of these can result in the perception of pain. Thus, clinically determining the underlying driver that maintains pain is critically important for effective treatment.

There are a number of potential risk factors and triggers that increase the risk for development of chronic pain after an acute injury (Fig. 3.11). These include acute pain associated with tissue insult; high levels of pain increase the risk of transition to chronic pain. Additionally, obesity and its associated systemic inflammation, physical inactivity, poor sleep, and psychological factors are all modifiable risk factors for the transition from acute to chronic pain. Furthermore, in people with chronic pain, sleep, fatigue, physical inactivity, and psychological factors are a consequence of the pain and can lead to poor outcomes for the development of chronic pain (Fig. 3.11). Thus, interventions and treatments aimed at modifying risk factors can improve outcomes for those with chronic pain.

Neural Mechanisms Underlying Pain Measures

There are a number of potential assessments that can provide insight into underlying mechanisms associated with acute and chronic pain. Local tissue injury with inflammation suggests there are peripheral drives to pain. Primary hyperalgesia is thought to reflect increased sensitivity of nociceptors to noxious input, i.e., peripheral sensitization. Although changes occur in the CNS within minutes after tissue injury, and central neurons show an enhanced response to application of noxious stimuli to the injured tissue, this central sensitization most likely reflects the increased activity of the nociceptors. Assessment of temporal summation, increased pain to the same repetitive stimuli, in human subjects is thought to reflect activity of dorsal horn neurons and is used experimentally to assess the sensitivity of the CNS. Several pain conditions, e.g. temporomandibular disorder, fibromyalgia, tension type headache, result in enhanced temporal summation when compared to controls (Ashina et al 2006; Sarlani et al 2007; Staud et al 1998). Referred pain is pain felt outside the site of tissue injury. It is not evoked by peripherally applied stimuli and reflects changes in central neurons. The *convergence-projection theory* is used to describe the mechanisms underlying referred pain. At the spinal level, neurons receive input from cutaneous as well as deep tissue such as muscles, joints or viscera. The increased activity from the site of injury is transmitted to the cortex where it is misinterpreted as pain from another structure. Secondary hyperalgesia is an increased pain response to stimuli outside the site of injury and reflects changes in central nociceptive neurons. This is thought to be the result of enlarged receptive fields of neurons after tissue injury, and/or enhanced activation of pain facilitatory pathways in the brainstem, and thus reflects an increased sensitivity in the central nervous system. Allodynia, a painful response to innocuous stimuli, most likely results from the increased responsiveness of dorsal horn neurons to innocuous stimuli, and is thus a central nervous system phenomenon. Changes in mood, sleep or fatigue are all symptoms that reflect changes in the central nervous system and can be used to detect nociplastic (central sensitization) pain in people with acute and chronic pain. Conditioned pain modulation is analgesia to a noxious stimulus applied outside of the testing site, and is a measure of the amount of central inhibition. In individuals with chronic pain, CPM is reduced (Correa et al 2015; Daenen et al 2013; Dailey et al 2013; Normand et al 2011; Peters et al 1992; Sandrini et al 2006).

Effects of Electrophysical Agents on Pain Mechanisms

Electrophysical agents have the ability to modulate peripheral and central mechanisms of pain to produce analgesia. The use of electrophysical agents for management of pain is often considered a self-management tool that allows the patient to reduce pain so they can participate in an active exercise programme and return to activities of daily living. The mechanisms underlying how these agents work to reduce pain will be briefly outlined below. In general, electrophysical agents can provide analgesia by 1) reducing nociceptor activity and sensitization through removing peripheral irritants, 2) activating peripheral inhibitory

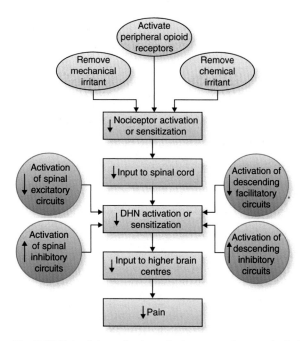

Fig. 3.12 Potential mechanisms for how non-pharmacological treatments can produce their effects on nociceptors and central neurons to inhibit pain. *DHN*, 5α-Dihydronandrolone Dorsal Horn Neuron.

mechanisms, and/or 3) activating spinal and supraspinal excitatory circuits and/or 4) activating spinal or supraspinal inhibitory circuits (Fig. 3.12). For more details, the reader is referred to additional sources (Sluka 2016).

Transcutaneous electrical nerve stimulation (TENS) The application of electrical current to the skin for pain control. Using animal models of pain, the mechanisms of action of TENS have been extensively studied. TENS reduces both primary and secondary hyperalgesia, and is effective in acute, chronic and neuropathic pain models (Ainsworth et al 2006; Chen et al 2014a,b; Cho et al 2014; Fang et al 2013; Gopalkrishnan & Sluka, 2000; Radhakrishnan et al 2003a; Resende et al 2004; Sluka et al 1998; Vance et al 2007). TENS primarily activates central inhibitory mechanisms that reduce central excitability using opioids, serotonin and GABA in a frequency-dependent manner. Both high and low frequency TENS activate the PAG, RVM and spinal cord inhibitory mechanisms to produce analgesia. A summary of the analgesic mechanisms of TENS is provided in Fig. 3.13.

High frequency TENS This increases release of β-endorphins in the bloodstream and cerebrospinal fluid, and increases methionine-enkephalin in the cerebrospinal fluid in human subjects (Han et al 1991; Salar et al 1981). In animals with knee joint inflammation, blockade of δ–opioid receptors in the spinal cord or the RVM reverses the

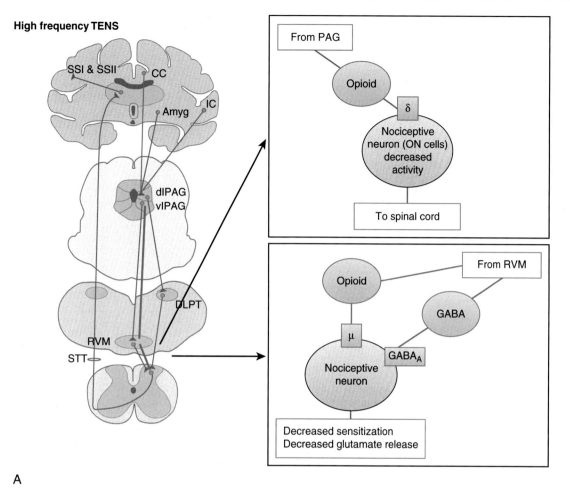

High frequency TENS

A

Fig. 3.13 The effects of (A) high frequency TENS or (B) low frequency TENS in supraspinal and spinal sites. *Amyg*, Amygdala; *CC*, cingulate cortex; *dlPAG*, dorsolateral PAG, *DLPT*, dorsolateral pontine nuclei; *GABA*, gamma-amino-butyric acid; *IC*, insular cortex; *PAG*, periaqueductal grey; *RVM*, rostral ventromedial medulla; *SSI*, *SSII*, somatosensory cortex I, II; *STT*, spinothalamic tract; *vlPAG*, ventrolateral PAG.

anti-hyperalgesia produced by high frequency TENS (Kalra et al 2001; Sluka et al 1999). Opioid effects of high frequency TENS have been confirmed in human subjects with chronic pain (Leonard et al 2010). The analgesic effects of high frequency TENS involve release of GABA and activation of the GABA$_A$ receptor, as well as activation of muscarinic receptors (M1, M3) in the spinal cord (Radhakrishnan & Sluka 2003). On the other hand, blockade of serotonin or noradrenergic receptors in the spinal cord has no effect on the antihyperalgesia produced by TENS.

In addition to its inhibitory mechanisms, high frequency TENS reduces enhanced release and expression of excitatory neurotransmitters glutamate and substance P in the spinal cord dorsal horn (Chen et al 2014b; Rokugo et al 2002; Sluka et al 2005), and reduces dorsal horn neuron sensitization

(Ma & Sluka 2001). The reduction in glutamate is prevented by blockade of δ−opioid receptors linking the effects of TENS on excitatory neurotransmitter release to activation of inhibitory pathways. High and mixed frequency TENS also reduces enhanced release of pro-inflammatory cytokines and prostaglandins in the spinal cord after tissue injury (Chen et al 2014b). Further phosphorylation of the intracellular messenger, extracellular signal-related kinase (ERK), is reduced by TENS (Fang et al 2013). Thus, high frequency TENS activates a complex endogenous inhibitory system that involves opioid, GABA and acetylcholine to reduce central excitability of nociceptive neurons.

Low frequency (<10 Hz) TENS activates classic descending inhibitory pathways that include the PAG, RVM and spinal cord (DeSantana et al 2009; Kalra et al 2001; Sluka

Low frequency TENS

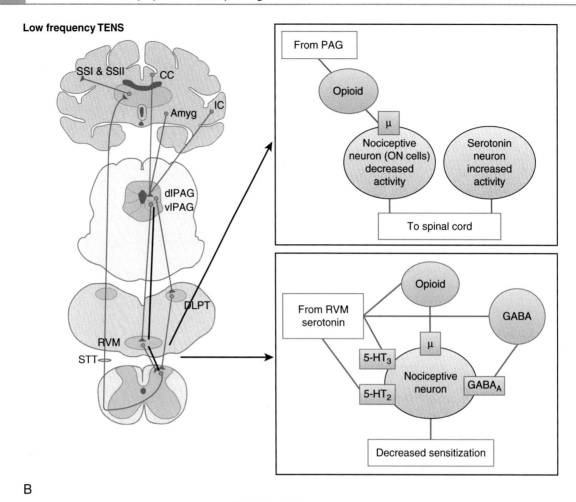

B

Fig. 3.13, cont'd

et al 1999). Low frequency TENS anti-hyperalgesia is prevented by blockade of μ-opioid receptors in the spinal cord or the RVM (Chandran & Sluka, 2003; Kalra et al 2001; Sluka et al 1999). The anti-hyperalgesia produced by low frequency TENS is also reduced by blockade of GABA$_A$, serotonin 5-HT$_{2A}$ and 5-HT$_3$, and muscarinic M1 and M3 receptors in the spinal cord (Radhakrishnan et al 2003b; Radhakrishnan & Sluka, 2003; Maeda et al 2007). Similarly, serotonin is released during low frequency TENS in animals with joint inflammation (Sluka et al 2006). In monkeys, positron emission tomography (PET) imaging studies show increases in the μ opioid receptor in multiple regions of the cortex involved in pain processing in response to low, but not high, frequency TENS: anterior cingulate cortex, caudate, putamen, somatosensory cortex and amygdala (Xiang et al 2014). Studies in human subjects confirm an opioid mediated effect of TENS (Sjolund & Eriksson 1979). Finally, low frequency TENS reduces dorsal horn neuron sensitization induced by peripheral inflammation (Ma & Sluka 2001). Taken together, these studies suggest that low frequency TENS utilizes classical descending inhibitory pathways involving the PAG-RVM pathway which utilize opioid, GABA, serotonin and muscarinic receptors in the spinal cord to reduce dorsal horn neuron activity, nociception and the consequent pain.

Photobiomodulation Also called low-level laser therapy, photobiomodulation uses light therapy with lasers or LEDs shone through the skin. Investigations of mechanisms for pain relief using animal models have shown that the majority of effects target the peripheral nervous system and are dependent on parameters used (Chow et al 2011). The mechanisms have been reviewed extensively and the reader is referred to these sources for additional details (Peplow et al 2010; Yadav et al 2016; Tsai & Hamblin 2017).

There is good experimental evidence showing that photobiomodulation improves tissue healing (Yadav et al 2016). Evidence suggests that photobiomodulation reduces neurophilic migration to a site of inflammation, increases expression of tumour growth factor, enhances collagen accumulation, activates intracellular signalling pathways and gene transcription (de Souza Costa et al 2018; Peplow et al 2010; Yadav et al 2016). Thus, through improved healing and reduction in inflammation, photobiomodulation would reduce activators of peripheral nociceptors with a subsequent reduction of input to the central nervous system and pain.

Recent evidence has begun to examine effects of photobiomodulation on pain mechanisms. Using low-level laser therapy over acupuncture points produced analgesia that was reversed by blockade of opioid and serotonin receptors systemically (Erthal et al 2013). Subsequent studies showed that blockade of spinal blockade of opioid receptors or RVM activity reversed analgesia produced by photobiomodulation (Ibrahim et al 2017). Thus, there is emerging evidence that low-level laser therapy may directly modulate central pain inhibitory pathways to produce analgesia.

Thermal agents Thermotherapies achieve their clinical effects by changing tissue temperatures, which ultimately alters cellular and physiological function. Heat therapies can be applied through use of warm baths, hot packs, diathermy or ultrasound with the goal of increasing tissue temperature. Cold therapies similarly can be applied with multiple methods with the goal of reducing tissue temperature. Thus, the majority of their effects are thought to be directed to peripheral sites and alter nociceptor sensitization. The mechanisms by which thermotherapies reduce pain are not well-studied.

Changes in blood flow are considered to be particularly important in terms of the pain relieving effects of heat and cold, with increases in blood flow thought to improve tissue healing, remove inflammatory irritants and consequently decrease activity of nociceptive afferents to ultimately decrease pain (Lehmann 1990). Ice can decrease conduction velocity of primary afferent fibres and if the temperature reaches 4°C conduction of afferent fibres is stopped (Algafly & George 2007; Lee et al 1978). Decreasing conduction velocity of afferent fibres thus would produce analgesia by decreasing firing of afferent fibres and consequently decreasing input to the central nervous system.

Heat is also used to help mobilize tissues and joints by increasing tissue extensibility and reducing muscle spasm. This would be expected to remove mechanical irritants from nociceptors and decrease input to the central nervous system. Heat-induced alterations in muscle spindle activity and in firing of Golgi tendon organs are thought to be responsible for the observed reductions in muscle tone. Type II spindle afferent fibres show a reduced activity and Golgi tendon organs show an increase in firing with increased tissue temperature (Mense 1978). Together these would decrease alpha-motor neuron firing through an interneuron circuit in the spinal cord.

SUMMARY

This section reviewed the underlying mechanisms of pain and how electrotherapeutic agents modulate pain mechanisms. Thermal agents and photobiomodulation produce the majority of their effects on the peripheral system indirectly by changing blood flow and improving healing. Cold can directly reduce nerve conduction velocity and heat can modulate muscle tone through its actions on primary afferent fibres. Emerging evidence suggests that photobiomodulation may activate central opioid inhibitory mechanisms. Electrical agents, such as TENS, produce the majority of their effects by increasing central inhibition and reducing central excitability. Understanding the contributions of peripheral and central mechanisms to an individual's pain condition will assist in determining which modalities will be most useful in the plan of care in an individual with pain. Electrotherapeutic modalities are useful agents in self-management and can be valuable tools to allow a person to participate in an active rehabilitation approach and participate in activities of daily living.

SOFT TISSUE HEALING AND REPAIR

INTRODUCTION

The inflammatory and repair processes are no longer simple events to describe owing to the ever-increasing knowledge in this field. This text is intended to provide a brief resume of the key events associated with tissue repair, with an emphasis on the musculoskeletal/soft tissues rather than a classic skin-wound approach, which is considered elsewhere in this text (see Chapters 10, 11 and 19). Examples of recent reviews can be found in Han and Ceilly (2017), Raffetto (2016), Serra et al (2017) and Sorg et al (2017), and the impact of chronic skin wounds is also usefully considered in Green et al (2014).

Tissue healing (or tissue repair) refers to the body's replacement of destroyed tissue by living tissue (Walter & Israel 1987) and comprises two essential components – regeneration and repair. The differentiation between the two is based on the resultant tissue. In regeneration, specialized tissues are replaced by the proliferation of surrounding undamaged specialized cells – in other words, new specialized tissue replaces that which has been damaged. In repair, lost tissue is replaced by granulation tissue, which matures to form scar tissue. This review concentrates on the events and processes associated with the repair process. The potential for stem cell-based therapy to dominate in this field at some point in the future raises the possibility of regeneration of the damaged tissue, which would be clinically preferable (e.g. Liu et al 2017; Lin et al 2017). This is a rapidly developing field, and there are numerous examples of electrophysical modality interventions being employed as a means to enhance the response of the implanted stem cells (e.g. Hernandez-Bule et al 2017; Priglinger et al 2018), which provides exciting future treatment potential.

Probably the most straightforward way to describe the healing process (repair) is to separate it into broad stages, which are not mutually exclusive and overlap considerably. The division into four phases is common and will be adopted here – these being *bleeding, inflammation, proliferation* and *remodelling*.

In addition to the historically established texts (Hardy 1989; Peacock 1984; Walter & Israel 1987) some more recent and detailed texts can be found at Broughton et al (2006), Granger and Senchenkova (2010), Pitzer (2006), Serhan et al (2010) and Stroncek and Reichert (2007). The key information in this section has been previously published in Watson (2003, 2006, 2016).

OVERVIEW

A brief overview of each phase is presented here before considering them in any detail. Fig. 3.14 refers to a general arrangement of the phases. Fig. 3.15 illustrates the physiological reality – in that the phases are not actually separated and the whole process is an integrated sequence of events with a continuous shift in emphasis rather than a sequence of discrete processes.

Bleeding Phase

This is a relatively short-lived phase, and will occur following injury, trauma or other similar insult, including surgery. Clearly if there has been no overt injury, this will be of little or no importance, but following soft tissue injury, there will have been some bleeding. The normal time for bleeding to stop will vary with the nature of the injury and the nature of the tissue in question. The more vascular tissues (e.g. muscle) will bleed for longer, and there will be a greater escape of blood into the tissues. Other tissues (e.g. ligament) will bleed less (both in terms of duration and volume). It is normally cited that the interval between injury and end of bleeding is a matter of a few hours (4–6 hours is often quoted) though this of course is the average duration after the average injury in the average patient. Some tissues may continue to bleed for a significantly longer period, albeit at a significantly reduced rate. Useful considerations of haemostasis can be found in Gale (2011) and Sira and Eyre (2016).

Tissue repair phases and timescale

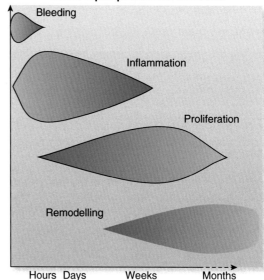

Fig. 3.14 Gross Representation of the Key Phases of the Tissue Repair Process The phases are shown as separate entities, though in reality, they are interlinked in a very deliberate way such that one phase acts as a stimulant or initiator for the following phase.

Tissue repair phases and timescale

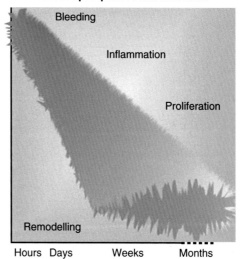

Fig. 3.15 The integrated reality of repair rather than the 'convenient' separate phase model.

Inflammatory Phase: Overview

The inflammatory phase is an *essential component* of the tissue repair process and is best regarded in this way rather than as an 'inappropriate reaction' to injury. There are, of course, numerous other initiators of the inflammatory process, though for the purpose of this paper, the single event injury model will be adopted. The inflammatory phase has a rapid onset (few hours at most) and swiftly increases in magnitude to its maximal reaction (1–3 days) before gradually resolving (over the next couple of weeks). It can result in several outcomes (see below), but in terms of tissue repair, it is both normal and essential. The onset and resolution are swifter in more vascular tissues and slower in the relatively poorly vascularized tissues (e.g. tendon, ligament). The alternative initiators of the inflammatory events include mechanical irritation, repeated minor trauma, excessive heating and cooling plus others that may be less significant in therapy, such as infection and a wide range of autoimmune disorders. The inflammatory events are essentially the same whichever 'route' is relevant for the initiation. The widely held belief that inflammation is something that must be stopped is inconsistent with current evidence (e.g. Yang et al 2018). Numerous papers identify the critical contribution that inflammation makes to the repair process. Managing it and facilitating its resolution would be consistent with current concepts. Trying to stop or arrest its progress would not (e.g. Gallo et al 2017; Serhan et al 2010). The concept that various musculoskeletal pathologies do not include an inflammatory component is losing ground (e.g. osteoarthritis: Silawal et al 2018; chronic tendinopathy: Mosca et al 2018).

Proliferation Phase: Overview

The proliferative phase essentially involves the generation of the repair material, which for the majority of musculoskeletal injuries involves the production of scar (collagen) material. The proliferative phase has a rapid onset (24–48 hours) but takes considerably longer to reach its peak reactivity, which is usually between 2–3 weeks post injury (the more vascular the tissue, the shorter the time taken to reach peak proliferative production). This peak in activity does not represent the time at which scar production (repair) is complete but the time phase during which the bulk of the scar material is formed. The production of a final product (a high quality and functional scar) is not achieved until later in the overall repair process. In general terms it is usually considered that proliferation runs from the first day or two post injury through to its peak at 2–3 weeks and decreases thereafter through to a matter of several months (typically 4–6) post trauma.

Remodelling Phase: Overview

The remodelling phase is an often-overlooked phase of repair in terms of its importance, especially in the context of therapy and rehabilitation. It is neither swift nor highly reactive, but does result in an organized, good quality and functional scar that is capable of behaving in a *similar* way to the parent tissue which it is replacing. The remodelling phase has been widely described as starting at around the same time as the peak of the proliferative phase (2–3 weeks post injury), but more recent evidence supports the proposal that the remodelling phase actually starts rather earlier than this, and it would be reasonable to consider the start point to be in the first week.

The final outcome of these combined events is that the damaged tissue will be repaired with a scar, which is not a 'like for like' replacement of the original, but does provide a functional, long-term repair that is capable of enabling good quality recovery from injury. For most patients, this is a process that will occur without the need for drugs, therapy or other intervention. The body has an intricately complex and balanced mechanism through which these events are controlled. It is possible, however, that in cases of inhibited response, delayed reactions, extensive injury or repeated trauma, therapeutic intervention is of value.

In cases where healing is compromised, the approach would be to *facilitate, promote or support* the normal tissue repair sequence, and thereby enhance the sequence of events that takes the tissues from their injured state to their recovered state. This is the argument that will be followed in this section – the promotion of normality, rather than trying to achieve a 'better' normality. The best of the available evidence would also support this approach. The techniques that are effective in the compromised healing situation are the same as those employed in a normally healing tissue, though a 'stronger' or 'more intense' intervention may be required in order to initiate a tissue response – the compromised healing tissue is typically more resistant to intervention.

In practice, our view of tissue repair is somewhat skewed by the patients that are seen (Fig. 3.16). The majority of patients whose tissues are repairing 'on track' do not need therapy help in order to achieve a quality result. The majority of the patients that arrive in the clinical environment are those for whom the normal repair sequence has been disturbed, therefore 'normal' musculoskeletal tissue repair is not routinely experienced by many therapists.

The mechanism through which therapy can be effective throughout the repair sequence is becoming better understood, though as a general comment, these effects appear to be achieved by 'stimulating' rather than 'changing' the events.

INFLAMMATORY EVENTS

Inflammation is a normal and necessary prerequisite to healing (Aller et al 2006; Hardy 1989; Medzhitov 2008; Serhan et al 2010) and recent insightful analyses are

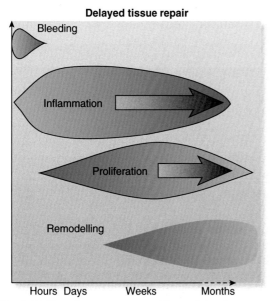

Fig. 3.16 The often-encountered 'delayed' healing seen by many therapists.

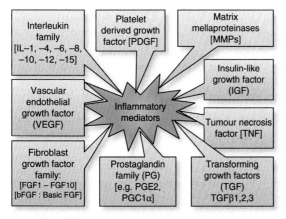

Fig. 3.17 Some of the major chemical mediation families involved in inflammation (modified from Watson 2016.)

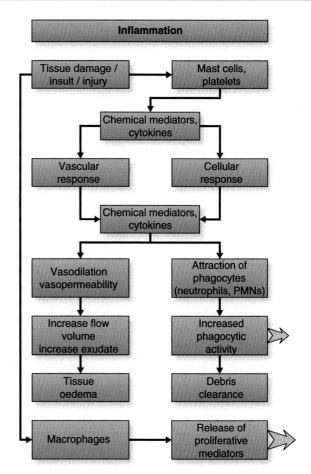

Fig. 3.18 Key Inflammatory Elements *PMNs*, polymorphonucleocytes.

provided by Dakin et al (2014) and Rees et al (2014). Following tissue bleeding, a number of substances remain in the tissues that make a contribution to the later phases. Fibrin and fibronectin form a substratum that is hospitable to the adhesion of various cells.

The complex *chemically mediated amplification cascade* (the sources of which are summarized in Fig. 3.17) that is responsible for both the initiation and control of the inflammatory response can be initiated by numerous direct and indirect events. The complexity and importance of the chemically mediated nature of the inflammatory events, together with links between this mediation system and the effects of therapeutic intervention, have been summarized in Watson (2016).

There are two essential elements to the inflammatory events, namely the *vascular* and *cellular* cascades. Importantly, these occur in parallel and are significantly interlinked. Fig. 3.18 summarizes the essential elements of the inflammatory cascade. The chemical mediators that make an active contribution to this process are myriad. They are usefully summarized in several reviews, including Jiminez and Jiminez (2004) and Singer and Clark (1999). Whilst these are clearly not the newest reviews, they do provide a useful background to the topic. Smith et al (2008) provide a useful review of the mediators associated with muscle injury, whilst Molloy et al (2003) have reviewed the role of these mediators in relation to ligament and tendon injury. Rutkowski et al (2010) review the role of the complement cascade in relation to growth and regeneration. A more detailed account can be found in Serhan et al (2010).

In recent years, the identification of numerous cytokines and 'growth factors' has led to several important discoveries and potential new treatment lines (e.g. Leung et al 2006; Wagner et al 2003). The effect of various therapies on the cytokine cascades is becoming more obvious with the increasing volume of research in this field (Watson 2016).

Vascular Events

In addition to the vascular changes associated with bleeding, there are also marked changes in the state of the intact vessels. There are changes in the calibre of the blood vessels, changes in the vessel wall and in blood flow. Vasodilation follows an initial but brief vasoconstriction and persists for the duration of the inflammatory response. Flow increases through the main channels and additionally, previously dormant capillaries are opened to increase the volume through the capillary bed.

The cause of this dilation is primarily by chemical means (e.g. histamine, prostaglandins and complement cascade components C3 and C5 and others) whilst the axon reflex and autonomic system may exert additional influences. There is an initial increase in blood flow velocity followed by a prolonged slowing of the stream. The white cells marginate, platelets adhere to the vessel walls and the endothelial cells swell.

In addition to the *vasodilation* response, there is an increase in the *vasopermeability* of the local vessels (also mediated by numerous chemical mediators), and thus the combination of vasodilation and vasopermeability means that there is an increased flow through vessels which are 'leakier', resulting in increased exudate production.

The flow and pressure changes in the vessels allow fluid and smaller solutes to pass into the tissue spaces. This can occur both at the arterial and venous ends of the capillary network as the increased hydrostatic pressure is sufficient to overcome the osmotic pressure of the plasma proteins. The vessels show a marked increase in permeability to plasma proteins. There are several phases to the permeability changes but essentially, there is a separation of the endothelial cells, particularly in the venules, and an increased escape of protein rich plasma to the interstitial tissue spaces. The chemical mediators responsible for the permeability changes include histamine, serotonin (5-HT), bradykinin and leukotrienes, together with a potentiating effect from the prostaglandins.

The *exudate* provides benefit in that it serves to dilute local irritants and its high fibrinogen content will result in a fibrin clot which provides an initial scaffold for the migrating cells to attach to in addition to a preliminary tissue union. Furthermore, the fibrin meshwork will trap debris and thus aids phagocytic activity (see below). Mast cells (Behzad et al 2013; Frenzel & Hermine 2013) in the damaged region release hyaluronic acid and other proteoglycans which bind with the exudate fluid and create a *gel*, which limits local fluid flow, and further traps various particles and debris (Hardy 1989).

Cellular Events

The cellular components of the inflammatory response include the early migration (within minutes) of phagocytes (neutrophils, polymorphonucleocytes or PMNs) from blood vessels. This is followed by several other species leaving the main flow, including monocytes, lymphocytes, eosinophils, basophils (Lorena et al 2002) and smaller numbers of red blood cells (though these leave the vessel passively rather than the active emigration of the white blood cells). In the tissue spaces, the monocytes modulate into macrophages (Forrest 1983; Hurst et al 2001). The main groups of chemical mediators responsible for chemotaxis are some components of the complement cascade, lymphokines, factors released for the PMNs and peptides released from the mast cells in the damaged tissue (Egozi et al 2003; Luster 1998; Rankin 2004; Vernon-Roberts 1988). Butterfield et al (2006) usefully consider the beneficial and the potentially detrimental effects of neutrophils and macrophages in inflammation whilst Snyder et al (2016) provide an excellent review considering macrophage roles in the inflammatory events.

The PMNs provide a means for early wound debridement. Numerous mediators have been identified as having a chemotactic role, for example platelet derived growth factor (PDGF) released from damaged platelets in the area. Components of the complement cascade (C3a and C5a), leukotrienes (released from a variety of white cells, macrophages and mast cells) and lymphokines (released from polymorphs) have been identified (see Dierich et al 1987; Smith et al 2008; Vernon-Roberts 1988; Walter & Israel 1987).

These cells exhibit a strong phagocytic activity and are responsible for the essential tissue debridement role. Dead and dying cells, fibrin mesh and clot residue all need to be removed. As a 'bonus', one of the chemicals released as an end product of phagocytosis is lactic acid, which is one of the stimulants of proliferation – the next sequence of events in the repair process.

The inflammatory response, therefore, results in a vascular response and a cellular and fluid exudate with resulting oedema and phagocytic activation. The complex interaction of the chemical mediators not only stimulates various components of the inflammatory phase, but also stimulates initiation of the proliferative phase. The course of the inflammatory response will depend upon the number of cells destroyed, the initiating event and the tissue condition at the time of insult.

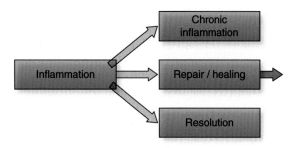

Fig. 3.19 Inflammatory Outcomes

Inflammatory Outcomes

Resolution is a possible outcome (Fig. 3.19) at this stage on condition that less than a critical number of cells have been destroyed. For most patients that present for therapy, this is an unlikely scenario unless tissue irritation rather than overt damage is the initiator. There is some considerable debate with regard to 'micro injury' or 'micro trauma' and whether it leads to a repair event or a resolution. If the body fails to mount a repair response to a micro injury, the resulting cumulative damage can result in longer term issues. This debate continues with interesting evidence, e.g. Frick and Murthy (2010), Lin et al (2004), Rompe et al (2008) and Taljanovic et al (2011). Widgerow (2012) authored an interesting paper looking at the naturally occurring 'stop' signals for inflammatory events.

Suppuration in the presence of infective microorganisms will result in pus formation. Pus consists of dead cell debris and living, dead and dying polymorphs suspended in an inflammatory exudate. Clearly, the presence of an infection will delay the healing of a wound (Zederfelt 1979) and in some areas of clinical practice, tissue infection is a key issue. Whilst not ignoring its importance, it will not be considered further in this chapter.

Chronic inflammation does not necessarily imply inflammation of long duration, and may follow a transient or prolonged acute inflammatory stage (Vernon-Roberts 1988). Essentially there are two forms of chronic inflammation: either the chronic reaction supervenes over the acute reaction or it may, in fact, develop slowly with no initial acute phase (ab initio) (Raftery (2011)). Chronic inflammation ab initio can have many causes, including local irritants, poor circulation, some microorganisms or immune disturbances. Chronic inflammation is usually more productive than exudative – it produces more fibrous material than inflammatory exudate. Frequently there is some tissue destruction, inflammation and attempted healing all occurring simultaneously (Raftery 2011; Metz et al 2007; Serhan et al 2010; Walters & Israel 1987).

Healing/repair by fibrosis will most likely be taking place in the tissue repair scenario considered in this chapter. The fibrin deposits from the inflammatory stage will be partly removed by the fibrinolytic enzymes (from the plasma and PMNs) and will be gradually replaced by granulation tissue, which becomes organized to form scar tissue. Macrophages are largely responsible for the removal of the fibrin, allowing capillary budding and fibroblastic activity to proceed (proliferation). The greater the volume of damaged tissue, the greater the extent of, and the greater the density of the resulting scar tissue. Chronic inflammation is usually accompanied by some fibrosis even in the absence of significant tissue destruction (e.g. Raftery (2011); Li et al 2007). There is significant evidence that chronic inflammation is a real element in pathologies previously ascribed as being non-inflammatory (e.g. Dakin et al 2017 for Achilles tendinopathy). Furthermore, pathologies that result in a chronic inflammatory state can give rise to secondary sequelae of relevance in rehabilitation – as in chronic obstructive pulmonary disease (COPD) or rheumatoid arthritis (e.g. Londhe & Gutteridge 2015).

The effects of acute inflammation are largely beneficial. The fluid exudate dilutes the toxins and escaped blood products, including antibodies (and systemic drugs). The fibrinogen forms fibrin clots providing a mechanical barrier to the spread of microorganisms (if present) and additionally assists phagocytosis. The gel-like consistency of the inflammatory exudate also makes a positive contribution by preventing the spread of the inflammatory mediators to surrounding intact tissues. Transportation of invading bacteria (if present) to the lymphatic system stimulates an immune response whilst the increased blood flow contributes to the increased cell metabolism necessary for the proliferative stage by increasing local oxygen content, supply of necessary nutrients and removal of waste products. The leucocytes provide a mechanism for the phagocytosis of foreign material, bacteria and dead cells, with the neutrophils (PMNs) and monocytes (becoming macrophages) making the greatest contribution.

There are several detrimental aspects of inflammation that deserve mention. Firstly, the increased local hydrostatic pressure from the oedema can restrict blood flow if the injured tissue space is limited, produce pain and therefore limit function and additionally reduce local oxygen levels. There have been suggestions that free radicals produced as a result of acute inflammatory responses may have detrimental effects on cell membrane processes, as may overproduction of lysosomal enzymes from PMN activity.

There are many aspects of the inflammatory events that can be influenced by therapeutic intervention, ranging from the mechanical to the biochemical. There is a growing body of evidence to support the effects of manual and exercise therapy on the 'soup' of chemical mediators, cytokines and growth factors. Various therapy modalities can also exert influence when applied at appropriate doses. Watson (2016) recently identified overt links between various therapy interventions and chemical mediation systems. There is insufficient space here to evaluate the literature on this topic more fully, but there are evidenced links cited in Watson (2016) for exercise, mechanical stress, massage, manual therapy, ultrasound, laser, shockwave, electrical stimulation (including microcurrent), radio frequency modalities, electroacupuncture and magnetic field based therapies. It appears that all these interventions (and inevitably others not yet fully investigated) have a common mode of action in that at least part of their mechanism of action is their capacity to influence the mediation systems of the inflammatory events.

PROLIFERATIVE EVENTS

The repair process restores tissue continuity by the deposition of repair tissue. This is initially granulation tissue, which matures to form scar tissue. Repair tissue is a connective tissue distinct from the onset in several ways from the connective tissue native to the site (Forrest 1983). Interesting recent developments have identified that in muscle there is a degree of regenerative activity post trauma, linked to the activation of a mechanosensitive growth factor and subsequent activation of muscle satellite (stem) cells (Hill et al 2003). A range of growth factors have been identified as being active in the processes of proliferation. The source of the majority of these cytokines is the inflammatory phase, thus 'turning off' or limiting the inflammatory events may have the unwanted effect of reducing the signal strength stimulating these proliferative events (e.g. Beck et al 2005; Boursinos et al 2009; Dimmen et al 2009; Radi et al 2005)

Fibroblasts also make a significant contribution to the mediator release (Charoenlarp et al 2017) mainly through the fibroblastic growth factor (FGF) family. Two fundamental processes involved in the repair are fibroplasia and angiogenesis (Fig. 3.20). The function of the fibroblast is to repair the connective tissue (Vanable 1989).

Fibroblasts migrate to the area from surrounding tissue. Fibroblastic activation is chemically mediated, particularly (but not exclusively) by chemicals released from the macrophages during the inflammatory stage. Fibroblasts migrate into the damaged area and proliferate within the first few days after the tissue damage. Macrophage derived growth factors (MGDFs) are a complex group of mediators responsible, at least in part, for the activation of fibroblasts (Li & Wang 2011).

Alongside the fibroblastic activation, capillaries bud and grow towards the repair zone. Loops and arcades are formed together with anastomoses, which re-establish

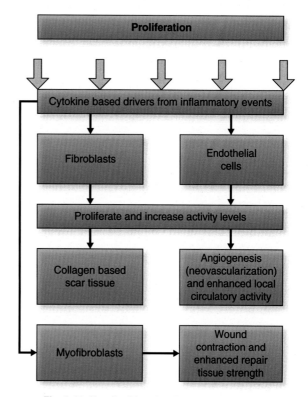

Fig. 3.20 Key Proliferative Elements EG MDGF

a blood flow through the region, providing oxygen and nutrients whilst removing metabolic and repair waste products. Oxygen is critical for many of the reparative processes, but especially for collagen production (Niinikoski 1979; Vanables 1989). A wide range of growth factors and chemical mediators have been identified that exert influences on the developing capillaries. These include macrophage derived factors, PDGF, lactic acid and fibroblast growth factor (Vernon-Roberts 1988). Some of these mediators are produced during the inflammatory phase, thus making an essential link between the inflammatory and proliferative phases. Li et al (2005) provide a review of the essential nature of the angiogenic events in the repair sequence. Numerous researchers (e.g. Oryan et al 2012) have illustrated that the healing rate varies between tissues – being slow, for example, in ligament, which given its relatively poor vascularity is predictable.

There is growing evidence that various therapies are able to positively influence these proliferative and angiogenic events, including ultrasound and LIPUS, shockwave, laser, exercise and manual therapies. As is the case with the inflammatory stage, the common mode of action of a wide range of therapeutic interventions appears to be

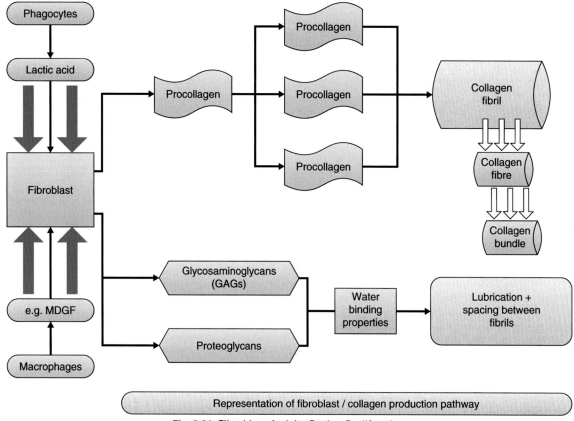

Fig. 3.21 Fibroblast Activity During Proliferation

their capacity to stimulate the mediation systems, thereby enhancing the normal proliferative events (Watson 2016).

Granulation tissue invasion follows the 'demolition' phase (when autolytic enzymes are released from PMNs and dead cells) (Walter & Israel 1987). The activation of fibroblasts and capillary budding would normally occur by about the third day after the tissue insult. The combination of capillary budding and collagen production results in a highly vascular repair site. The fibroblasts initially produce predominantly type III collagen, which will become type I collagen as the repair matures – during remodelling (Walter & Israel 1987).

Fibroblasts also produce glycosaminoglycans, fibronectins and proteoglycans, which are essential components of the ground substance (Fig. 3.21) (Forrest 1983; Hardy 1989; Walter & Israel 1987).

Myofibroblasts are derived from fibroblasts activated by a variety of chemical mediators, and are responsible for wound contraction and the early strength of the repair. They draw the edges of the wound/damaged area together, thus reducing the size of the final scar (Gabbiani 2003; Hardy 1989; Lorena et al 2002; McAnulty 2007; Peacock 1984; Wipff et al 2007).

Granulation tissue matures with lymphatic development (in much the same way as capillary development), nerve fibre ingrowth and mast cell invasion. Collagen fibres are oriented in response to local stress thus providing tensile strength in the required directions (see Forrest (1983) and Hardy (1989) for useful collagen reviews). As the granulation tissue matures, there is a process of devascularization with obliteration of the lumen of the vessels.

REMODELLING EVENTS

The remodelling phase primarily involves the refinement of the collagen and its associated extracellular matrix (Fig. 3.22). The primary importance of remodelling, from a therapy perspective, is that the scar tissue effecting the repair improves in quality over time and its resulting organization results in enhanced functional capacity.

The initial deposition of collagen produces relatively weak fibrils with random orientation. With maturity, the collagen becomes more obviously oriented in line with local stresses (Culav et al 1999; Gomez et al 1991).

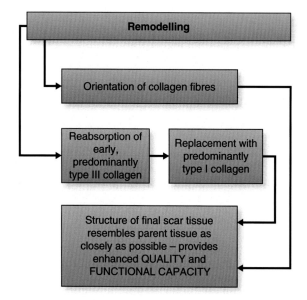

Fig. 3.22 Principal Events of Remodelling

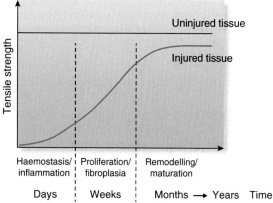

Fig. 3.23 Representation of Regained Tissue Strength (Modified from Lin et al 2004.)

A proportion of the original fine (type III) collagen is reabsorbed (due to the action of collagenases) and is replaced with type I collagen with more cross links and greater tensile strength (Forrest 1983; Huisman et al 2014; Vanables 1989). Collagen synthesis and lysis both occur at a greater rate in repairing tissue when compared with non-wounded tissue as old fibrous tissue is removed and new scar tissue is laid down. The maturing scar is therefore a dynamic system rather than a static one. Snyman and Niesler (2015) provide some interesting insight into the role of the MMP mediator family and their role in remodelling following muscle injury, extending concepts outlined by Page-McCaw et al (2007).

There are several influential factors during this long phase, including physical stress. This remodelling process is initiated whilst the proliferative stage proceeds, therefore providing a considerable overlap between the phases. Current evidence suggests that remodelling begins within the first week of the repair sequence, thus remodelling is underway before the proliferative phase reaches peak activity. The older concept of remodelling starting after proliferation is completed has been abandoned. Final remodelling will continue for months, and typically at least a year from the initial damage: see Hardy (1989) for a comprehensive consideration of collagen behaviour in remodelling and Culav et al (1999) for an excellent review of collagen and its roles. The potential mechanism by which physical stress can influence cell and tissue behaviour is usefully considered by Ingber (2003, 2008). Kahn and Scott (2009) and Killian et al (2012) provide more recent papers linking

mechanical stress and tissue repair, as do Bring et al (2007) and Ogawa (2011), whilst Mackey et al (2008) also provide a valuable review. Dunn and Olmedo (2015) have revitalized this topic to useful effect.

It is suggested that the strength of the final repair, whilst impressive, will not match that of the pre-injury strength, as illustrated in Fig. 3.23 (after Lin et al (2004)).

Factors Known to Delay Healing

Factors known to delay healing are divided into general and local:

General: Age, protein deficiency, low vitamin C levels, steroids and NSAIDs (inhibitory effect), temperature (lower rate when colder).

Local: Poor blood supply/ischaemia, adhesion to bone or other underlying tissue, prolonged inflammation, excessive movement or mechanical stress (restarts inflammation).

THERAPY INFLUENCES

Clearly the effects of the whole range of therapies cannot be considered in any significant detail here, but in principle a therapy that is beneficial to the repair events is a therapy which stimulates rather than 'changes' the natural sequence. Promoting or stimulating the inflammatory events is not intended to achieve a 'bigger' inflammatory response, but to maximize its efficiency. Similarly, if delivering therapy during the proliferative phase, there would be no benefit in simply creating a bigger volume of scar tissue. The advantage of appropriate intervention is that it stimulates a maximally efficient response, and therefore the required repair material is generated with best quality and minimal time. In the remodelling phase, the aim is refinement of the scar tissue and the use of therapy can

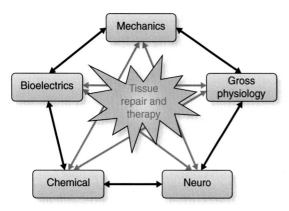

Fig. 3.24 The Concept of Multiple Influences of Therapy on the Tissue Repair Events (From Watson 2011.)

have a significant effect, especially given the growing body of evidence relating the effects of mechanical stress and collagen behaviour.

Inappropriate therapy at any stage is perfectly capable of inhibiting these events and therefore can result in a poorer quality repair or one that progresses at a slower rate. Therapy is not guaranteed to be beneficial – one has to be mindful of the events needed at a particular stage and be selective of the most appropriate (evidenced) therapy at each stage.

The mode of action of these therapies, historically employed, is actually a lot more complex than was originally conceived and hitherto understood and is summarized in Fig. 3.24 (after Watson (2011)).

An interesting recent development is that there is an increasing body of knowledge which supports the concept that existing therapies have an effect on the chemical environment of the repairing tissue (Fig. 3.25; Watson 2011, 2016). Exercise therapy, manual therapy and various electrophysical modalities are now known to exert such effects. This need not 'replace' the current explanations for the mode of action of therapy, but offers an extended effects model in which there are mechanical, neurological, gross physiological, chemical and bioelectric effects of therapy. Whilst this is a strongly reductionist approach, it is supported by a growing body of evidence (Watson 2016). Further details can be found in the modality chapters of this text. If one looks, for example, at the effect of various therapies in stimulating bone growth – something that is common to many therapy modes – and looks at the commonality of the chemical pathways, the degree of overlap is highly significant. It is, of course, distinctly possible that therapy A might be more effective than therapy B, but the fact that more than one therapy mode stimulates the same chemically mediated pathway is of potential value.

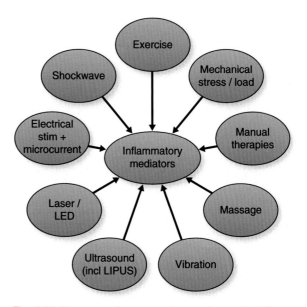

Fig. 3.25 Numerous therapy modes are known to influence chemical mediation systems associated with inflammation and repair.

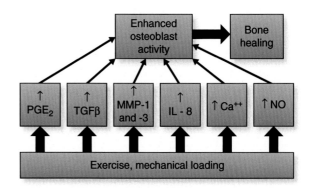

Fig. 3.26 Example of different therapies stimulating common chemical mediation pathways – in this example, for enhanced bone healing (From Watson 2016.)

An example of this common mode of action is shown in Fig. 3.26, taken from Watson (2016).

Stem Cell-Based Therapy – Potential Impact on Musculoskeletal Tissue Repair

Stem cell research has developed at a phenomenal rate over the last 20 years. The state of this research and the advances in the field of stem cell-based therapies are beyond the remit of this chapter; however, the potential impact of stem cell science on musculoskeletal rehabilitation merits a brief discussion. As mentioned at the start of this chapter, tissue regeneration rather than repair is a remarkably attractive idea. Imagine damaged ligamentous tissue being replaced with 'new' ligament: there would be a clear advantage – with potentially a higher quality outcome and improved functional capacity for the patient.

Stem cells present in the tissues have the potential to differentiate into a range of cell types and specialist cell types. There are multiple sources of stem cells (e.g. embryonic stem cells, non-embryonic (adult) stem cells, etc.) and historically these were thought to be present only in embryonic tissue. The recognition of their presence in many adult tissues has boosted further developments in this field. In addition, the harvesting of stem cells from tissue A and implanting them into damaged tissue B offers significant possibilities (Fong et al 2011). Numerous reviews provide insight for the interested reader, including in osteoarthritic knees (Pas 2017), in tendon repair (Liu 2017), and in cartilage repair Lee and Wang (2017).

Electrophysical modalities (e.g. laser, radiofrequency energy) may have a significant role to play in this developing field. Stem cells need a 'signal' to initiate their differentiation. Much research has evaluated chemical based signal systems (drugs), but recent work has recognized that various external energy sources can facilitate differentiation, including radiofrequency energy (Hernandez-Bule 2014), laser (Amaroli 2018), shockwave (Zhang 2018) and ultrasound (Zhang 2017). The possibility for future musculoskeletal and rehabilitation medicine is that stem cells will be 'inserted' into the damaged tissue and the therapist will then employ an appropriate electrophysical energy to facilitate cell differentiation.

Establishing optimal energy delivery and 'dose' parameters will be critical and is likely to open up an entire new field of research in electrophysical agents. It may transpire that drug-based differentiation systems will prove to be more effective, but the clearly demonstrated beneficial effects of electrophysical modalities in this field merit their consideration as an effective differential trigger.

SUMMARY

Tissue healing is a complex and dynamic system, which enables effective repair of damaged tissue. The repair control system and links between its various components are complex, and there is an ever-increasing volume of literature that continues to identify new mediators, cytokines and variants. Whilst this knowledge base continues to expand, the links between the effects of therapy and these chemical control systems are also growing.

There is little doubt that appropriate therapy has the capacity to influence the process in a positive way and the most logical and best evidenced approach to intervention is to stimulate or promote the 'normal' events rather than trying to change them to something better. If repair is underway, then keep it moving. If it is delayed, then stimulate it in order to help get it back on track. Whilst there are myriad approaches, those that are most effective appear to follow this philosophy.

REFERENCES

Abdelhamid, R. E., & Sluka, K. A. (2015). ASICs mediate pain and inflammation in musculoskeletal diseases. *Physiology, 30,* 449–459.

Ainsworth, L., Budelier, K., Clinesmith, M., et al. (2006). Transcutaneous electrical nerve stimulation (TENS) reduces chronic hyperalgesia induced by muscle inflammation. *Pain, 120,* 182–187.

Algafly, A. A., & George, K. P. (2007). The effect of cryotherapy on nerve conduction velocity, pain threshold and pain tolerance. *British Journal of Sports Medicine, 41,* 365–369; discussion 369.

Aller, M. A., Arias, J. L., Sanchez-Patan, F., & Arias, J. (2006). The inflammatory response: An efficient way of life. *Medical Science Monitor: International Medical Journal of Experimental and Clinical Research, 12*(10), RA225–234.

Amano, T., Yamakuni, T., Okabe, N., Sakimura, K., & Takahashi, Y. (1991). Production of nerve growth factor in rat skeletal muscle. *Neuroscience Letters, 132,* 5–7.

Amaroli, A., Agas, D., Laus, F., et al. (2018). The effects of photobiomodulation of 808 nm diode laser therapy at higher fluence on the in vitro osteogenic differentiation of bone marrow stromal cells. *Frontiers in Physiology, 9,* 123.

Appelgren, A., Applegren, B., Eriksson, S., et al. (1991). Neuropeptides in temporomandibular joints with rheumatoid arthritis: A clinical study. *Scandinavian Journal of Dental Research, 99,* 519–521.

Ashina, S., Bendtsen, L., Ashina, M., Magerl, W., & Jensen, R. (2006). Generalized hyperalgesia in patients with chronic tension-type headache. *Cephalalgia, 26,* 940–948.

Baba, H., Ji, R. R., Kohno, T., et al. (2003). Removal of GABAergic inhibition facilitates polysynaptic A fiber-mediated excitatory transmission to the superficial spinal dorsal horn. *Molecular and Cellular Neurosciences, 24,* 818–830.

Barbaro, N. M., Hammond, D. L., & Fields, H. L. (1985). Effects of intrathecally administered methysergide and yohimbine on microstimulation-produced antinociception in the rat. *Brain Research, 343,* 223–229.

Basbaum, A. I., Bautista, D. M., Scherrer, G., & Julius, D. (2009). Cellular and molecular mechanisms of pain. *Cell, 139,* 267–284.

Basbaum, A. I., & Fields, H. L. (1984). Endogenous pain control systems: Brainstem spinal pathways and endorphin circuitry. *Annual Review of Neuroscience, 7,* 309–338.

Beck, A., Salem, K., Krischak, G., Kinzl, L., Bischoff, M., & Schmelz, A. (2005). Nonsteroidal anti-inflammatory drugs (NSAIDs) in the perioperative phase in traumatology and orthopedics effects on bone healing. *Operative Orthopädie und Traumatologie, 17*(6), 569–578.

Behzad, H., Sharma, A., Mousavizadeh, R., Lu, A., & Scott, A. (2013). Mast cells exert pro-inflammatory effects of relevance to the pathophyisology of tendinopathy. *Arthritis Research and Therapy, 15*(6), R184.

Beitz, J. M. (2017). Pharmacologic impact (aka "Breaking Bad") of medications on wound healing and wound development: A literature-based overview. *Ostomy Wound Management, 63*(3), 18–35.

Black, J. A., Liu, S., Tanaka, M., Cummins, T. R., & Waxman, S. G. (2004). Changes in the expression of tetrodotoxin-sensitive sodium channels within dorsal root ganglia neurons in inflammatory pain. *Pain, 108*, 237–247.

Bouhassira, D., Chitour, D., Villanueva, L., & Le, B. D. (1993). Morphine and diffuse noxious inhibitory controls in the rat: Effects of lesions of the rostral ventromedial medulla. *European Journal of Pharmacology, 232*, 207–215.

Boursinos, L. A., Karachalios, T., Poultsides, L., & Malizos, K. N. (2009). Do steroids, conventional non-steroidal anti-inflammatory drugs and selective Cox-2 inhibitors adversely affect fracture healing? *Journal of Musculoskeletal and Neuronal Interactions, 9*(1), 44–52.

Brain, S. D., & Williams, T. J. (1985). Inflammatory oedema induced by synergism between calcitonin gene-related peptide (CGRP) and mediators of increased vascular permeability. *British Journal of Pharmacology, 86*, 855–860.

Bring, D. K., Kreicbergs, A., Renstrom, P. A., & Ackermann, P. W. (2007). Physical activity modulates nerve plasticity and stimulates repair after Achilles tendon rupture. *Journal of Orthopaedic Research: Official Publication of the Orthopaedic Research Society, 25*(2), 164–172.

Brito, R. G., Rasmussen, L. A., & Sluka, K. A. (2017). Regular physical activity prevents development of chronic muscle pain through modulation of supraspinal opioid and serotonergic mechanisms. *Pain Reports, 2*, e618.

Brodie, M. S., & Proudfit, H. K. (1986). Antinociception induced by local injections of carbachol into the nucleus raphe magnus in rats: Alteration by intrathecal injection of monoaminergic antagonists. *Brain Research, 371*, 70–79.

Broughton, G., 2nd., Janis, J. E., & Attinger, C. E. (2006). The basic science of wound healing. *Plastic and Reconstructive Surgery, 117*(Suppl. 7), 12S–34S.

Burgess, S. E., Gardell, L. R., Ossipov, M. H., et al. (2002). Time-dependent descending facilitation from the rostral ventromedial medulla maintains, but does not initiate, neuropathic pain. *Journal of Neuroscience, 22*, 5129–5136.

Butterfield, T. A., Best, T. M., & Merrick, M. A. (2006). The dual roles of neutrophils and macrophages in inflammation: A critical balance between tissue damage and repair. *Journal of Athletic Training, 41*(4), 457–465.

Cairns, B. E., Svensson, P., Wang, K., et al. (2003). Activation of peripheral NMDA receptors contributes to human pain and rat afferent discharges evoked by injection of glutamate into the masseter muscle. *Journal of Neurophysiology, 90*, 2098–2105.

Cairns, B. E., Svensson, P., Wang, K., et al. (2006). Ketamine attenuates glutamate-induced mechanical sensitization of the masseter muscle in human males. *Experimental Brain Research, 169*, 467–472.

Calcutt, N. A., & Chaplan, S. R. (1997). Spinal pharmacology of tactile allodynia in diabetic rats. *British Journal of Pharmacology, 122*, 1478–1482.

Calejesan, A. A., Kim, S. J., & Zhuo, M. (2000). Descending facilitatory modulation of a behavioral nociceptive response by stimulation in the adult rat anterior cingulate cortex. *European Journal of Pain, 4*, 83–96.

Cameron, A. A., Khan, I. A., Westlund, K. N., & Willis, W. D. (1995). The efferent projections of the periaqueductal gray in the rat: A Phaseolus vulgaris-leucoagglutinin study. II. Descending projections. *The Journal of Comparative Neurology, 351*, 585–601.

Carlton, S. M., Hargett, G. L., & Coggeshall, R. E. (1995). Localization and activation of glutamate receptors in unmyelinated axons of rat glabrous skin. *Neuroscience Letters, 197*, 25–28.

Carruba, M. O., Nisoli, E., Garosi, V., Sacerdote, P., Panerai, A. E., & Da Prada, M. (1992). Catecholamine and serotonin depletion from rat spinal cord: Effects on morphine and footshock induced analgesia. *Pharmacological Research: The Official Journal of the Italian Pharmacological Society, 25*, 187–194.

Castrillon, E. E., Cairns, B. E., Ernberg, M., et al. (2007). Effect of a peripheral NMDA receptor antagonist on glutamate-evoked masseter muscle pain and mechanical sensitization in women. *Journal of Orofacial Pain, 21*, 216–224.

Castro-Lopes, J. M., Tavares, I., Tolle, T. R., Coito, A., & Coimbra, A. (1992). Increase in GABAergic cells and GABA levels in the spinal-cord in unilateral inflammation of the hindlimb in the rat. *European Journal of Neuroscience, 4*, 296–301.

Chandran, P., & Sluka, K. A. (2003). Development of opioid tolerance with repeated transcutaneous electrical nerve stimulation administration. *Pain, 102*, 195–201.

Chapman, V., & Dickenson, A. H. (1995). Time-related roles of excitatory amino acid receptors during persistent noxiously evoked responses of rat dorsal horn neurones. *Brain Research, 703*, 45–50.

Charoenlarp, P., Rajendran, A. K., & Iseki, S. (2017). Role of fibroblast growth factors in bone regeneration. *Inflammation and Regeneration, 37*(1), 10.

Chen, Y. W., Tzeng, J. I., Lin, M. F., Hung, C. H., & Wang, J. J. (2014a). Transcutaneous electrical nerve stimulation attenuates postsurgical allodynia and suppresses spinal substance P and proinflammatory cytokine release in rats. *Physical Therapy, 95*(1), 76–85.

Chen, Y. W., Tzeng, J. I., Lin, M. F., Hung, C. H., Hsieh, P. L., & Wang, J. J. (2014b). High-frequency transcutaneous electrical nerve stimulation attenuates postsurgical pain and inhibits excess substance P in rat dorsal root ganglion. *Regional Anesthesia and Pain Medicine, 39*, 322–328.

Chimenti, R. L., Frey-Law, L. A., & Sluka, K. A. (2018). A mechanism-based approach to physical therapist management of pain. *Physical Therapy, 98*, 302–314.

Cho, H. Y., Suh, H. R., & Han, H. C. (2014). A single trial of transcutaneous electrical nerve stimulation reduces chronic neuropathic pain following median nerve injury in rats. *Tohoku Journal of Experimental Medicine, 232*, 207–214.

Chow, R., Armati, P., Laakso, E. L., Bjordal, J. M., & Baxter, G. D. (2011). Inhibitory effects of laser irradiation on peripheral mammalian nerves and relevance to analgesic effects: A systematic review. *Photomedicine and Laser Surgery, 29*, 365–381.

Clark, F. M., & Proudfit, H. K. (1991). The projection of locus coeruleus neurons to the spinal cord in the rat determined by anterograde tracing combined with immunocytochemistry. *Brain Research, 538*, 231–245.

Coderre, T. J., Fisher, K., & Fundytus, M. E. (1997). The role of ionotropic and metabotropic glutamate receptors in persistent nociception. In T. S. Jensen, J. A. Turner, Z. Wiesenfeld-Hallin (Eds.), *Proceedings of the 8th World Congress on Pain* (pp. 259–275). Seattle: IASP Press.

Coderre, T. J., Katz, J., Vaccarino, A. L., & Melzack, R. (1993). Contribution of central neuroplasticity to pathological pain: Review of clinical and experimental evidence. *Pain, 52*, 259–285.

Coderre, T. J., & Melzack, R. (1985). Increased pain sensitivity following heat injury involves a central mechanism. *Behavioural Brain Research, 15*, 259–262.

Coderre, T. J., & Melzack, R. (1987). Cutaneous hyperalgesia: Contributions of the peripheral and central nervous systems to the increase in pain sensitivity after injury. *Brain Research, 404*, 95–106.

Coderre, T. J., & Melzack, R. (1992). The role of NMDA receptor-operated calcium channels in persistent nociception after formalin-induced tissue injury. *Journal of Neuroscience: The Official Journal of the Society for Neuroscience, 12*, 3671–3675.

Coghill, R. C., Talbot, J. D., Evans, A. C., et al. (1994). Distributed processing of pain and vibration by the human brain. *Journal of Neuroscience: The Official Journal of the Society for Neuroscience, 14*, 4095–4108.

Colpaert, F. C., Donnerer, J., & Lembeck, F. (1983). Effects of capsaicin on inflammation and on substance P content of nervous tissues in rats with adjuvant arthritis. *Life Sciences, 32*, 1827–1834.

Institute of Medicine. 2011. Relieving Pain in America: A Blueprint for Transforming Prevention, Care, Education, and Research. Washington, DC: The National Academies Press.

Correa, J. B., Costa, L. O., de Oliveira, N. T., Sluka, K. A., & Liebano, R. E. (2015). Central sensitization and changes in conditioned pain modulation in people with chronic nonspecific low back pain: A case-control study. *Experimental Brain Research, 233*, 2391–2399.

Coutinho, S. V., Urban, M. O., & Gebhart, G. F. (1998). Role of glutamate receptors and nitric oxide in the rostral ventromedial medulla in visceral hyperalgesia. *Pain, 78*, 59–69.

Crock, L. W., Kolber, B. J., Morgan, C. D., Sadler, K. E., Vogt, S. K., Bruchas, M. R., et al. (2012). Central amygdala metabotropic glutamate receptor 5 in the modulation of visceral pain. *Journal of Neuroscience: The Official Journal of the Society for Neuroscience, 32*, 14217–14226.

Culav, E. M., Clark, C. H., & Merrilees, M. J. (1999). Connective tissues: Matrix composition and its relevance to physical therapy. *Physical Therapy, 79*(3), 308–319.

Cummins, T. R., Sheets, P. L., & Waxman, S. G. (2007). The roles of sodium channels in nociception: Implications for mechanisms of pain. *Pain, 131*, 243–257.

Cunha, F. Q., Poole, S., Lorenzetti, B. B., & Ferreira, S. H. (1992). The pivotal role of tumour necrosis factor alpha in the development of inflammatory hyperalgesia. *British Journal of Pharmacology, 107*, 660–664.

da Silva, L. F. S., DeSantana, J. M., & Sluka, K. A. (2010a). Activation of NMDA receptors in the brainstem, rostral ventromedial medulla, and nucleus reticularis gigantocellularis mediates mechanical hyperalgesia produced by repeated intramuscular injections of acidic saline in rats. *Pain, 11*, 378–387.

da Silva, L. F. S., Walder, R. Y., Davidson, B. L., Wilson, S. P., & Sluka, K. A. (2010b). Changes in expression of NMDA-NR1 receptor subunits in the rostral ventromedial medulla modulates pain behaviors. *Pain, 151*, 155–161.

da Silva, M. D., Bobinski, F., Sato, K. L., Kolker, S. J., Sluka, K. A., & Santos, A. R. (2015). IL-10 cytokine released from M2 macrophages is crucial for analgesic and anti-inflammatory effects of acupuncture in a model of inflammatory muscle pain. *Molecular Neurobiology, 51*, 19–31.

Daenen, L., Nijs, J., Roussel, N., Wouters, K., Van Loo, M., & Cras, P. (2013). Dysfunctional pain inhibition in patients with chronic whiplash-associated disorders: An experimental study. *Clinical Rheumatology, 32*, 23–31.

Dailey, D. L., Rakel, B. A., Vance, C. G., et al. (2013). Transcutaneous electrical nerve stimulation reduces pain, fatigue and hyperalgesia while restoring central inhibition in primary fibromyalgia. *Pain, 154*, 2554–2562.

Dakin, S. G., Dudhia, J., & Smith, R. K. (2014). Resolving an inflammatory concept: The importance of inflammation and resolution in tendinopathy. *Veterinary Immunology and Immunopathology, 158*(3–4), 121–127.

Dakin, S. G., Newton, J., Martinez, F. O., et al. (2017). Chronic inflammation is a feature of Achilles tendinopathy and rupture. *British Journal of Sports Medicine, 52*(6), 359.

Dawes, J. M., Andersson, D. A., Bennett, D. L. H., Bevan, S., & McMahon, S. B. (2013). Inflammatory mediators and modulators of pain. In S. B. McMahon, M. Koltzenburg, I. Tracey, & D. C. Turk (Eds.), *Melzack and Wall's textbook of pain* (6th ed.) (p. 48). Philadelphia: Elsevier.

De Resende, M. A., Silva, L. F., Sato, K., Arendt-Nielsen, L., & Sluka, K. A. (2011). Blockade of opioid receptors in the medullary reticularis nucleus dorsalis, but not the rostral ventromedial medulla, prevents analgesia produced by diffuse noxious inhibitory control in rats with muscle inflammation. *The Journal of Pain: Official Journal of the American Pain Society, 12*, 687–697.

de Souza Costa, M., Teles, R. H. G., Dutra, Y. M., et al. (2018). Photobiomodulation reduces neutrophil migration and oxidative stress in mice with carrageenan-induced peritonitis. *Lasers in Medical Science*.

Deakin, J. F., & Dostrovsky, J. O. (1978). Involvement of the periaqueductal grey matter and spinal 5-hydroxytryptaminergic pathways in morphine analgesia: Effects of lesions and 5-hydroxytryptamine depletion. *British Journal of Pharmacology, 63*, 159–165.

DeSantana, J. M., da Silva, L. F., De Resende, M. A., & Sluka, K. A. (2009). Transcutaneous electrical nerve stimulation at both high and low frequencies activates ventrolateral periaqueductal grey to decrease mechanical hyperalgesia in arthritic rats. *Neuroscience, 163,* 1233–1241.

DeSantana, J. M., & Sluka, K. A. (2008). Central mechanisms in the maintenance of chronic widespread noninflammatory muscle pain. *Current Pain and Headache Reports, 12,* 338–343.

Dib-Hajj, S. D., Cummins, T. R., Black, J. A., & Waxman, S. G. (2007). From genes to pain: Na v 1.7 and human pain disorders. *Trends in Neurosciences, 30,* 555–563.

Dib-Hajj, S. D., Rush, A. M., Cummins, T. R., et al. (2005). Gain-of-function mutation in Nav1.7 in familial erythromelalgia induces bursting of sensory neurons. *Brain, 128,* 1847–1854.

Dierich, M. P., Forster, O., Grunicke, H., Guder, W. G., & Lang, H. (1987). In flammation and phagocytosis. *Journal of Clinical Chemistry & Clinical Biochemistry, 25,* 785–793.

Dimmen, S., Nordsletten, L., Engebretsen, L., Steen, H., & Madsen, J. E. (2009). The effect of parecoxib and indometacin on tendon-to-bone healing in a bone tunnel: An experimental study in rats. *Journal of Bone and Joint Surgery American Volume, 91*(2), 259–263.

Dougherty, P. M., Palecek, J., Paleckova, V., Sorkin, L. S., & Willis, W. D. (1992). The role of NMDA and non-NMDA excitatory amino-acid receptors in the excitation of primate spinothalamic tract neurons by mechanical, chemical, thermal, and electrical stimuli. *Journal of Neuroscience: The Official Journal of the Society for Neuroscience, 12,* 3025–3041.

Dougherty, P. M., & Willis, W. D. (1991). Enhancement of spinothalamic neuron responses to chemical and mechanical stimuli following combined micro-iontophoretic application of N-methyl-D-aspartic acid and substance P. *Pain, 47,* 85–93.

Drenth, J. P., & Waxman, S. G. (2007). Mutations in sodium-channel gene SCN9A cause a spectrum of human genetic pain disorders. *Journal of Clinical Investigation, 117,* 3603–3609.

Du, J., Koltzenburg, M., & Carlton, S. M. (2001). Glutamate-induced excitation and sensitization of nociceptors in rat glabrous skin. *Pain, 89,* 187–198.

Dunn, S. L., & Olmedo, M. L. (2015). Mechanotransduction: Relevance to physical therapist practice-understanding our ability to affect genetic expression through mechanical forces. *Physical Therapy, 96*(5), 712–721.

Eccleston, C., Fisher, E., Craig, L., Duggan, G. B., Rosser, B. A., & Keogh, E. (2014). Psychological therapies (Internet-delivered) for the management of chronic pain in adults. *Cochrane Database of Systematic Reviews, 2,* CD010152.

Egozi, E. I., Ferreira, A. M., Burns, A. L., Gamelli, R. L., & Dipietro, L. A. (2003). Mast cells modulate the inflammatory but not the proliferative response in healing wounds. *Wound Repair and Regeneration: Official Publication of the Wound Healing Society [and] the European Tissue Repair Society, 11*(1), 46–54.

Erthal, V., da Silva, M. D., Cidral-Filho, F. J., Santos, A. R., & Nohama, P. (2013). ST36 laser acupuncture reduces pain-related behavior in rats: Involvement of the opioidergic and serotonergic systems. *Lasers in Medical Science, 28,* 1345–1351.

Fang, J. F., Liang, Y., Du, J. Y., & Fang, J. Q. (2013). Transcutaneous electrical nerve stimulation attenuates CFA-induced hyperalgesia and inhibits spinal ERK1/2-COX-2 pathway activation in rats. *BMC Complementary and Alternative Medicine, 13,* 134.

Feldmann, M., Brennan, F. M., Elliott, M. J., Williams, R. O., & Maini, R. N. (1995). TNF alpha is an effective therapeutic target for rheumatoid arthritis. *Annals of the New York Academy of Sciences, 766,* 272–278.

Ferreira, S. H., Lorenzetti, B. B., Bristow, A. F., & Poole, S. (1988). Interleukin-1 beta as a potent hyperalgesic agent antagonized by a tripeptide analogue. *Nature, 334,* 698–700.

Fields, H. L., Basbaum, A. I., & Heinricher, M. M. (2006). Central nervous system mechanisms of pain modulation. In S. B. McMahon & M. Koltzenburg (Eds.), *Textbook of pain* (5th ed.) (pp. 125–142). Philadelphia: Elsevier.

Fleetwood-Walker, S. M., Mitchell, R., Hope, P. J., El-Yassir, N., Molony, V., & Bladon, C. M. (1990). The involvement of neurokinin receptor subtypes in somatosensory processing in the superficial dorsal horn of the cat. *Brain Research, 519,* 169–182.

Flor, H. (2014). Psychological pain interventions and neurophysiology: Implications for a mechanism-based approach. *American Psychologist, 69,* 188–196.

Fong, E. L., Chan, C. K., & Goodman, S. B. (2011). Stem cell homing in musculoskeletal injury. *Biomaterials, 32*(2), 395–409.

Forrest, L. (1983). Current concepts in soft connective tissue wound healing. *British Journal of Surgery, 70,* 133–140.

American Pain Foundation. Voices of Chronic Pain Survey. Baltimore, MD, American Pain Foundation, 2006

Frenzel, L., & Hermine, O. (2013). Mast cells and inflammation. *Joint Bone Spine: Revue du Rhumatisme, 80*(2), 141–145.

Frick, M. A., & Murthy, N. S. (2010). Imaging of the elbow: Muscle and tendon injuries. *Seminars in Musculoskeletal Radiology, 14*(4), 430–437.

Fu, K. Y., Light, A. R., Matsushima, G. K., & Maixner, W. (1999). Microglial reactions after subcutaneous formalin injection into the rat hind paw. *Brain Research, 825,* 59–67.

Gabbiani, G. (2003). The myofibroblast in wound healing and fibrocontractive diseases. *The Journal of Pathology, 200*(4), 500–503.

Gale, A. J. (2011). Continuing education course #2: Current understanding of hemostasis. *Toxicologic Pathology, 39*(1), 273–280.

Gallo, J., Raska, M., Kriegova, E., & Goodman, S. B. (2017). Inflammation and its resolution and the musculoskeletal system. *Journal of Orthopaedic Translation, 10,* 52–67.

Garrison, C. J., Dougherty, P. M., Kajander, K. C., & Carlton, S. M. (1991). Staining of glial fibrillary acidic protein (GFAP) in lumbar spinal cord increases following a sciatic nerve constriction injury. *Brain Research, 565,* 1–7.

Gaskin, D. J., & Richard, P. (2012). The economic costs of pain in the United States. *The Journal of Pain: Official Journal of the American Pain Society, 13,* 715–724.

Gebhart, G. F. (1996). Visceral polymodal receptors. *Progress in Brain Research, 113,* 101–112.

Gebhart, G. F., Sandkuhler, J., Thalhammer, J. G., & Zimmermann, M. (1983). Quantitative comparison of inhibition in spinal cord nociceptive information by stimulation in periaqueductal gray or nucleus raphe magnus of the cat. *Journal of Neurophysiology, 50,* 1433–1445.

Gerdle, B., Ghafouri, B., Ernberg, M., & Larsson, B. (2014). Chronic musculoskeletal pain: Review of mechanisms and biochemical biomarkers as assessed by the microdialysis technique. *Journal of Pain Research, 7,* 313–326.

Goldin, S. M., Subbarao, K., Sharma, R., et al. (1997). Neuroprotective use-dependent blockers of Na+ and Ca2+ channels controlling presynaptic release of glutamate. *Annals of the New York Academy of Sciences,* 210–229.

Gold, M. S., Weinreich, D., Kim, C. S., et al. (2003). Redistribution of Na(V)1.8 in uninjured axons enables neuropathic pain. *Journal of Neuroscience: The Official Journal of the Society for Neuroscience, 23,* 158–166.

Gomez, M. A., Woo, S. L., Amiel, D., Harwood, F., Kitabayashi, L., & Matyas, J. R. (1991). The effects of increased tension on healing medical collateral ligaments. *The American Journal of Sports Medicine, 19*(4), 347–354.

Gopalkrishnan, P., & Sluka, K. A. (2000). Effect of varying frequency, intensity and pulse duration of TENS on primary hyperalgesia in inflamed rats. *Archives of Physical Medicine and Rehabilitation, 81,* 984–990.

Granger, D. N., & Senchenkova, E. (2010). *Inflammation and the microcirculation.* San Francisco: Morgan and Claypool.

Green, J., Jester, R., McKinley, R., & Pooler, A. (2014). The impact of chronic venous leg ulcers: A systematic review. *Journal of Wound Care, 23*(12), 601–612.

Guan, Y., Guo, W., Zou, S. P., Dubner, R., & Ren, K. (2003). Inflammation-induced upregulation of AMPA receptor subunit expression in brain stem pain modulatory circuitry. *Pain, 104,* 401–413.

Hammond, D. L., & Drower, E. J. (1984). Effects of intrathecally administered THIP, baclofen, and muscimol on nociceptive threshold. *European Journal of Pharmacology, 103,* 121–125.

Han, G., & Ceilley, R. (2017). Chronic wound healing: A review of current management and treatments. *Advances in Therapy, 34*(3), 599–610.

Han, J. S., Chen, X. H., Sun, S. L., et al. (1991). Effect of low and high frequency TENS on Met-enkephalin-Arg-Phe and dynorphin A immunoreactivity in human lumbar CSF. *Pain, 47,* 295–298.

Hardy, M. A. (1989). The biology of scar formation. *Physical Therapy, 69*(12), 1014–1024.

Hayashi, K., Ozaki, N., Kawakita, K., et al. (2011). Involvement of NGF in the rat model of persistent muscle pain associated with taut band. *The Journal of Pain: Official Journal of the American Pain Society, 12,* 1059–1068.

Heinricher, M. M. (1997). Organizational characteristics of supraspinally mediated responses to nociceptive input. In T. L. Yaksh (Ed.), *Anesthesia: Biologic foundations.* Philadelphia: Lippincott-Raven Publishers.

Hernandez-Bule, M. L., Angeles Trillo, M., Martinez Garcia, M. A., Abilahoud, C., & Ubeda, A. (2017). Chondrogenic differentiation of adipose-derived stem cells by radiofrequency electric stimulation. *Journal of Stem Cell Research & Therapy, 7*(12), 7–12.

Hernández-Bule, M. L., Paíno, C. L., Trillo, M. Á., & Úbeda, A. (2014). Electric stimulation at 448 kHz promotes

proliferation of human mesenchymal stem cells. *Cellular Physiology and Biochemistry, 34*(5), 1741–1755.

Hill, M., Wernig, A., & Goldspink, G. (2003). Muscle satellite (stem) cell activation during local tissue injury and repair. *Journal of Anatomy, 203,* 89–99.

Hofbauer, R. K., Rainville, P., Duncan, G. H., & Bushnell, M. C. (2001). Cortical representation of the sensory dimension of pain. *Journal of Neurophysiology, 86,* 402–411.

Hoheisel, U., Mense, S., Simons, D. G., & Yu, X.-M. (1993). Appearance of new receptive fields in rat dorsal horn neurons following noxious stimulation of skeletal muscle: A model for referral of muscle pain? *Neuroscience Letters, 153,* 9–12.

Hoheisel, U., Unger, T., & Mense, S. (2007). Sensitization of rat dorsal horn neurons by NGF-induced subthreshold potentials and low-frequency activation. A study employing intracellular recordings in vivo. *Brain Research, 1169,* 34–43.

Holden, J. E., Schwartz, E. J., & Proudfit, H. K. (1999). Microinjection of morphine in the A7 catecholamine cell group produces opposing effects on nociception that are mediated by alpha1- and alpha2-adrenoceptors. *Neuroscience, 91,* 979–990.

Huisman, E., Lu, A., McCormack, R. G., & Scott, A. (2014). Enhanced collagen type I synthesis by human tenocytes subjected to periodic in vitro mechanical stimulation. *BMC Musculoskeletal Disorders, 15*(1), 386.

Hurst, S. M., Wilkinson, T. S., McLoughlin, R. M., et al. (2001). IL-6 and its soluble receptor orchestrate a temporal switch in the pattern of leukocyte recruitment seen during acute inflammation. *Immunity, 14*(6), 705–714.

Ibrahim, M. M., Patwardhan, A., Gilbraith, K. B., et al. (2017). Long-lasting antinociceptive effects of green light in acute and chronic pain in rats. *Pain, 158,* 347–360.

Ingber, D. E. (2003). Mechanobiology and diseases of mechanotransduction. *Annals of Medicine, 35,* 564–577.

Ingber, D. E. (2008). Tensegrity and mechanotransduction. *Journal of Bodywork and Movement Therapies, 12*(3), 198–200.

Jackson, D. L., Graff, C. B., Richardson, J. D., & Hargreaves, K. M. (1995). Glutamate participates in the peripheral modulation of thermal hyperalgesia in rats. *European Journal of Pharmacology, 284,* 321–325.

Jimenez, P. A., & Jimenez, S. E. (2004). Tissue and cellular approaches to wound repair. *The American Journal of Surgery, 187,* 56S–64S.

Ji, R. R., Samad, T. A., Jin, S. X., Schmoll, R., & Woolf, C. J. (2002). p38 MAPK activation by NGF in primary sensory neurons after inflammation increases TRPV1 levels and maintains heat hyperalgesia. *Neuron, 36,* 57–68.

Johannes, C. B., Le, T. K., Zhou, X., Johnston, J. A., & Dworkin, R. H. (2010). The prevalence of chronic pain in United States adults: Results of an Internet-based survey. *The Journal of Pain: Official Journal of the American Pain Society, 11,* 1230–1239.

Jones, S. L., & Gebhart, G. F. (1987). Spinal pathways mediating tonic, coeruleospinal, and raphe-spinal descending inhibition in the rat. *Journal of Neurophysiology, 58,* 138–159.

Kalra, A., Urban, M. O., & Sluka, K. A. (2001). Blockade of opioid receptors in rostral ventral medulla prevents antihyperalgesia produced by transcutaneous electrical nerve stimulation

(TENS). *Journal of Pharmacology and Experimental Therapeutics, 298*, 257–263.

Kaneko, S., Satoh, T., Chiba, J., Ju, C., Inoue, K., & Kagawa, J. (2000). Interleukin-6 and interleukin-8 levels in serum and synovial fluid of patients with osteoarthritis. *Cytokines, Cellular & Molecular Therapy, 6*, 71–79.

Kaneyama, K., Segami, N., Nishimura, M., Suzuki, T., & Sato, J. (2002). Importance of proinflammatory cytokines in synovial fluid from 121 joints with temporomandibular disorders. *British Journal of Oral and Maxillofacial Surgery, 40*, 418–423.

Khan, K. M., & Scott, A. (2009). Mechanotherapy: How physical therapists' prescription of exercise promotes tissue repair. *British Journal of Sports Medicine, 43*(4), 247–252.

Killian, M. L., Cavinatto, L., Galatz, L. M., & Thomopoulos, S. (2012). The role of mechanobiology in tendon healing. *Journal of Shoulder and Elbow Surgery, 21*(2), 228–237.

Kolber, B. J., Montana, M. C., Carrasquillo, Y., Xu, J., Heinemann, S. F., Muglia, L. J., et al. (2010). Activation of metabotropic glutamate receptor 5 in the amygdala modulates pain-like behavior. *Journal of Neuroscience: The Official Journal of the Society for Neuroscience, 30*, 8203–8213.

Kulshreshtha, P., & Deepak, K. K. (2013). Autonomic nervous system profile in fibromyalgia patients and its modulation by exercise: A mini review. *Clinical Physiology and Functional Imaging, 33*, 83–91.

Kuraishi, Y., Hirota, N., Sato, Y., Satou, M., & Takagi, H. (1985). Noradrenergic inhibition of the release of substance P from primary afferents in the rabbit spinal cord dorsal horn. *Brain Research, 359*, 177–182.

Lam, F. Y., & Ferrell, W. R. (1989). Capsaicin suppresses substance P-induced joint inflammation in the rat. *Neuroscience Letters, 105*, 155–158.

Lam, F. Y., & Ferrell, W. R. (1991). Specific neurokinin receptors mediate plasma extravasation in the rat knee joint. *British Journal of Pharmacology, 103*, 1263–1267.

Larsson, J., Ekblom, A., Henriksson, K., Lundeberg, T., & Therdorsson, E. (1989). Immunoreactive tachykinins, calcitonin gene-related peptide and neuropeptide Y in human synovial fluid from inflamed knee joints. *Neuroscience Letters, 100*, 326–330.

Lawand, N. B., McNearney, T., & Westlund, K. N. (2000). Amino acid release into the knee joint: Key role in nociception and inflammation. *Pain, 86*, 69–74.

Lawand, N. B., Willis, W. D., & Westlund, K. N. (1997). Excitatory amino acid receptor involvement in peripheral nociceptive transmission in rats. *British Journal of Pharmacology, 324*, 169–177.

Lee, W. Y., & Wang, B. (2017). Cartilage repair by mesenchymal stem cells: Clinical trial update and perspectives. *Journal of Orthopaedic Translation, 9*, 76–88.

Lee, J. M., Warren, M. P., & Mason, S. M. (1978). Effects of ice on nerve conduction velocity. *Physiotherapy, 64*, 2–6.

Lehmann, J. F. (1990). *Therapeutic heat and cold* (4th ed.). Baltimore, MD: Williams and Wilkins.

Leonard, G., Goffaux, P., & Marchand, S. (2010). Deciphering the role of endogenous opioids in high-frequency TENS using low and high doses of naloxone. *Pain, 151*, 215–219.

Leung, A., Gregory, N. S., Allen, L. A., & Sluka, K. A. (2016). Regular physical activity prevents chronic pain by altering resident muscle macrophage phenotype and increasing IL-10 in mice. *Pain, 157* 79–79.

Leung, M. C., Ng, G. Y., & Yip, K. K. (2006). Therapeutic ultrasound enhances medial collateral ligament repair in rats. *Ultrasound in Medicine and Biology, 32*(3), 449–452.

Levine, J. D., Moskowitz, M. A., & Basbaum, A. I. (1985). The contribution of neurogenic inflammation in experimental arthritis. *The Journal of Immunology, 135*, 843s–847s.

Li, B., & Wang, J. H. C. (2011). Fibroblasts and myofibroblasts in wound healing: Force generation and measurement. *Journal of Tissue Viability, 20*(4), 108–120.

Li, J., Chen, J., & Kirsner, R. (2007). Pathophysiology of acute wound healing. *Clinics in Dermatology, 25*(1), 9–18.

Li, W. W., Talcott, K. E., Zhai, A. W., Kruger, E. A., & Li, V. W. (2005). The role of therapeutic angiogenesis in tissue repair and regeneration. *Clinics in Dermatology, 18*(9), 491–500.

Liebeskind, J. C., Guilbaud, G., Besson, J. M., & Oliveras, J. L. (1973). Analgesia from electrical stimulation of periaqueductal grey matter in the cat: Behavioral observations and inhibitory effects on spinal cord interneurons. *Brain Research, 50*, 441–446.

Lin, Q., Peng, Y. B., & Willis, W. D. (1996). Inhibition of primate spinothalamic tract neurons by spinal glycine and GABA is reduced during central sensitization. *Journal of Neurophysiology, 76*, 1005–1014.

Lin, T. W., Cardenas, L., & Soslowsky, L. J. (2004). Biomechanics of tendon injury and repair. *Journal of Biomechanics, 37*(6), 865–877.

Lin, W., Xu, L., Zwingenberger, S., Gibon, E., Goodman, S. B., & Li, G. (2017). Mesenchymal stem cells homing to improve bone healing. *Journal of Orthopaedic Translation, 9*, 19–27.

Liu, L., Hindieh, J., Leong, D. J., & Sun, H. B. (2017). Advances of stem cell based-therapeutic approaches for tendon repair. *Journal of Orthopaedic Translation, 9*, 69–75.

Londhe, P., & Guttridge, D. C. (2015). Inflammation induced loss of skeletal muscle. *Bone, 80*, 131–142.

Lorena, D., Uchio, K., Costa, A. M. A., & Desmouliere, A. (2002). Normal scarring: Importance of myofibroblasts. *Wound Repair and Regeneration, 10*(2), 86–92.

Luster, A. D. (1998). Chemokines – chemotactic cytokines that mediate inflammation. *New England Journal of Medicine, 338*(7), 436–445.

Ma, Y. T., & Sluka, K. A. (2001). Reduction in inflammation-induced sensitization of dorsal horn neurons by transcutaneous electrical nerve stimulation in anesthetized rats. *Experimental Brain Research, 137*, 94–102.

Machelska, H., & Stein, C. (2006). Leukocyte-derived opioid peptides and inhibition of pain. *Journal of Neuroimmune Pharmacology: The Official Journal of the Society on NeuroImmune Pharmacology, 1*, 90–97.

Mackey, A. L., Heinemeier, K. M., Koskinen, S. O., & Kjaer, M. (2008). Dynamic adaptation of tendon and muscle connective tissue to mechanical loading. *Connective Tissue Research, 49*(3), 165–168.

Maeda, Y., Lisi, T. L., Vance, C. G., & Sluka, K. A. (2007). Release of GABA and activation of GABAA receptors in the spinal cord mediates the effects of TENS in rats. *Brain Research, 1136*, 43–50.

Mao, J., Price, D. D., Hayes, R. L., Lu, J., & Mayer, D. J. (1992). Differential roles of NMDA and non-NMDA receptor activation in induction and maintenance of thermal hyperalgesia in rats with painful peripheral mononeuropathy. *Brain Research, 598*, 271–288.

Mapp, P. I., Kidd, B. L., Gibson, S. J., et al. (1990). Substance P-, calcitonin gene-related peptide- and C-flanking peptide of neuropeptide Y-immunoreactive fibres are present in normal synovium but depleted in patients with rheumatoid arthritis. *Neuroscience, 37*, 143–153.

McAnulty, R. J. (2007). Fibroblasts and myofibroblasts: Their source, function and role in disease. *The International Journal of Biochemistry & Cell Biology, 39*(4), 666–671.

McNearney, T., Baethge, B. A., Cao, S., Alam, R., Lisse, J. R., & Westlund, K. N. (2004). Excitatory amino acids, TNF-alpha, and chemokine levels in synovial fluids of patients with active arthropathies. *Clinical and Experimental Immunology, 137*, 621–627.

McNearney, T., Speegle, D., Lawand, N., Lisse, J., & Westlund, K. N. (2000). Excitatory amino acid profiles of synovial fluid from patients with arthritis. *Journal of Rheumatology, 27*, 739–745.

Medzhitov, R. (2008). Origin and physiological roles of inflammation. *Nature, 454*(7203), 428–435.

Melzack, R., & Casey, K. L. (1968). Sensory, motivational, and central control determinants of pain: A new conceptual model. In D. Kenshalo (Ed.), *The skin senses* (pp. 423–439). Springfield, IL: Thomas.

Mense, S. (1978). Effects of temperature on the discharges of muscle spindles and tendon organs. *Pflugers Archiv: European Journal of Physiology, 374*, 159–168.

Metz, M., Grimbaldeston, M. A., Nakae, S., Piliponsky, A. M., Tsai, M., & Galli, S. J. (2007). Mast cells in the promotion and limitation of chronic inflammation. *Immunological Reviews, 217*, 304–328.

Metz, M., & Maurer, M. (2007). Mast cells – key effector cells in immune responses. *Trends in Immunology, 28*(5), 234–241.

Millan, M. J. (1999). The induction of pain: An integrative review. *Progress in Neurobiology, 57*, 1–164.

Millan, M. J. (2002). Descending control of pain. *Progress in Neurobiology, 66*, 355–474.

Molloy, T., Wang, Y., & Murrell, G. A. C. (2003). The roles of growth factors in tendon and ligament healing. *Sports Medicine, 33*(5), 381–394.

Mosca, M. J., Rashid, M. S., Snelling, S. J., Kirtley, S., Carr, A. J., & Dakin, S. G. (2018). Trends in the theory that inflammation plays a causal role in tendinopathy: A systematic review and quantitative analysis of published reviews. *BMJ Open Sport & Exercise Medicine, 4*(1).

Murase, S., Terazawa, E., Queme, F., Ota, H., Matsuda, T., Hirate, K., et al. (2010). Bradykinin and nerve growth factor play pivotal roles in muscular mechanical hyperalgesia after exercise (delayed-onset muscle soreness). *Journal of Neuroscience: The Official Journal of the Society for Neuroscience, 30*, 3752–3761.

Nahin, R. L., Hylden, J. L., Iadarola, M. J., & Dubner, R. (1989). Peripheral inflammation is associated with increased dynorphin immunoreactivity in both projection and local circuit neurons in the superficial dorsal horn of the rat lumbar spinal cord. *Neuroscience Letters, 96*, 247–252.

Neugebauer, V., & Li, W. (2003). Differential sensitization of amygdala neurons to afferent inputs in a model of arthritic pain. *Journal of Neurophysiology, 89*, 716–727.

Neugebauer, V., Lucke, T., & Schaible, H. G. (1993). N-methyl-D-aspartate (NMDA) and non-NMDA receptor antagonists block the hyperexcitability of dorsal horn neurons during development of acute arthritis in rats knee joint. *Journal of Neurophysiology, 70*, 1365–1377.

Neugebauer, V., Ruemenapp, P., & Schaible, H.-G. (1996). Calcitonin gene-related peptide is involved in the spinal processing of mechanosensory input from the rat's knee joint and in the generation and maintenance of hyperexcitability of dorsal horn neurons during development of acute inflammation. *Neuroscience, 71*, 1095–1109.

Neugebauer, V., & Schaible, H.-G. (1988). Peripheral and spinal components of the sensitization of spinal neurons during an acute experimental arthritis. *Agents & Actions, 25*, 234–236.

Neugebauer, V., Weiretter, F., & Schaible, H.-G. (1995). Involvement of substance P and neurokinin-1 receptors in the hyperexcitability of dorsal horn neurons during development of acute arthritis in rat's knee joint. *Journal of Neurophysiology, 73*, 1574–1583.

Niinikoski, J. (1979). *Current concepts in wound nutrition. Paper presented at the Symposium on Wound Healing.* Helsinki: Finland.

Normand, E., Potvin, S., Gaumond, I., Cloutier, G., Corbin, J. F., & Marchand, S. (2011). Pain inhibition is deficient in chronic widespread pain but normal in major depressive disorder. *Journal of Clinical Psychiatry, 72*, 219–224.

Nuseir, K., & Proudfit, H. K. (2000). Bidirectional modulation of nociception by GABA neurons in the dorsolateral pontine tegmentum that tonically inhibit spinally projecting noradrenergic A7 neurons. *Neuroscience, 96*, 773–783.

O'Neill, S., Manniche, C., Graven-Nielsen, T., & Arendt-Nielsen, L. (2007). Generalized deep-tissue hyperalgesia in patients with chronic low-back pain. *European Journal of Pain, 11*, 415–420.

Ogawa, R. (2011). Mechanobiology of scarring. *Wound Repair and Regeneration: Official Publication of the Wound Healing Society [and] the European Tissue Repair Society, 19*(Suppl. 1), s2–9.

Oryan, A., Moshiri, A., & Meimandi-Parizi, A. H. (2012). Short and long terms healing of the experimentally transverse sectioned tendon in rabbits. *Sports Med Arthrosc Rehabil Ther Technol, 4*(1), 14.

Ozaktay, A. C., Cavanaugh, J. M., Asik, I., DeLeo, J. A., & Weinstein, J. N. (2002). Dorsal root sensitivity to interleukin-1 beta, interleukin-6 and tumor necrosis factor in rats. *European Spine Journal: Official Publication of the European Spine Society, the European Spinal Deformity Society, and the European Section of the Cervical Spine Research Society, 11*, 467–475.

Page-McCaw, A., Ewald, A. J., & Werb, Z. (2007). Matrix metalloproteinases and the regulation of tissue remodelling. *Nature Reviews Molecular Cell Biology, 8*(3), 221–233.

Palecek, J., Dougherty, P. M., Kim, S. H., et al. (1992). Responses of spinothalamic tract neurons to mechanical and thermal stimuli in an experimental model of peripheral neuropathy in primates. *Journal of Neurophysiology, 68*, 1951–1965.

Pas, H. I., Winters, M., Haisma, H. J., Koenis, M. J., Tol, J. L., & Moen, M. H. (2017). Stem cell injections in knee osteoarthritis: A systematic review of the literature. *British Journal of Sports Medicine, 51*(15), 1125.

Peacock, E. E. (1984). *Wound repair* (3rd ed.). WB Saunders.

Peplow, P. V., Chung, T. Y., & Baxter, G. D. (2010). Laser photobiomodulation of wound healing: A review of experimental studies in mouse and rat animal models. *Photomedicine and Laser Surgery, 28*, 291–325.

Pereira da Silva, J. A., & Carmo-Fonseca, M. (1990). Peptide containing nerves in human synovium: Immunohistochemical evidence for decreased innervation in rheumatoid arthritis. *Journal of Rheumatology, 17*, 1592–1599.

Peters, M. L., Schmidt, A. J., Van den Hout, M. A., Koopmans, R., & Sluijter, M. E. (1992). Chronic back pain, acute postoperative pain and the activation of diffuse noxious inhibitory controls (DNIC). *Pain, 50*, 177–187.

Pitzer, J. A. (2006). *Progress in inflammation research.* Nova Science Pub Inc.

Priglinger, E., Maier, J., Chaudary, S., et al. (2018). Photobiomodulation of freshly isolated human adipose tissue-derived stromal vascular fraction cells by pulsed light-emitting diodes for direct clinical application. *Journal of Tissue Engineering and Regenerative Medicine, 12*(6), 1352–1362.

Proudfit, H. K. (1988). Pharmacologic evidence for the modulation of nociception by noradrenergic neurons. *Progress in Brain Research, 77*, 357–370.

Radhakrishnan, V., & Henry, J. L. (1991). Novel substance P antagonist, CP-96345, blocks responses of cat spinal dorsal horn neurons to noxious cutaneous stimulation and substance P. *Neuroscience Letters, 132*, 39–43.

Radhakrishnan, V., & Henry, J. L. (1995). Antagonism of nociceptive responses of cat spinal dorsal horn neurons in vivo by the NK-1 receptor antagonists CP-96,345 and CP-99,994, but not by CP-96,344. *Neuroscience, 64*, 943–958.

Radhakrishnan, R., Moore, S. A., & Sluka, K. A. (2003a). Unilateral carrageenan injection in muscle or joint induces chronic bilateral hyperalgesia in rats. *Pain, 104*, 567–577.

Radhakrishnan, R., King, E. W., Dickman, J., et al. (2003b). Blockade of spinal 5-HT receptor subtypes prevents low, but not high, frequency TENS-induced antihyperalgesia in rats. *Pain, 105*, 205–213.

Radhakrishnan, R., & Sluka, K. A. (2003). Spinal muscarinic receptors are activated during low or high frequency TENS-induced antihyperalgesia in rats. *Neuropharmacology, 45*, 1111–1119.

Radhakrishnan, R., & Sluka, K. A. (2009). Increased glutamate and decreased glycine release in the rostral ventromedial medulla during induction of a pre-clinical model of chronic widespread muscle pain. *Neuroscience Letters, 457*, 141–145.

Radi, Z. A., & Khan, N. K. (2005). Effects of cyclooxygenase inhibition on bone, tendon, and ligament healing. *Inflammation Research: Official Journal of the European Histamine Research Society...[et al.], 54*(9), 358–366.

Raffetto, J. D. (2016). Pathophysiology of wound healing and alterations in venous leg ulcers-review. *Phlebology, 31*(Suppl. 1), 56–62.

Raftery, A.T. Applied Basic Science for Basic Surgical Training. 2nd Edition. 2011. Churchill Livingstone. Chapter 2 : Inflammation

Rainville, P., Duncan, G. H., Price, D. D., Carrier, B., & Bushnell, M. C. (1997). Pain affect encoded in human anterior cingulate but not somatosensory cortex. *Science, 277*, 968–971.

Rankin, J. A. (2004). Biological mediators of acute inflammation. *AACN Clinical Issues: Advanced Practice in Acute and Critical Care, 15*(1), 3–17.

Rees, H., Sluka, K. A., Westlund, K. N., & Willis, W. D. (1994). Do dorsal root reflexes augment peripheral inflammation? *NeuroReport, 5*, 821–824.

Rees, H., Sluka, K. A., Westlund, K. N., & Willis, W. D. (1995). The role of glutamate and GABA receptors in the generation of dorsal root reflexes by acute arthritis in the anaesthetized rat. *The Journal of physiology, 484*(2), 437–445.

Rees, J. D., Stride, M., & Scott, A. (2014). Tendons – time to revisit inflammation. *British Journal of Sports Medicine, 48*(21), 1553–1557.

Ren, K., Williams, G. M., Hylden, J. L. K., Ruda, M. A., & Dubner, R. (1992). The intrathecal administration of excitatory amino-acid receptor antagonists selectively attenuated carrageenan-induced behavioral hyperalgesia in rats. *European Journal of Pharmacology, 219*, 235–243.

Resende, M. A., Sabino, G. G., Candido, C. R. M., Pereira, L. S. M., & Francischi, J. N. (2004). Transcutaneous electrical stimulation (TENS) effects in experimental inflammatory edema and pain. *European Journal of Pharmacology, 504*, 217–222.

Reynolds, D. V. (1969). Surgery in the electrical analgesia induced by focal brain stimulation. *Science, 164*, 444–445.

Ringkamp, M., Raja, S. N., Campbell, J. N., & Meyer, R. A. (2013). Peripheral mechanisms of cutaneous nociception. In S. B. McMahon, M. Koltzenburg, I. Tracey, & D. C. Turk (Eds.), *Melzack and Wall's textbook of pain* (6th ed.). Philadelphia: Elsevier.

Rokugo, T., Takeuchi, T., & Ito, H. (2002). A histochemical study of substance P in the rat spinal cord: Effect of transcutaneous electrical nerve stimulation. *Journal of Nippon Medical School = Nihon Ika Daigaku Zasshi, 69*, 428–433.

Rompe, J. D., Furia, J. P., & Maffulli, N. (2008). Mid-portion Achilles tendinopathy – current options for treatment. *Disability & Rehabilitation, 30*(20–22), 1666–1676.

Rutkowski, M. J., Sughrue, M. E., Kane, A. J., Ahn, B. J., Fang, S., & Parsa, A. T. (2010). The complement cascade as a mediator of tissue growth and regeneration. *Inflammation Research: Official Journal of the European Histamine Research Society... et al.], 59*(11), 897–905.

Sabharwal, R., Rasmussen, L., Sluka, K. A., & Chapleau, M. W. (2016). Exercise prevents development of autonomic dysregulation and hyperalgesia in a mouse model of chronic muscle pain. *Pain, 157*, 387–398.

Salar, G., Job, I., Mingrino, S., Bosio, A., & Trabucchi, M. (1981). Effect of transcutaneous electrotherapy on CSF b-endorphin content in patients without pain problems. *Pain, 10*, 169–172.

Sandrini, G., Rossi, P., Milanov, I., Serrao, M., Cecchini, A. P., & Nappi, G. (2006). Abnormal modulatory influence of diffuse noxious inhibitory controls in migraine and chronic tension-type headache patients. *Cephalalgia, 26*, 782–789.

Sarlani, E., Garrett, P. H., Grace, E. G., & Greenspan, J. D. (2007). Temporal summation of pain characterizes women but not men with temporomandibular disorders. *Journal of Orofacial Pain, 21*, 309–317.

Schaible, H. G., Hope, P. J., Lang, C. W., & Duggan, A. W. (1992). Calcitonin gene-related peptide causes intraspinal spreading of substance P released by peripheral stimulation. *European Journal of Neuroscience, 4*, 750–757.

Schaible, H.-G., & Schmidt, R. F. (1985). Effects of an experimental arthritis on the sensory properties of fine articular afferent units. *Journal of Neurophysiology, 54*, 1109–1122.

Schaible, H.-G., & Schmidt, R. F. (1988). Direct observation of the sensitization of articular afferents during an experimental arthritis. In R. Dubner, G. F. Gebhart, & M. R. Bond (Eds.), *Proceedings of the Vth World Congress on Pain* (pp. 44–50). Amsterdam: Elsevier.

Schaible, H.-G., Schmidt, R. F., & Willis, W. D. (1987). Enhancement of the responses of ascending tract cells in the cat spinal cord by acute inflammation of the knee joint. *Experimental Brain Research, 66*, 489–499.

Schmidt, R., Schmelz, M., Forster, C., Ringkamp, M., Torebjork, E., & Handwerker, H. (1995). Novel classes of responsive and unresponsive C nociceptors in human skin. *Journal of Neuroscience: The Official Journal of the Society for Neuroscience, 15*, 333–341.

Schneider, S. P., & Perl, E. R. (1985). Selective excitation of neurons in the mammalian spinal dorsal horn by aspartate and glutamate in vitro: Correlation with location and synaptic input. *Brain Research, 360*, 339–343.

Schneider, S. P., & Perl, E. R. (1988). Comparison of primary afferent and glutamate excitation of neurons in the mammalian spinal dorsal horn. *Journal of Neuroscience: The Official Journal of the Society for Neuroscience, 8*, 2062–2073.

Serhan, C. N., Ward, P. A., & Gilroy, D. W. (2010). *Fundamentals of inflammation.* Cambridge; New York: Cambridge University Press.

Serra, M. B., Barroso, W. A., da Silva, N. N., et al. (2017). From inflammation to current and alternative therapies involved in wound healing. *International Journal of Inflammation*, 3406215.

Shah, J. P., Phillips, T. M., Danoff, J. V., & Gerber, L. H. (2005). An in vivo microanalytical technique for measuring the local biochemical milieu of human skeletal muscle. *Journal of Applied Physiology, 99*, 1977–1984.

Silawal, S., Triebel, J., Bertsch, T., & Schulze-Tanzil, G. (2018). Osteoarthritis and the complement cascade. *Clinical Medicine Insights: Arthritis and Musculoskeletal Disorders, 11*, 1179544117751430.

Singer, A. J., & Clark, A. F. (1999). Mechanisms of disease: Cutaneous wound healing. *New England Journal of Medicine, 341*(10), 738–746.

Sira, J., & Eyre, L. (2016). Physiology of haemostasis. *Anaesthesia and Intensive Care Medicine, 17*(2), 79–82.

Sjolund, B. H., & Eriksson, M. B. E. (1979). The influence of naloxone on analgesia produced by peripheral conditioning stimulation. *Brain Research, 173*, 295–301.

Skyba, D. A., King, E. W., & Sluka, K. A. (2002). Effects of NMDA and non-NMDA ionotropic glutamate receptor antagonists on the development and maintenance of hyperalgesia induced by repeated intramuscular injection of acidic saline. *Pain, 98*, 69–78.

Sluka, K. A. (2016). *Mechanisms and management of pain for the physical therapist* (2nd ed.). Philadelphia: Wolters Kluwer.

Sluka, K. A., Bailey, K., Bogush, J., Olson, R., & Ricketts, A. (1998). Treatment with either high or low frequency TENS reduces the secondary hyperalgesia observed after injection of kaolin and carrageenan into the knee joint. *Pain, 77*, 97–102.

Sluka, K. A., & Clauw, D. J. (2016). Neurobiology of fibromyalgia and chronic widespread pain. *Neuroscience, 338*, 114–129.

Sluka, K. A., Danielson, J., Rasmussen, L., & Dasilva, L. F. (2012). Exercise-induced pain requires NMDA receptor activation in the medullary raphe nuclei. *Medicine & Science in Sports & Exercise, 44*, 420–427.

Sluka, K. A., Deacon, M., Stibal, A., Strissel, S., & Terpstra, A. (1999). Spinal blockade of opioid receptors prevents the analgesia produced by TENS in arthritic rats. *Journal of Pharmacology and Experimental Therapeutics, 289*, 840–846.

Sluka, K. A., & Gregory, N. S. (2015). The dichotomized role for acid sensing ion channels in musculoskeletal pain and inflammation. *Neuropharmacology, 94*, 58–63.

Sluka, K. A., Kalra, A., & Moore, S. A. (2001). Unilateral intramuscular injections of acidic saline produce a bilateral, long-lasting hyperalgesia. *Muscle & Nerve, 24*, 37–46.

Sluka, K. A., Lawand, N. B., & Westlund, K. N. (1994). Joint inflammation is reduced by dorsal rhizotomy and not by sympathectomy or spinal cord transection. *Annals of the Rheumatic Diseases, 53*, 309–314.

Sluka, K. A., Lisi, T. L., & Westlund, K. N. (2006). Increased release of serotonin in the spinal cord during low, but not high frequency TENS in rats with joint inflammation. *Archives of Physical Medicine and Rehabilitation, 87*, 1137–1140.

Sluka, K. A., Milton, M. A., Westlund, K. N., & Willis, W. D. (1997). Differential roles of neurokinin 1 and neurokinin 2 receptors in the development and maintenance of heat hyperalgesia induced by acute inflammation. *British Journal of Pharmacology, 120*, 1263–1273.

Sluka, K. A., O'Donnell, J. M., Danielson, J., & Rasmussen, L. A. (2013). Regular physical activity prevents development of chronic pain and activation of central neurons. *Journal of Applied Physiology, 114*, 725–733.

Sluka, K. A., Rees, H., Westlund, K. N., & Willis, W. D. (1995). Fiber types contributing to dorsal root reflexes induced by joint inflammation in cats and monkeys. *Journal of Neurophysiology, 74*, 981–989.

Sluka, K. A., Vance, C. G. T., & Lisi, T. L. (2005). High-frequency, but not low-frequency, transcutaneous electrical nerve stimulation reduces aspartate and glutamate release in the spinal cord dorsal horn. *Journal of Neurochemistry, 95*, 1794–1801.

Sluka, K. A., & Westlund, K. N. (1993). Centrally administered non-NMDA but not NMDA receptor antagonists block peripheral knee joint inflammation. *Pain, 55*, 217–225.

Smith, C., Kruger, M. J., Smith, R. M., & Myburgh, K. H. (2008). The inflammatory response to skeletal muscle injury: Illuminating complexities. *Sports Medicine, 38*(11), 947–969.

Snider, W. D., & McMahon, S. B. (1998). Tackling pain at the source: New ideas about nociceptors. *Neuron, 20*, 629–632.

Snyder, R. J., Lantis, J., Kirsner, R. S., Shah, V., Molyneaux, M., & Carter, M. J. (2016). Macrophages: A review of their role in wound healing and their therapeutic use. *Wound Repair and Regeneration, 24*(4), 613–629.

Snyman, C., & Niesler, C. U. (2015). MMP-14 in skeletal muscle repair. *Journal of Muscle Research & Cell Motility, 36*(3), 215–225.

Sorg, H., Tilkorn, D. J., Hager, S., Hauser, J., & Mirastschijski, U. (2017). Skin wound healing: An update on the current knowledge and concepts. *European Surgical Research, 58*(1–2), 81–94.

Sousa-Valente, J., & Brain, S. D. (2018). A historical perspective on the role of sensory nerves in neurogenic inflammation. *Seminars in Immunopathology, 40*, 229–236.

Staud, R., Vierck, C. J., Mauderli, A., & Cannon, R. (1998). Abnormal temporal summation of second pain (wind-up) in patients with the fibromyalgia syndrome. *Arthritis & Rheumatism, 41* S353–S353.

Stein, C. (1995). The control of pain in peripheral tissue by opioids. *Mechanisms of Disease, 332*, 1685–1690.

Stein, C., Hassan, A. H., Przewlocki, R., Gramsch, C., Peter, K., & Herz, A. (1990). Opioids from immunocytes interact with receptors on sensory nerves to inhibit nociception in inflammation. *Proceedings of the National Academy of Sciences of the United States of America, 87*, 5935–5939.

Stroncek, J. D., & Reichert, W. M. (2007). Overview of wound healing in different tissue types. In W. M. Reichert (Ed.), *Indwelling neural implants: Strategies for contending with the in vivo environment.* CRC Press.

Suzuki, R., Morcuende, S., Webber, M., Hunt, S. P., & Dickenson, A. H. (2002). Superficial NK1-expressing neurons control spinal excitability through activation of descending pathways. *Nature Neuroscience, 5*, 1319–1326.

Svensson, P., Cairns, B. E., Wang, K., & Arendt-Nielsen, L. (2003a). Injection of nerve growth factor into human masseter muscle evokes long-lasting mechanical allodynia and hyperalgesia. *Pain, 104*, 241–247.

Svensson, P., Cairns, B. E., Wang, K., et al. (2003b). Glutamate-evoked pain and mechanical allodynia in the human masseter muscle. *Pain, 101*, 221–227.

Sweitzer, S. M., Colburn, R. W., Rutkowski, M., & DeLeo, J. A. (1999). Acute peripheral inflammation induces moderate glial activation and spinal IL-1beta expression that correlates with pain behavior in the rat. *Brain Research, 829*, 209–221.

Taljanovic, M. S., Nisbet, J. K., Hunter, T. B., Cohen, R. P., & Rogers, L. F. (2011). Humeral avulsion of the inferior glenohumeral ligament in college female volleyball players caused by repetitive microtrauma. *The American Journal of Sports Medicine, 39*(5), 1067–1076.

Terayama, R., Guan, Y., Dubner, R., & Ren, K. (2000). Activity-induced plasticity in brain stem pain modulatory circuitry after inflammation. *NeuroReport, 11*, 1915–1919.

Tillu, D. V., Gebhart, G. F., & Sluka, K. A. (2008). Descending facilitatory pathways from the RVM initiate and maintain bilateral hyperalgesia after muscle insult. *Pain, 136*, 331–339.

Tsai, S. R., & Hamblin, M. R. (2017). Biological effects and medical applications of infrared radiation. *Journal of Photochemistry and Photobiology B: Biology, 170*, 197–207.

Tsuruoka, M., & Willis, W. D. (1996). Descending modulation from the region of the locus coeruleus on nociceptive sensitivity in a rat model of inflammatory hyperalgesia. *Brain Research, 743*, 86–92.

Urban, M. O., Zahn, P. K., & Gebhart, G. F. (1999). Descending facilitatory influences from the rostral medial medulla mediate secondary, but not primary hyperalgesia in the rat. *Neuroscience, 90*, 349–352.

Vance, C. G., Radhakrishnan, R., Skyba, D. A., & Sluka, K. A. (2007). Transcutaneous electrical nerve stimulation at both high and low frequencies reduces primary hyperalgesia in rats with joint inflammation in a time-dependent manner. *Physical Therapy, 87*, 44–51.

Vanable, J. (1989). Integumentary potentials and wound healing. Electric Fields in Vertebrate Repair. R. Borgens. New York, Alan Liss Inc: 171-224.

Vera-Portocarrero, L. P., Xie, J. Y., Kowal, J., Ossipov, M. H., King, T., & Porreca, F. (2006). Descending facilitation from the rostral ventromedial medulla maintains visceral pain in rats with experimental pancreatitis. *Gastroenterology, 130*, 2155–2164.

Vernon Roberts, B. (1988). Inflammation 1987; an overview. *Agents & Actions Supplements, 24*, 1–18.

Wagner, S., Coerper, S., Fricke, J., et al. (2003). Comparison of inflammatory and systemic sources of growth factors in acute and chronic human wounds. *Wound Repair and Regeneration, 11*(4), 253–260.

Walter, J. B., & Israel, M. S. (1987). *General pathology* (6th ed.). Churchill Livingstone.

Watkins, L. R., & Maier, S. F. (2002). Beyond neurons: Evidence that immune and glial cells contribute to pathological pain states. *Physiological Reviews, 82*, 981–1011.

Watkins, L. R., Maier, S. F., & Goehler, L. E. (1995). Immune activation: The role of pro-inflammatory cytokines in inflammation, illness responses and pathological pain states. *Pain, 63*, 289–302.

Watkins, L. R., Milligan, E. D., & Maier, S. F. (2001). Glial activation: A driving force for pathological pain. *Trends in Neurosciences, 24*, 450–455.

Watkins, L. R., Wiertelak, E. P., Goehler, L. E., Smith, K. P., Martin, D., & Maier, S. F. (1994). Characterization of cytokine-induced hyperalgesia. *Brain Research, 654*, 15–26.

Watson, T. (2016). *Expanding our understanding of the inflammatory process and its role in pain & tissue healing.* Paper presented at the IFOMPT 2016, Glasgow.

Watson, T. (2003). Soft tissue healing. *In Touch, 104*, 2–9.

Watson, T. (2006). Tissue repair: The current state of the art. *Sportex-Medicine, 28*, 8–12.

Westlund, K. N., Lu, Y., Coggeshall, R. E., & Willis, W. D. (1992). Serotonin is found in myelinated axons of the dorsolateral funiculus in monkeys. *Neuroscience Letters, 141*, 35–38.

White, D. M., & Helme, R. D. (1985). Release of substance P from peripheral nerve terminals following electrical stimulation of the sciatic nerve. *Brain Research, 336*, 27–31.

Widgerow, A. D. (2012). Cellular resolution of inflammation – catabasis. *Wound Repair and Regeneration: Official Publication of the Wound Healing Society [and] the European Tissue Repair Society, 20*(1), 2–7.

Wilcox, G. L. (1988). Pharmacological studies of grooming and scratching behavior elicited by spinal substance P and excitatory amino acids. *Annals of the New York Academy of Sciences, 525*, 228–236.

Willis, W. D., & Coggeshall, R. E. (2004). *Sensory mechanisms of the spinal cord* (3rd ed.). New York: Springer.

Wipff, P. J., Rifkin, D. B., Meister, J. J., & Hinz, B. (2007). Myofibroblast contraction activates latent TGF-beta1 from the extracellular matrix. *The Journal of Cell Biology, 179*(6), 1311–1323.

Wong, H., Kang, I., Dong, X. D., et al. (2014). NGF-induced mechanical sensitization of the masseter muscle is mediated through peripheral NMDA receptors. *Neuroscience, 269*, 232–244.

Woolf, C. J., & Wall, P. D. (1986). Relative effectiveness of C primary afferent fibers of different origins in evoking a prolonged facilitation of the flexor reflex in the rat. *Journal of Neuroscience: The Official Journal of the Society for Neuroscience, 6*, 1433–1442.

Woolf, C., & Wiesenfeld-Hallin, Z. (1986). Substance P and calcitonin gene-related peptide synergistically modulate the gain of the nociceptive flexor withdrawal reflex in the rat. *Neuroscience Letters, 66*, 226–230.

Wu, C., Erickson, M. A., Xu, J., Wild, K. D., & Brennan, T. J. (2009). Expression profile of nerve growth factor after muscle incision in the rat. *Anesthesiology, 110*, 140–149.

Xiang, X. H., Chen, Y. M., Zhang, J. M., Tian, J. H., Han, J. S., & Cui, C. L. (2014). Low- and high-frequency transcutaneous electrical acupoint stimulation induces different effects on cerebral mu-opioid receptor availability in rhesus monkeys. *Journal of Neuroscience Research, 92*, 555–563.

Yadav, A., Gupta, A., Keshri, G. K., Verma, S., Sharma, S. K., & Singh, S. B. (2016). Photobiomodulatory effects of super-pulsed 904nm laser therapy on bioenergetics status in burn wound healing. *Journal of Photochemistry and Photobiology B: Biology, 162*, 77–85.

Yaksh, T. L. (1988). Substance P release from knee joint afferent terminals: Modulation by opioids. *Brain Research, 458*, 319–324.

Yaksh, T. L. (2006). Central pharmacology of nociceptive transmission. In S. B. McMahon & M. Koltzenburg (Eds.), *Textbook of pain* (5th ed.) (pp. 371–414). Philadelphia: Elsevier.

Yang, W., & Hu, P. (2018). Skeletal muscle regeneration is modulated by inflammation. *Journal of Orthopaedic Translation, 13*, 25–32.

Yarnitsky, D., Crispel, Y., Eisenberg, E., et al. (2008). Prediction of chronic post-operative pain: Pre-operative DNIC testing identifies patients at risk. *Pain, 138*, 22–28.

Yashpal, K., Radhakrishnan, V., Coderre, T. J., & Henry, J. L. (1993). CP-96,345, but not its stereoisomer, CP-96,344, blocks the nociceptive responses to intrathecally administered substance P and to noxious thermal and chemical stimuli in the rat. *Neuroscience, 52*, 1039–1047.

Zederfeldt, B. (1979). *Factors influencing wound healing. Paper presented at the Symposium on Wound Healing.* Helsinki: Finland.

Zhang, N., Chow, S. K., Leung, K. S., & Cheung, W. H. (2017). Ultrasound as a stimulus for musculoskeletal disorders. *Journal of Orthopaedic Translation, 9*, 52–59.

Zhang, H., Li, Z. L., Yang, F., et al. (2018). Radial shockwave treatment promotes human mesenchymal stem cell self-renewal and enhances cartilage healing. *Stem Cell Research & Therapy, 9*(1), 54.

Zhao, Z.-Q., & Duggan, A. W. (1988). Idazoxan blocks the action of noradrenaline but not spinal inhibition from electrical stimulation of the locus coeruleus and nucleus Kolliker-Fuse of the cat. *Neuroscience, 25*, 997–1005.

4

Foundations of Electrical Stimulation

David M. Selkowitz

INTRODUCTION

This chapter introduces concepts and material that serve as the foundation for the clinical application of electrical stimulation (ES). This includes pertinent terminology, basic neurophysiology underlying ES, parameters of ES, and the manipulation of these parameters to produce the desired neurophysiologic responses.

BASICS OF ELECTRICITY

Electrical current is the flow of charged particles. A battery or a power station are power sources that can generate an electric current. A patient-device circuit is formed by a battery, lead wires connecting the battery to electrodes, and electrodes attached to the body (Fig. 4.1). The battery has a negative pole connected to the negative electrode, called the cathode, and a positive pole connected to the positive electrode, called the anode. In metals, e.g., the lead wires of a patient stimulation device, current is the flow of negatively charged electrons from cathode to anode. In solution (as in the human body), electrical current comprises the flow of charged particles (ions) which, by convention, are designated as moving from positive to negative poles; in fact, ions move in both directions, in accordance with their charges and those of the electrodes. The cathode and anode repel ions that are similarly charged and attract those that are oppositely charged.

The flow of electrons in the circuit occurs because of the charge difference between the poles of the battery, which creates a 'potential difference' or voltage that in turn creates an electromotive force to move the electrons. Conductance, capacitance, resistance, and impedance are terms used to characterize electrical current. Conductance is a measure of the ease of flow through substances and resistance is a measure of the difficulty of flow. Capacitance is the ability of substances to store charge. Impedance comprises resistance and capacitance, and is a measure of the difficulty of flow through human tissues.

The flow of ions in the body has relevance to the effects of ES that will be discussed later in the chapter. Electrotherapeutic devices are engineered to convert the incoming current from power stations (to line-powered devices) or from batteries (to portable devices) into characteristics appropriate for clinical use.

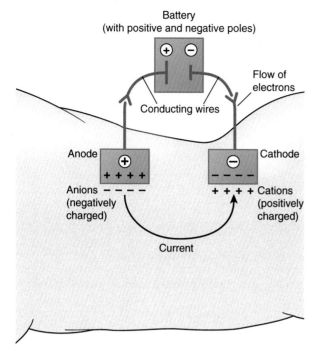

Fig. 4.1 Patient-device (battery-powered) electrical circuit. Note, by convention, the direction of current (ion flow) ion flow is opposite to that of electrons.

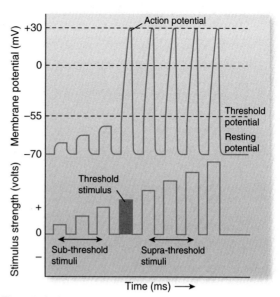

Fig. 4.2 Action potential (AP) generation illustrating the all-or-none principle. Sub-threshold stimuli do not produce an AP. Each supra-threshold stimulus does not produce a stronger AP, or more than one AP on that same nerve fibre.

BASICS OF NERVE EXCITATION

Electrical stimulation is used to stimulate nerves and muscles, and to affect other biological substrates. This section will include a basic and cursory description of the process of exciting a nerve to create an action potential (AP) along that nerve. A nerve has more sodium ions outside the cell membrane and more potassium ions inside. This concentration gradient, as well as active transport via the sodium-potassium pump, results in a resting electrical potential (or charge difference) of approximately -70 millivolts (mV) across the nerve membrane. To create an AP, a stimulus must be of adequate magnitude to cause the nerve to depolarize to its threshold potential, which is approximately -55 mV. The stimulus causes sodium ion channels in the membrane to open such that the sodium ions diffuse into the nerve through the membrane faster than the potassium ions can diffuse out. At this point, the process is self-sustaining such that the charge inside changes from negative to positive. When the nerve membrane becomes depolarized to about +30 mV, an AP is generated. Then, the membrane permeability to sodium decreases, and increases to potassium, resulting in a repolarization of the nerve to its resting potential, including a late, brief hyperpolarization

(i.e. more negative than resting potential). If the stimulus is not of adequate magnitude to depolarize the nerve to the threshold, an AP will not be generated. This is the 'all-or none' principle. There is no such thing as a partial or lower magnitude AP, nor is there a higher magnitude AP (Fig. 4.2). A stimulus of a higher magnitude than that needed to generate an AP will not generate an AP that is 'stronger', nor will it generate more than one AP along that same nerve simultaneously. Generating more than one AP along a nerve fibre requires additional stimuli, delivered in succession, each reaching the necessary threshold for depolarization. However, a stronger stimulus may excite APs on multiple nerve fibres simultaneously.

The process of AP generation described above lasts approximately 1 millisecond (ms), depending on the nerve (Fig. 4.3). During this time, no other AP can be created, regardless of the magnitude or number of stimuli. This is called the absolute refractory period. Immediately following this period is the 'relative refractory period' (approximately 10 ms), during which time it is possible to generate another AP with another stimulus (Koester 2013). However, during the relative refractory period, the threshold for depolarization for AP generation is elevated, requiring a stimulus of higher magnitude. The process of AP generation is influenced by the parameters of ES; in particular, current amplitude and duration, frequency, and time-modulated medium frequency currents.

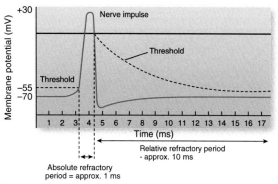

Fig. 4.3 Absolute and relative refractory periods after a stimulus depolarizes a nerve to its threshold. A lower resting potential and a higher threshold potential would make it more difficult for an AP to be created.

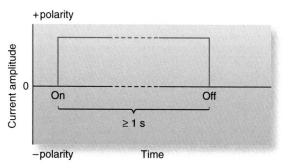

Fig. 4.4 Direct Current (DC). Note, current is shown as going on and off abruptly; in practice, this is typically more gradual. Zero current line is also called a dielectric line.

PARAMETERS OF ELECTRICAL STIMULATION

The main parameters that need to be considered are as follows: type of current/waveform; current amplitude, duration, frequency, and modulation; on and off times/cycling, ramp-up and -down times, total treatment times; and electrode set-up. These parameters are manipulated for different treatment purposes. Specific effects and manipulations related to treatment purposes will be discussed in other chapters.

There are three neurophysiologic responses to electrical stimulation – sensory, motor, and noxious/nociceptive (pain), as well as other biological responses. Deciding which response to elicit depends on the impairment or treatment purpose; then, the ES parameters can be manipulated to achieve the desired response. Deciding which device to use depends on the range of parameter settings that are offered by a given device. Purchasing decisions might be based on typical patient populations or impairments that one encounters in practice, and the range of parameter settings available on particular devices (Selkowitz 1999).

Devices may be small and portable, usable in the clinic or by patients at home, or they may be large devices intended for in-clinic use only. Either may provide only a single type of current or they may be multi-modal, having different types of current. Regardless of how a manufacturer may label a device (e.g. transcutaneous electrical nerve stimulation (TENS), neuromuscular electrical stimulation (NMES), interferential current (IFC), 'Russian', etc.), frequently it can be used for more than just what the marketing name implies (Selkowitz 1999).

Type of Current/Waveform

The three types of current most commonly used are pulsatile/pulsed current (PC), alternating current (AC), and direct current (DC). These currents are typically depicted on a graph (Fig. 4.4) that shows the current amplitude on the y-axis and time on the x-axis. The x-axis is also used as the zero-current baseline (also known as the dielectric line) and, by convention, the portion of the graph that is above the baseline represents the amount of positive charge and the portion below the line is the amount of negative charge.

Direct Current

DC is typically defined as unidirectional current that is uninterrupted for at least 1 second (s). It flows in this manner until it is programmed to turn off. It should be noted that after flowing for 1 s, the direction of DC can reverse/alternate and can also be interrupted with on and off cycling. With DC, there is no waveform, per se (see Fig. 4.4). The electrodes will remain at their set polarities for the entire delivery time, unless polarity is reversed or current is interrupted by the clinician. This means that oppositely charged ions will accumulate continuously under each electrode. This can result in discomfort or pain due to irritation of the skin under the electrodes. Nonetheless, DC can be used for stimulating muscle that has lost its nerve supply, for biological effects used in promoting wound healing, and for iontophoresis.

DC is the typical current used for iontophoresis, which is the delivery of ions (such as from medicinal compounds) through the skin. The compound comprises positively and negatively charged ions, but it must be applied to the electrode of the same polarity as the therapeutic ion so that the ion will be repelled by that electrode (i.e. the 'treatment electrode') and driven into the body. For example, if the therapeutic ion is negatively charged, the compound must be applied to the cathode. Unidirectional uninterrupted DC is preferred because it provides adequate electromotive force to drive the ions. Discomfort due to accumulation of ions under the electrodes can be limited by decreasing the current amplitude and extending the delivery time. In addition, there are iontophoresis electrodes with a built-in battery that deliver current at very low levels over a period of hours, which are typically not uncomfortable.

DC is one of the current types used for healing open wounds (e.g. diabetic, venous, or pressure ulcers) (see Chapter 19). It influences movement of ions that are substrates of the different phases of healing, based on the polarity of the tissue ions and that of the treatment electrode; a process called galvanotaxis. With wound healing, the current amplitude of DC is in the microamperage range (i.e. less than 1 milliampere), and is called 'microcurrent' or low intensity direct current (LIDC). This amperage is too low to produce APs or neurophysiological responses, but it has biological effects on cells and substrates of healing.

DC has also been used for stimulating muscles that have lost their nerve supply due to a lower motor neuron injury, i.e. denervated muscles. It can be used for this purpose primarily because of its long, uninterrupted duration and unidirectional nature. Typically, the cathode is used as the target electrode over the muscle because it stimulates more forceful contractions (Cummings 1991; Seckel 1988). Further rationale for using DC will be discussed later in this chapter.

Alternating Current

AC is a continuous current that is bidirectional such that the electrodes repeatedly switch polarity. In its most common form, AC is symmetrical, meaning that the shape of the waveform looks identical on both sides of the dielectric line. Thus, AC has no net polarity; neither electrode is considered an anode or cathode. The completion of one consecutive positive and negative period is called a cycle. Each positive and negative component is called a phase; thus, a cycle has two phases (biphasic), with the current amplitude passing through zero between the phases, but there is no interruption between the phases (Fig. 4.5). In contrast, DC has a net polarity that is negative at one electrode and positive at the other.

The shape of the phase of an AC waveform can vary. Most commonly, it is a sine wave (see Fig. 4.5), but it may take other forms such as triangular or rectangular. A phase is characterized by a rise time and a decay time (see Fig. 4.5). The rise time is the amount of time it takes for the phase amplitude to increase from zero to its maximum value, and the decay time is the time for the amplitude to return to zero. The significance of rise time is that if it is too slow, the nerve will accommodate such that the threshold for depolarization will increase too high and an AP will not be produced, i.e. the nerve will not respond to the stimulation (Fig. 4.6) (Hill 1936). Rise time cannot be

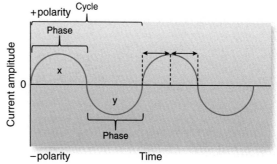

Fig. 4.5 Alternating Current (AC). A pair of consecutive positive and negative phases is called a cycle. Charge of each phase is represented by area under the curve; x is the positive phase's charge and y is the negative phase's charge. With symmetrical AC, x = y. Rise time from zero to peak and decay time from peak to zero are shown by the *double-arrowed lines*. Unlike ramp-up time (see Fig. 4.18), rise time applies to a single stimulus.

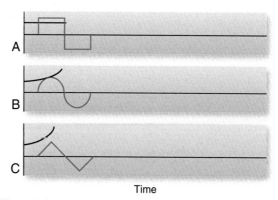

Fig. 4.6 Accommodation and the effect of stimulus rise time on the ability to generate an action potential (AP) along a nerve fibre. The *black line* represents depolarization threshold. (A) Fast rise time reaches depolarization threshold, generating an AP. (B) Gradual rise time meets a slightly elevated depolarization threshold, generating an AP. (C) Slow rise time results in sharply elevated depolarization threshold and, thus, no AP.

manipulated by the clinician; however, it is engineered into the waveform of AC such that the amplitude rises at a rate too fast for nerves to accommodate.

The area under the curve (i.e. the area bounded by the waveform shape) of each phase of a cycle represents the phase charge (see Fig. 4.5). The two phases together comprise the cycle charge. AC has symmetrical phases; thus, the charges of the positive and negative phases of the cycle are equal and, therefore, balanced (referred to as 'zero net charge'). When a current is charge-balanced, there is no accumulation of ions under the electrodes.

For therapeutic applications, AC is commonly interrupted, creating millisecond bursts of cycles separated by a brief interval; in this form AC is more versatile, and in some respects more like symmetrical biphasic pulsed current. These are called time modulations and will be discussed later in the chapter.

Pulsed Current

PC is always interrupted and comprises phases that can be biphasic/bidirectional (like AC), or monophasic/unidirectional (like DC). The interruption between pulses is called the interpulse interval (Fig. 4.7). In biphasic PC, the positive and negative phases may immediately follow each other or may be separated by a brief interphase (sometimes called intrapulse) interval. There is evidence that the presence of an interphase interval in rectangular biphasic symmetrical PC may increase electrically stimulated isometric contraction force (Laufer 2013). The term for a pair of positive and negative phases is 'pulse' (not 'cycle', as in AC).

Biphasic PC can be symmetrical, in which case it would, by definition, be charge-balanced (Fig. 4.8A), which avoids possible deleterious effects of charge build-up associated with unbalanced currents. However, biphasic PC can also be asymmetrical such that the phases of the pulse would be different in shape; in which case it could be charge-balanced or unbalanced (see Fig. 4.8B,C). If there were an imbalance in charge between the phases of the pulse, then there would be an imbalance in charge between the electrodes such that one would be the cathode and the other would be the anode. The shapes of PC waveforms can vary similarly to those of AC, and can include phases with brief peaks and sloped or curved rise and/or decay times (see Fig. 4.8B).

Symmetrical biphasic PC can be used for a variety of treatment purposes, including muscle strengthening, pain control, and blood flow enhancement (Selkowitz 1999). This current with a rectangular waveform and long pulse duration has also been shown to have positive effects in treating denervated muscle (Boncompagni et al 2007; Kern et al 2005; Modlin et al 2005; Valencic et al 1986), and its symmetrical nature avoids ion accumulation under the electrodes; however, for denervated muscle the stimulators must have long pulse duration capabilities (tens to hundreds of milliseconds) and are not commonly available. Additionally, triangular waveforms with slow rise times could be used for denervated muscle. Slowly rising, long duration pulses cause any intact sensory or nociceptive fibres in the area to accommodate (remain unresponsive), thereby limiting pain perception; importantly, muscle fibres do not readily accommodate.

Asymmetrical balanced biphasic PC is typically found in TENS devices, but may also be found in other devices

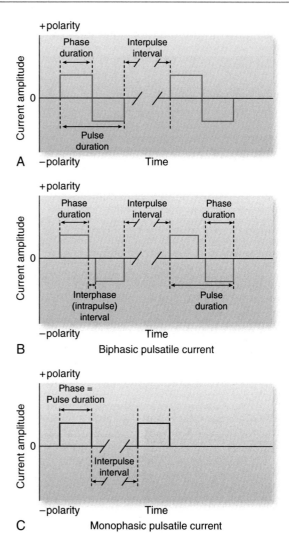

Fig. 4.7 Pulsed Currents (PC) (A) Biphasic PC showing phase and cycle duration (on the order of tens to hundreds of microseconds). The break in the zero current line represents the typically long interpulse interval relative to the pulse duration (on the order of tens to hundreds of *milli*seconds). During the interpulse interval, the current is at the zero baseline because there is no stimulus. (B) Biphasic PC with interphase interval. (C) Monophasic PC with interphase interval: a pulse consists of one phase, so phase and pulse are the same. This illustrates the rectangular low-volt type of monophasic PC.

(e.g. portable NMES and large multi-modal devices). Symmetrical and asymmetrical *balanced* biphasic PCs can be used for similar therapeutic purposes. Biphasic asymmetrical *unbalanced* PC is not typically used in therapeutic ES. Note that slight charge imbalances may occur with asymmetrical balanced biphasic PCs due to the long decay

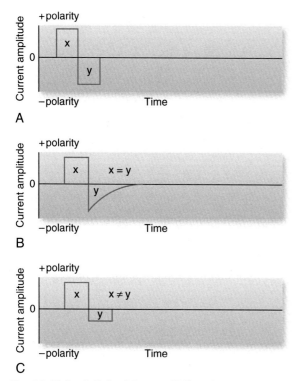

A

B

C

Fig. 4.8 Biphasic Pulsed Current (PC) (A) Symmetrical biphasic PC; the phases are shaped identically, so phase charges x and y are equal. (B) Asymmetrical balanced biphasic PC; the phases are shaped differently, but the charges of the paired phases are equal (x = y). (C) Asymmetrical unbalanced biphasic PC, the phases are shaped differently, and the charges of the paired phases are unequal (x ≠ y). In this case, one electrode would be the cathode and the other would be the anode.

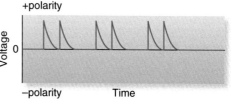

Fig. 4.9 High-volt monophasic PC, commonly known as HVPC. Note HVPC's twin peaks paired phases, with their exponential decay. The paired phases comprise a pulse, which is typically of short duration (100 μs or less, often as low as 20 μs). With HVPC, the magnitude of the stimulus is typically recorded in mV.

current (i.e. sub-sensory-level), it may be called microcurrent electrical nerve stimulation (MENS). MENS has been used clinically for improving muscle function (Kwon 2014, 2017), wound healing (Nair 2018), and for pain control with a variety of tissue injuries, but there is conflicting and questionable evidence for its effectiveness (Allen 1999; Bonacci 1997; Curtis 2010; Gossrau 2011; Ho 2007; Johnson 1997; Koopman 2009; Poltawski 2009). The problematic aspects of the evidence relate to quality and research design, methodological differences and outcome measures; most of the favourable studies used no control, sham or comparison group, small sample sizes, or had results that were of questionable clinical relevance (Atya 2002; Korelo 2012; Lee 2013; Nair 2018; Park 2011; Poltawski 2011).

High-volt monophasic PC, commonly known as HVPC, or twin-peaked monophasic PC, is characterized by pulses comprising two spiked phases of equal amplitude and polarity (Fig. 4.9). These phases may or may not be separated by an *interphase* interval that is very brief, relative to the phase duration. There is an *interpulse* interval between each set of paired spiked phases. Thus, even though HVPC contains two phases in a pulse, it is considered a type of monophasic PC because the two phases are of the same polarity and any interval between them is very brief.

HVPC is recommended for acute-stage oedema control because this purpose requires a constant difference in polarity of the electrodes (Bettany 1990; Fish 1991; Snyder 2010; Taylor 1997). HVPC is also used for wound healing. As with DC, the constant polarity difference between the electrodes influences movement of ions and cells involved in healing.

HVPC can be used for many other treatment purposes, even those not requiring a constant polarity difference between electrodes (Selkowitz 1999). However, it is not typically used for strengthening, likely due to the fixed, short pulse durations, although this has only been tested in uninjured persons (Mohr 1985). It is also not used for iontophoresis or stimulating denervated muscle because of the short pulse durations and long interpulse intervals.

times (see Fig. 4.8B), but the imbalance and any ion accumulation are insignificant because of the long interpulse intervals relative to the pulse durations.

Monophasic PC is unidirectional, asymmetrical and charge-unbalanced because there is only one phase to a pulse (Fig.4.7C). Therefore, the current is delivered with a constant polarity difference between electrodes. There is an interpulse interval between these single-phase pulses, which differentiates it from DC. Although the current is not charge-balanced, the interpulse interval limits the accumulation of ions under the electrodes because the interval is much longer proportionally than the pulse duration in typical therapeutic devices.

There are numerous shape options for monophasic pulses, as for AC and biphasic PC. In addition, there are two types of monophasic PC: low-volt and high-volt. The low-volt type typically consists of rectangular pulses (see Fig. 4.7C). When used with microamperage levels of

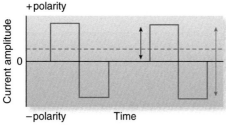

Fig. 4.10 Measures of Current Amplitude The *black arrowed line* represents peak amplitude; the *grey arrowed line* represents peak-to-peak amplitude; the *green dashed dotted line* shows total or average current (per second), which depends on the pulse frequency and size of pulses, and it factors in the interpulse intervals, which contain no current.

The characteristics of rise and decay times, and the property of accommodation, apply to the phases of PC as well as AC. The common rectangular and twin-spiked shapes of PCs have sharp rises that limit accommodation (see Figs 4.7C and 4.9). The concept of charge as discussed for the phases and cycles of AC also applies to the phases and pulses of PC.

Amplitude

Current amplitude is the magnitude of the current. The units are given in amperes (amps), but the amounts of current used in therapeutic ES are typically in the milliamps (mA) or, less often, microamps (μA) range. Less frequently, voltage is used as a measure of magnitude but, technically, voltage is the magnitude of the potential difference between the two poles of the circuit.

There are different measures of current amplitude, including peak amplitude, peak-to-peak amplitude, and total or average current (Fig. 4.10). Peak amplitude – the maximum amplitude per phase – is the commonly used term, and the amplitude factor that impacts depolarization of nerves. Peak amplitude is the measure referred to in this chapter unless otherwise stated.

Pulse or Cycle Duration

Pulse duration is the term used with PC, and cycle duration is the term used with AC; phase duration is applicable to both current types (see Figs 4.5 and 4.7). 'Width' is sometimes used to describe duration, and may appear as a label on therapeutic devices, but 'duration' is more appropriate as a term denoting time. With DC there are no pulses, so one can only appropriately use the term current duration.

Phase duration is measured from the beginning of the increase in amplitude from the zero baseline until it declines back to zero (see Figs 4.5 and 4.7). There is inconsistency as to whether the duration of an interphase interval is included when reporting the duration of a biphasic pulse. Note that the effective stimulus with respect to depolarizing nerves does not include the interphase interval. Thus, one should be clear in all circumstances whether interphase interval has been included in the pulse duration calculation.

Relationships Between Amplitude, Duration, and Charge

Current amplitude and current duration are the parameters comprising charge. Charge is expressed in coulombs (in ES, typically in microcoulombs). Charge is the foremost factor for determining the types of neurophysiological responses that ES will produce. As stated previously, these responses are sensation, muscle contraction and nociception. Electrical stimulation can also induce direct biological effects in addition to or independent of exciting nerve or muscle fibres (e.g. galvanotaxis for wound healing). The magnitude of the charge will determine the magnitude of the response. For example, as charge increases (via increasing amplitude and/or duration), more motor nerve fibres and motor units are activated, and force output increases (Alon 1983; Gregory 2007; Medeiros 2017; Parker 2005; Scott 2009; Selkowitz 1999; Selkowitz 2009; Ward 2001, 2004). Similarly, greater charge will result in a perception of greater tingling and/or pain.

Phase charge is affected by the shape of the waveform. As stated previously, phase charge is the area bounded by the phase shape. For rectangular phases, the charge is the product of the amplitude and duration. For sinusoidal shapes, the phase charge is the integral of the amplitude multiplied by the phase duration (Alon 1991). Thus, given phases of equal amplitude and duration, charge for a rectangular phase is greater than that of a sinusoidal phase and will, therefore, produce a greater magnitude of response. This may contribute to the greater muscular forces produced using symmetrical rectangular biphasic PC and burst-modulated rectangular PC compared with 'Russian' current, which incorporates a sinusoidal waveform (discussed later in the chapter).

A schematic of the strength–duration (S-D) curve (Fig. 4.11) illustrates the relationship between amplitude and duration with regard to stimulating sensory-, motor-, and noxious-level responses. The y-axis shows current amplitude (in mA) and the x-axis shows current duration (in ms or μs); some sources show voltage on the y-axis. As shown, sensory nerve fibres are closest to the left on the x-axis and lowest on the y-axis. Therefore, sensory fibres are easiest to stimulate, requiring less amplitude and duration than motor fibres. The nerve fibres that require the most charge to stimulate are the nociceptive fibres, furthest to the right and highest on the graph.

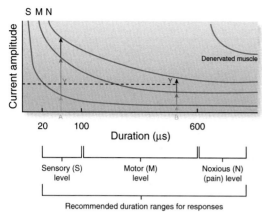

Fig. 4.11 A schematic strength–duration (S-D) curve for each of the three nerve fibre types, and for denervated muscle. Note that: 1. For a given magnitude of duration, it requires less amplitude to stimulate sensory nerve fibres than motor or nociceptive fibres (see *vertical arrows at A or B*). 2. More amplitude is needed to stimulate a given type of nerve fibre at a shorter duration than a longer one (compare *like-coloured vertical arrows at A versus B*). 3. At a shorter duration (*A*) it will be easier, i.e., require less amplitude to stimulate a sensory response without exciting the other responses; e.g. at the same amplitude, A–Y produces a moderate sensory response and B–Y produces a moderate motor response. 4. The curve for denervated muscle is displaced much higher and to the right, indicating that skeletal muscle is much less excitable than nerve and requires much more current amplitude and duration to stimulate a response. At durations less than approximately 1–10 ms, amplitude cannot be increased high enough to produce a contraction in denervated muscle. Recommended ranges of pulse (or cycle) duration are shown for stimulating each type of nerve while minimizing excitation of the other responses.

Ease of stimulation is related to speed of conduction and ease of depolarization, which are related to fibre size (less internal resistance to current flow) and myelination (Lloyd 1948). Sensory and motor nerve fibres are generally large-diameter fibres, thus, are more easily stimulated and conduct stimuli faster than the smaller, lesser myelinated nociceptive fibres (e.g. C-fibres). In addition, larger-diameter motor nerve fibres, sub-serving larger motor units and fast-twitch (type II) muscle fibres, are more easily stimulated than smaller-diameter motor nerve fibres sub-serving type 1 muscle fibres (Garnett 1981). Thus, ES may preferentially recruit fast-twitch muscle fibres, which are more easily fatigued but capable of producing greater force. This is different from the order of recruitment with voluntary contractions, i.e. from small to large (Henneman 1965, 1981; Stein 1981). However, it has been theorized that recruitment of motor units with ES is not due to a reversal of the volitional recruitment order but, rather, due to a more random, non-selective, spatially fixed, temporally synchronous recruitment (Bickel 2011; Brown 1981; Gregory 2005; Knaflitz 1990). Nonetheless, adequate charge is an important factor in recruitment. Failure to produce high force levels at low amounts of charge is likely due to recruiting too few motor units to create complete tetany, even when using stimulation frequencies appropriate for tetanic contractions (see later section on Frequency).

Another factor impacting nerve fibre response is proximity to the surface of the body and, therefore, to the electrodes (Alon 1983; Selkowitz 1999). In general, sensory nerve fibres are closest to the surface; the SD curve reflects the ease of stimulating sensory nerves. Some larger nociceptive fibres (A-delta) may also be close to the surface, but their higher resistance makes them more difficult to stimulate than motor fibres. Some exceptions other than those previously stated include areas where tissues overlying muscle or motor nerves are thinner, such as the forearm, where motor fibres may respond simultaneously with sensory fibres. Similarly, nociceptive fibres may be stimulated before motor fibres in areas where there is minimal overlying tissue, such as near bones (e.g. ankle). Also, motor fibres might not be stimulated if there is excessive overlying adipose tissue.

The S-D curve can also be used to illustrate the difference between nerve fibres and skeletal muscle fibres for ease of stimulation (see Fig. 4.11). Muscle fibres are only stimulated directly when they have lost their nerve supply (i.e. denervated muscle). Muscle fibres are less excitable and much more difficult to depolarize using ES than are nerves, primarily due to the greater impedance and lower resting potential of the muscle fibre membrane. Denervated muscle stimulation could be very uncomfortable if there are intact sensory and nociceptive fibres in the area of the electrodes due to the large amount of charge needed, as well as the accumulation of ions under the electrodes if monophasic current is used.

Recommended ranges for current (pulse, cycle) duration settings are noted in Fig. 4.11 for stimulating sensory nerves relatively easily without recruiting motor nerves as current amplitude is increased, and for stimulating motor nerves relatively easily to produce a reasonably forceful contraction while limiting a noxious-level response (Alon et al 1983; Selkowitz 1999). It is important to note that even if the current duration does not fall within these recommended ranges, it is still possible to obtain the desired response by manipulating current amplitude (Selkowitz 1999). For example, one could create a sensory-level response with a duration of 400 µs (0.4 ms) by limiting the current amplitude to a level below that which would produce muscle contraction. A specific setting or range of settings for current amplitude cannot be recommended because tissue and nerve characteristics vary within the electrical field across body regions and between individuals, as does the experience, perception and tolerance of ES. Responses may even vary by day or time of day (Selkowitz 1985). It is noteworthy that portable devices have been shown to be comparable to clinic devices in their charge-generating capabilities (Laufer 2001; Lyons 2005).

In summary thus far, the type and magnitude of the neurophysiological response depends in part on rise time, charge and the location of the nerves in relation to the electrodes. Thus, the operator primarily needs to consider the current amplitude and duration, and electrode location. Other aspects of the electrode set-up that impact the responses to ES will be discussed later in the chapter.

Frequency

Frequency is the term for number of stimuli (e.g. pulses) or APs per second; the term 'rate' is also used on devices. By convention (in physical therapy), frequencies up to 1000 are called 'low', from 1000 to 10,000 are 'medium', and over 10,000 are 'high'. However, these are non-specific terms and the specific frequency should be identified. The units of frequency depend on the type of current: pps (pulses per second) for PC; Hz (Hertz) or cycles per second for AC; bursts/s or beats/s for modulated currents (e.g. 'Russian' and interferential currents, respectively). Frequencies found on therapeutic devices are typically 1–250 pps (or bursts/s or beats/s) in the low-frequency range and 1000–5000 Hz in the medium frequency AC range. High frequency AC is not typically delivered in ES treatments discussed in this chapter.

Frequency does not determine the type of neurophysiological response produced (it does not factor into the S-D curve). Once there is enough charge to produce a sensory, motor or noxious level response, frequency affects the quality, i.e. pattern of that response (Selkowitz 1999). For example, a sensory-level response (typical frequencies are in the range of 50–200 pps) can be manipulated using a higher frequency to produce a 'fine' tingling sensation, while a lower frequency will produce a slower, 'coarse' tingling sensation. Comfort level of different frequencies varies among individuals.

When using motor-level stimulation, frequency can be manipulated to produce either tetanic or sub-tetanic contractions. A tetanic contraction can be described as smooth or continuous, with no discernible interruption between pulses. If the current is not cycled on and off, the muscle will eventually fatigue and cease to contract. A sub-tetanic contraction can be described as intermittent or twitch-like. Although the time periods between the twitches are relatively short (typically between 50 ms and 1 second), the patient will be able to perceive the separation between the stimuli and the twitch-like contractions will continue until the current is turned off. Tetanic contractions are typically produced with

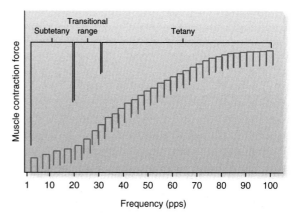

Fig. 4.12 Relationship Between Frequency and Contraction Force Approximate ranges for producing sub-tetanic (up to about 20 pps) and tetanic contractions (starting around 30 pps) are shown. Note, the units for frequency can also be cycles or bursts or beats per second, depending on the type of current used.

frequencies of 30 pps or higher, and sub-tetanic contractions with frequencies of 20 or lower (Fig. 4.12).

In practice, initially, as the first motor units are recruited, the contraction may appear to be sub-tetanic, but it is actually incomplete fusion of the muscle contraction. With increasing current amplitude, thereby stimulating more motor units, the muscle contraction will become more fused.

Relationships Between Frequency, Force, and Fatigue

Another property of frequency important in motor-level stimulation is that as frequency increases, more contractile force is created (see Fig. 4.12) (Baker 2000; Basmajian 1985; Ghez 1991; Gregory 2007; Kramer 1987; Milner-Brown 1973; Moreno-Aranda 1981c). When the interpulse interval becomes shorter than the duration of the muscle fibre contraction-relaxation time, the muscle does not return to its relaxed state; the twitches overlap and superimpose on each other until the intermittent contractions become indistinguishable and fuse together into a smooth continuous contraction and their forces summate (Ghez 1991). However, there comes a point of diminishing returns where force plateaus, in spite of further increasing frequency. This occurs at around 80–100 stimuli per second (Baker 2000; Ghez 1991; Gregory 2007; Russ 2002b). However, as frequency increases, so does fatigue, which may manifest as a faster decrease in force over successive contractions or during a sustained contraction (Fig. 4.13A,B) (Baker 2000; Bigland-Ritchie 1979; Binder-Macleod 1990, 1992; Gorgey 2009; Gregory 2007; Jones 1979; Moritani 1985; Selkowitz 1985). By itself, the higher force associated with higher frequencies may also play a role in the fatigue demonstrated at higher frequencies (Russ 2002a). As with force, there is little change in fatigue at about 80–100 pps (Russ 2002b), although this has not been tested at higher frequencies. Thus, the need for greater forces must be balanced with the inevitable by-product of greater fatigue with higher frequencies (Selkowitz 1999).

Electrical stimulation recruits motor units to fire synchronously, unlike volition, so it is more fatiguing than volition (Baker 2000; Bickel 2011; Kloth 1991). Also, as stated previously, ES may preferentially stimulate fast-twitch fibres, which are more fatigable than slow-twitch fibres.

Thus, ES can result in fatigue and associated decline in muscle force with time and number of contractions more quickly than with voluntary contractions (Fig. 4.14A) (Baker 2000; Currier 1983, Gregory 2007; Russ 2002a, 2002b; Selkowitz 1985, 1989). At lower forces, there is some evidence that increasing frequency preserves force output over successive contractions more than does pulse duration (Kesar 2008). However, this has not been tested with high-force contractions; nor have these parameters been compared with current amplitude for force preservation. At higher forces, increasing current amplitude has been reported to preserve

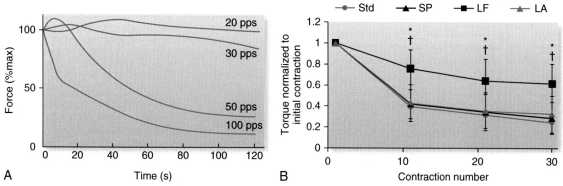

Fig. 4.13 Relationship between frequency and fatigue (A) over a sustained 120-second contraction. Lowest frequencies preserved force output better over time. (From Baker et al 2000). (B) Normalized torque output over 30 successive contractions. The lower frequency preserved torque output at a higher level. *LA,* Low amplitude (100 pps, 450 µs); *LF,* low frequency (20 pps, 450 µs); *SP, short pulse* (100 pps, 150 µs); *Std,* standard (100 pps, 45 µs). (From Gorgey et al 2009.)

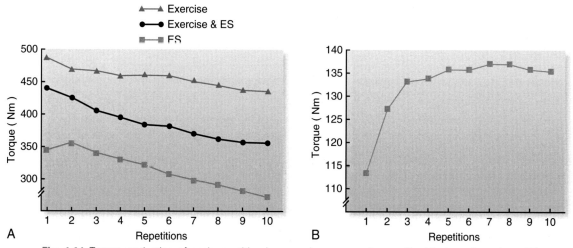

Fig. 4.14 Torque production of each repetition in a session, averaged over all subjects and sessions. (A) Current amplitude was not altered during the session: note the steady decline of voluntary and electrically stimulated contraction torque. (From Currier & Mann 1983). (B) Current amplitude was increased as tolerated during the session: note the preservation of electrically stimulated contraction torque over successive repetitions. (From Selkowitz 1985). ES, electrical stimulation

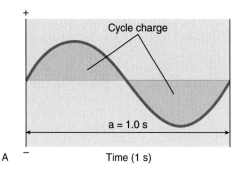

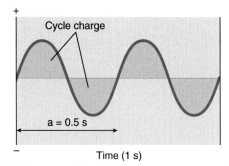

Fig. 4.15 The inverse relationship between frequency and duration for AC. The frequencies are 1 Hz and 2 Hz, in graphs (A) and (B), respectively; (B) is twice the frequency of (A). However, the cycle duration 'a' in graph (A) is 1 s, while in graph (B), a= 0.5 s; (A) is twice the duration of (B). Note, the amplitude is the same in both graphs. Thus, cycle charge in graph (A) is twice that of graph (B), so the lower AC frequency of graph (A) will produce a greater neurophysiological response.

force output over successive contractions (see Fig. 4.14B) (Selkowitz 1985). Manipulation of ES parameters to limit force decline will be discussed in depth in Chapter 16.

Relationship Between Frequency and Duration

The relationship between frequency and duration depends on whether the type of current is AC or PC. With AC, frequency and duration are interdependent because there are no inter-cycle intervals: as frequency increases, duration necessarily decreases; for more cycles to fit into a second, each cycle will need to be shorter. Similarly, if one increases the cycle duration, fewer cycles will fit into a second, which means that the frequency will decrease (Fig. 4.15). Cycle duration can be calculated if frequency is known; conversely, frequency can be calculated if duration is known (see Box 4.1). It is important to recognize that with AC, because of the inverse relationship between cycle frequency and duration, there is necessarily an inverse relationship between cycle frequency and charge. This has clinical relevance when using medium frequency AC such as 'Russian' and IFC.

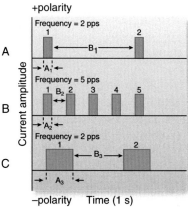

Fig. 4.16 The independent relationship between frequency and duration for PC. (A) Example of a frequency of 2 pps with a pulse duration of A_1 and interpulse interval of B_1. (B) An increase in frequency (to 5 pps) would result in a decrease in the interpulse interval (from B_1 to B_2) to allow pulse duration to remain unchanged ($A_2=A_1$). (C) An increase in pulse duration (from A_1 to A_3) would result in a decrease in the interpulse interval (from B_1 to B_3) to allow the frequency to remain unchanged. Note, pulse durations and interpulse intervals not drawn to scale.

BOX 4.1

The equation describing the relationship between AC frequency and duration is: f=1/d if one knows the duration and wishes to solve for frequency; and d=1/f if one knows the frequency and wishes to solve for duration. Most commonly, one will know the frequency and need to calculate the duration.

Example: solving for cycle duration if frequency is given as 100 Hz (cycles/s)

$d = 1/f = 1/100 = .01$ s

Example: solving for frequency if duration is given as .01 s

$f = 1/d = 1/.01 = 100$ Hz

The units for frequency and duration in the equation are given in seconds, which need to be converted to ms or µs units for practical application.

The relationship between frequency and duration is an independent one for PC; i.e. a change in one of these parameters does not automatically cause a change in the other. This is because there are interpulse intervals, which automatically adjust in duration with a change in either frequency or pulse duration (Fig. 4.16). This allows great flexibility in parameter setting to obtain the desired neurophysiological response. The duration of the interpulse interval can be calculated if pulse duration and frequency are known; however, it is not essential information for setting up a device that uses pulsed current.

Modulation

Modulation is the automatic, sequential variation of amplitude, duration, or frequency, alone or in combination, over a series of stimuli (Fig. 4.17). For example, the initial amplitude set by the operator would decrease and then increase to the initial level over several seconds in a repetitive pattern until the stimulation period ends. The time over which the parameter is modulated can sometimes be set by the operator, but is often unalterable.

Portable TENS devices may allow modulation of a parameter by about 50% of the initial setting. For example, after setting the frequency to 100 pps, the device would modulate frequency between 50–100 pps. Multi-modal devices typically allow modulation of frequency for certain modes, e.g. IFC, biphasic PC, HVPC, in a flexible manner, allowing one to set the precise frequencies between which the stimulation can vary. For example, one could set the maximum level at 100 pps and the minimum at 30 pps; it can pass through each frequency in the range over a period lasting a few seconds, or, can switch abruptly delivering pulses at only the highest and lowest selected frequencies, alternating between them every few seconds. Some of these devices use the term 'sweep' for frequency modulation, and use Hz as the units (which is incorrect).

Modulation is used to limit the possibility of adaptation, which may occur when nerves are stimulated at the same parameter settings without change for a period of time, such that the frequency of APs decrease. This may progress to the point where the nerves stop responding entirely (Vander 1994). It is as if the nerves become accustomed to the stimulus, 'become bored' and 'fall asleep' (a phenomenon completely unheard of when studying electrical stimulation).

Many resources confuse the terms adaptation and accommodation. Adaptation is the correct term to describe an already present but diminishing neurophysiological response to a series of unchanging stimuli (pulses or cycles, etc.), as discussed above, while accommodation refers to a process (described earlier in the chapter) involving a single stimulus with a slow rise time, to which the nerves never respond with an AP (Selkowitz 1999).

Some devices modulate amplitude and duration to mimic the pattern of sensory nerve fibre response as shown on the SD curve; i.e. magnitudes of amplitude and duration vary in opposite directions simultaneously. However, there is no evidence that this is more effective at limiting adaptation or accomplishing the treatment purpose. Modulation is typically not used with motor-level stimulation, wound healing, acute-stage oedema control or iontophoresis.

On and Off Times (On/Off Cycling; or, Duty Cycle)

On and off times (hereafter referred to as on/off times when appropriate) (Fig. 4.18) are programmed by the clinician to allow the current to automatically turn on and off in a repetitive pattern throughout a treatment session. They refer to the durations of and intervals between series (trains) of stimuli (pulses, cycles, bursts or beats). During 'on time', the current is at the amplitude set by the clinician; during 'off time', no current is delivered. On/off times may be thought of as 'macro' times because they are measured in seconds. On and off times should not be confused with pulse duration and interpulse interval, which are very brief and measured in milli- or microseconds (i.e. 'micro' times).

Duty cycle is another way to express on/off times. By definition, a duty cycle is the on time divided by the total of the on plus off time, then multiplied by 100 to express it in terms of the percentage of time that the current is delivered out of the total time.

$$\text{Duty cycle} = [(\text{on time}) / (\text{on} + \text{off time})] \times 100$$

Any regular succession of on and off times can be expressed as a duty cycle, whether they are 'macro' or 'micro' times. Duty cycles with PCs are typically very small

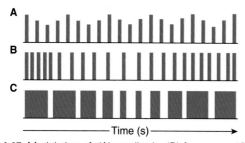

Fig. 4.17 Modulation of: (A) amplitude; (B) frequency; (C) duration. The series of stimuli (pulses, in this illustration) continuously decreases and increases over several seconds.

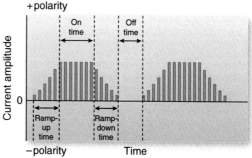

Fig. 4.18 On and off times (on/off cycling or duty cycle) and ramp-up and ramp-down times. On and ramp times involve series (also called 'trains') of stimuli; e.g. pulse trains.

(less than 1%) and seldom reported because there is no setting for it on a device; pulse duration is the important parameter to set and report with PC. Duty cycles are larger and are clinically relevant when describing time-modulated currents, such as Russian current; clinicians must specifically set duty cycle when using such currents.

On/off times can be described in terms of a ratio or duty cycle (e.g. an on time of 1 second and an off time of 1 second would be expressed as 1:1, or a 1 to 1 ratio, or as a 50% duty cycle); however, without the actual/specific times and units, this could be misleading, e.g. a 50% duty cycle could also be 10 seconds on and 10 seconds off [(10)/(10 + 10)) × 100 = 50%]. Thus, it is more appropriate to report the specific on/off times (Fig. 4.19).

Setting on/off times is important when using tetanic contractions, to provide rest intervals to limit fatigue (neural and muscular) and preserve force output between contractions (see Fig. 4.19), as for volitional contractions. On/off cycling is typically not necessary with sub-tetanic contractions, (e.g., as used in AL-TENS, see Chapter 15) because of the discrete, albeit brief, interruptions between contractions, which minimize the effects of fatigue. Application of on/off times in therapy will be discussed in later chapters.

Constant Stimulation

There may be a setting on the device called 'constant' or 'continuous' for holding the stimulation in a continuous mode whilst setting the initial current amplitude before starting on/off cycling. In addition, for certain treatment purposes, the ES should remain on and the series of pulses be delivered continuously throughout the treatment session until turned off by the operator or the device timer: for example, when using sensory-level or sub-tetanic motor-level stimulation in treatments for pain control, oedema control, wound healing, iontophoresis and circulation enhancement.

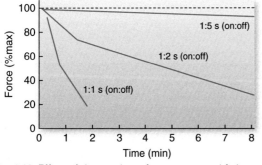

Fig. 4.19 Effect of duty cycle on force output and fatigue: 1 s on and 5 s off = 16.67% duty cycle [1/(1+5) = 1/6]; 1 s on and 1 s off = 50% duty cycle. Therefore, a lower duty cycle is better for preserving force output over time. (From Baker et al 2000.)

Ramp-Up/ Ramp-Down Times

If on/off cycling times are set, then ramp times are needed. Ramp-up is the time for a series of pulses to increase from the zero baseline to the current amplitude set by the operator (in contrast to rise time which applies to a single pulse). Ramp-down is the time for the series of pulses to decrease to zero amplitude (see Fig. 4.18). Ramp-up immediately precedes the on time. Ramp-down immediately follows the on time. Less commonly, ramp times are included in the on-cycle time (e.g. with ramp-up and ramp-down times set to 2 seconds each, and the on time to 10 seconds, the current amplitude is at maximum for only 6 of 10 seconds): thus, it is critical to consult the device manual. Furthermore, in some devices the ramp-up and ramp-down times cannot be set separately. Ramps are necessary with tetanic contractions to prevent the sudden increase and decrease in current amplitude and, hence, contraction force when current goes on and off. Another relevant factor is that if maximum amplitude is increased without increasing the ramp-up time, the ramp-up *rate* will increase. In this case, it might be necessary to increase the ramp-up time for patient comfort.

Ramp-up is unrelated to accommodation or adaptation.

As a special case, when applying iontophoresis, ramps are not set by the operator; they are engineered into the device and typically last between 30–60 seconds.

Total Treatment Time

Total treatment time is simply the total time devoted to the application of ES during a therapeutic session (i.e. not the 'on' time). It will depend on many factors, primarily patient status and treatment purpose. Treatment times will be covered in later chapters devoted to specific types of current.

Electrode Set-Up

Note that the information on electrodes in this chapter is not all-inclusive; more information regarding electrodes is presented in other chapters covering the different types of electrical stimulation.

Electrode Types, Conductive (Coupling) Media

There are different types of electrodes: this chapter refers only to surface electrodes, carbon-silicon rubber type or self-adhesive pre-gelled type; not indwelling needle or fine-wire electrodes.

The most commonly used conductive agents with carbon-silicone electrodes include aqueous conductive gel, water-moistened sponges on which the electrodes are placed, and water by itself, such as a non-metallic tub of water in which the electrode is submerged. Keep in mind that the electrode then comprises the entire submerged area so that the larger the submerged area, the more the current amplitude will need to be increased due to the

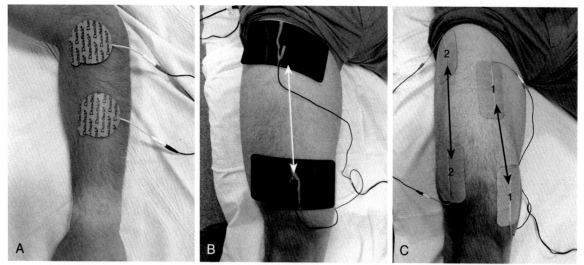

Fig. 4.20 Electrode sizes based on size of target tissue area. (A) Equal size small electrodes over the same small target tissue area, called a bipolar electrode placement. (B) Equal size large electrodes for large target tissue area – a bipolar arrangement. The *white line* shows the direction current will travel, i.e. along a line that is parallel to the course of the muscle fibres. (C) Use of two electrodes on each of two channels (1 and 2) for a large target tissue area, to maximize coverage; *black lines* show configuration of electrodes on each channel approximately parallel to course of muscle fibres.

lower current density. Either one or both electrodes may be submerged unless a polarity difference between electrodes is needed, in which case only the treatment electrode with the desired polarity should be placed in the water, with the other (larger) electrode acting as a dispersive electrode placed at a convenient, remote (i.e. away from the target) site.

Electrode Size, Shape, and Configuration

Electrode size, shape, and configuration (number, location and orientation) are important to focus the effect at a target area. Small electrodes should be used for small areas (e.g. hand muscles, etc.) and large electrodes for large areas (e.g. large muscle groups, etc.) (Fig. 4.20A,B). If the area is larger than both electrodes, two channels each with two electrodes can be used to maximize muscle coverage, e.g. for quadriceps femoris contraction (see Fig. 4.20C). There are separate amplitude controls for each channel. When two electrodes of equal size and shape from one channel are placed over the same target area, it is called a bipolar placement (see Fig. 4.20A,B), and both are considered treatment electrodes.

Charge density is the amount of charge per unit area. Thus, if the surface area of an electrode is small, the charge delivered at that electrode will be spread over a smaller area, increasing the charge density. If the target area is small and both electrodes will not fit within its boundaries without causing overflow to adjacent unwanted areas, a small

electrode can be placed over the target area and a larger one at a remote area. Unequal electrode size will produce a greater effect for the same amount of charge at the smaller electrode due to its higher charge density; although there may still be a response at the larger electrode. Unequal electrode size is also used when a difference in electrode polarity is required: a smaller treatment electrode is applied over the target area and a larger electrode is applied at a remote area. Care should be taken when increasing current amplitude in this case as stimulation could become uncomfortable with high amounts of charge at the small electrode (Alon 1994; Lyons 2004). There are also electrodes with very small surface areas, called 'point stimulators' (Fig. 4.21), typically used to find motor points of an innervated muscle or the most easily stimulated part of a muscle that has been denervated; or for noxious-level stimulation for pain control. When two electrodes of unequal size are used in the above ways, it is called a monopolar electrode placement (Fig. 4.22). Two electrodes of the same shape and size may also be placed on different areas to affect those different areas (e.g. one on the low back and one on the calf), and this would also be a monopolar set-up.

Innervated muscles are often stimulated via their supplying nerve by placing the electrode(s) over the motor point(s) (Gobbo 2011). The motor point is the area of a muscle where its subserving nerve stimulates the most motor units. The nerve has least resistance at this point and will require

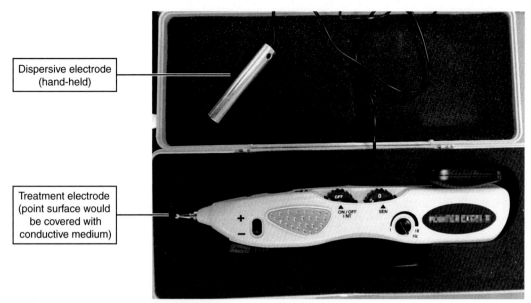

Dispersive electrode (hand-held)

Treatment electrode (point surface would be covered with conductive medium)

Fig. 4.21 Point Stimulator Electrode

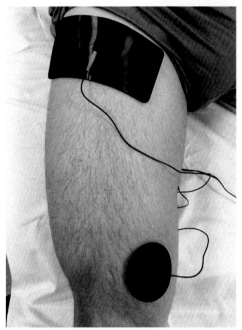

Fig. 4.22 Monopolar electrode placement, with a smaller electrode at the target site and the dispersive electrode remote to the target area.

less current amplitude to stimulate. With denervated muscle, there is no motor point. The location of least resistance can be determined by moving the treatment electrode (cathode) to search for the site that yields the greatest response for a given level of amplitude. However, studies have been successful in improving muscle and skin characteristics using two large electrodes over the denervated quadriceps femoris muscle when using symmetrical biphasic PC with long pulse durations (Albertin 2018; Modlin 2005).

Other aspects of electrode configuration to consider are electrode spacing and orientation. The closer together that electrodes of the same channel are placed, the more superficial the current. If they are placed too close together (e.g. closer than about 2 cm), the current density could be increased in the superficial tissues between the electrodes, causing skin burns. For deeper targets, such as deeper muscles, the electrodes should be placed further apart using care that unwanted muscles, e.g. antagonists, are not being activated. Electrodes can be placed on targets that are separated by a considerable distance (e.g. on the low back and lower limb). The greatest effect of stimulation is directly under or near the electrodes.

Electrode configuration or orientation also refers to the placement of the electrodes relative to the target area. Apart from following the principles that have already been presented, 'treatment' electrode(s) should usually be placed over areas that are anatomically, neurophysiologically or biologically related to the area to be treated (e.g. injured tissues, areas of symptom referral, etc.) (Dean 2006; Selkowitz 1999) (see Chapters 3 and 15). Additionally, with stimulation of large muscles where the electrode size might not provide complete muscle coverage, arranging the electrodes (such that the current will travel) along a line that is parallel to the course of the muscle fibres (see Fig. 4.20B,C) will produce contraction force most efficiently (Barnett 1991; Brooks 1990; Ferguson 1989). With acute-stage oedema control, a monopolar set-up with the (smaller) cathode

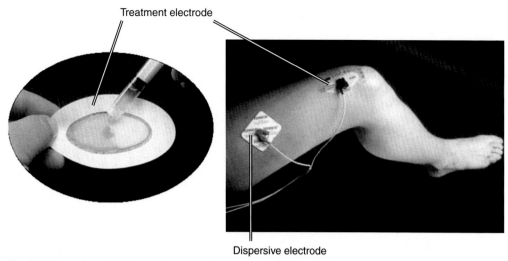

Treatment electrode

Dispersive electrode

Fig. 4.23 Iontophoresis 2-electrode set-up: the treatment ('delivery') electrode with the pad to which the water-soluble, liquid chemical compound is applied (using a needle-less syringe), and the dispersive (or non-treatment) electrode.

placed over the site of injury is most appropriate, with the dispersive electrode placed over a remote, convenient site. Electrode placements for TENS, wound healing and NMES will be discussed in the relevant chapters.

With iontophoresis, the chemical compound containing the therapeutic ion is applied to the smaller of a pair of electrodes, i.e. the 'treatment' or 'delivery' electrode, which is then placed over the target site (for example, the base of the thumb over tendons of abductor pollicis longus and extensor pollicis brevis to treat De Quervain's disease). The treatment electrode is set to the same polarity as the therapeutic ions in order to drive them into the tissues (recall that like charges repel). For example, under the influence of the current, the compound dexamethasone disodium phosphate dissociates into the anti-inflammatory agent dexamethasone phosphate (a corticosteroid), which is negatively charged. In the example given, the cathode would deliver the drug. The treatment electrode may have a reservoir or pad to which the chemical compound is applied (Fig. 4.23). The larger dispersive (or 'non-treatment') electrode should be placed over a remote, convenient site. Unfortunately, some manufacturers make the dedicated pair of iontophoresis electrodes of equal size. There are also single-use disposable electrodes/patches consisting of adjacent but distinct negative and positive polarity conductive surfaces (one of which would be the 'treatment electrode'), with a small battery to deliver the current.

Skin and Tissue Conductivity

Conductivity of tissues influences the ability to deliver the current. Bone, skin and fat are poor conductors, while nerves, muscles and water are good conductors. Thus, greater charge will be required to stimulate nerves where there is thicker skin or more overlying adipose tissue (Medeiros 2015; Petrofsky 2008). For example, in obese clients, it might not be possible to achieve the desired magnitude of muscle contraction.

Adequate skin preparation will assist in lowering the skin's resistance to the electrical current. Procedures for safe treatment and improving current penetration are discussed in Chapter 22.

TIME-MODULATED MEDIUM FREQUENCY CURRENTS

Timing modulations are applied most frequently to medium frequency AC to produce burst-modulated medium frequency AC, which is typically referred to as 'Russian' current (RC), and beat-modulated medium frequency AC, which is commonly known as interferential current or IFC. These currents are sometimes referred to as polyphasic currents. In this chapter, the terms RC and IFC will be used. Timing modulations as applied to AC are methods of modifying AC into forms that allow it to more closely mimic biphasic symmetrical PC's effects on nerve stimulation and make it easier and less restrictive for therapeutic use than unmodulated AC. Key considerations to be discussed with these currents include carrier frequency, burst frequency (with RC) and beat frequency (with IFC), cycle duration, burst duration, and duty cycle (with RC) and how each of these impacts the nerve response.

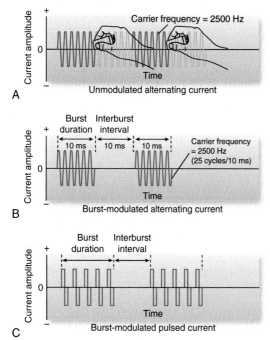

Fig. 4.24 Burst-modulated medium frequency AC (figures not drawn to scale). (A) The original unmodulated 2500-Hz AC becomes interrupted to produce a burst-modulated current. (B) The original burst-modulated 2500-Hz Russian current: burst frequency = 50 bursts/s, duty cycle = 50%, yielding a burst duration of 10 ms and an interburst interval of 10 ms. The frequency within each burst is the same as the original carrier frequency, i.e. 2500-Hz, just with a few cycles for the shorter period of time; e.g. a frequency within the burst of 25 cycles/10 ms = 2500 cycles/1000 ms (or 1 s). Cycle duration can be calculated: d = 1/f = 1/2500 = 0.0004 s = 0.4 ms (or 400 μs). Therefore, in a 10-ms burst duration there are 10/0.4 ms = 25 cycles. (C) Burst-modulated biphasic PC. This example shows a series of five pulses in each burst.

Russian Current

The development of RC has been attributed to Yakov Kots, a researcher from the Soviet Union, in the 1970s (Babkin 1977; Ward 2002). The derivation of RC is illustrated in Fig 4.24A,B. The underlying current is AC, typically with a sinusoidal waveform. The carrier frequency is the underlying uninterrupted AC frequency, which for RC is fixed, commonly at 2500 Hz. Recent devices may offer a range of settings for carrier frequency between 1000–5000 Hz. Australian authors tested a range of carrier frequencies and recommended using a carrier frequency of 1000 Hz, naming this variation of RC 'Aussie' current.

The continuous AC cycles are modulated into bursts by interrupting the current; it is as if some of the cycles were

erased in a recurring pattern during the period of the current delivery. The burst frequency describes the number of bursts per second. The rate of cycles *within* each burst is not changed by interrupting the current, i.e. it is the same as that of the underlying AC carrier frequency. The original RC is a 2500-Hz carrier frequency interrupted such that there is a burst frequency of 50 bursts/second, with each burst duration lasting 10 ms followed by a 10-ms *interburst interval* (see Fig. 4.24).

One important question regarding the response of nerves to the parameters of medium frequency currents is, how do carrier frequency and burst frequency impact the neurophysiological responses? Nerves will respond to the burst frequency of RC in the same manner as to the pulse frequency of PC; i.e. current delivered at both 50 bursts/second and 50 pps will initiate 50 APs per second. A carrier frequency of 2500 Hz will not trigger 2500 APs per second because some of the current cycles would be delivered during the absolute refractory period (and some during the relative refractory period) of stimulated nerves. Thus, with RC, *the firing pattern of nerves reflects the burst frequency* not the carrier frequency of the current (Selkowitz 1999, 2009). Under certain conditions, the nerves may fire in a harmonic, multiple pattern, such as 2–3 times that of the burst frequency (e.g. 2 x 50 bursts/s or 100 APs/second), but this is still not nearly the rate of the carrier frequency. Further explanation for nerve responses to medium frequency currents can be found in the appendix to this chapter.

Burst duration in RC, comprising the summed duration of all the cycles in a burst, is dependent on the burst frequency and the duty cycle. There is no control with which to set burst duration on devices; however, there are controls to set burst frequency and duty cycle. With RC, duty cycle refers to the relationship between burst duration and interburst interval (see Box 4.2 for calculations).

If burst frequency and duty cycle settings are known, the burst duration can be calculated. Knowing this duration is not necessary for treatment set-up; however, it may enhance understanding of how the duty cycle setting affects the stimulation of APs and neuromuscular responses.

Duty cycle settings typically range between 10% and 50% in increments of 10% (Fig 4.25). Studies in uninjured humans have shown that for RC with a 2500-Hz carrier frequency and a burst frequency of 50 burst/second, 10–20% duty cycles were more efficient at force production than higher percent duty cycles (Liebano 2013; McLoda 2000; Moreno-Aranda 1981a; Parker 2011; Selkowitz 1999; Ward 2004).

There is no direct setting on devices for cycle duration of the AC carrier current because of the inverse relationship between frequency and duration with AC. When

BOX 4.2   Determination of duty cycle, burst duration and interburst interval for a current with a frequency of 50 bursts/s:

Each burst is paired with an interburst interval; thus, there are 50 pairs of bursts and interburst intervals in 1 second (i.e. 1000 ms), and the total time for each pair is 1000/50 = 20 ms. The specific time periods for the separate burst and interburst interval are then determined by the duty cycle.

Determination of duty cycle:
Example for a current delivered with 10-ms burst duration and 10-ms interburst interval:
  Duty cycle = [burst duration/(burst duration + interburst interval)] × 100
  Duty cycle = [10/(10 + 10)] × 100 = [10/20] × 100 = 50%

Determination of burst duration and interburst interval:
Example: If a 10% duty cycle had been selected, then of the total 20 ms, 10% of that would be burst duration, i.e., 20 ms × .10 = 2 ms, and interburst interval would be 20 − 2 ms = 18 ms.

carrier frequency is known, cycle duration can be calculated (see Box 4.1). It is noteworthy that the inverse relationship between cycle frequency and duration ensures that the typical therapeutic medium frequency currents (i.e. 1000–5000 Hz) produce cycle durations of 200–1000 μs (including RC at 2500 Hz producing a 400-μs cycle duration), which are within the recommended range for motor-level stimulation.

Given that RC includes two types of durations, another important question is, how do burst and cycle durations impact nerve responses? Nerves will respond to the cycle duration of an AC carrier current in the same manner as to the pulse duration setting of a PC; i.e. both a cycle duration of 400 μs (from a 2500-Hz AC) and a pulse duration of 400 μs (from a PC) will produce the same amount of charge and cause the same number of nerve fibres to be activated, thus producing the same type and magnitude of neurophysiologic response. In terms of producing a motor-level response, a lower carrier frequency (e.g. 1000 Hz versus 5000 Hz) would be more appropriate because it would produce a longer cycle duration and would, therefore, require less amplitude to produce a given amount of force (Gregory 2007; Medeiros 2017; Moreno-Aranda 1981b; Parker 2005; Scott 2009; Selkowitz 2009; Ward 2004).

RC burst durations consist of multiple, short, medium frequency AC cycles, such as the original RC's 10-ms burst durations containing 400-μs cycles. Some of these cycles occur during the absolute refractory period and some during the relative refractory period of the nerves; thus, the nerves do not respond to all the cycles in a burst. Therefore, it can be stated that the nerves do not respond to the burst duration.

Further explanation for nerve responses to medium frequency currents can be found in the appendix to this chapter.

Interferential Current (IFC)

IFC The derivation of IFC is depicted by the diagram in Fig. 4.26. IFC, as with RC, includes a carrier frequency which is the underlying continuous, uninterrupted AC frequency. The continuous AC is modulated into beats by 'interfering' two medium frequency ACs with each other. True IFC is characterized by using two channels on a device, each delivering AC with a different medium frequency (offset from each other typically by up to 200 Hz), with the electrodes from the two channels set in a crossing pattern (Fig. 4.27). The result is a combination of the two carrier frequencies to produce a beat frequency, the value of which is the difference between the two carrier frequency values (see Fig. 4.26).

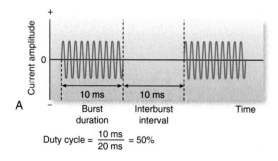

Duty cycle = $\dfrac{10\ ms}{20\ ms}$ = 50%

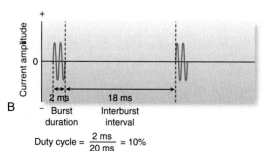

Duty cycle = $\dfrac{2\ ms}{20\ ms}$ = 10%

Fig. 4.25 Illustration of duty cycles used with Russian current. A lower duty cycle means there is a shorter burst duration.

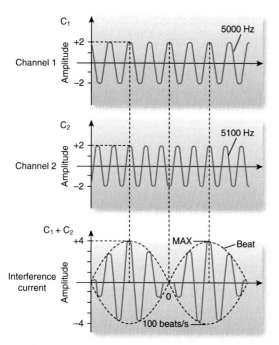

Fig. 4.26 **Interferential Current** Beat frequency derivation from the two carrier frequencies. When the carrier frequency on channel 1 interferes (i.e. overlaps in the tissues) with that of channel 2, the resulting beat frequency is the subtraction of the two carrier frequencies: 5100 Hz – 5000 Hz = 100 beats/s (see bottom graph). Note, the amplitude of the interference current (bottom graph) is more than the current amplitudes of either contributing channel (up to the sum of the two amplitudes). (Adapted from May H-U, Hansjürgens A. Nemectrodyn Model 7 Manual of Nemectron GmbH, Daimlerstr.15, Karlsruhe, Germany, 1984.)

Where the electrical fields of the two carrier frequencies overlap, their cycles overlap at these offset frequencies such that some cycles are completely out of phase and cancel each other's amplitudes resulting in zero current for that moment; some are completely in phase such that they are completely superimposed, and the amplitude of the combined cycles is the sum of the two amplitudes; and some are partially overlapped (or partially cancelled) resulting in amplitudes somewhere between zero and the fully superimposed, summed value. The beat duration is the time from one zero-amplitude point to the next (see Fig. 4.26).

When charge is adequate, APs will be triggered. This may occur only when cycles are fully superimposed (i.e. at the highest amplitude), or at the lower amplitudes of partially superimposed cycles if there is enough charge,

or summation occurs. The amplitude that is ultimately delivered to the tissues is greater than the setting of either channel alone, so, in that sense, it is more efficient. For example, if each channel's amplitude is set to 10 mA, the tissues in the area where the two channel fields intersect and are fully superimposed may receive up to 20 mA. Thus, less amplitude may be required on each channel to achieve a desired magnitude of neurophysiological response. IFC is considered an amplitude modulated current, but not in the sense as presented earlier where amplitude modulation is used to counteract adaptation to ES.

With IFC we have similar questions regarding frequency and duration as with RC: How do IFC beat frequency and beat duration impact nerve response? The nerves respond to the beat frequency of IFC in the same manner as to the pulse frequency of PC; i.e. both a beat frequency of 50 beats/second and a pulse frequency of 50 pps will produce 50 APs/second. An IFC carrier frequency of 2500 Hz will not cause a nerve to fire 2500 times a second. Thus, the nerves respond to the beat frequency, not the carrier frequency, with respect to firing pattern; in practice, if 100 stimuli/second are desired, then one should set 100 beats/second.

To determine the impact of the two duration parameters in IFC on nerve response – the cycle duration of the underlying medium frequency AC and the beat duration – it is important to remember that frequency and duration of AC cycles are inversely related. With IFC, two channels are applied with slightly different carrier frequencies. If the carrier frequency of the fixed channel is 5000 Hz and the other channel is 5100 Hz, the resultant carrier frequency of the combined channels is 5050 Hz. One could reasonably (for ease of calculation) consider duration of the individual cycles to be about 200 µs (i.e. 1/5000 Hz = 0.2 ms/cycle), based on the fixed carrier frequency. With a beat frequency of 200 beats/second, the beat duration would be 5 ms (1/200 = 5.0 ms/beat) (even longer with a lower beat frequency); so, as with RC, the nerves will not respond to the beat duration or all of the carrier frequency cycles within a beat due to the absolute and relative refractory periods. Thus, nerves respond to the cycle duration (of the carrier frequency) of IFC in the same manner as to the pulse duration of a PC. The cycle duration needed for a given purpose will determine the choice of AC carrier frequency, which is the inverse of the duration. There is no setting on a device for cycle duration, only carrier frequency. Further explanation for nerve responses to medium frequency currents can be found in the appendix to this chapter.

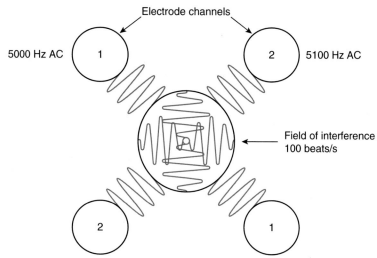

Fig. 4.27 Classic illustration of electrical field interference pattern and location. Note that this is an idealized geometric illustration that does not represent the actual distribution of the individual and interference fields due to various factors including homogeneity of tissues in a given region.

In practice, a device may have choices for the fixed carrier frequency delivered on one channel; otherwise, it will be pre-set by the manufacturer (usually at 4000 Hz). The carrier frequency on the second channel is usually automatically adjusted in the device depending on the beat frequency selected by the therapist. Thus, if the fixed carrier frequency on channel one is 5000 Hz and the clinician set a beat frequency of 100 beats/s, the device will deliver a carrier frequency of 5100 Hz on the second channel (see Fig. 4.26). If a device provides options for the fixed carrier frequency, the type and magnitude of the desired response (sensory versus motor) should determine the appropriate choice.

Applying the electrodes of the two channels in a crossing pattern causes their electrical current fields to overlap which, because of the difference between the two carrier frequencies, results in amplitude modulation where the carrier frequencies interfere with each other. This is commonly represented by the pattern in Fig. 4.27. However, the electrical fields, their points of intersection, and the patient's perception of the stimulation are not predictable. Fig. 4.27 assumes that in the area under the electrodes and within the IFC field, the volume, orientation and types of tissues (including nerve fibres, muscle, tendon, etc) are all perfectly symmetrical and/or homogenous. In reality, the electrical fields may overlap anywhere within the area circumscribed by the electrodes and possibly some distance beyond. Typically, the most pronounced effect and the one perceived by the patient is immediately under the electrodes.

In order to more 'evenly' affect the tissues within the treatment area, IFC technology provides an option commonly called 'scan' (labels may vary by manufacturer), which redistributes the area of 100% amplitude summation. Scan alters the amplitude on one channel relative to the other. Amplitude is typically set simultaneously on the two channels to levels that produce the required response from the patient. When the electrical stimulation is set to scan, amplitude on one channel automatically decreases from, then returns to, the set level, typically over a few seconds, while amplitude on the second channel remains the same; then, the process switches with the second channel sequentially decreasing and increasing. This continuously changing offset in amplitude has the effect on the electric field of moving the direction of the 100% amplitude summation around so that nerves in different parts of the area circumscribed by the electrodes are maximally stimulated at different times. In fact, it has the effect of favouring the path created by the electrodes of one channel, then the other, so the patient should be able to discern which electrodes are being preferentially stimulated (Fig. 4.28). Devices typically 'scan' by decreasing the set amplitude by 40% or 100%. For example, if the amplitude is initially set to 10 mA on both channels, at the 40% setting one channel decreases to 6 mA while the other remains at 10 mA. At the 100% setting, channels in turn decrease to 0 mA. This would have the effect of completely abolishing the stimulation along one channel so that it would

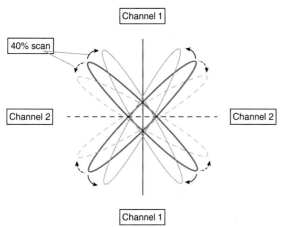

Fig. 4.28 'Scan' amplitude modulation illustration. The black solid and dashed straight lines represent the electrical field directions for channels 1 and 2, respectively. The dark green ovals are the theoretical interference field based on equal, unchanging amplitudes on both channels. If the amplitude were 'scanned' 40%, the electrical field direction would always favour (i.e., rotate towards) the channel with the higher amplitude and rotate away from the channel reduced to 40% of the set amplitude, then would switch to favour the second channel as its input increased to 100% of the set amplitude, as represented by the solid and dashed light green ovals, respectively. The short black arched solid and dashed arrow lines show the changing orientation of the field towards the respective channels in all quadrants. (Adapted from Kloth LC: Interference current (1991). In Nelson RM, Currier DP (eds): *Clinical Electrotherapy*, 2nd ed. Norwalk, CT: Appleton & Lange.)

momentarily receive no stimulation; which would also have the effect of abolishing the interference effect and delivering unmodulated AC at the carrier frequency of the active channel. Thus, a 100% scan setting may be less productive.

The premise of 'scan' – for example, with sensory-level pain control – is that if the area is large and/or the symptoms are vague or generalized, the stimulation will engage different areas. However, it is not clear that this is more beneficial than keeping the field in one place. Some present-day devices allow the amplitudes on each channel to be set at different levels but kept constant at those levels. Thus, the field of stimulation would favour the area closer to the channel with the higher amplitude for the duration of the treatment session. Ultimately, there is no evidence that any of these methods of altering the IFC field improves treatment effectiveness.

'Scan' might have an additional effect of limiting adaptation because it modulates the amplitude, but limiting

adaptation is not the main purpose of scan. Most IFC devices allow one to modulate the beat frequency to limit adaptation. This is called 'sweep' based on the original term used when IFC was created. 'Sweep' is a synonym for beat frequency modulation, but it complicates the electrical stimulation 'dictionary', which is further confounded by the use of 'sweep' by some manufacturers with other types of current on multimodal devices. Sweep on most IFC devices permits specific upper and lower bounds of beat frequencies to be set, e.g. burst frequency modulation of 10–150 bursts/second.

There is also a type of current called premodulated IFC (often referred to as 'premod' or bipolar). This is similar to 'true' IFC in that it comprises an amplitude modulated waveform similar to the beat of IFC, but it is engineered 'within the device' rather than created by the currents of two channels interfering in the tissues. In fact, only one channel (two electrodes) is used with 'premod', making it similar in practice to a symmetrical biphasic PC. Thus, there is no interference and no additive effect of current amplitude from using two channels with different frequencies of AC, as with 'true IFC'. The convention of referring to it as a form of IFC is, therefore, misrepresentative and may be confusing.

IFC is typically marketed and most often used clinically for sensory-level pain control. However, both IFC and 'premod' can be used for the same treatment purposes as biphasic PC and RC; this includes the production of muscle force that would be appropriate for strengthening (Bellew 2012, 2014), although it has not been specifically tested in strength-training studies.

It should be noted that one may place electrodes from two different channels in a crossing pattern when using biphasic PC or RC. However, because the frequencies delivered are identical the frequencies do not interfere and there is no amplitude modulation, so it would not be true IFC. Rather, the two identical frequencies are delivered as they normally would be to the areas where the two fields overlap.

Burst Modulated Pulsed Currents

Pulsed currents can be modified to deliver a burst of pulses (see Fig. 4.24C). This may be seen in TENS devices (called 'burst mode') delivered at fixed, low burst frequencies (e.g. 2–5 burst/second), or in multimodal devices with greater flexibility of range. The pulses within the burst are very close together, with interpulse intervals that may be only 0.1 ms. With such short interpulse intervals, successive pulses will fall within the absolute

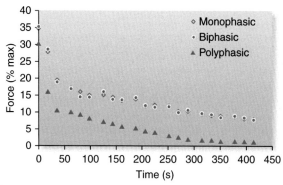

Fig. 4.29 Fatigue (decrease in force over multiple contractions) was shown to be greater with Russian current (polyphasic) than biphasic PC and monophasic PC. (From Laufer et al 2001.)

refractory period of the nerves. Therefore, as with RC and IFC, the nerves are not likely to be responding to all of the pulses within the burst, so the nerves would not be responding to the pulse frequency within the burst (i.e. the PC carrier frequency) or to the entire burst duration. Instead, the nerves are likely responding to the burst frequency and the pulse duration of the PC carrier current. Burst-modulated PC can be appropriately used for the same treatment purposes as biphasic PC, RC, IFC and 'premod'.

Muscular fatigue effects on force output have been found to vary among different types of therapeutic currents. Laufer et al (2001) found that polyphasic currents (i.e. RC) fatigue more readily than pulsed currents (Fig. 4.29). This may be due to the effects of the characteristic multiple cycles within the bursts of AC, including the potential occurrence of harmonic frequencies that increase the effective frequency of the burst. Although burst-modulated PC can also be considered polyphasic, it typically uses shorter burst durations than RC and, therefore, has fewer pulses within a burst.

It should also be noted that studies have reported greater force output using burst-modulated PC, IFC, and symmetrical biphasic PC when compared with RC (Adams 2018; Bellew 2012, 2014, 2018; Laufer et al 2001; Ward et al 2006). However, this can be attributed either to the larger pulse or cycle durations, lower duty cycles (burst or pulse frequencies relative to interburst or interpulse intervals), or the rectangular waveforms used in the non-RC current types. In contrast, a systematic review of studies comparing symmetrical biphasic PC to RC performed a meta-analysis demonstrating that there was no significant difference between these two current types for torque produced or for self-reported discomfort (da Silva 2015). However, there were also confounding factors in the studies surveyed in this review, including differences between some studies in sex of subjects, electrode size and burst duty cycle, and between studies and groups within studies, in burst versus pulse frequency and phase duration. In addition, no studies reported having matched subjects based on body composition (e.g. percent body fat), or having controlled for the effects of menstrual cycle (da Silva 2015). Sex of subjects can confound torque and tolerance results because some studies have reported that males produce more torque and tolerate more phase charge than females (Alon 2005; Kramer 1987; Laufer 2001); however, it has also been reported that there is no difference between the sexes when the stimulated torque is expressed in percent of maximum voluntary isometric torque (Kramer 1987). In addition, some subjects have been reported to reach the maximum output of the device before reaching maximum patient tolerance (Kramer 1987). Subject tolerance may also depend on magnitude of torque produced, which may be the result of differences in parameters. Possible evidence of this is from a study that found only 13 of 32 subjects produced their greatest torque with their preferred (most comfortable) waveform (Adams 2018). Thus, studies comparing parameters between groups of subjects on torque produced or tolerance to stimulation are vulnerable to differences in characteristics of the subjects as well as those of the parameter settings.

SUMMARY

This chapter began with the terminology and basic elements of electricity and neurophysiology necessary to understand electrical stimulation. Next, the essential ES parameters were described – including current type (DC, AC and variations of PC), amplitude, duration, frequency, on/off times, including duty cycle, ramp-up and ramp-down times, modulation (of current amplitude, frequency and duration, alone or in combination), electrode characteristics (type, conductive media, size, placement, polarity) and treatment time. Manipulating these parameters produces sensory-level, motor-level and noxious-level stimulation and their associated neurophysiological responses (sensation, contraction and nociception), as well as other biological responses (e.g. galvanotaxis, iontophoresis). The key parameters determining the type and magnitude of responses are the amount of charge (i.e. current amplitude and duration), electrode characteristics, such as size and location/configuration, and proximity of nerve fibres to the electrodes. Frequency affects the pattern of response and as such, the type of contraction; and can augment force output but also fatigue. On/off cycling is used to moderate fatigue, and ramps up and down assist patient comfort. Both on/off cycling and ramps are necessary with tetanic contractions, not with sub-tetanic contractions or sensory-level stimulation. In addition, time modulations of medium frequency AC, creating RC and IFC, were discussed, along with the neurophysiological theory to explain how they work. With time-modulated medium frequency currents, nerves essentially respond to the cycle duration of the carrier current (not the burst or beat duration) and the frequency of the burst (not the carrier frequency).

The treatment purpose will determine what neurophysiological response is required, which, in turn, will inform the selection of appropriate parameter settings. Then, one must evaluate the available electrical stimulation devices to determine, based on the range of parameter settings available on each device, which device(s) can be appropriately used for a given treatment purpose. Similarly, given a specific device, one should be able to determine the treatment purpose(s) for which that device may be appropriately used.

APPENDIX

Factors Underlying Nerve Response to Time-Modulated Medium Frequency Currents

As stated previously, with RC, nerves respond to the frequency of the burst and the duration of cycles within the burst (i.e. cycle duration of the carrier frequency).

As a reminder, an AP lasts approximately 1 ms, and this period is known as the absolute refractory period.

Traditional RC, with a frequency of 2500 Hz, delivers bursts of cycles whereby each cycle has a duration of 0.4 ms (400 μs). Thus, three cycles within the burst will be initiated during the absolute refractory period of the stimulated nerve. If the first cycle was of sufficient charge to generate an AP, the next two will not cause an AP because they will occur during the *absolute* refractory period. Only the ensuing cycles that fall within the *relative* refractory period have a chance to initiate an AP, if their charge is sufficient to reach the elevated depolarization threshold (Fig. 4.30). Therefore, a frequency of 2500 Hz cannot create 2500 APs per second (e.g. 2500 'tingles' per second with sensory-level stimulation). This has been referred to as stimulus-asynchronous depolarization (Kloth 1991). This is the case for any medium frequency current, whether or not it is burst-modulated. With RC at 50 bursts/second, at least one cycle with adequate charge within each of the 50 bursts will generate an AP, i.e. 50 APs/second.

However, it is possible that during the relative refractory period, with high enough amplitude, or with summation of charges, additional APs would be generated. Thus, each burst could initiate multiple APs, increasing the effective firing rate to more than 50 APs/second. For example, with a burst frequency of 50 bursts/second, if two APs were generated during each burst, the nerve would respond 100 times a second and with three APs per burst, 150 times per second. A multiple of the originally set burst frequency is considered a harmonic frequency, (i.e. the burst frequency setting multiplied by the number of APs generated during the burst). The number of APs that are generated within a burst is also determined by the burst duration. The longer the burst duration (i.e. with higher duty cycles), the more likely that a harmonic of the burst frequency will be produced (see Fig. 4.30). However, this can be counterproductive because higher effective frequencies (i.e. above 50–80

Fig. 4.30 The absolute and relative refractory periods of an action potential (AP) showing the elevated depolarization threshold during the latter period. Comparison between medium frequency burst modulated AC and biphasic PC with different duty cycles; with reference to refractory periods and AP generation. (A) "Russian" current (2500-Hz carrier frequency, 50 bursts/s, 50% duty cycle). The AP is overlaid with a 10-ms burst of AC with 25 cycles in each 10-ms burst, three of which would occur during the absolute refractory period, with one of those producing an AP. One (or more) of the next 22 cycles could produce another AP if they were of sufficient charge to reach the elevated depolarization threshold during the relative refractory period. This would create an increased effective frequency, a harmonic of the burst frequency setting. This illustrates the multiple, ineffective cycles that are delivered with medium frequency burst-modulated AC. (B) Current as in (A) with 10% duty cycle which would produce five cycles in each 2-ms burst, three of which would occur during the absolute refractory period, and two during the relative refractory period. This would make it highly unlikely that another cycle in the burst would stimulate an AP; so there would be no harmonic frequency, although the multiple cycles could still contribute to fatigue. (C) Biphasic PC (50 pps, 0.4-ms pulse duration, 19.6-ms interpulse interval, i.e. 2% duty cycle), which would deliver a single pulse and generate only one AP. As such, it is less fatiguing than burst-modulated medium frequency AC.

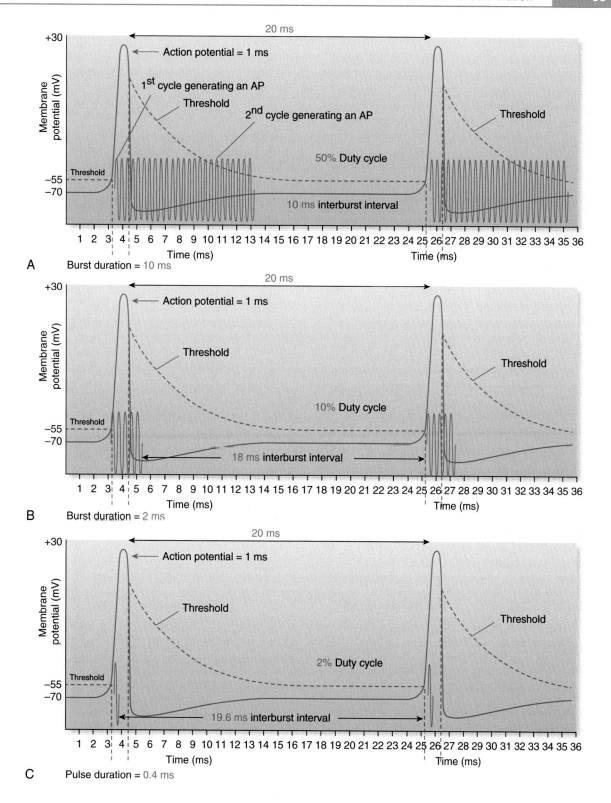

APs/second) can increase fatigue with little if any increase in force output.

Although more research is needed, this might explain why some studies (previously noted in the chapter) found that the original RC with its 50% duty cycle produced less force and greater fatigue than RC with shorter burst durations (e.g. 10% duty cycles), or than non-burst symmetrical biphasic PCs at equivalent amplitudes, pulse frequencies and pulse durations (see Fig. 4.30). Further, any number of multiple ineffective stimuli delivered during the nerves' refractory periods, as occurs with RC, would likely create more fatigue than non-burst symmetrical biphasic PC, which does not deliver successive stimuli during refractory periods and has lower duty cycles than RC. In addition, Bowman and McNeal (1986) found that there is a progressive decrease in firing rate of nerves leading to complete conduction block with unmodulated AC medium frequencies (and frequencies between 100–1000 Hz), which occurs faster as frequency increases. Ward and Robertson (2001) found evidence of this same phenomenon with RC. Thus, higher frequencies, including those leading to successive stimuli during refractory periods, appear to produce greater fatigue. This may be due to presynaptic failure and decreased sensitivity of the postsynaptic membrane, and/or decreased neurotransmitter release (Brown 1949; Krnjevic 1958).

REFERENCES

Adams, C., Scott, W., Basile, J., et al. (2018). Electrically elicited quadriceps muscle torque: A comparison of 3 waveforms. *The Journal of Orthopaedic and Sports Physical Therapy*, 48(3), 217–224.

Albertin, G., Kern, H., Hofer, C., et al. (2018). Two years of functional electrical stimulation by large surface electrodes for denervated muscles improve skin epidermis in SCI. *European Journal of Translational Myology*, 28(1), 7373.

Allen, J. D., Mattacola, C. G., & Perrin, D. H. (1999). Effect of microcurrent stimulation on delayed-onset muscle soreness: A double-blind comparison. *Journal of Athletic Training*, 34(4), 334–337.

Alon, G. (1991). Principles of electrical stimulation. In R. M. Nelson & D. P. Currier (Eds.), *Clinical electrotherapy* (2nd ed.). Norwalk, CT: Appleton & Lange.

Alon, G., Allin, J., & Inbar, G. F. (1983). Optimization of pulse duration and pulse charge during transcutaneous electrical nerve stimulation. *The Australian Journal of Physiotherapy*, 29(6), 195–201.

Alon, G., Kantor, G., & Ho, H. S. (1994). Effects of electrode size on basic excitatory responses and on selected stimulus parameters. *The Journal of Orthopaedic and Sports Physical Therapy*, 20(1), 29–35.

Alon, G., & Smith, G. V. (2005). Tolerance and conditioning to neuro-muscular electrical stimulation within and between sessions and gender. *Journal of Sports Science & Medicine*, 4(4), 395–405.

Atya, A. M. (2002). Efficacy of microcurrent electrical stimulation on pain, proprioception accuracy and functional disability in subacromial impingement: RCT. *Indian Journal of Physiotherapy & Occupational Therapy*, 6(1), 15–18.

Babkin, D., & Timtsenko, N. (1977). *Electrostimulation: Notes from Dr. YM Kots' (USSR) lectures and laboratory periods. Canadian-Soviet Exchange Symposium on Electrostimulation of Skeletal Muscles*. Montreal, Quebec, Canada: Concordia University. December 6-15.

Baker, L. L., Wederich, C. L., McNeal, D. R., Newsam, C. J., & Waters, R. L. (2000). *Neuromuscular electrical stimulation – a practical guide* (4th ed.). Downey, CA: Los Amigos Research and Educational Institute.

Barnett, S., Cooney, K., & Johnston, R. (1991). Electrically elicited quadriceps femoris muscle torque as a function of various electrode placements. *Journal Clinical Electrophysiology*, 3, 5–8.

Basmajian, J. V., & De Luca, C. J. (1985). *Muscles alive* (5th ed.). Baltimore: Williams & Wilkins.

Bellew, J. W., Allen, M., Biefnes, A., Grantham, S., Miglin, J., & Swartzell, D. (2018). Efficiency of neuromuscular electrical stimulation: A comparison of elicited force and subject tolerance using three electrical waveforms. *Physiotherapy Theory and Practice*, 34(7), 551–558.

Bellew, J. W., Beiswanger, Z., Freeman, E., Gaerte, C., & Trafton, J. (2012). Interferential and burst-modulated biphasic pulsed currents yield greater muscular force than Russian current. *Physiotherapy Theory and Practice*, 28(5), 384–390.

Bellew, J. W., Sanders, K., Schuman, K., & Barton, M. (2014). Muscle force production with low and medium frequency burst modulated biphasic pulsed currents. *Physiotherapy Theory and Practice*, 30(2), 105–109.

Bettany, J. A., Fish, D. R., & Mendel, F. C. (1990). Influence of cathodal high voltage pulsed current on acute edema. *Journal Clinical Electrophysiology*, 2, 5–8.

Bickel, C. S., Gregory, C. M., & Dean, J. C. (2011). Motor unit recruitment during neuromuscular electrical stimulation: A critical appraisal. *European Journal of Applied Physiology*, 111, 2399–2407.

Bigland-Ritchie, B., Jones, D. A., & Woods, J. J. (1979). Excitation frequency and muscle fatigue: Electrical responses during human voluntary and stimulated contractions. *Experimental Neurology*, 64, 414–427.

Binder-MacLeod, S. A., & Guerin, T. (1990). Preservation of force output through progressive reduction of stimulation frequency in human quadriceps femoris muscle. *Physical Therapy*, 70, 619–625.

Binder-MacLeod, S. A., & McDermond, L. R. (1992). Changes in the force-frequency relationship of the human quadriceps femoris muscle following electrically and voluntarily induced fatigue. *Physical Therapy*, 72, 95–104.

Bonacci, J. A., & Higbie, E. J. (1997). Effects of microcurrent treatment on perceived pain and muscle strength following eccentric exercise. *Journal of Athletic Training*, 32(2), 119–123.

Boncompagni, S., Kern, H., Rossini, K., et al. (2007). Structural differentiation of skeletal muscle fibres in the absence of innervation in humans. *Proceedings of the National Academy of Sciences of the United States of America*, 104(49), 19339–19344.

Bowman, B. R., & McNeal, D. R. (1986). Response of single alpha motoneurons to high-frequency pulse trains. *Applied Neurophysiology, 49*, 121–138.

Brooks, M. E., Smith, E. M., & Currier, D. P. (1990). Effect of longitudinal versus transverse electrode placement on torque production by the quadriceps femoris muscle during neuromuscular electrical stimulation. *The Journal of Orthopaedic and Sports Physical Therapy, 11*, 530–534.

Brown, G. L., & Burns, B. D. (1949). Fatigue and neuromuscular block in mammalian skeletal muscle. *Proceedings of the Royal Society of London Biological Sciences, 136*(883), 182–195.

Brown, W. F., Kadrie, H. A., & Milner-Brown, H. S. (1981). Rank order of recruitment of motor units with graded electrical stimulation of median or ulnar nerves in normal subjects and in patients with entrapment neuropathies. In J. E. Desmedt (Ed.), *Motor unit types, recruitment and plasticity in health and disease: Progress in clinical neurophysiology*. Basel: Karger.

Cummings, J. (1991). Electrical stimulation of healthy muscle and tissue repair. In R. M. Nelson & D. P. Currier (Eds.), *Clinical electrotherapy* (2nd ed.). Norwalk, CT: Appleton & Lange.

Currier, D. P., & Mann, R. (1983). Muscular strength development by electrical stimulation in healthy individuals. *Physical Therapy, 63*, 915–921.

Curtis, D., Fallows, S., Morris, M., & McMakin, C. (2010). The efficacy of frequency specific microcurrent therapy on delayed onset muscle soreness. *Journal of Bodywork and Movement Therapies, 4*(3), 72–279.

da Silva, V. Z. M., Durigan, J. L., Arena, R., de Noronha, M., Gurney, B., & Cipriano, G., Jr. (2015). Current evidence demonstrates similar effects of kilohertz-frequency and low-frequency current on quadriceps evoked torque and discomfort in healthy individuals: A systematic review with meta-analysis. *Physiotherapy Theory and Practice, 31*(8), 533–539.

Dean, J., Bowsher, D., & Johnson, M. I. (2006). The effects of unilateral transcutaneous electrical nerve stimulation of the median nerve on bilateral somatosensory thresholds. *Clinical Physiology and Functional Imaging, 26*(5), 314–318.

Ferguson, J. P., Blackley, M. W., Knight, R. D., Sutlive, T. G., Underwood, F. B., & Greathouse, D. G. (1989). Effects of varying electrode site placements on the torque output of an electrically stimulated involuntary quadriceps femoris muscle contraction. *The Journal of Orthopaedic and Sports Physical Therapy, 11*, 24–29.

Fish, D. R., Mendel, F. C., Schultz, A. M., & Gottstein-Yerke, L. M. (1991). Effect of anodal high voltage pulsed current on edema formation in frog hind limbs. *Physical Therapy, 71*, 724–730.

Garnett, R., & Stephens, J. A. (1981). Changes in the recruitment threshold of motor units produced by cutaneous stimulation in man. *Journal of Physiology (Land), 311*, 463–473.

Ghez, C. (1991). Muscles: Effectors of the motor systems. In E. R. Kandel, J. H. Schwartz & T. M. Jessel (Eds.), *Principles of neural science* (3rd ed.). New York: Elsevier.

Gobbo, M., Gaffurini, P., Bissolotti, L., Esposito, F., & Orizio, C. (2011). Transcutaneous neuromuscular electrical stimulation: Influence of electrode positioning and stimulus amplitude settings on muscle response. *European Journal of Applied Physiology, 111*(10), 2451–2459.

Gorgey, A. S., Black, C. D., Elder, C. P., & Dudley, G. A. (2009). Effects of electrical stimulation parameters on fatigue in skeletal muscle. *The Journal of Orthopaedic and Sports Physical Therapy, 39*(9), 684–692.

Gossrau, G., Wahner, M., Kuschke, M., et al. (2011). Microcurrent transcutaneous electric nerve stimulation in painful diabetic neuropathy: A randomized placebo-controlled study. *Pain Medicine, 12*, 953–960.

Gregory, C. M., & Bickel, C. S. (2005). Recruitment patterns in human skeletal muscle during electrical stimulation. *Physical Therapy, 85*, 358–364.

Gregory, C. M., Dixon, W., & Bickel, C. S. (2007). Impact of varying pulse frequency and duration on muscle torque production and fatigue. *Muscle & Nerve, 35*(4), 504–509.

Henneman, E. (1981). The size principle of motoneuron recruitment. In J. E. Desmedt (Ed.), *Motor unit types, recruitment and plasticity in health and disease: Progress in clinical neurophysiology*. Basel: Karger.

Henneman, E., Somjen, G., & Carpenter, D. O. (1965). Functional significance of cell size in spinal motoneurons. *Journal of Neurophysiology, 28*, 560–580.

Hill, A. V. (1936). Excitation and accommodation in nerve. *Proceedings of the Royal Society of London, Bl 19*, 305–355.

Ho, L. O. L., Kwong, W. L., & Cheing, G. L. Y. (2007). Effectiveness of microcurrent therapy in the management of lateral epicondylitis: A pilot study. *Hong Kong Physiotherapy Journal, 25*, 14–20.

Johnson, M. I., Penny, P., & Sajawal, M. A. (1997). Clinical technical note: An examination of the analgesic effects of microcurrent electrical stimulation (MES) on cold-induced pain in healthy subjects. *Physiotherapy Theory & Practice, 13*(4), 293–301.

Jones, D. A., Bigland-Ritchie, B., & Edwards, R. H. T. (1979). Excitation frequency and muscle fatigue: Mechanical responses during voluntary and stimulated contractions. *Experimental Neurology, 64*, 401–413.

Kern, H., Salmons, S., Mayr, W., Rossini, K., & Carraro, U. (2005). Recovery of long-term denervated human muscles induced by electrical stimulation. *Muscle & Nerve, 31*(1), 98–101.

Kesar, T., Chou, L.-W., & Binder-Macleod, S. A. (2008). Effects of stimulation frequency versus pulse duration modulation on muscle fatigue. *Journal of Electromyography and Kinesiology, 18*(4), 662–671.

Kloth, L. C. (1991). Interference current. In R. M. Nelson & D. P. Currier (Eds.), *Clinical electrotherapy* (2nd ed.). Norwalk, CT: Appleton & Lange.

Knaflitz, M., Merletti, R., & De Luca, C. J. (1990). Inference of motor unit recruitment order in voluntary and electrically elicited contractions. *Journal of Applied Physiology, 68*, 1657–1667.

Koester, J., & Siegelbaum, S. A. (2013). Propagated signaling: The action potential. In E. R. Kandel, J. H. Schwartz, T. M. Jessel, S. A. Siegelbaum & A. J. Hudspeth (Eds.), *Principles of neural science* (5th ed.). New York: Elsevier.

Koopman, J. S., Vrinten, D. H., & van Wijck, A. J. (2009). Efficacy of microcurrent therapy in the treatment of chronic nonspecific back pain: A pilot study. *The Clinical Journal of Pain, 25*(6), 495–499.

Korelo, R. I. G., Valderramas, S., Ternoski, B., et al. (2012). Microcurrent application as analgesic treatment in venous ulcers: A pilot study. *Rev. Latino-Am. Enfermagem, 20*(4), 753–760.

Kramer, J. F. (1987). Effect of electrical stimulation current frequencies on isometric knee extension torque. *Physical Therapy, 67*, 31–38.

Krnjevic, K., & Miledi, R. (1958). Failure of neuromuscular propagation in rats. *Journal of Physiology, 140*, 440–461.

Kwon, D. R., Kim, J., Kim, Y., An, S., Kwak, J., Lee, S., et al. (2017). Short-term microcurrent electrical neuromuscular stimulation to improve muscle function in the elderly: A randomized, double-blinded, sham-controlled clinical trial. *Medicine, 96*, 26 (e7407).

Kwon, D. R., & Park, G. Y. (2014). Efficacy of microcurrent therapy in infants with congenital muscular torticollis involving the entire sternocleidomastoid muscle: A randomized placebo-controlled trial. *Clinical Rehabilitation, 28*(10), 983–991.

Laufer, Y. (2013). A brief interphase interval interposed within biphasic pulses enhances the contraction force of the quadriceps femoris muscle. *Physiotherapy Theory and Practice, 29*(6), 461–468.

Laufer, Y., Ries, J. D., Leininger, P. M., et al. (2001). Quadriceps femoris muscle torques and fatigue generated by neuromuscular electrical stimulation with three different waveforms. *Physical Therapy, 81*, 1307–1316.

Lee, J.-W., Kang, J.-S., Park, S.-J., et al. (2013). Effects of inter-electrode distance on delayed onset muscle soreness in microcurrent therapy. *Journal of Physical Therapy Science, 25*, 1451–1454.

Liebano, R. E., Waszczuk, S., Jr., & Corrêa, J. B. (2013). The effect of burst-duty-cycle parameters of medium-frequency alternating current on maximum electrically induced torque of the quadriceps femoris, discomfort, and tolerated current amplitude in professional soccer players. *The Journal of Orthopaedic and Sports Physical Therapy, 43*(12), 920–926.

Lloyd, D. P. C., & Chang, H. T. (1948). Afferent fibres in muscle nerves. *Journal of Neurophysiology, 11*, 199–207.

Lyons, G. M., Leane, G. E., Clarke-Moloney, M., O'Brien, J. V., & Grace, P. A. (2004). An investigation of the effect of electrode size and electrode location on comfort during stimulation of the gastrocnemius muscle. *Medical Engineering & Physics, 26*(10), 873–878.

Lyons, C. L., Robb, J. B., Irrgang, J. J., & Fitzgerald, G. K. (2005). Differences in quadriceps femoris muscle torque when using a clinical electrical stimulator versus a portable electrical stimulator. *Physical Therapy, 85*, 44–51.

McLoda, T. A., & Carmack, J. A. (2000). Optimal burst duration during a facilitated quadriceps femoris contraction. *Journal of Athletic Training, 35*(2), 145–150.

Medeiros, F. V., Bottaro, M., Vieira, A., et al. (2017). Kilohertz and low-frequency electrical stimulation with the same pulse duration have similar efficiency for inducing isometric knee extension torque and discomfort. *American Journal of Physical Medicine & Rehabilitation, 96*, 388–394.

Medeiros, F. V. A., Vieira, A., Carregaro, R. L., Bottaro, M., Maffiuletti, N. A., & Durigan, J. L. Q. (2015). Skinfold thickness affects the isometric knee extension torque evoked by neuromuscular electrical stimulation. *Brazilian Journal of Physical Therapy, 19*(6), 466–472.

Milner-Brown, H. S., Stein, R. B., & Yemm, R. (1973). Changes in firing rate of human motor units during linearly changing voluntary contractions. *Journal of Physiology (Land), 230*, 371–390.

Modlin, M., Forstner, C., Hofer, C., et al. (2005). Electrical stimulation of denervated muscles: First results of a clinical study. *Artificial Organs, 29*(3), 203–206.

Mohr, T., Carlson, B., Sulentic, C., & Landry, R. (1985). Comparison of isometric exercise and high volt galvanic stimulation on quadriceps femoris muscle strength. *Physical Therapy, 65*, 606–612.

Moreno-Aranda, J., & Seireg, A. (1981a). Electrical parameters for over-the-skin electrical muscle stimulation. *Journal of Biomechanics, 14*, 579–585.

Moreno-Aranda, J., & Seireg, A. (1981b). Investigation of over-the-skin electrical stimulation parameters for different normal muscles and subjects. *Journal of Biomechanics, 14*, 587–593.

Moreno-Aranda, J., & Seireg, A. (1981c). Force response to electrical stimulation of canine skeletal muscle. *Journal of Biomechanics, 14*, 595–599.

Moritani, T., Muro, M., & Kijima, A. (1985). Electromechanical changes during electrically induced and maximal voluntary contractions: Electrophysiologic responses of different muscle fibre types during stimulated contractions. *Experimental Neurology, 88*, 471–483.

Nair, H. K. R. (2018). Microcurrent as an adjunct therapy to accelerate chronic wound healing and reduce patient pain. *Journal of Wound Care, 27*(5), 296–306.

Parker, M. G., Broughton, A. J., Larsen, B. R., et al. (2011). Electrically induced contraction levels of the quadriceps femoris muscles in healthy men: The effects of three patterns of burst-modulated alternating current and volitional muscle fatigue. *American Journal of Physical Medicine & Rehabilitation, 90*, 999–1011.

Parker, M. G., Keller, L., & Evenson, J. (2005). Torque responses in human quadriceps to burst-modulated alternating current at 3 carrier frequencies. *The Journal of Orthopaedic and Sports Physical Therapy, 35*, 239–245.

Park, R. J., Son, H., Kim, K., Kim, S., & Oh, T. (2011). The effect of microcurrent electrical stimulation on the foot blood circulation and pain of diabetic neuropathy. *Journal of Physical Therapy Science, 23*, 515–518.

Petrofsky, J., Prowse, M., Bain, M., et al. (2008). Estimation of the distribution of intramuscular current during electrical stimulation of the quadriceps muscle. *European Journal of Applied Physiology, 103*, 265–273.

Poltawski, L., Johnson, M., & Watson, T. (2011). Microcurrent therapy in the management of chronic tennis elbow: Pilot studies to optimize parameters. *Physiotherapy Research International, 17*(3), 157–166.

Poltawski, L., & Watson, T. (2009). Bioelectricity and microcurrent therapy for tissue healing – a narrative review. *Physical Therapy Reviews, 14*(2), 104–114.

Russ, D. W., Vandenborne, K., & Binder-Macleod, S. A. (2002a). Factors in fatigue during intermittent electrical stimulation of human skeletal muscle. *Journal of Applied Physiology, 93*, 469–478.

Russ, D. W., Vandenborne, K., Walter, G. A., Elliott, M., & Binder-Macleod, S. A. (2002b). Effects of muscle activation on fatigue and metabolism in human skeletal muscle. *Journal of Applied Physiology, 92*, 1978–1986.

Scott, W. B., Causey, J. B., & Marshall, T. L. (2009). Comparison of maximum tolerated muscle torques produced by 2 pulse durations. *Physical Therapy, 89*, 851–857.

Seckel, B. R. (1988). Discussion. Of: Beveridge JA, Politis MJ: Use of exogenous electric current in the treatment of delayed lesions in peripheral nerves. *Plastic and Reconstructive Surgery, 82*, 578–579.

Selkowitz, D. M. (1985). Improvement in isometric strength of the quadriceps femoris muscle after training with electrical stimulation. *Physical Therapy, 65*, 186–196.

Selkowitz, D. M. (1989). High-frequency electrical stimulation in muscle strengthening. *The American Journal of Sports Medicine, 17*, 103–111.

Selkowitz, D. M. (1999). Electrical currents. In M. H. Cameron (Ed.), *Physical agents: From research to practice* (1st ed.). Philadelphia, PA: WB Saunders.

Selkowitz, D. M., Rossman, E., & Fitzpatrick, S. (2009). Effect of burst-modulated alternating current carrier frequency on current amplitude required to produce maximally-tolerated electrically-stimulated quadriceps femoris knee extension torque. *American Journal of Physical Medicine & Rehabilitation, 88*, 973–978.

Snyder, A. R., Perotti, A. L., Lam, K. C., & Bay, R. C. (2010). The influence of high-voltage electrical stimulation on edema formation after acute injury: A systematic review. *Journal of Sport Rehabilitation, 19*, 436–451.

Stein, R. B., & Bertoldi (1981). The size principle: A synthesis of neurophysiological data. In J. E. Desmedt (Ed.), *Motor unit types, recruitment and plasticity in health and disease: Progress in clinical neurophysiology*. Basel: Karger.

Taylor, K., Mendel, F. C., Fish, D. R., Hard, R., & Burton, H. W. (1997). Effect of high-voltage pulsed current and alternating current on macromolecular leakage in hamster cheek pouch microcirculation. *Physical Therapy, 77*, 1729–1740.

Valencic, V., Vodovnik, L., Stefancic, M., & Jelnikar, T. (1986). Improved motor response due to chronic electrical stimulation of denervated tibialis anterior muscle in humans. *Muscle & Nerve, 9*, 612–617.

Vander, A. J., Sherman, J. H., & Luciano, D. S. (1994). Human Physiology. In *The mechanisms of body function* (6th ed.). New York: McGraw-Hill.

Ward, A. R., Oliver, W. G., & Buccella, D. (2006). Wrist extensor torque production and discomfort associated with low-frequency and burst-modulated kilohertz-frequency currents. *Physical Therapy, 86*(10), 1360–1367.

Ward, A. R., & Robertson, V. J. (2001). The variation in motor threshold with frequency using kHz-frequency alternating current. *Muscle & Nerve, 24*, 1303–1311.

Ward, A. R., Robertson, V. J., & Ioannou, H. (2004). The effect of duty cycle and frequency on muscle torque production using kilohertz frequency range alternating current. *Medical Engineering & Physics, 26*, 569–579.

Ward, A. R., & Shkuratova, N. (2002). Russian electrical stimulation: The early experiments. *Physical Therapy, 82*, 1019–1030.

Thermal and Microthermal Modalities

5

Biophysical Effects of Heating and Cooling

Tim Watson

INTRODUCTION

Chapter 2 presented the basic scientific principles of thermal energy. This chapter examines in more detail the effects that are produced in biological materials, particularly when these are part of a functioning body. The clinical effects of heating and cooling are considered in later chapters (see Chapter 6: Superficial heating, Chapter 7: Pulsed and continuous shortwave and radiofrequency therapies, Chapter 8: Cryotherapy).

THERMAL HOMOEOSTASIS

In health, humans preserve a constant body temperature by means of a highly efficient thermoregulatory system. This process involves close temperature regulation of the deep body (core) temperature, with more varied but managed temperature regulation of the peripheral (shell) layers (Fig. 5.1).

Core Temperature

Core temperature is maintained at approximately 37°C despite marked variations in the ambient temperature (International Union of Physiological Sciences 1987).

Variation of ±2°C defines clinical hyperthermia (core temperature >39°C) and hypothermia (core temperature <35°C). At rest, and in a neutral environment, core temperature can be kept within a narrow band of control (±0.3°C). Additionally, core temperature varies with the body's intrinsic diurnal temperature rhythm.

Shell Temperature

Whereas the core temperature is stable, the shell – at the interface between the body and the environment – is subject to greater variations in temperature. Across approximately 1 cm of the body shell, from the skin surface to the superficial layer of muscle, the temperature gradient varies according to the temperature of the external environment (demonstrated for the forearm in Fig. 5.2). The gradient is not uniform and changes with the thermal conductivity of the tissue layers and the rate of blood flow in the different regions. Additionally, skin temperatures differ widely over the body surface, especially in hot or cold conditions. When an individual is in a comfortable environment of, say, 24°C, the skin of the toes might be 27°C, that of the upper arms and legs 31°C and the forehead 34°C while the core is maintained at 37°C.

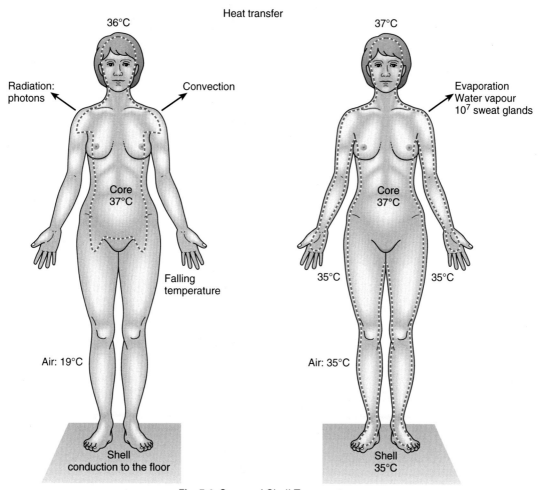

Fig. 5.1 Core and Shell Temperatures

Diurnal (Circadian) Core Temperature Rhythm

The diurnal (circadian) core temperature rhythm is one of the most stable of biological rhythms, with a well-marked intrinsic component (Fig. 5.3). Body temperature is typically lowest in the early morning and highest in the evening. The diurnal range of variation is usually about 0.5–1.5°C in adults, depending on other external factors, such as the effects of meals, activity, sleep and ambient temperature. Various intrinsic biological rhythms may be in or out of phase with each other, and there is evidence that when they are out of phase, synchronization function is compromised. For example, desynchronization of the sleep–wake cycle and the core temperature cycle by continuous light exposure can bring about impairment of thermoregulatory function (Moore-Ede & Sulzman 1981). Other rhythms, which are not daily (e.g. the female menstrual cycle), also affect core temperature.

Body Temperature Measurement

Core temperature is measured conventionally by a mercury-in-glass or electrical thermometer placed in the mouth; both are quick and accurate. Errors occur with mouth breathing or talking during measurement or following hot or cold drinks. Alternatives are rectal or urinary measurement of core temperature (more reliable but generally less practical), which give results that are on average about 0.5°C higher than mouth temperatures. For accurate and fast recording, the most commonly used method in clinical practice is to measure the ear canal temperature with an infrared based thermometer. Several useful comparisons have been published in relation to clinical temperature measurement, (e.g. Mangat et al 2010).

Thermal Balance

For the core temperature to remain constant there needs to be a balance (equilibrium) between internal heat production, heat gain from the environment and external heat loss. This is illustrated in Fig. 5.4 and expressed in the form of a *heat balance equation* (Box 5.1).

Metabolic heat production (M) is the heat produced during the work of metabolism. Basal metabolic rate, which occurs during complete physical and mental rest, is about 45 W/m² (i.e. watts per square metre of body surface) for an adult male of 30 years and 41 W/m² for a female of the same age. These values can be almost doubled during strenuous physical work and might be as high as 900 W/m² for brief periods. A small increase in M follows the eating of a meal; M is also increased by shivering.

Heat loss or gain by *conduction* (K) depends on the temperature difference between the body and the surrounding environment, on thermal conductivity

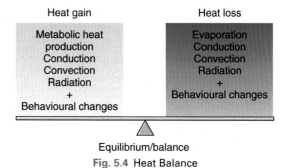

Fig. 5.4 Heat Balance

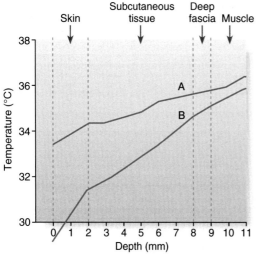

Fig. 5.2 Temperature gradients in the forearm between the skin surface and deep tissues in A, comfortably warm conditions and B, cold conditions.

BOX 5.1   Heat Balance Equation

$$M \pm w = \pm K \pm C \pm R - E \pm S$$

where:

M is the rate of metabolic heat production

w is the external work performed by or on the body

K, C and R are the loss or gain of heat by conduction, convection and radiation, respectively

E is the evaporative heat loss from the skin and respiratory tract

S is the rate of change of body heat storage (resultant = 0 at thermal equilibrium).

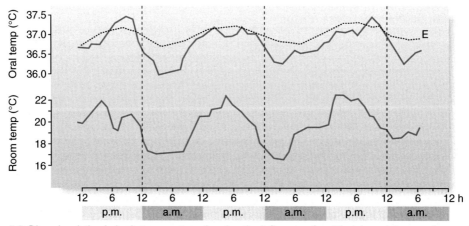

Fig. 5.3 Diurnal variation in body temperature showing the influence of ambient (room) temperature on the oral temperature when meals and physical activity are kept constant. E, intrinsic temperature rhythm.

between the two and on the area of contact. Little heat is normally lost by conduction to the air because air is a poor thermal conductor. Immersion in cold water, e.g. during open-water swimming, can lead to rapid cooling. Subcutaneous fat is important in determining the level of cooling because it provides effective insulation.

Convective heat exchange (C) depends on the fluid (most commonly air) surrounding the body, and its flow patterns. Normally, an individual's surface temperature is higher than the temperature of the surrounding air, so that heated air close to the body moves upwards by convection and colder air takes its place, thus cooling the body.

Radiant heat transfer (R) depends on the nature of the surfaces involved, their temperature and the geometrical relationship between them. Extending the arms and legs effectively increases the surface area over which convective and radiant heat exchange can take place.

Evaporative heat loss (E): at rest in a comfortable ambient temperature, an individual loses water by evaporation through the skin and from the respiratory tract. This is described as insensible water loss. It occurs at a rate of about 30 g per hour and produces a heat loss of about 10 W/m². Sweating (sensible water loss) contributes a much greater potential heat loss. Complete evaporation of 1 litre of sweat from the body surface in 1 hour will dissipate about 400 W/m².

Rate of heat storage (S): the specific heat of the human body is 3.5 kJ/kg. If a person of 65 kg increases mean core temperature by 1°C over a period of 1 hour, S becomes 230 kJ/h, or 64 W. S can be positive or negative.

Control of Body Temperature

The factors that contribute to changes in body temperature, and control of these processes (thermoregulation) is essential for survival. Good health requires that very limited variation occurs, despite the need to function in environments of very different temperatures.

Complete texts have been published describing the complexity of human thermoregulation (e.g. Flouris 2009) as have numerous models (e.g. Foda et al 2011). Morrison and Nakamura (2011) provide a comprehensive review of the neural control of thermoregulation. A brief summary is provided here.

Thermoregulation is integrated by a controlling mechanism in the central nervous system (CNS) that responds to the heat of the tissues, detected by thermoreceptors. These receptors are sensitive to heat and cold information arising in the skin, the deep tissues and within the CNS. They provide feedback signals to CNS structures, which are situated mainly in the hypothalamus of the brain, via a servo- or loop system (Fig. 5.5). The temperature of the blood perfusing the hypothalamus also provides a major thermoregulatory drive. The hypothalamus monitors ambient temperature and initiates appropriate physiological responses (vasodilatation and sweating in hot conditions, or vasoconstriction and shivering in cold) that counteract any deviation in the core temperature (Fig. 5.6). Apart from these involuntary responses, thermal information is transmitted by afferent nerves to regions of the brain that control endocrine functions and to the cerebral cortex, which makes individuals aware of their thermal sensations by inducing behavioural changes such as moving away from/towards heat sources.

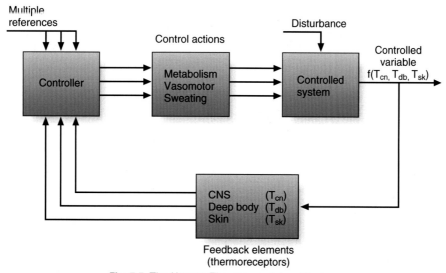

Fig. 5.5 The Human Thermoregulatory System

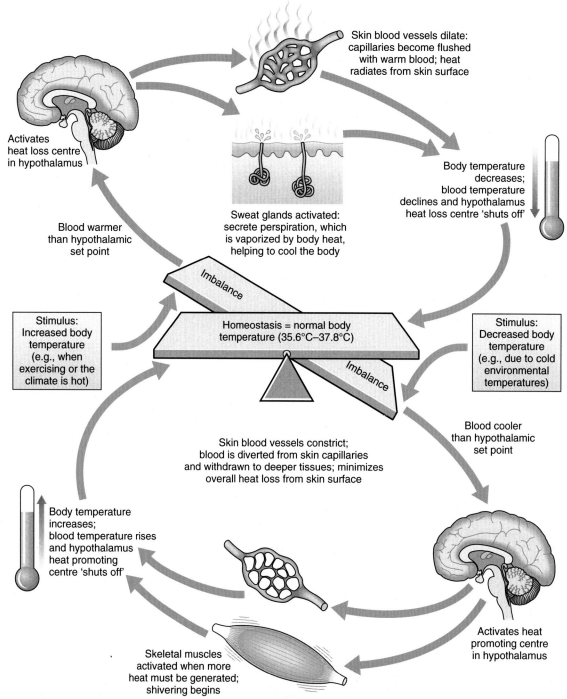

Skin blood vessels dilate: capillaries become flushed with warm blood; heat radiates from skin surface

Activates heat loss centre in hypothalamus

Body temperature decreases; blood temperature declines and hypothalamus heat loss centre 'shuts off'

Blood warmer than hypothalamic set point

Sweat glands activated: secrete perspiration, which is vaporized by body heat, helping to cool the body

Imbalance

Stimulus: Increased body temperature (e.g., when exercising or the climate is hot)

Homeostasis = normal body temperature (35.6°C–37.8°C)

Imbalance

Stimulus: Decreased body temperature (e.g., due to cold environmental temperatures)

Skin blood vessels constrict; blood is diverted from skin capillaries and withdrawn to deeper tissues; minimizes overall heat loss from skin surface

Blood cooler than hypothalamic set point

Body temperature increases; blood temperature rises and hypothalamus heat promoting centre 'shuts off'

Activates heat promoting centre in hypothalamus

Skeletal muscles activated when more heat must be generated; shivering begins

Fig. 5.6 The Role of the Hypothalamus in Thermoregulation (From E N Marieb and K N Hoehn. Human Anatomy and Physiology Page 1014 Pearson New International Edition.)

An essential role in processing thermal signals is ascribed to the preoptic region of the anterior hypothalamus and to a region in the posterior hypothalamus, described respectively as the 'heat loss' and 'heat gain' centres. These are considered to exert primary thermoregulatory control. The integration of incoming and outgoing information, and the 'set-point' from which the hypothalamic centres operate, is the basis on which present views on thermoregulatory control are constructed (Collins 1992; Hensel 1981).

PHYSIOLOGICAL EFFECTS OF THERMAL CHANGES

The general physiological effects of heating and cooling of tissue are described in some detail here; the chapters following highlight issues related to individual modalities.

Physiological Effects of Cold

This overview is necessarily succinct, and readers are referred to Chapter 8 (Cryotherapy) and the cited literature for further detail.

Local Effects

Once cooling has occurred, how this was brought about is largely immaterial. Therefore the issues discussed here are dependent on the actual temperature change rather than the process of cooling. The effects of cooling are the consequence of factors such as the:

- volume of tissue
- composition of the tissue
- capacity of tissue to moderate the effects of cooling: largely a factor of blood supply
- rate of temperature fall
- temperature to which the tissue is lowered.

The general local effects (cell activity, blood flow, collagen behaviour) are summarized in following sections while the clinically relevant effects of tissue cooling are considered in Chapter 8 (Cryotherapy).

Cell activity. It is generally, but not universally, true that chemical and biological processes slow down with decreasing temperature. As most enzyme systems operate at an optimal temperature, lowering the temperature generally results in a slowing of activity. Cell viability is critically dependent on membrane transport systems involving active biochemical pumps and passive leaks in membranes, which maintain intracellular ionic composition. The failure of pumps at low temperatures relative to the leaks brings about a gain in Na^+ and Ca^{++}, and a loss of K^+ from cells: that is, membranes lose their selective permeability in cold conditions.

Freezing damage to cells occurs when the local temperature drops to zero. Viscosity increases, ice crystals form and the remaining solution in the cells is reduced in volume as water leaks into the interstitial space. A characteristic feature of cold injury is the vascular damage that occurs with intravascular aggregation of platelets and red blood cells to form blockages in vessels.

Blood flow. Cooling skin causes immediate vasoconstriction, diminishing heat loss. Thermoreceptors in the skin are stimulated and produce vasoconstriction over the body surface through a vasoconstrictive reflex (Paine 2010). In addition, there is a direct constrictor effect of cold on the smooth muscle of arterioles and venules. Countercurrent heat exchange between blood vessels helps to reduce heat loss. This is most effective in the limbs because of the relatively long parallel pathways between the deep arteries and veins. Body core temperature is therefore prevented from falling rapidly. Arteriovenous anastomoses that open to allow more blood flow to the skin in hot conditions are constricted in cold conditions.

A further effect is seen, for example, in the hand. Immersion of the hands in water at 0–12°C initially causes the expected vasoconstriction, which is followed after a delay of 5 minutes or more by a marked vasodilatation. This is then interrupted by another burst of vasoconstriction and subsequent waves of increased and decreased local blood flow. This phenomenon is known as cold-induced vasodilatation (CIVD) (Daanen 2003; 2009) and demonstrates a hunting reaction of the vessels (Fig. 5.7). CIVD is most likely to be due to the direct effect of low temperature causing paralysis of smooth muscle contraction in the blood vessels (Keatinge 1978). The reaction provides protection to tissues from damage caused by prolonged cooling and relative ischaemia (Flouris et al 2008).

Muscle blood flow is primarily determined by local muscle metabolic rate. Muscle cooling takes a more prolonged period: muscles are insulated from temperature changes at the skin surface by a layer of subcutaneous tissue (Jutte et al 2001, 2012; Otte et al 2002).

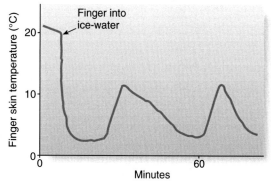

Fig. 5.7 Cold vasodilatation in the finger immersed in ice-water, measured by skin temperature changes.

Collagen behaviour. Although most studies examining stretch in collagen focus on the effects of heat (e.g. Rigby et al 1959, 1964; Warren et al 1971), it is expected that collagen tends to become stiffer when cooled. Some recent research (e.g. Sefiddashti et al 2018) demonstrated significant benefit when stretch is combined with cooling, which appears counter intuitive. It is likely however that a neural mechanism is activated rather than a stiffening of the collagen tissue. Weppler and Magnusson (2010) usefully consider the relationship between mechanical and sensory aspects of tissue extensibility and stretch. Cryostretch has achieved clinical uptake on this basis and appears effective (e.g. Gkrilias et al 2017). Some concerns are raised with regard to the potential to diminish the protective pain responses while applying stretch. The clinician should therefore be mindful of reduced tissue protection when employing these techniques.

Nerve conduction. Reducing the temperature of a nerve will have a marked effect on nerve conduction characteristics. Algafly and George (2007) demonstrated a reduction in nerve conduction velocity as a result of local tissue cooling with a reduction of over 30% with progressive cooling to 10°C. There are also significant changes in pain threshold and pain tolerance. It is proposed that at least part of the beneficial effects of cryotherapy may be attributed to this physiological response.

Herrera et al (2010) also identified a clear alteration in nerve conduction velocity, further identifying a possible difference between different modes of cryo application, though this aspect of the study had some limitations. There have also been concerns with regard to a possible detrimental effect of this change with, for example, a reduction in joint position sense, reviewed in Costello and Donnelly (2010) who were unable to identify a consistent and clinically meaningful response. The influence of cryo applications on motor nerves may be partly responsible for alterations in muscle tone noted with this intervention and are further considered in Chapter 8.

Pain relief. Cold applied to the skin initially stimulates both cold and pain sensations. If the cold is sufficiently intense, both sensations are suppressed because of inhibition of nerve conduction and decreasing the activation threshold of tissue nociceptors (Malanga et al 2015). The reduction in pain that accompanies cooling can be due to either direct (e.g. spinal gating) or indirect factors (e.g. reduced nerve conduction velocity) and are further considered in Chapter 8 (Cryotherapy).

Muscular performance. The effect of temperature on muscle performance is complex, involving the effects of cold on the contractile process, neuromuscular transmission and circulatory oxygen. Some muscle properties have a large thermal dependence (e.g. power, velocity, maximal isometric force by stimulation at high frequencies) whereas others are barely influenced by temperatures between 25 and 37°C (e.g. maximal isometric force by stimulation at low frequencies) (Jones et al 2004). The time to peak and time to half relaxation of an isometric twitch increases with cooling, suggesting a slowing of contraction and relaxation.

Maximum tetanic tension is relatively stable between temperatures of 25 and 35°C, which is within the normal physiological range; more pronounced effects are seen below 25°C. With cooling, therefore, muscle contractions tend to slow, but a reasonably normal level of force can be generated, provided the cooling is within reasonable limits. The ability to sustain a maximal muscle contraction is also temperature dependent and is optimal at 27°C. Temperatures below this might reduce muscle performance.

Muscle tone. Although the underlying physiology is not totally understood, cold can reduce muscle tone. The neural effects might be due to changes in the activity of muscle spindles, Ia and secondary afferents, α motor neurons, γ fibres, neuromuscular junctions or the muscle tissue itself. Muscle spindles respond more rapidly than other neural and muscular structures as smaller reductions in temperatures are required to achieve this effect.

With reduced temperatures, muscle spindle sensitivity drops in proportion to the degree of cooling, possibly as a result of a direct effect on the sensory terminal, or as the firing rate of Ia afferents is decreased, or both (Eldred et al 1960; Ottoson 1965). It is also possible that the cooling influences muscle spasm by inhibiting a spinal reflex loop (Malanga et al 2015). Many muscles are well insulated, and thorough cooling is necessary to achieve a muscle spindle response as the spindles are embedded in the muscle structure. Miglietta (1973) and Trnavsky (1983) showed that prolonged cooling was needed to reduce clonus. This was confirmed by Price et al (1993), who demonstrated a significant reduction in spasticity at the ankle (secondary to head injury) following the application of liquid ice in a bag to the gastrocnemius muscle after cooling for 20 minutes. Again, the work of Jutte et al (2001) demonstrates that it is likely that prolonged cooling (up to an hour) is necessary to produce cooling of 7°C in muscle beneath a skin-fold thickness of 30–40 mm.

In addition to spindle changes on cooling, it is also possible that greater degrees of cooling can affect other tissues. Effects might be the result of a slowing of conduction in both the muscle and motor nerves or impaired conduction in the γ or α efferents. However, because rapid responses are also seen on skin cooling (30 seconds after the application of ice) other explanations have also been sought. It is postulated that reflexes from the cold skin might inhibit the dominant excitatory stimuli that operate in the region of the anterior horn neurons of the spinal cord (Lehmann & De Lateur 1990b).

In addition, following an acute injury, a reduction in muscle spasm in response to cooling could in part be attributed to the reduction of pain (as a secondary effect).

Despite all these inhibitory effects, it is important to note that cooling can result in an immediate increase in tone for a short period. Clinically, increases in tone have been noted in response to cold application for patients with CNS lesions: Lehmann and de Lateur (1999) suggest that evidence points to an initial increase in excitability of α motor neurons. An increase in tone has also been demonstrated with the use of ice massage.

Thus it is important to use an appropriate method of cooling to produce either excitation (e.g. a brief stimulus such as ice massage) or inhibition (more prolonged cooling such as with an ice pack). The response to cold might be rapid, occurring in a matter of seconds, but to obtain muscle cooling treatments must be at appropriate temperatures and adequate times (30 minutes or more).

Systemic Effects

These are summarized in Box 5.2.

Generalized vasoconstriction develops over the skin surface when a cold stimulus is applied and can produce large changes in heat transfer (e.g. 60 W/m^2 transferred across the shell of the body with peripheral vasodilation; 10 W/m^2 with vasoconstriction). Skin vasoconstriction and increased blood viscosity raise peripheral resistance and produce an increase in arterial blood pressure. As the skin temperature decreases, the drive to internal heat production grows. This is brought about by an involuntary increase in muscle tone (preshivering tone) that eventually develops into shivering. Voluntary movement and muscular exercise tend to inhibit shivering, primarily by helping to raise the body temperature, and reduce the central nervous drive.

Physiological Effects of Heat
Local Effects

Once energy is absorbed, it is largely immaterial as to how the heat was delivered. There are no *different* heats, only different means of generating the same heat, discussed in

---

BOX 5.2   Systemic Effects of Cooling

Generalized vasoconstriction
Increased blood viscosity
Increased arterial blood pressure
Shivering, including preshivering
Voluntary activity
Altered (contracted) posture
Behavioural changes
Tissue injury, nerve paralysis and 'hypothermia'

---

the relevant chapters. The effects of heating are the consequence of such factors as the:
- volume of tissue absorbing the energy
- composition of the absorbing tissue
- capacity of the tissue to dissipate heat, which is largely a factor of blood supply
- rate of temperature rise
- temperature to which the tissue is raised.

Cell activity. Chemical reactions involved in metabolic activity are increased by a rise in temperature (Van't Hoff's law). Metabolic rate increases by about 13% for each 1°C rise in tissue temperature, with a corresponding increase in tissue demands for oxygen and nutrients and an enhanced output of metabolic waste products. While this is a widely cited 'fact', there is little by way of direct *in vivo* evidence.

An increase in temperature can produce beneficial effects, as it increases activity in most cells. However, with rising temperature, a point is reached when it is detrimental. For example, enzyme systems are heat sensitive: rising tissue temperature first produces an increase in enzyme activity to a peak value, followed by a decline, and then finally abolition of activity. As an example, an increase in temperature to 36°C brings about an increase in the destructive enzyme collagenase when compared with that at 30°C in tissue experiments (Harris & McCroskery 1974). Clinically, it has been demonstrated that the healthy knee joint has a temperature of 30.5–33°C (Oosterveld & Rasker 1994), whereas joints with active synovitis have temperatures between 34 and 37.6°C. Raising the joint temperature to, say, 40–45°C, might render inactive the destructive collagenase but may destroy other essential enzymes, hence posing a risk to the patient.

Heat-shock proteins accumulate in cells and tissues exposed to high temperatures (Whitley et al 1999), the function of which is thought to be to confer a degree of protection to cells upon subsequent heat exposure. While originally identified in response to thermal stress, their expression has since been demonstrated in response to multiple stimuli including cold, ultraviolet and during the normal repair sequence. Heat-shock proteins are said to act as an intracellular chaperone, assisting with protein folding and conformation (Walter 2002). Infrared radiation has been shown to cause an alteration in the amino acid composition of proteins which develop thermal tolerance (Westerhof et al 1987). Heat-shock proteins may confer some protection against this effect. This effect is overcome by allowing between 36 and 72 hours to elapse between applications.

At temperatures of 45°C or greater, the magnitude of protein damage results in destruction of cells and tissues. At this temperature, skin burns also occur if contact is maintained for long enough. Cell membranes are particularly sensitive: the lipoprotein structure of membranes may become more fluid with increasing temperature and cause a breakdown in permeability (Bowler 1987). Whereas healthy cells are unaffected by mild heating, the effects of temperatures of around 40°C on cancer cells can include the inhibition of the synthesis of RNA, DNA and proteins (Westerhof et al 1987). This can cause irreversible structural damage to cell membranes and the disruption of organelles, hence the developing field of deliberate hyperthermia as a means to treat some cancers (Sethi & Chakravarti 2015).

Blood flow. Heat can induce changes both in the superficial and deep tissues. When the skin is heated, blood vessels become vasodilated resulting in increased blood flow. Vasodilatation may be due to: (1) a direct effect on the smooth muscle of arterioles and venules; (2) a local axon reflex; and (3) increased levels of certain metabolites in the blood. Historically, the axon reflex was ascribed as being the primary mechanism, but various mediators (such as nitric oxide, NO) are now thought to be primary stimulants of this response (e.g. Brunt et al 2016).

If local tissue damage occurs, further dilatation may be produced by histamine-like mediators, such as bradykinin. Increased skin blood flow occurs in areas remote from the heated tissue owing to long spinal nervous reflexes (Kerslake & Cooper 1950). There is a complex response in deeper tissues, involving a balance between vasodilatation due directly to heating and increased blood flow due to increased metabolic activity (e.g. in skeletal muscle) on the one hand and a reduced blood flow because of a relative vasoconstriction brought about by thermoregulation as blood is directed towards the surface to enable heat loss, on the other. In addition, heat exchange occurs between arterial and venous vessels, with heat flow from the arterial to the cooler venous blood. Vasodilatation of the large superficial veins can have considerable effects of heat loss, as can the opening of the arteriovenous anastomoses deep below the skin capillaries.

Slight differences in circulatory changes occur with superficial (e.g. infrared irradiation or contact methods) and deep methods of heating (e.g. shortwave), although only due to relative depth of penetration. Infrared radiation (see Chapter 6) has been shown to cause an increase in blood flow in the cutaneous circulation, whereas shortwave therapy (see Chapter 7) achieves a deeper effect (Wyper & McNiven 1976). Local heat in the early stages of injury should be avoided. Some increased blood flow and the presence of chemical mediators such as bradykinin and histamine, which are associated with heating, can detrimentally affect capillary and postcapillary venule permeability. This, together with the increase in capillary hydrostatic pressure, may result in increased oedema. Clinical and laboratory research has demonstrated an increase in oedema together with a prolonged healing time in acute injuries treated with heat (e.g. Feibel & Fast 1976; Wallace et al 1979).

Collagen behaviour. The properties of collagen change with heat. Thus the viscoelastic properties of tendon, ligament and, to some degree, muscle can be influenced. Early work examined the behaviour of animal collagen tissue under passive stretch with and without heat. Gersten (1955) initially showed an increase in the extensibility of frog Achilles tendons following heating with ultrasound. In a series of key studies, Rigby and colleagues (1959, 1964) showed that the viscoelastic properties of tendon are temperature dependent between 37 and 40°C, with an increase in the stress–relaxation relationship. Changes were reversible with loads of less than 4% and at temperatures below 40°C, and it was shown that repeated stress could be applied at temperatures of below 37°C with no change in stress–strain curves. Lehmann et al (1970) and Warren et al (1971, 1976), using rat-tail collagen heated in a water bath to temperatures between 41 and 45°C, showed reduced tensile strength and residual elongation following the application of force at temperatures of 45°C, and the need for lower forces to produce rupture (30–50% of normal). A temperature of 39°C relates to the transition phase of collagen. All this suggests that normal body temperatures could allow collagen to perform optimally, although when permanent elongation is required, such as to mobilize a stiff joint, a raised temperature of over 39°C in the target tissue is needed. This is unlikely to be achieved clinically with superficial heating mechanisms given the 3–4°C rise in temperature required to achieve significant benefit and to elongate shortened tissue. If heat is a significant contributor to changes in tissue extensibility, when combined with stretch (Weppler 2010) then the essential principle is the need to raise the target tissue temperature by 3–4°C using a heating mechanism that is capable of reaching sufficient tissue depth to make the intervention worthwhile.

Owing to the large number of confounding factors that can affect results, few studies have examined the effect of heat on stretch of collagenous tissues such as ligaments and tendons in vivo. Recent work by Draper (2011, 2014) has examined the effect of heating collagenous tissue to a known temperature of around 40°C prior to specific stretch. This material is considered further in Chapter 7; however, there is some indication that adequate heating does facilitate stretch.

Nerve conduction. In nerve conduction tests in healthy participants, Kramer (1984) demonstrated an increase in nerve conduction velocity with increasing tissue temperature. More recently, increases in median nerve conduction velocity were demonstrated following heating (Laymon et al 2015).

Pain relief. Heat is often used to relieve pain (e.g. Igwea et al 2016). Various mechanisms may be responsible, including activation of antinociceptive descending pathways (Palazzo et al 2008). Pain may also be relieved by reducing secondary muscle spasm and increasing local tissue circulation, thereby influencing presence and concentration of metabolites, cytokines and inflammatory mediators. Heat has also been claimed to act as a 'counterirritant' though this is not widely supported from the research literature.

Muscle performance. Few studies have looked at the effect of an increase in temperature on muscle in situ beyond that in normal physiological ranges, and certainly not much beyond 40°C, as above this temperature tissue damage occurs rapidly. The principles governing temperature changes are discussed in previous sections relative to the effects of cold. However, a number of studies have indicated some points for consideration. Strength and endurance might be affected by an increase in temperature. Following immersion of the lower limbs in a water bath at 44°C for 45 minutes (actual temperature of muscle not known), Edwards et al (1970) demonstrated a reduction in the ability of subjects to sustain an isometric contraction. Similarly, an immediate reduction in the strength of the quadriceps muscle following the application of heat through the use of shortwave diathermy has also been demonstrated (Chastain 1978). In this study, a temperature of 42.4°C at a depth of 3.22cm was reported. However, Chastain (1978) also noted that over the ensuing 2 hours the muscle strength increased and remained above pretreatment levels. These findings are important for clinical practice and should be considered both when making objective measurements of muscle strength in order to evaluate treatment efficacy and when implementing exercise programmes.

Muscle tone. It is evident from practice that increased muscle tone can sometimes be relieved by heat, and some research supports this view. Lehmann and de Lateur (1990a), for example, describe work that shows that heating to temperatures of between 40 and 45°C results in a reduction of spasm. Although the physiological basis for this is still unclear, a number of possibilities have been considered.

The responses of muscle spindles, secondary afferents and Golgi tendon organs to heating have all been investigated. The Ia afferents of muscle spindles have been shown to increase their firing rate with a moderate rise in temperature (Mense 1978), whereas most (although not quite all) secondary afferents demonstrate decreased firing with temperature increases (Lehmann & de Lateur 1999). In addition, there is increased firing from Golgi tendon organs, resulting in increased inhibition. These factors are likely to reduce tone, assuming that secondary muscle spasm is largely a tonic phenomenon. There is also some evidence that heating of the skin results in reduced tension, probably due to γ fibre activity affecting the muscle spindles (Fischer & Solomon 1965). Thus superficial heating, such as hot packs and infrared, can reduce tone as well as the deeper-penetrating modalities. While the research supporting these changes is not new, it is methodologically sound and largely not replicated on that basis.

Increased tone associated with upper motor neuron lesions can be reduced to some degree by heating. These effects tend to be short term, however, and the use of cold may be a more effective method of treatment as the temperature of muscle returns to normal less rapidly following cooling than following heating.

Systemic Effects

These are summarized in Box 5.3.

Local heating causes a rise in temperature of tissues and reflex vasodilatation in remote areas of the body and, if heating is extensive and prolonged, a general rise in core temperature can ensue. The immediate systemic response is a generalized skin vasodilatation, which serves to transport heat by conduction and convection from the core to the shell. There is a concomitant reduction in splanchnic blood flow resulting in reduced hepatic clearance rate and reduction in urine flow.

If the heat stress is great, the skin temperature rises and approaches 35°C over the entire body. At or near this point, the body temperature becomes stabilized by the stimulation of sweat glands, which secrete hypotonic sweat on to the body surface so that increased evaporative cooling can take place. High radiant temperatures can be tolerated for many minutes if the environment is dry. An increase in ambient humidity makes these conditions immediately unbearable as it reduces the possibility of evaporation of sweat (which simply runs off the body).

BOX 5.3   Systemic Effects of Heat

Reflex vasodilation remote to site of heating
Increase in core temperature
Reduced renal function
Sweating
Heat illness:
    swelling of feet and ankles
    prickly heat
    water deficiency
Heat stroke and death

Heat illness may occur with sudden increases in heat stress, most readily in those who are not adapted (acclimatized) to heat. Generalized skin vasodilatation may cause swelling of the feet and ankles (heat oedema) or syncope during postural change or prolonged standing. Prickly heat, a papulovesicular rash accompanied by a dermal prickling sensation when sweating is provoked, occurs in some people when areas of the skin are continuously wetted by sweat. More serious heat illnesses, such as heat exhaustion from water deficiency or salt deficiency, are due to imbalance of body water and salt, respectively, with excessive sweating, and lead to collapse. Left untreated, they may result in potentially fatal heat stroke when the core temperature reaches high levels of 41°C and above and the central heat-regulatory mechanisms fail (Khogali & Hales 1983).

SUMMARY

The core physiological effects of thermal energy (both those arising from an increase or a decrease of tissue temperature) are well established. Although there are some areas of controversy, which have been highlighted, the responses of the tissues are reasonably well understood. These physiological changes will give rise to a range of therapeutic effects, which are discussed in each of the relevant modality chapters.

MICROTHERMAL LOW ENERGY EFFECTS

Introduction

The body is a complex mechanism, and the ways in which the various electrophysical agents (EPAs) discussed in this text interact with it continue to be researched. In particular, the relationship between the thermal and so-called 'non-thermal' effects that can arise constitute an ongoing investigation area.

The physiological changes that occur as a result of the application of heat are considered earlier in this chapter. Although these effects are significant, heating is not the only way in which physiological changes can be brought about in the tissues by EPAs. Some modalities, such as ultrasound, pulsed shortwave therapy and laser, are commonly used by practitioners at very low doses, often employing a pulsed delivery mode, to facilitate tissue repair and reduce pain.

The term 'non-thermal' is frequently used in clinical practice to mean a treatment that does not result in the patient being conscious of any warming. Critically, however, all forms of energy can degrade ultimately into heat energy, although the level may be extremely low. The delivery and subsequent absorption of electrophysical energy to the tissues will inevitably result in a thermal change – however small – giving rise to the concept of microthermal effects. This is certainly a preferred term to the oft used 'non-thermal' or 'athermal' phrases employed in therapy. The thermal changes may be at a micro level, and considerably below anything detectable by the recipient, but they do exist (Dyson 2006; Foster & Glaser 2007).

Although there is clear evidence of the non-thermal effects of agents such as ultraviolet irradiation and visible light, there has been considerable controversy surrounding the possible existence of such effects from the use of low-intensity, non-ionizing radiations and mechanical waves in therapy practice. It is argued that even ultraviolet and light based therapies may exert a (secondary) thermal influence by increasing local tissue metabolism in response to the treatment. One active, linked area of research is concerned with the environmental exposure to low-level EM fields (such as those from mobile phones, power lines and equipment such as televisions and microwaves) and whole texts are devoted to this topic (e.g. Barnes & Greenebaum 2018) though the details are beyond the remit of this chapter.

Arguments for and against the existence of microthermal effects arose early in clinical practice (e.g. with ultrasound and pulsed shortwave diathermy) and controversies have continued. For example, in 1990 Frizzell and Dunn believed there to be no evidence of biological effects arising with the use of low-energy ultrasound. By contrast, Mortimer and Dyson (1988) reported changes in the permeability of the cell membrane to calcium ions, while Dyson et al (1974) noted the temporary banding at half-wavelength intervals of blood cells and endothelial cell damage within blood vessels exposed to ultrasound in a stationary wave field in vivo.

More recently, the use of low-intensity pulsed ultrasound (LIPUS) (see Chapter 9) involves the delivery of mechanical energy at very low levels (typically 1/3 of the lowest power density employed with traditional ultrasound) yet the tissue healing response appears to be significantly influenced (reviewed in Bayat et al 2018; Harrison et al 2016). The energy levels employed are below those required to bring about perceptible tissue heating.

Similarly, Barker and Freestone (1985) and Barker (1993) expressed reservations with respect to pulsed shortwave diathermy, and many people have doubted the benefits of therapeutic laser. Although for many years the American Food and Drug Administration (FDA) was unconvinced of the clinical efficacy of low-level laser therapy (LLLT)/ photobiomodulation (PBM), this has now changed due to an increase in scientifically valid clinical trials. In 2002 the FDA granted approval for some LLLT devices to be marketed for specific indications, such as 'adjunctive use in providing temporary relief of minor chronic neck and shoulder pain of musculoskeletal origin' and for 'adjunctive use in the temporary relief of hand and wrist pain associated with carpal tunnel syndrome' (Swedish Laser Medical Society 2004).

A variety of suggestions has been made about the underlying ways in which predominantly non-thermal effects may occur. Many of those postulated are based on the suggestion that electrophysical energy can influence the mechanisms that lead to cell communication. Tsong (1989) suggested that cells communicate both directly through chemical means and indirectly through the influence of electrical, physical and acoustic signals. It seems that electrophysical energy may produce physiological changes through these mechanisms.

Work in this area has gained momentum recently, particularly as knowledge of growth factors and their role in tissue repair and function increases (Watson 2016). Researchers have examined the possible effects derived from using electromagnetic fields to stimulate cell activity (Cifra et al 2011) and recent work, using a variety of EM field parameters, has examined changes in growth-factor production, signalling pathways (e.g. Ca^{2+} mediated), cell growth and survival, cell cycle distribution, Cyclic adenosine monophosphate (cAMP) content and gap-junction-mediated communication between cells (e.g. Morabito et al 2017; Ross et al 2017; Tong et al 2017).

For any agent to be effective, the applied energy will need to have one or more identified targets in the tissue. These targets are most commonly described at the cellular or subcellular level, though energy transduction within extracellular molecules, such as collagen, might also be involved and result in the activation of these intracellular sites, here termed interactive targets.

INTERACTIVE TARGETS

'Interactive targets' are cellular components that may be receptive to energy-based interventions. These interactive targets include the cell membrane and intracellular structures, such as the intracellular membranes, microtubules, mitochondria, chromophores, cell-associated ions and the nucleus, each of which is briefly considered below.

Cell Membrane

The cell (plasma) membrane consists of a bilayered, phospholipid structure which surrounds the cell and is studded with transmembranous proteins (Alberts et al 1994; Hall 2011). These proteins have a number of functions: they strengthen the membrane; they transport substances such as proteins, sugars, fats and ions across the membrane;

and they form specialist receptor sites for hormones, neurotransmitters and enzymes. In addition, the cell membrane is electrically charged, possessing a negative charge on its internal surface and a positive charge on its external surface. The resulting potential difference of approximately 70 mV is maintained through the passive and active movement of ions across the cell membrane.

A number of EPAs are thought to effect changes at the level of the cell membrane. While much of the early work was reported in the 1980s (e.g. Adey 1988; Tsong 1989) more recent work, utilizing advanced cell techniques, has confirmed the capacity of EM energy to influence the behaviour of the cell membrane (e.g. Frey et al 2006; Krutakova et al 2016; Lucia 2016; Ross 2017). The general consensus among these researchers is that the membrane is the primary site of interaction between the EM energy and the cell. The membrane effectively achieves an amplification of a weak trigger achieved by conformational change, binding behaviour and channel/gating mechanisms resulting in membrane transport changes. It is further proposed that the strength and frequency of the applied EM field could be critical for optimal influence (Tsong 1989).

Mechanical energy might also effect changes in cell membrane behaviour; such changes have been shown to occur when therapeutic levels of ultrasound are applied to cells in vitro. Acoustic cavitation and its associated microstreaming results in membrane permeability changes, which in turn leads to enhanced cell activity levels. Hill and ter Haar (1982), Repacholi (1970) and Repacholi et al (1971) provided early reports of this phenomenon with Louw et al (2013), Whitney et al (2012) and Zhao et al (2016) providing more recent confirmation.

Mechanotransduction is receiving significant research attention as a means to describe how other mechanical energy applications, including ultrasound and shockwave, can bring about physiological responses in the tissue. The cell membrane is a primary target for these effects (Dunn 2016; Huang 2013).

While numerous researchers have identified the effects of laser light at mitochondrial level, there are numerous reports stretching back to the 1980s which identify the cell membrane as an evidenced target. Kujawa et al (2004), Lubart et al (1997) and Smith (1991) provided some of the seminal research followed by Karu et al (2005) and more recently, de Freitas and Hamblin (2016), Hamblin and Huang (2013) and Sassoli et al (2016). The modification of light sensitive Ca ion channels in the membrane has been demonstrated.

The cell membrane, therefore, is a target for electromagnetic, mechanical and light-based energies. Changing the behaviour, especially the permeability, of the membrane can initiate a cascade of intracellular effects, resulting in altered cell activity levels and, in turn, facilitated physiological responses.

Intracellular Membranes

Intracellular membranes surround the internal organelles of the cell and exhibit similar electrical characteristics to cell membranes (Hall 2011). One of their functions is to exercise control over the movement of substances into and out of these structures (Alberts et al 1994, Frohlich 1988) and thereby control the behaviour and actions of the organelles and ultimately of the entire cell. Similar effects to those induced at the cell surface may occur across these internal membranes, resulting in changes in activity of the organelles. Light-based therapies (de Freitas 2016; Hamblin 2018) are strongly evidenced as targeting the mitochondrial membrane and Keczan et al (2016) identify the influence of pulsed EM fields on the endoplasmic reticulum.

Microtubules

Microtubules are elongated cylinders made of protein that are present within cells and act as a cytoskeleton. Electrically, they consist of dimers, which are charged dipole units, their internal ends being negatively charged relative to the periphery. This arrangement results in the cell having similar electrical properties to electrets, which are insulators carrying a permanent charge analogous to permanent magnets. These properties include the ability to exhibit piezoelectric and electropiezo effects and, in addition, such dipole units rotate under the influence of oscillating fields. However, they do not respond equally to all frequencies of energy, but instead have preferred resonant frequencies, which are governed by their moment of rotation (Frohlich 1988).

Such dipole units may respond to the alternating magnetic and electrical fields produced by radiofrequency applications. The resulting dipole rotation motion will likely give rise to microthermal changes (see Chapter 7), and the absorption of energy (Muller 1983). More recently, these relations have been further explored in relation to EM fields (Lil 2019) magnetic fields (Dadras 2015) and ultrasound/vibration (Kucera 2017; Udroiu 2018) with positive findings which support the contention that microtubules can be added to the EPA energy target list.

Mitochondria

It has been suggested that mitochondria may be stimulated directly by the application of electrophysical energy. Laser (photobiomodulation) is a strong contender in this area, and a number of researchers have suggested that certain laser wavelengths may initiate changes at the mitochondria. Karu (1988) has postulated the following sequence of events: certain wavelengths of red light, when absorbed by components of the respiratory chain within the mitochondria, cause a brief activation of that chain; oxidation of the nicotinamide adenine dinucleotide (NAD) pool occurs, leading to changes in the redox status of the mitochondria and cytoplasm; these changes lead to altered membrane permeability and consequently to changes in the transport of ions across the cell wall. Hamblin (2018) and de Freitas and Hamblin (2016) add updated explanations that support the seminal evidence from 15 or more years ago.

Ions

Ions are electrically charged particles that are present in both intracellular and extracellular fluids. Being electrically charged, they respond to oscillating electrical fields and ionic vibration is likely to occur (Frohlich 1988). Such movement again may lead to changes in ionic distribution within the cells, affecting cell activity. A wide range of EPAs could achieve their effects, in part at least, by exerting a direct influence on ions in the extra and intracellular environment, Belayev and Markov (2015) clearly reporting this process in relation to RF applications and Cifra et al (2011) for EM field applications. Alternating electric currents and fields can be expected to influence ion movement and migration, though the frequencies at which they are employed in therapy would preclude sufficient vibration to achieve thermal activity.

Cells

If free to move and subjected to ultrasonically induced standing waves, entire cells can be transported in a predominantly non-thermal fashion to pressure nodes spaced at half-wavelength intervals (Dyson 1974). Most cell movement that occurs as a result of EPA application is now ascribed as a galvanotaxis (movement in response to an electric field) or chemotaxis (movement in response to a chemical gradient). While these are critical in some areas of EPA effects and mechanisms, their importance in terms of thermal and microthermal effects is not currently strongly evidenced.

THE EFFECT OF DOSAGE

While there are clearly evidenced effects of energy interactions at all levels (subcellular, cellular, tissue) there is a distinct 'dose' response at each. The amount of energy required to have a meaningful response clinically is considered in the specific modality chapters in this text. The evidence for cell and subcellular dose-response is also evidence, and while it may not directly relate to therapy applications, it is worthy of brief consideration.

Many forms of energy (including electrical, mechanical and chemical) may initiate changes in cell behaviour and it is clear that the dosage parameters of the energy imparted to the cell are likely to affect the end result. For example, Frohlich (1988) has suggested that ion oscillation and dipole rotation are dependent upon the frequency and amplitude of an applied electrical field. In the EPA realm, this proposal was extended (Watson 2010) with examples across several modalities.

Recent in vitro work using RF electric currents on cells in culture clearly showed that at lower energy levels, the cell level effects were positive, while at higher energy levels, they were detrimental (Hernandez-Bule 2007). Additionally, the same study clearly demonstrated the energy levels that were thermal and 'non-thermal' – the latter being employed in subsequent research in which a non-thermal cell-level effect was being investigated (e.g. Hernandez-Bule 2017), further evidencing that energy delivery to cells in culture at a level insufficient to instigate a thermal change was nevertheless able to bring about significant cellular change.

Tsong (1989) states that 'in principle, each class of protein is adapted to respond to an oscillating force field (electrical, sonic or chemical potential) of a defined frequency and strength'. Smith (1991) has suggested that laser radiations of different wavelengths may affect different structures; he postulates that radiation at 633 nm may initiate activity at the mitochondrial level, as suggested by Karu (1987), whereas at 904 nm it may initiate reactions at the cell membrane level, possibly through photophysical effects on calcium channels.

Takashima et al (2006) demonstrated the importance of dosage. Cells were exposed to EMFs (2.45 GHz) ranging from 0.05 to 1500 W/kg. Results varied from suppression of activity (continuous, 200 W/kg), through no effect (continuous application, 0.05–100 W/kg; intermittent application, 300, 900, 1500 W/kg peak (100 W/kg mean)) to an effect (continuous application, 50 W/kg for 2 hours). This final effect appeared to occur as a result of thermal changes. George et al (2002) specify that they selected their intervention based on the 'mitogenic' (i.e. cell-cycle-stimulating) properties of a specific spatial–temporal conformation of low-level, confined, high-frequency electromagnetic field. Li et al (1999) highlight the dose – and time-dependent nature of the effects seen in fibroblasts with the application of electromagnetic energy.

There is still relatively little information about the precise dosage parameters of many of these agents which are most likely to achieve therapeutic effects in clinical practice. The Arndt–Schultz law applies with ultrasound and light, too little energy having no measurable effect, too much being damaging, while energy levels between these extremes can be therapeutic. It appears that this 'rule' applies at cell, tissue and body segment levels – thereby constituting a stable construct.

CONCLUSION

This material has provided an overview that identifies both the microthermal (non-thermal) construct and provides a summary of the potential sites at which energy delivered at levels insufficient to generate measurable thermal change, can exert an effect. The terms 'non-thermal' and 'athermal' are not strictly correct, and although the use of 'microthermal' may appear pedantic, it is likely to be closer to reality.

The dose-response relationships demonstrated in many of these cell level studies reflects the situation when delivering electrophysical energy in the clinical setting. In modern practice, the delivery of energy at levels below the sensory thermal threshold (i.e. the level at which a patient will be able to determine a change in temperature) is amply demonstrated to have significant benefit. This in no way obviates the benefits of heat-based therapy applications – they have value and are clinically evidenced. It does, however, support the contention that it is not necessary to heat a tissue in order for meaningful therapeutic effects to be achieved.

REFERENCES

Adey, W. R. (1988). Physiological signalling across cell membranes and co-operative influences of extremely low frequency electromagnetic fields. In H. Frohlich (Ed.), *Biological coherence and response to external stimuli*. Heidelberg: Springer-Verlag.

Alberts, B., Bray, D., Lewis, J., et al. (1994). *Molecular biology of the cell* (2nd ed.). New York: Garland Publishing.

Algafly, A. A., & George, K. P. (2007). The effect of cryotherapy on nerve conduction velocity, pain threshold and pain tolerance. *British Journal of Sports Medicine*, 41(6), 365–369.

Barker, A. T. (1993). Electricity magnetism and the body. *IEE Science, Education and Technology Division December*, 249–256.

Barker, A. T., & Freestone, I. L. (1985). Medical applications of electric and magnetic fields. *IEE Electronics and Power*, 757–760.

Barnes, F. S., & Greenebaum, B. (2018). *Biological and medical aspects of electromagnetic fields*. CRC Press.

Bayat, M., Virdi, A., Jalalifirouzkouhi, R., & Rezaei, F. (2018). Comparison of effects of LLLT and LIPUS on fracture healing in animal models and patients: A systematic review. *Progress in Biophysics and Molecular Biology*, 132, 3–22.

Belyaev, I., & Markov, M. S. (2015). Biophysical mechanisms for nonthermal microwave effects. In M. S. Markov (Ed.), *Electromagnetic fields in biology and medicine*. Boca Raton: CRC Press.

Bowler, K. (1987). Cellular heat injury: Are membranes involved? In K. Bowler & B. J. Fuller (Eds.), *Temperature and animal cells* (pp. 157–185). Cambridge: Company of Biologists.

Brunt, V. E., Eymann, T. M., Francisco, M. A., Howard, M. J., & Minson, C. T. (2016). Passive heat therapy improves cutaneous microvascular function in sedentary humans via improved nitric oxide-dependent dilation. *Journal of Applied Physiology (1985)*, *121*(3), 716–723.

Chastain, P. B. (1978). The effect of deep heat on isometric strength. *Physical Therapy*, *58*, 543.

Cifra, M., Fields, J. Z., & Farhadi, A. (2011). Electromagnetic cellular interactions. *Progress in Biophysics and Molecular Biology*, *105*(3), 223–246.

Collins, K. J. (1992). Regulation of body temperature. In J. Tinker & W. M. Zapol (Eds.), *Care of the critically ill patient* (2nd ed.) (pp. 155–173). London: Springer-Verlag.

Costello, J. T., & Donnelly, A. E. (2010). Cryotherapy and joint position sense in healthy participants: A systematic review. *Journal of Athletic Training*, *45*(3), 306–316.

Daanen, H. A. (2003). Finger cold-induced vasodilation: A review. *European Journal of Applied Physiology*, *89*(5), 411–426.

Daanen, H. (2009). Cold-induced vasodilation. *European Journal of Applied Physiology*, *105*(4), 663–664.

Dadras, A., Naghshineh, A., Atarod, D., Liaghi, A., Riazi, G. H., & Afrasiabi, A. (2015). *Static magnetic fields can diminish neuron spines through microtubule dynamicity disruption*. 2015 Sixth International Conference of Cognitive Science (ICCS).

de Freitas, L. F., & Hamblin, M. R. (2016). Proposed mechanisms of photobiomodulation or low-level light therapy. *IEEE Journal of Selected Topics in Quantum Electronics*, *22*(3).

Draper, D. O. (2011). Injuries restored to ROM using PSWD and mobilizations. *International Journal of Sports Medicine*, *32*(4), 281–286.

Draper, D. O. (2014). Pulsed shortwave diathermy and joint mobilizations for achieving normal elbow range of motion after injury or surgery with implanted metal: A case series. *Journal of Athletic Training*, *49*(6), 851–855.

Dunn, S. L., & Olmedo, M. L. (2016). Mechanotransduction: Relevance to physical therapist practice-understanding our ability to affect genetic expression through mechanical forces. *Physical Therapy*, *96*(5), 712–721.

Dyson, M. (2006). *Primary, secondary, and tertiary effects of phototherapy: A review. Mechanisms for low-light therapy*. International Society for Optics and Photonics.

Dyson, M., Pond, J., Woodward, B., et al. (1974). The production of blood cell stasis and endothelial damage in the blood vessels of chick embryos treated with ultrasound in a stationary wave field. *Ultrasound in Medicine and Biology*, *1*, 133–148.

Edwards, R., Harris, R., Hultman, E., et al. (1970). Energy metabolism during isometric exercise at different temperatures of M. quadriceps femoris in man. *Acta Physiologica Scandinavica*, *80*, 17–18.

Eldred, E., Lindsey, D. F., & Buchwald, J. S. (1960). The effects of cooling on the mammalian muscle spindle. *Experimental Neurology*, *2*, 144–157.

Feibel, H., & Fast, H. (1976). Deep heating of joints: A reconsideration. *Archives of Physical Medicine and rehabilitation*, *57*, 513–514.

Fischer, E., & Solomon, S. (1965). Physiological responses to heat and cold. In S. Licht (Ed.), *Therapeutic heat and cold* (2nd ed.) (pp. 126–169). New Haven, CT: E Licht.

Flouris, A. (2009). *On the functional architecture of the human thermoregulatory system: A guide to the biological principles and mechanisms underlying human thermoregulation*. VDM Publishing.

Flouris, A. D., Westwood, D. A., Mekjavic, I. B., & Cheung, S. S. (2008). Effect of body temperature on cold induced vasodilation. *European Journal of Applied Physiology*, *104*(3), 491–499.

Foda, E., Almesri, I., Awbi, H. B., & Sirén, K. (2011). Models of human thermoregulation and the prediction of local and overall thermal sensations. *Building and Environment*, *46*(10), 2023–2032.

Foster, K. R., & Glaser, R. (2007). Thermal mechanisms of interaction of radiofrequency energy with biological systems with relevance to exposure guidelines. *Health Physics*, *92*(6), 609–620.

Frey, W., White, J. A., Price, R. O., Blackmore, P. F., Joshi, R. P., Nuccitelli, R., et al. (2006). Plasma membrane voltage changes during nanosecond pulsed electric field exposure. *Biophysical Journal*, *90*(10), 3608–3615.

Frizzell, L. A., & Dunn, F. (1990). Biophysics of ultrasound. In J. F. Lehmann (Ed.), *Therapeutic heat and cold* (4th ed.) (pp. 362–397). Baltimore, MD: Williams and Wilkins.

Frohlich, H. (1988). *Biological coherence and response to external stimuli*. Heidelberg: Springer-Verlag.

George, F. R., Lukas, R. J., Moffett, J., & Ritz, M. C. (2002). In vitro mechanisms of cell proliferation induction: A novel bioactive treatment for accelerating wound healing. *Wounds*, *14*, 107–115.

Gersten, J. W. (1955). Effect of ultrasound on tendon extensibility. *American Journal of Physical Medicine & Rehabilitation / Association of Academic Physiatrists*, *34*, 362–369.

Gkrilias, P. D., Tsepis, E. M., & Fousekis, K. A. (2017). The effects of hamstrings' cooling and cryostretching on sit and reach flexibility test performance in healthy young adults. *British Journal of Medicine and Medical Research*, *19*, 1–11.

Hall, J. E. (2011). *Guyton and Hall textbook of medical physiology*. Philadelphia: Saunders Elsevier.

Hamblin, M. R. (2018). Mechanisms and mitochondrial redox signaling in photobiomodulation. *Journal of Photochemistry and Photobiology B: Biology*, *94*(2), 199–212.

Hamblin, M. R., & Huang, Y. (2013). *Handbook of photomedicine*. Taylor & Francis.

Hardy, M., & Woodall, W. (1998). Therapeutic effects of heat, cold, and stretch on connective tissue. *Journal of Hand Therapy: Official Journal of the American Society of Hand Therapists*, *11*(2), 148–156.

Harris, E. D., Jr., & McCroskery, P. A. (1974). The influence of temperature and fibril stability on degradation of cartilage collagen by rheumatoid synovial collagenase. *New England Journal of Medicine*, *290*, 1–6.

Harrison, A., Lin, S., Pounder, N., & Mikuni-Takagaki, Y. (2016). Mode & mechanism of low intensity pulsed ultrasound (LIPUS) in fracture repair. *Ultrasonics, 70*, 45–52.

Hensel, H. (1981). *Thermoreception and temperature regulation. Monographs of the Physiological Society no. Vol. 38.* London: Academic Press.

Hernandez-Bule, M. L., Angeles Trillo, M., Martinez Garcia, M. A., Abilahoud, C., & Ubeda, A. (2017). Chondrogenic differentiation of adipose-derived stem cells by radiofrequency electric stimulation. *Journal of Stem Cell Research & Therapy, 7*(12), 7–12.

Hernandez-Bule, M. L., Trillo, M. A., Cid, M. A., Leal, J., & Ubeda, A. (2007). In vitro exposure to 0.57-MHz electric currents exerts cytostatic effects in HepG2 human hepatocarcinoma cells. *International Journal of Oncology, 30*(3), 583–592.

Herrera, E., Sandoval, M. C., Camargo, D. M., & Salvini, T. F. (2010). Motor and sensory nerve conduction are affected differently by ice pack, ice massage, and cold water immersion. *Physical Therapy, 90*(4), 581–591.

Hill, C. R., & ter Haar, G. (1982). Ultrasound. In M. J. Suess & D. A. Benwell-Morison (Eds.), *Nonionizing radiation protection series no. 10 199–228* (2nd ed.). Geneva: World Health Organization.

Huang, C., Holfeld, J., Schaden, W., Orgill, D., & Ogawa, R. (2013). Mechanotherapy: Revisiting physical therapy and recruiting mechanobiology for a new era in medicine. *Trends in Molecular Medicine, 19*(9), 555–564.

Igwea, S. E., Tabansi-Ochuogu, C. S., & Abaraogu, U. O. (2016). TENS and heat therapy for pain relief and quality of life improvement in individuals with primary dysmenorrhea: A systematic review. *Complementary Therapies in Clinical Practice, 24*, 86–91.

International Union of Physiological Sciences. (1987). Commission for thermal physiology. A glossary of terms for thermal physiology. *Pflugers Archiv: European Journal of Physiology, 410*, 567–587.

Jones, D., Round, J., & de Haan, A. (2004). *Skeletal muscle from molecules to movement.* London: Churchill Livingstone.

Jutte, L. S., Hawkins, J., Miller, K. C., Long, B. C., & Knight, K. L. (2012). Skinfold thickness at 8 common cryotherapy sites in various athletic populations. *Journal of Athletic Training, 47*(2), 170–177.

Jutte, L. S., Merrick, M. A., Ingersoll, C. D., & Edwards, J. E. (2001). The relationship between intramuscular temperature, skin temperature and adipose thickness during cryotherapy and rewarming. *Archives of Physical Medicine and Rehabilitation, 82*, 845–850.

Karu, T. I. (1987). Photobiological fundamentals of low power laser therapy. *IEEE Journal of Quantum Electronics, 23*, 1703–1717.

Karu, T. I. (1988). Molecular mechanism of the therapeutic effects of low intensity laser radiation. *Lasers in the Life Sciences, 2*, 53–74.

Karu, T. I., Pyatbrat, L. V., & Afanasyeva, N. I. (2005). Cellular effects of low power laser therapy can be mediated by nitric oxide. *Lasers in Surgery and Medicine, 36*, 307–314.

Keatinge, W. R. (1978). *Survival in cold water.* Oxford: Blackwell, 39–50.

Keczan, E., Keri, G., Banhegyi, G., & Stiller, I. (2016). Effect of pulsed electromagnetic fields on endoplasmic reticulum stress. *Canadian Journal of Physiology and Pharmacology, 67*(5), 769–775.

Kerslake, D. McK, & Cooper, K. E. (1950). Vasodilatation in the hand in response to heating the skin elsewhere. *Clinical Science, 9*, 31–47.

Khogali, M., & Hales, J. R. S. (1983). *Heat stroke and temperature regulation.* London: Academic Press.

Kramer, J. F. (1984). Ultrasound: Evaluation of its mechanical and thermal effects. *Archives of Physical Medicine and Rehabilitation, 65*, 223–227.

Krutáková, M., Matáková, T., Halašová, E., Šarlinová, M., Špánik, P., & Janoušek, L. (2016). *Analysis of electromagnetic field effect on cell plasma membrane potential.* 2016 ELEKTRO.

Kučera, O., Havelka, D., & Cifra, M. (2017). Vibrations of microtubules: Physics that has not met biology yet. *Wave Motion, 72*, 13–22.

Kujawa, J., Zavodnik, L., Zavodnik, I., et al. (2004). Effect of low-intensity (3.75–27 J/cm2) near-infrared (810 nm) laser radiation on red blood cell ATPase activities and membrane structure. *Journal of Clinical Laser Medicine and Surgery, 22*, 111–117.

Laymon, M., Petrofsky, J., McKivigan, J., Lee, H., & Yim, J. (2015). Effect of heat, cold, and pressure on the transverse carpal ligament and median nerve: A pilot study. *Medical Science Monitor: International Medical Journal of Experimental and Clinical Research, 21*, 446–451.

Lehmann, J. F., & de Lateur, B. J. (1990a). Therapeutic heat. In J. F. Lehmann (Ed.), *Therapeutic heat and cold* (4th ed.) (p. 444). Baltimore, MD: Williams & Wilkins.

Lehmann, J. F., & de Lateur, B. J. (1990b). Cryotherapy. In J. F. Lehmann (Ed.), *Therapeutic heat and cold* (4th ed.) (pp. 590–632). Baltimore, MD: Williams & Wilkins.

Lehmann, J. F., & de Lateur, B. (1999). Ultrasound, shortwave, microwave, laser, superficial heat and cold in the treatment of pain. In P. D. Wall & R. Melzack (Eds.), *Textbook of pain* (4th ed.) (pp. 1383–1397). New York: Churchill Livingstone.

Lehmann, J. F., Masock, A. J., Warren, C. G., & Koblanski, J. N. (1970). Effects of therapeutic temperatures on tendon extensibility. *Archives of Physical Medicine and Rehabilitation, 51*, 481–487.

Li, R., Ritz, M. C., Lukas, R. J., et al. (1999). Cell proliferation induction (CPI); dose- and time-dependent effects on fibroblast proliferation in vitro. *The FASEB Journal: Official Publication of the Federation of American Societies for Experimental Biology, 13*, 351.

Li, S., Wang, C., & Nithiarasu, P. (2019). Electromechanical vibration of microtubules and its application in biosensors. *Journal of The Royal Society Interface, 16*(151), 20180826.

Louw, T. M., Budhiraja, G., Viljoen, H. J., & Subramanian, A. (2013). Mechanotransduction of ultrasound is frequency dependent below the cavitation threshold. *Ultrasound in Medicine and Biology, 39*(7), 1303–1319.

Lubart, R., Friedmann, H., Sinyakov, M., et al. (1997). Changes in calcium transport in mammalian sperm mitochondria and plasma membranes caused by 780 nm irradiation. *Lasers in Surgery and Medicine, 21*, 493–499.

Lucia, U. (2016). Electromagnetic waves and living cells: A kinetic thermodynamic approach. *Physica A: Statistical Mechanics and Its Applications, 461*, 577–585.

Malanga, G. A., Yan, N., & Stark, J. (2015). Mechanisms and efficacy of heat and cold therapies for musculoskeletal injury. *Postgraduate Medical, 127*(1), 57–65.

Mangat, J., Standley, T., Prevost, A., Vasconcelos, J., & White, P. (2010). A comparison of technologies used for estimation of body temperature. *Physiological Measurement, 31*(9), 1105–1118.

Mense, S. (1978). Effects of temperature on the discharges of motor spindles and tendon organs. *Pflugers Arch, 374*, 159–166.

Miglietta, O. (1973). Action of cold on spasticity. *American Journal of Physical Medicine, 52*, 198–205.

Moore-Ede, M. C., & Sulzman, F. M. (1981). Internal temporal order. In J. Aschoff (Ed.), *Handbook of behavior neurobiology* (pp. 215–241). New York: Plenum Press.

Morabito, C., Steimberg, N., Rovetta, F., Boniotti, J., Guarnieri, S., et al. (2017). Extremely low-frequency electromagnetic fields affect myogenic processes in c2c12 myoblasts: Role of gap-junction-mediated intercellular communication. *BioMed Research International, 2017*, 2460215.

Morrison, S. F., & Nakamura, K. (2011). Central neural pathways for thermoregulation. *Frontiers in Bioscience (Landmark Ed), 16*, 74–104.

Mortimer, A. J., & Dyson, M. (1988). The effect of therapeutic ultrasound on calcium uptake in fibroblasts. *Ultrasound in Medicine and Biology, 14*, 499–506.

Muller, A. W. J. (1983). Thermoelectric energy conversion could be an energy source of living organisms. *Physics Letters A, 96*, 319–321.

Oosterveld, F. G., & Rasker, J. J. (1994). Effects of local heat and cold treatment on surface and articular temperature of arthritic knees. *Arthritis & Rheumatism, 37*(11), 1578–1582.

Otte, J. W., Merrick, M. A., Ingersoll, C. D., & Cordova, M. L. (2002). Subcutaneous adipose tissue thickness alters cooling time during cryotherapy. *Archives of Physical Medicine and Rehabilitation, 83*, 1501–1505.

Ottoson, D. (1965). The effects of temperature on the isolated muscle spindle. *Journal of Physiology, 180*, 636–648.

Paine, R. (2010). Rehabilitation and therapeutic modalities. Language of exercise and rehabilitation. In J. C. DeLee, D. Drez & M. D. Miller (Eds.), *DeLee and Drez's orthopaedic sports medicine principles and practice* (pp. 221–331). Philadelphia: Elsevier.

Palazzo, E., Rossi, F., & Maione, S. (2008). Role of TRPV1 receptors in descending modulation of pain. *Molecular and Cellular Endocrinology, 286*(1–2 Suppl. 1), S79–S83.

Price, R., Lehmann, J. F., Boswell-Bessette, S., et al. (1993). Influence of cryotherapy on spasticity at the human ankle. *Archives of Physical Medicine and Rehabilitation, 74*, 300–304.

Repacholi, M. H. (1970). Electrophoretic mobility of tumour cells exposed to ultrasound and ionising radiation. *Nature, 227*, 166–167.

Repacholi, M. H., Woodcock, J. P., Newman, D. L., & Taylor, K. J. W. (1971). Interaction of low intensity ultrasound and ionising radiation with the tumour cell surface. *Physics in Medicine and Biology, 16*, 221–227.

Rigby, B. J. (1964). The effect of mechanical extension upon the thermal stability of collagen. *Biochem Biophys Acta, 79*, 634–636.

Rigby, B. J., Hirai, N., & Spikes, J. D. (1959). The mechanical behaviour of rat tail tendon. *The Journal of General Physiology, 43*, 265–283.

Ross, C. L. (2017). The use of electric, magnetic, and electromagnetic field for directed cell migration and adhesion in regenerative medicine. *Biotechnology Progress, 33*(1), 5–16.

Sassoli, C., Chellini, F., Squecco, R., et al. (2016). Low intensity 635 nm diode laser irradiation inhibits fibroblast-myofibroblast transition reducing TRPC1 channel expression/activity: New perspectives for tissue fibrosis treatment. *Lasers in Surgery and Medicine, 48*(3), 318–332.

Sefiddashti, L., Ghotbi, N., Salavati, M., Farhadi, A., & Mazaheri, M. (2018). The effects of cryotherapy versus cryostretching on clinical and functional outcomes in athletes with acute hamstring strain. *Journal of Bodywork and Movement Therapies, 22*(3), 805–809.

Sethi, M., & Chakarvarti, S. (2015). Hyperthermia techniques for cancer treatment: A review. *International Journal of PharmTech Research, 8*(6), 292–299.

Smith, K. C. (1991). The photobiological basis of low level laser radiation therapy. *Laser Therapy, 3*, 19–24.

Swedish Laser Medical Society. (2004). Online. Available: http://www.laser.nu/lllt/fda.htm

Takashima, Y., Hirose, H., Koyama, S., et al. (2006). Effects of continuous and intermittent exposure to RF fields with a wide range of SARs on cell growth, survival and cell cycle distribution. *Bioelectromagnetics, 27*, 392–400.

Tong, J., Sun, L., Zhu, B., Fan, Y., Ma, X., Yu, L., & Zhang, J. (2017). Pulsed electromagnetic fields promote the proliferation and differentiation of osteoblasts by reinforcing intracellular calcium transients. *Bioelectromagnetics, 38*(7), 541–549.

Trnavsky, G. (1983). Die beeinflussing des Hoffman-reflexes durch kryoangzeittherapie. *Wiener Medizinische Wochenschrift, 11*, 287–289.

Tsong, T. Y. (1989). Deciphering the language of cells. *Trends in Biochemical Sciences, 14*, 89–92.

Udroiu, I., Marinaccio, J., Bedini, A., Giliberti, C., Palomba, R., & Sgura, A. (2018). Genomic damage induced by 1-MHz ultrasound in vitro. *Environmental and Molecular Mutagenesis, 59*(1), 60–68.

Wallace, L., Knortz, K., & Esterton, P. (1979). Immediate care of ankle injuries. *Journal of Orthopaedic & Sports Physical Therapy, 1*, 46.

Walter, S., & Buchner, J. (2002). Molecular chaperones – cellular machines for protein folding. *Angewandte Chemie International Edition, 41*(7), 1098–1113.

Warren, C. G., Lehmann, J. F., & Koblanski, J. N. (1971). Elongation of rat tail tendon: Effect of load and temperature. *Arch Physical Medicine and Rehabilitation, 52,* 465–475.

Warren, C. G., Lehmann, J. F., & Koblanski, J. N. (1976). Heat and stretch procedures: An evaluation using rat tail tendon. *Archives of Physical Medicine and Rehabilitation, 57,* 122–126.

Watson, T. (2010). Narrative review: Key concepts with electrophysical agents. *Physical Therapy Reviews, 15*(4), 351–359.

Watson, T. (2016). *Expanding our understanding of the inflammatory process and its role in pain & tissue healing.* Glasgow: IFOMPT 2016.

Weppler, C. H., & Magnusson, S. P. (2010). Increasing muscle extensibility: A matter of increasing length or modifying sensation? *Physical Therapy, 90*(3), 438–449.

Westerhof, W., Siddiqui, A. H., Cormane, R. H., & Scholten, A. (1987). Infrared hyperthermia and psoriasis. *Archives of Dermatological Research, 279,* 209–210.

Whitley, D., et al. (1999). Heat shock proteins: A review of the molecular chaperones. *Journal of Vascular Surgery: Official Publication, the Society for Vascular Surgery [and] International Society for cardiovascular Surgery, North American Chapter, 29*(4), 748–751.

Whitney, N. P., Lamb, A. C., Louw, T. M., & Subramanian, A. (2012). Integrin-mediated mechanotransduction pathway of low-intensity continuous ultrasound in human chondrocytes. *Ultrasound in Medicine and Biology, 38*(10), 1734–1743.

Wyper, D. J., & McNiven, D. R. (1976). Effects of some physiotherapeutic agents on skeletal muscle blood flow. *Physiotherapy, 62,* 83–85.

Zhao, L., Feng, Y., Hu, H., Shi, A., Zhang, L., & Wan, M. (2016). Low-intensity pulsed ultrasound enhances nerve growth factor-induced neurite outgrowth through mechanotransduction-mediated ERK1/2-CREB-Trx-1 signaling. *Ultrasound in Medicine and Biology, 42*(12), 2914–2925.

6

Superficial Heating

Binoy Kumaran

HISTORY

Heat has probably been used to manage pain and other symptoms relating to physical ailments for as long as humans have had access to usable sources such as hot springs and pools, hot rocks, or simply wrapping body parts in blankets. Heat can be an effective form of treatment, for example to manage pain, stiffness, oedema and spasticity. This chapter discusses the use of agents that produce a temperature rise through direct physical contact with tissues and through radiation.

Two main methods of heating are used in contemporary clinical practice: contact heating, commonly delivered via hot packs, paraffin wax and hydrotherapy, and radiant heating – infrared radiation (IR).

PHYSICAL PRINCIPLES

The concepts of heat and temperature are clearly defined and distinguished in physics. This distinction is maintained for electrophysical agents, as identified in Chapter 2. Both contact and radiant heating cause a rise in tissue temperature, but through dissimilar mechanisms. Radiant heating transmits electromagnetic (EM) energy to the body initiating heat production in the tissues. Heat transfer from heated agents during contact occurs because of 'conduction' via direct molecular collision. Energy exchange occurs between regions of different temperature, with thermal transfer from hotter to colder regions. The transferred energy increases molecular vibration, which in turn is transmitted to adjacent molecules. The rate of energy transfer depends on the temperature difference, surface area of contact and thermal conductivity of the treated tissue.

A radiant energy source, such as an IR lamp, emits electromagnetic waves, primarily in the IR band, when its surface temperature is above absolute zero. The rate of radiation emission depends on the nature of the lamp material and its surface temperature. IR is produced as a result of molecular motion (vibration or rotation of molecules within matter). The temperature of the radiating body affects the wavelength of the radiation, with the mean frequency of emission rising with an increase in temperature. Thus, the higher the temperature of the radiating body the higher the mean frequency of the output and, consequently, the shorter the wavelength. However, most radiating bodies do not emit IR of a single waveband – a number of different wavelengths may be emitted (e.g. luminous and non-luminous IR lamps) due to interplay between the emission and absorption of radiations affecting the behaviour of molecules. While some radiant energy is reflected from an object it encounters and some is transmitted through the object, some energy gets absorbed, resulting in heat production and hence a temperature rise.

BIOPHYSICAL EFFECTS

The general principles of heat–tissue interactions and their effects on pain and tissue repair are described in Chapter 5 and relate to both contact and radiant heating. It is important to remember that both types of heating produce only relatively superficial (primarily skin and subcutaneous tissues) thermal changes and that the effects will be minimal in the deeper tissues (e.g. muscle). Important effects include changes in cell function, vasodilatation (increased rate of blood flow), collagen production, neurological function (pain, spasm), muscle activity (contraction rates and power) and tissue repair. This section will identify the specific physiological mechanisms, issues, responses and interactions that pertain to superficial heat and will discuss recent research.

Heat induces changes in the tissues at local cellular and systemic levels. There is evidence from contemporary literature that application of superficial heat improves cutaneous microcirculation, either with moist heat (Binzoni et al 2012; Brunt et al 2016; Lohman et al 2011; Petrofsky et al 2010, 2012a & 2012b) or with dry heat (Clijsen et al 2008; Heinonen et al 2011; Kubo 2011; Song 2008). It can increase the extensibility of tendon and ligaments (connective tissue compliance) when the tissues are relatively superficial, such as in the hands and feet, and to some extent reduce the tone and spasm of muscles, the mechanism of which is likely sedation of pain nerve endings in the skin and superficial structures (Lehmann & de Lateur 1990; Petrofsky et al 2013; Robertson et al 2005). Heat is also cited as reducing the energy needed for muscle contraction by reducing the internal friction. In other words, warming the muscle reduces its internal energy costs (Jarosch 2008, 2011). Increase in local muscle temperature (in vastus lateralis) secondary to a hot pack was also shown to increase glycogenesis in a study by Slivka et al (2012).

The moisture levels in the skin influence the thermal response and heat transfer to deeper tissues. Petrofsky et al (2010) suggested that a substantial portion of the increase in skin blood flow associated with warm water therapy is probably connected with moisturizing of the skin rather than the heat itself. In their experiment the change in skin blood flow was significantly greater when the body was exposed to moist heat when compared with dry heat. However, this study was conducted on a small sample of young asymptomatic adults. The authors point out that older people and people with conditions such as diabetes may respond differently. Reducing moisture in the skin might have the effect of altering ionic flux through skin

thermal receptors (believed to be temperature sensitive calcium gated channels in endothelial cells which couple calcium influx to a release of nitric oxide (NO)). The 'bio heat' model first described by Pennes states that heat flow to or from tissues is proportional to the product of the perfusion rate of blood and the difference of arterial and tissue temperature (Brink and Werner 1994; Pennes 1948). Petrofsky et al (2009a) suggested that the Pennes model, which was intended to predict the temperature in resting skin and deeper tissues, should take the heat moisture content into consideration.

Skin is a barrier acting as a medium for heat exchange between the body's core and the external environment. When local heat is applied to the skin a bimodal response ensues. The initial response is linked to substance P and other vasoactive compounds, such as calcitonin gene-related peptide (CGRP) (Holwatz 2003; Minson et al 2001; Petrofsky et al 2009a). However, this initial increase in skin blood flow lasts only a few seconds and is replaced by a sustained increase in skin blood flow mediated by the release of NO (Charkoudian 2002, Holwatz 2003, Minson et al 2001). A full description of this process is beyond the scope of this text. Greater vasodilatation can be obtained with fast heating compared with slower heating (this could be achieved, for example, by increasing the temperature of the heat source): the difference is due to greater endothelial activity following fast heating compared to slow heating, suggesting that the rate of skin heating may alter the mechanisms contributing to cutaneous vasodilatation (Del Pozzi et al 2016).

The reflective and absorptive responses of skin to heat energy sources such as IR are not uniform due to its anatomical complexity (Moss et al 1989). Radiation must be absorbed to facilitate changes within the tissues, and absorption depends on the structure and type of tissue, vascularity and pigmentation. Penetration of IR energy into a medium is dependent upon the intensity of the source of IR, the wavelength/frequency, the angle of radiation to the surface and the coefficient of absorption of the material. The greatest penetration occurs when the rays are incident at 90° to the surface, and with wavelengths of 1.2 mm, whereas the skin is virtually opaque to wavelengths of 2 mm and more (Moss et al 1989). Research has shown that at least 50% of radiations of 1.2 mm penetrated to a depth of 0.8 mm, allowing interaction with capillaries and nerve endings (Hardy 1956). While almost all energy is absorbed by a depth of 2.5 mm (Selkins & Emery 1990), it is observed that long IR wavelengths penetrate to depths of 0.1 mm and shorter wavelengths up to 3 mm (Harlen 1980). In addition, because energy penetration decreases exponentially with depth, the greatest heating will occur most superficially. Some heating occurs at greater depths owing to the transfer of heat from the superficial tissue by conduction between layers of tissue, convection through the local circulation and increased blood flow. Infrared should, however, be regarded as a surface heating modality.

The temperature of the body is at a higher level than the shell and is finely regulated. The cooler temperature of the shell establishes a thermal gradient, thereby making heat exchange possible between the core and the external environment. The shell tissue itself has two thermal gradients: the skin surface being cooler than the deeper tissues (across approximately one centimetre), and the proximal part of the limb shell being warmer than the distal part (Kenney & Hodgson 1987; Singer 2007). The increased insulation resulting from subcutaneous fat will alter heat transfer to the deeper tissue when surface heat is applied. Impaired heat transfer may be found in overweight people; however, different heat modalities may affect heat transfer differently depending on their moisture content (Ducharme et al 1991; Igaki et al 2014; Petrofsky & Lind 1975a, 1975b; 1988). The typical Pennes model of heat transfer (Pennes 1948) does not account for the thickness of subcutaneous fat. If subcutaneous fat causes a time delay in heat transfer to and from the deep tissues, then a modality applied to the skin for a longer period of time would be better because the deep tissue temperature would eventually come to equilibrium at the applied higher temperature. A rapid heat modality, such as the whirlpool, may not be applied for long enough to overcome the insulation of the fat layer. The study by Petrofsky et al (2009b) showed that for heating modalities that are maintained in skin contact for long periods of time, such as dry heat packs (in place for 6 hours), subcutaneous fat did not impair the change in deep muscle temperature (measured at 25 mm below the skin surface). In contrast, when rapid heat modalities were used, such as the hydrocollator and the whirlpool (15 minutes of sustained skin contact), the transfer of heat from the skin to deep muscle was significantly impaired in people with thicker subcutaneous fat layers. At the same time as muscle heating was reduced, greater skin temperature increase was observed: this is probably explained by heat storage in the skin as a result of reduced heat transfer through the insulating fat layer. The skin temperature increase was proportional to the extent of impairment in the heat transfer from skin to muscle.

Individual factors, such as the presence of pathology, body composition and age, will affect the above mechanisms. Ageing skin will dissipate heat with reduced efficacy when there are deficits in circulation and thinning of the dermis, thereby reducing skin's ability to remove heat from the epidermis (McLellan et al 2009b; Petrofsky et al 2011): reduced subcutaneous fat as well as water content of

the skin may further affect heat dissipation in the elderly. The age-related reduction in skin's ability to dissipate heat secondary to reduced circulation and thinning of dermis is overall greater than the potential increase in heat dissipation due to reduced fat. It is proposed that the reduction in the blood flow response to heat with ageing may be linked to reduced skin moisture (Petrofsky et al 2012b). Similarly, in the presence of pathology, the body responds differently to heat. For example, in people with diabetes there is an increase in the amount of subcutaneous fat, reduction in capillary density and a reduction in dermal thickness: these changes cause people with diabetes to be more susceptible to heat stress and heat burns (McLellan et al 2009a, 2009b).

CLINICAL EVIDENCE

This section provides a critical summary of contemporary clinical research on the use of superficial and conduction heating. Numerous studies and reviews in the past have underlined the effect of superficial heat, mainly on conditions that cause pain and inflammation (Brosseau et al 2002; Chou & Huffman 2007; Dellhag et al 1992; French 2006; Nuhr et al 2004; Robinson et al 2002) and on stretching and range of movement (ROM) (Bleakley & Costello 2013; Henricson et al 1984; Lentell et al 1992; Nakano et al 2012).

In the last 10 years numerous studies have been published relating to effectiveness of thermotherapy in musculoskeletal conditions and some studies in non-musculoskeletal conditions. While most of these studies have employed various contact heating methods, some have employed IR heat as the energy source. Many studies used heating modalities as an adjuvant together with other physiotherapy treatments (Alptekin et al 2016; Aytar et al 2015; Benjaboonyanupap et al 2015; Cetin et al 2008; Gunay Ucurum et al 2018; Homayouni et al 2013; Köroğlu et al 2017; Ojoawo et al 2017; Satpute et al 2015; Tüzün et al 2017). Although it is not possible to determine the effect of heat treatments alone from these studies, as they formed part of an inclusive joint intervention, they inform the reader on the widespread use of superficial heat in therapy.

Musculoskeletal Conditions
Arthritis
Various studies on arthropathies, mainly osteoarthritis (OA) of the knee and hands, were identified and they formed the largest cohort of studies involving musculoskeletal conditions. Spa therapy of 1–2 weeks could significantly reduce pain and improve function of knee and hip joints according to Vaht and colleagues (2008). Patients received traditional Estonian spa therapy daily (Day 1 – mud treatment or paraffin–ozocerite treatment (42–45°C, 15 min); Day 2 – pearl bath or underwater shower massage

(35–37°C, 10–15 min), plus daily massage (20 min) and gym and pool exercises (30 min). Although this was a large study with 296 participants, it lacked a sufficiently robust study design and lacked any follow-up assessments. Similarly, Evcik et al (2007) compared effects of three superficial heating techniques on pain and function in 80 patients with OA knee, mostly females. All groups attended 10 sessions over 2 weeks, 20 minutes per session: balneotherapy (bathing in mineral water pools at 36°C), mud pack therapy (42°C) or hot pack therapy (42°C). All groups showed significantly reduced pain and improved physical function up to 12 weeks after treatment (all $p<0.05$). Balneotherapy and mud pack therapy were found to be significantly more beneficial for improving the quality of life, whereas hot pack therapy showed no benefit ($p>0.05$). The trial was neither randomized nor blinded, neither did it employ a control group.

In a more rigorously designed randomized controlled trial (RCT) involving patients with bilateral knee OA, Gungen et al (2012) compared 23 patients receiving mud pack treatment (45°C) with 21 patients receiving hot packs (42–45°C) for 12 sessions over 2 weeks at 20 minutes per session. Outcome measures were local inflammation, biological markers and cartilage degeneration. While both therapies were beneficial ($p<0.05$), the effects of mud pack treatment were more pronounced and sustained. The improvement in the biological markers were not sustained in the hot packs group ($p<0.017$). Similar findings about mud pack therapy when compared with hot packs (both applied at 42°C) were also reported by Sarsan et al (2012). Although the latter study employed a smaller sample (27 participants), the follow-up was longer (6 months as opposed to 3 months). These studies suggest that in comparison, mud pack therapy potentially provides greater benefits for patients with OA when compared with hot pack.

In a three-arm RCT of 45 patients with knee OA, superficial heat (dry hot pack at 40°C) when combined with transcutaneous electrical nerve stimulation (TENS) immediately improved knee pain during standing and walking, and improved dynamic balance and gait (Maeda et al 2017). The effects were significantly better than that of TENS alone or TENS combined with cold therapy. The study was single-session only, hence it is difficult to conclude the long-term clinical relevance.

Dilek et al (2013) investigated the effects of paraffin therapy on pain, function and muscle strength in 56 patients with hand OA. Paraffin (50°C) was applied for 15 sessions over 3 weeks. The authors reported a significant decrease in visual analogue scale (VAS) pain score and an improvement in hand muscle strength compared with the control group (advice and education) after 3 weeks, with the effects maintained for 12 weeks. This was a well-designed trial except that it was underpowered, and the participants were mostly females. Myrer et al (2011) compared the effects of two paraffin baths (at 52–57°C), one containing 100% wax by volume and the other containing 80% wax and 20% topical analgesic by volume, on patients with hand OA. Treatment consisted of 12 sessions over 4 weeks. Both groups registered significant reductions in pain but there was no difference between groups, indicating that added analgesics did not enhance the outcome. The trial did not employ a control group or any follow-up assessment. Similarly, paraffin therapy (52°C, 10 sessions over 2 weeks) when combined with 15 minutes of twice daily home exercises improved pain control, strength and function among patients with hand OA when compared with home exercises alone (Kasapoğlu Aksoy & Altan 2018). Benefit was seen up to 6 weeks post intervention; however, it is unclear if the patients continued with their exercises during the 6 weeks. The study was adequately powered, but potentially the paraffin group participants were more compliant with the exercises as they received more clinician contact.

Only a single study was identified on radiant heat, a pilot study by Oosterveld et al (2008), which suggested that IR treatment has significant short-term yet clinically relevant benefits in rheumatoid arthritis (RA) and ankylosing spondylitis. Eighteen patients with either RA or ankylosing spondylitis were treated in a whole-body IR cabin twice weekly, 30 minutes a session at 55°C, for 4 weeks. Clinically relevant improvements were noted in perceptions of pain, stiffness and fatigue by all patients after the intervention. Being a pilot cohort study, it lacked robustness in its methodology.

Tissue Compliance

There are several recent studies on the effect of superficial heat on tissue compliance and ROM. Bleakley and Costello (2013) performed a systematic review on the effect of various thermal agents (year range of identified studies was 1981 to 2011) and concluded that superficial heat (moist/dry hot pack, IR) immediately increases ROM in a variety of joints, and that a combination of heat and stretch is more effective than stretch alone. The authors recommended heat as an adjunct to therapeutic stretching. The review noted a high risk of bias in the included studies; however, there was clearer evidence for heat to increase ROM than for cold. Although it is generally accepted that heat is beneficial for improving joint ROM, its mechanism of action is not fully understood. One theory proposes that temperature change reduces pain responses thereby allowing patients to move through greater ROM without eliciting a protective response and co-contraction (Bleakley & Costello 2013). Muscle relaxation resulting from an increase in the sensitivity of neurotendinous organs, and a decrease in pain as a consequence of increased stretching and pain tolerance, also may allow a greater ROM (Garcia et al 2014; Nakano et al 2012).

Recently, Szekeres et al (2017a) reported a greater immediate increase in wrist ROM with whirlpool than with hot pack among patients undergoing rehabilitation after distal radius fracture. Sixty patients (mostly females) were randomized to receive either whirlpool therapy at 40°C or hot pack from a hydrocollator (water temperature at 73°C) for 15 minutes, in three consecutive weekly sessions. At the end of 3 weeks both groups had made similar progress in wrist ROM relative to baseline. One advantage of whirlpool is that it allows movements during heating unlike hot pack. The added benefit of performing motion during heating may be the reason for the finding of greater improvement in the whirlpool group. Unfortunately, the authors only measured active ROM (passive ROM unknown). A further study by Szekeres et al (2017b) employed similar methods, except that they measured hand volume and that both groups additionally underwent hand therapy for 30 minutes after the heating and were assessed a third time. There was a significant difference between groups immediately after heat application, as patients in the whirlpool group experienced an initial volume increase greater than those who received a hot pack ($p<0.001$). The group difference in volume change was no longer significant at the third assessment after the 30-minute hand therapy indicating that the oedema was temporary. The overall change in volume from enrolment in the study to completion of the study 3 weeks later was not statistically different between groups. There was no control group or follow-up assessments in either study.

The effects of paraffin wax and joint mobilization were tested on 37 patients with post traumatic stiff ankle in a study by Rashid et al (2013). Half the group were treated by wax bath followed by joint mobilization, and the other half by mobilization alone (60 sessions over 10 weeks). Mobilization performed after wax bath resulted in greater improvements in ROM and function ($p<0.05$). The number of treatment sessions employed in this study was significantly higher than that in most other studies. Potentially, it greatly exceeds what may be available to patients in the clinical settings of many countries.

Carpal Tunnel Syndrome

Paraffin wax may be a suitable treatment option to deliver superficial heat to the extremities for conditions like carpal tunnel syndrome (CTS); however, there are few recent studies on this topic. Horng et al (2011) treated 53 patients with CTS in three groups. Two groups received nightly splinting and paraffin treatment in addition to either nerve or tendon gliding exercises performed three times daily (paraffin at 55°C, twice a week for 8 weeks). The third group (control) received only paraffin and splinting. Pain and function improved significantly for all groups, including the control group, with no significant difference between groups for pain and symptom severity. Neither tendon nor nerve gliding exercises added benefit over the effects of using wax and splint alone for these outcomes. In a study by Chang et al (2014), involving 47 patients randomized to two groups, the efficacy of paraffin treatment (55°C for 20 minutes twice a week for 8 weeks) and splinting was compared to that of ultrasound therapy (1 MHz, 1 W/cm^2, 20% output, 5 cm^2 treatment head, 5 minutes twice a week for 8 weeks) and splinting. After 8 weeks, although both groups improved significantly in all the outcomes – pain, symptom severity and function – the effects of ultrasound were more pronounced. The drop-out rate was high and there was no follow-up assessment in either of the CTS studies discussed above. Moreover, it is difficult to determine how much of the improvement was due to paraffin and how much was due to splinting in either study.

In contrast, more recently Ordahan and Karahan (2017) compared a combination of paraffin, home exercise and splinting with splinting and exercise alone in 70 female patients with CTS (paraffin applied at 50°C, 5 days per week for 3 weeks, 15 minutes per session; splint worn throughout the day for 3 weeks). Based on pain, function and electrophysiological (EMG) outcomes, the authors concluded that splinting and exercise is an effective treatment for CTS, but the addition of paraffin therapy can significantly enhance the outcome ($p<0.05$). This was an adequately powered study; however, like the studies previously mentioned, there was no follow-up assessment. The paraffin group attended a significantly greater number of clinical sessions during the study; therefore, treatment compliance and therapist exposure may not have been equivalent across groups.

Other Studies

In a multi-centre blinded RCT Freiwald et al (2018) investigated the effects of supplemental heat therapy on strength and flexibility in multimodal treated patients with chronic low back pain (LBP) and concluded that thermotherapy for several hours a day additional to individualized multimodal treatment can enhance strength parameters. Within a multimodal treatment concept (interdisciplinary treatment under supervision of physicians, physiotherapists, sports therapists and psychologists), 176 patients, randomized chronologically into two equal groups, were treated either with or without a supplemental 40°C heat wrap worn on the lower back for 8 hours. The multimodal treatment was carried out in two phases of 6 weeks, with two 90-minute therapy sessions per week (all patients underwent warm-up, stretching, equipment-based training, cooling down and extension followed by treatment with paraffin heat carriers at 50–60°C for 20 minutes over the entire length of the spine). The range of movement and strength parameters of the trunk (flexion, extension, lateral flexion and rotation measured in a biomechanical measurement device) were measured before and after 12 weeks of treatment. Patients receiving additional thermotherapy showed a greater but non-significant improvement in strength in extension ($p=0.09$) and rotation ($p=0.09$) compared with those receiving only the multimodal treatment. No group differences were detected in flexibility. The study did not measure outcomes on pain or quality of life. Also, long-term benefits of this treatment approach are unknown as there were no follow-ups.

In another study on patients with chronic LBP, Lewis et al (2012) reported that the use of heat wrap is associated with a decrease in muscle activity and a short-term improvement in certain aspects of well-being (perceived disability, pain-related anxiety, catastrophizing and self-efficacy) ($p<0.05$), indicating a link between the biomechanical and psychological factors. Twenty-four participants with chronic LBP and 11 asymptomatic participants (controls) were assessed on two occasions for changes in muscle activity (using EMG), stature (using a standing standiometer), pain and function. On the second occasion, a heat wrap (40°C) was given to the participants in advance, with instructions to put it on 2 hours before the time of the assessment. The heat wrap was then worn throughout the testing session. When compared to participants with chronic LBP, the control group participants demonstrated no change. As noted in the Freiwald et al (2018) study, the longer-term effects are unknown.

It is thought that superficial heat may have potential to diminish arthrogenic muscle inhibition in the quadriceps, as therapeutic heat can modulate pain by stimulating sensory receptors. This was however contradicted in the study by Warner et al (2013), where a 15-minute superficial moist heat pack (stored in a commercial unit at 77°C) applied to the knee joint did not change quadriceps central activation or maximal isometric knee-extension torque in individuals with history of knee injury. Twelve subjects were measured on an isokinetic dynamometer in a three-arm crossover RCT (heat, no heat, control) where they either performed a maximal voluntary isometric contraction (with or without heat) or rested. This was a single-session study mostly comprising young adults. As stated previously, the response could be different in older adults with different pathology, and especially with longer-term treatment.

The potential benefit of superficial heat has been investigated in a variety of other conditions. The clinical efficacy of immediate rewarming after application of vapocoolant spray in patients with myofascial pain syndrome was investigated by Bahadir et al (2010). Eighty female patients with myofascial pain in upper trapezius muscle were studied in two groups. Patients were treated on three consecutive days with either conventional spray and stretch or with spray and stretch and rewarming with a moist hot pack for 60 seconds. Improvements in pain and cervical ROM were significantly higher in the hot pack group. Leung and Cheing (2008) reported that in patients with frozen shoulder, the addition of superficial heat (electrical hot pack set at 63°C) to stretch was more effective than stretch alone, but less effective than deep heat (obtained using short-wave therapy) combined with stretch in improving shoulder pain and function ($p \leq 0.016$). Thirty patients (mostly females) were treated in three groups involving 12 sessions over 4 weeks at 20 minutes per session. The control group (stretching only) attended the clinic less frequently than the other two groups raising concerns about equivalent treatment compliance between groups. Also, the sample size was potentially too small to give the study sufficient statistical power.

Two thermal baths daily (at 36± 1°C for 20 minutes) for 2 weeks (balneotherapy) in addition to usual medication and exercise was found to improve the symptoms and function in women affected by fibromyalgia when compared with medication and exercise only (significance levels not reported) (Ozkurt et al 2012). The study included 50 participants randomized to two groups, however, the study had limited statistical power. Also, the control group participants had significantly less contact with the researchers compared to the balneotherapy group. Bagdatli et al (2015) examined the effects of adding balneotherapy to patient education on the symptoms of fibromyalgia. Thirty-five female patients in the balneotherapy group received 10 heated baths at 38°C for 20 minutes. Immediately after the immersion, mud packs at 45°C were applied to the back region of the patients for 20 minutes. Thirty-five female patients in the control group (education) continued with their standard care. Similar to the study above, the balneotherapy group showed greater and more significant improvements in pain ($p=0.002$) and function ($p<0.05$).

Non-Musculoskeletal Conditions

A recent Cochrane Review (Smith et al 2018) showed that treatment using hot or warm packs may have a role in reducing pain, reducing length of labour and improving women's sense of control and emotional experience of labour in primiparous women. Warm packs were associated with reduced pain in the first stage of labour and reduced length of labour. The quality of evidence, however, was poor. The review included three recent studies where heat therapies were employed (Behmanesh et al

2009; Ganji et al 2013; Taavoni et al 2013). All three trials employed comparable study methods by applying a warm pack to the low back, sacrum and/or perineal area (except that Ganji et al (2013) also used an ice pack intermittently) during various stages of labour. Although greater and statistically significant benefits in pain and duration of labour were reported with the addition of heat therapy, it is unclear if these benefits were clinically meaningful. Potentially, the results were further affected by participant selection bias, lack of assessor blinding and the absence of a placebo group. Moreover, it was likely that the participants in the warm pack group received a greater duration of care.

The study by Denton et al (2018) demonstrated that bilateral application of gel-filled hot packs and an insulating wrap (neoprene) to the leg muscles for 30 minutes significantly improved walking speed and foot tap time in hereditary and spontaneous spastic paraparesis in the short term (1 hour after application). On one occasion the insulating wrap was maintained for a further 30 minutes after the hot pack application and on the other occasion it was removed with the hot pack after the initial 30 minutes of application. This was a randomized crossover study on 21 patients with a relatively rare medical condition. There was no control group, and the assessment was not blinded. With only one session per treatment condition, it is unclear whether the results would have any bearing in the long term or on other neurological conditions.

Previous studies have also demonstrated the effects of heat on nerve conduction velocity and muscle spindle excitability. The anti spastic effects of thermotherapy were reported by Matsumoto et al (2006) in a single-session experimental study involving 10 male patients with post-stroke spastic hemiparesis and 10 healthy controls. The patients, who were not on any anti spasticity medication, were immersed in water at 41°C for 10 minutes and their F-wave parameters studied (amplitude and duration) from recordings made over the abductor hallucis muscle; F-waves can be used to study long pathway nerve conduction and motor neuron excitability. The patients whose F-wave parameters were higher on the affected side prior to thermotherapy showed significant reduction after treatment in contrast to the healthy controls for whom there was no change. Similar results were repeated in a later study by Matsumoto et al (2010): identical methods were employed, except that only the affected leg was immersed up to the knee in warm water at 41°C for 15 minutes using a foot bath. Being cohort studies lacking a robust design, both studies were limited in their scope; in addition, being a single-session study the longer-term benefits and comparative efficacy in relation to usual care could not be determined.

In another study, Gu et al (2016) demonstrated significant warming effects using superficial heating methods in people with hand hypothermia due to Raynaud's disease. Forty-two participants were enrolled in two groups – group 1 participants suffered from Raynaud's and demonstrated hand hypothermia; group 2 were a normothermic control group with no hand hypothermia. The treatment methods used were hot pack (tank set at 80°C), paraffin bath (55°C) and IR lamp (250 W at 50 centimetres), with each heat treatment applied for 20 minutes to both groups. Significantly greater change in skin temperature was noted in the hypothermic group when compared to the control group. Among the three modalities, hot pack appeared to bring the greatest change for the hypothermic group compared to the other two methods ($p<0.05$). However, it is normal for skin temperature to increase after the application of therapeutic heat. Whether it is sustained for longer periods and whether it helps clinically to alleviate the symptoms of Raynaud's disease remains to be seen.

The use of a heating pad with far-infrared radiation improved blood flow and autonomic nervous system function in patients with diabetes, thereby improving and alleviating the symptoms of diabetes-related complications, according to a recent study by Lung et al (2019). Ten patients with diabetes and four people without diabetes were recruited for this study. The participants were assessed for their microvascular function before and after the interventions in each month for three consecutive months. The results showed that surface temperature increased by 2°C after using the pad in the first and third months; and blood flow increased on the plantar foot but not on the dorsal foot. The increase in blood flow may serve to alleviate diabetes-related complications.

Summary of the Evidence

This review of recent literature has focused on individual RCTs involving the use of superficial heat. In a Cochrane Review, French et al (2006) concluded that there is moderate evidence that heat wrap therapy provides small short-term reduction in pain and disability in populations with a mix of acute and sub-acute LBP, and that the addition of exercise further reduces pain and improves function. The review by Chou and Huffman (2007) suggested that superficial heat is the only non-pharmacologic therapy with good evidence of efficacy for acute LBP among other therapies, such as massage, yoga, exercise and manipulation. Furthermore, past studies have also highlighted the usefulness of superficial heat combined with stretch in improving ROM of joints such as the hip (Henricson et al 1984), knee (Lin 2003) and shoulder (Lentell et al 1992), and for pain and other symptoms of arthritis (Ayling & Marks 2000; Brosseau et al 2002; Dellhag et al 1992; Yurtkuran et al

2006) and for the treatment of post-exercise delayed onset muscle soreness (Mayer et al 2006). For a more detailed analysis of the earlier literature, the reader is advised to refer to older texts and literature.

Various arthropathies, mainly OA of the knee and hands, comprised the largest cohort of recent studies. In general, the studies across all conditions, despite their identified methodological limitations, recommended the application of some form of heat as the main or as an adjunct treatment. Superficial heat for knee OA is also recommended in clinical guidelines (McAlindon et al 2014), in conditions such as CTS that benefit from pain relief, and for conditions where increasing the tissue extensibility is the principal aim. In these cases the heat may play a significant role by reducing pain and inflammation, thereby allowing other therapies, such as passive stretching, to be applied, or exercises performed (fibromyalgia) more effectively (providing a treatment window).

The preceding review should be considered in the context of the overall volume and varying quality of the studies. Not many studies were published in the last 10 years and robustness and integrity of methodological designs were often lacking. Where the treatment doses were reported adequately, the rationale for selection was unclear. Additionally, most studies either did not report statistical power and clinical significance of their findings, or they fell short of enough power to detect a statistically significant treatment effect. Participant drop-outs, which were sometimes high, were not accounted for in the final analysis in most studies (no intention-to-treat analysis) as would be the norm in high quality studies. Owing to the varied nature of heating methods, outcomes and intervention protocols in the identified studies, it has not been possible to compare and draw any commonalities between them or to identify and draw any conclusions on treatment protocol and dosing. Wider and further research is needed to establish which superficial heating modality would provide the maximum benefits and for which conditions.

THERAPEUTIC USES

Heat therapy is used in clinical practice to relieve subacute pain and inflammation; reducing pain and inflammation will enable patients to do their exercises more effectively. Changes arising in tissues from an increase in the blood flow, oxygen uptake and chemical reaction rates are believed to be the physiological mechanisms underpinning the effects of heat on pain and tissue repair. Although heating alone can be of significant benefit, when used in combination (e.g. heating prior to stretching of tight tissue structures using manual therapy or exercise therapy) it enhances the effectiveness of the overall treatment outcome. In other instances, heat has a palliative effect on patients suffering from pain and stiffness due to conditions such as degenerative joint disease. It is also used widely as an adjunct to stretching to improve joint ROM (Bleakley & Costello 2013).

Maximal elevation of the temperature of the skin and very superficial tissues will occur within 6–8 minutes of application of a heat source. The underlying muscle will respond to a lesser extent and more slowly, and, at tolerable skin temperatures, muscle temperature can be expected to be raised by about 1°C at a depth of 3 cm. However, where subcutaneous fat is present, heating of deeper tissues is less because of insulation. Where a greater depth of penetration is required, deep-heating modalities, such as radiofrequency-based therapies or ultrasound, should be employed. Considering the fact that a higher level of temperature rise (3–4 °C) is required at depth (at the joint level) to enhance tissue extensibility, any increase in ROM secondary to superficial heating may only be due to muscle relaxation and/or pain relief.

It is not the primary aim of this chapter to provide the reader with a recipe for treatment where superficial heat can be used. Where appropriate, superficial heat should be used as an adjunct to other treatment methods to reduce pain and inflammation that are sub-acute or chronic in nature. This may include conditions such as (but not limited to) OA, RA, CTS and chronic LBP. Superficial heat is also recommended combined with stretching where reducing stiffness and increasing the ROM is a treatment aim (e.g. post trauma stiffness). Such treatment may be considered also for non-musculoskeletal conditions, such as labour pain. As a general rule, acute conditions (e.g. acute sprain with swelling) and infected tissues are not suitable for such treatment due to the risk of further swelling, aggravation of inflammation due to vasodilatation and potential spread of infection. Similarly, heating avascular tissues and areas that lack sensation should be avoided to prevent burns.

Heating modalities often tend to be overused by patients while it is unnecessary or even inappropriate. Patient education is therefore imperative, because superficial heating modalities such as electrical/microwaveable heating pads and hot-water bottles are commonly used by patients at home. Precautions and contraindications are covered in detail in Chapter 22.

APPLICATION

Contact Techniques

Surface heat can be applied using various approaches. All raise superficial tissue temperatures, but some may be more suitable in given situations owing to the material used (e.g. wet or dry heat) and practicalities. The most common methods are considered here. Before any application, the body part should be inspected for any contraindications and washed; an explanation and safety warnings should be given.

Wet Versus Dry Heat

An important factor to be considered when selecting thermal treatments is that of choosing between wet and dry contact techniques. The relative efficacy of one compared with the other is still debated; however, it is suggested that dry heat can elevate surface temperature to a slightly greater degree, whereas wet heat can lead to rises in temperature at slightly deeper levels (Abramson 1967; Brunt et al 2016; Heinonen et al 2011; Petrofsky et al 2009b, 2010). Thus either can be used for closed injuries, with choice largely dependent on pragmatic considerations. Wet techniques have the potential to introduce infection into an open wound and to waterlog tissues. Drying, for example with IR heating, can be detrimental to wound repair but has been demonstrated to be effective in the management of some skin conditions.

Hot Packs and Pads

A variety of heated pads/packs may be used to provide heat to small areas.

Dry pads/packs. These are the most common, vary greatly, and include many that can be bought over the counter or are home made. They include those that contain heat-retentive gels, hot water (hot water bottles), grains, such as wheat, electrical elements or heat-producing chemicals. They can be heated in microwave ovens, by electrical means or through mixing chemical components within a sachet (often by simply crushing). The temperature of the final pack should be around 40–42°C. Gradual cooling of the pack will occur. If the pack comes with a one-sided insulating layer, or if an insulating layer can be wrapped around the body part (e.g. neoprene sleeve), heat loss will be slowed down.

Moist pads/packs. These are hydrocollator packs used to provide moist heat. The pack normally consists of a fabric envelope with silica gel or bentonite as filling. They are prepared for application using a hydrocollator unit with hot water typically maintained at 71–74°C. After immersion in the hot water for about 20 minutes the pack reaches around 41°C and is applied to the skin with several layers of towelling for about 15–20 minutes. They perform a similar function to the dry packs above but tend to cool more quickly because the surface of the pack exposed to room air is usually covered only by cotton towelling.

Application. The type of pack is selected based on the comments above. The part to be treated must be able to tolerate the pressure of the pack, besides its temperature. Replenishment of the packs during treatment can prolong heating, however, no additional significant differences are found in subcutaneous temperatures due to prolonging the heating (Lehmann et al 1966).

Paraffin Wax

Paraffin wax, with a melting point of approximately 54°C, is combined with a mineral oil, such as liquid paraffin, to produce a temperature-controlled bath of between 42° and 50°C. These temperatures are slightly higher than would be tolerated if the body part were placed in hot water. This is because the specific heat of paraffin wax is less than that of water (2.72 kJ/kg per °C for wax and 4.2 kJ/kg per °C for water). Wax therefore releases less energy than water while the wax cools. The amount of heat imparted to the tissue due to the solidification of the wax – the latent heat of fusion – is small (Selkins & Emery 1990). At the same time, heat loss is prevented owing to the insulating nature of the wax coating. The net result is a well-insulated, low-temperature method of heating tissue. Slightly higher temperatures may be used for the upper extremities than for the lower extremities and newly healed tissue (Burns & Conin 1987; Head & Helms 1977).

Application. In the dip and wrap method, the part is first immersed in the warm wax, then withdrawn and the wax allowed to set. The procedure is repeated, normally 6 to 12 times, to develop a 'wax glove'. The whole is then wrapped in plastic or waxed paper, and finally enclosed in an insulating layer of material, such as towelling. Alternatively, the part may be retained in the bath following the development of the wax glove – the dip and re-immerse method. This technique results in a greater increase in temperature (Abramson et al 1964; Abramson et al 1965).

Hydrotherapy

The use of hot water to heat tissues is an effective way of increasing temperature, and both still-water baths and – less often – whirlpool baths may be used for local treatment. Temperatures are usually between 36 and 41°C (lower than wax temperatures for the reasons discussed above). Treatment at these temperatures results in an increase in cutaneous/subcutaneous temperature. The motion of the water in whirlpool baths may, in addition, stimulate receptors in the skin surface, giving rise to pain relief through the pain gate mechanism (Borell et al 1980).

Application. This treatment should only be used when a wet application is appropriate; see above. Movement of the body part can occur during heating, which could be encouraged in the form of ROM exercises, where appropriate, to reduce dependency oedema.

TABLE 6.1	Characteristics of Luminous and Non-Luminous Generators		
Generator	Peak Wavelength Emitted	Power Levels Emitted	Comments
Luminous	1 mm IR and visible radiations emitted	250 and 1500 W	Red filters used; minimal warm-up period required (few minutes)
Non-luminous (resistance wire embedded in insulating material)	4 mm IR radiation emitted; wider spectrum of emission	250 and 1000 W	No filter; warm-up period required (approximately 15 minutes)

IR, Infrared.

Radiant Techniques

Infrared Radiation

All hot bodies emit IR to varying degrees and sources can be either natural (e.g. the sun) or artificial. Artificial IR is generally produced by passing an electrical current through a coiled resistance wire, and therapeutically both luminous generators (radiant heaters) and non-luminous generators are available. Their characteristics are shown in Table 6.1. Many sources that emit visible light or ultraviolet (UV) radiation also emit IR. The International Commission on Illumination (CIE) describes IR in terms of three biologically significant bands, which differ in the degree to which they are absorbed by biological tissues and therefore in their effect upon those tissues. The wavelengths mainly used in clinical practice are between 0.7 mm (700 nm) and 1.5 mm (1500 nm) and are concentrated in the IRA band.

Application. Before treatment, the body part should be inspected for any contraindications and an explanation and safety warnings given (see Chapter 22 for contraindications). The following procedure should be used when applying IR therapy:

1. Select and warm up equipment.
2. Patient preparation: a comfortable, supported position is required to allow the subject to remain still. The skin should be uncovered, clean and dry, all liniments and creams having been removed.
3. Lamp position: at a right-angle to the skin to facilitate maximum absorption of energy but not directly above a part to avoid burns should the lamp fall. A distance of between 50 and 75 cm is suggested, although this should be adjusted depending on patient sensation.
4. Dosage: this is determined in clinical practice by the response of the subject. It is essential, therefore, that the patient is advised of the appropriate level of heating and understands the importance of reporting any unexpected heating sensation or adverse response, such as pain or sweating.

Dosage. The amount of energy received by the patient will be governed by:

1. Intensity of the lamp output.
2. Distance between the lamp and the patient.
3. Duration of treatment.

A gradual rise in temperature is noted during the first 10 minutes of irradiation, with the return to normal taking an average of 35 minutes (Crockford & Hellon 1959). The intensity is altered either by changing the distance of the lamp from the body part or by altering the output of the generator. By the end of a treatment, a mild dose should generate skin temperatures in the region of 36–38°C, and a moderate dose should produce temperatures of between 38 and 40°C. Infrared treatment is normally continued for a period of between 10 and 20 minutes, depending on the size and vascularity of the body part, and the type and chronicity of the lesion.

SUMMARY

Heat has been used for centuries to manage symptoms from physical ailments. This chapter discussed the biophysical effects, evidence base and methods of use of superficial heat in clinical practice. While contact methods cause tissue heating primarily by conduction, radiant heating transmits electromagnetic energy causing heat production in the tissues. The main methods of contact heating (moist or dry) are hot packs, paraffin wax and hydrotherapy. Radiant heat is normally applied using IR lamps. Both contact and radiant heating methods produce only relatively superficial (primarily skin and subcutaneous tissues) thermal changes, hence the effects will be minimal in the deeper tissues (e.g. muscle). Heat can induce changes in the tissues at local cellular and systemic levels, leading to numerous therapeutic benefits. It is argued that the amount of moisture in the skin influences the depth of heat penetration. Individual factors, such as the presence of pathology, body composition and age, will affect the body's response.

A review of literature published in the past decade on the use of superficial heat in clinical practice identified a modest number of studies. The methodological quality of these was varied. Various studies on arthropathies (mainly OA of knee and hands) formed the largest cohort. Heat may play a significant role by reducing pain and inflammation, thereby enhancing tissue healing and helping to enhance stretching and ROM. An increase in tissue temperature by about 1°C will help to relieve mild inflammation whereas an increase of 2–3°C will lead to reduction in pain and muscle spasm. It is recommended that superficial heat is best used in combination with other treatment methods (e.g. adjunct to manual therapy or exercise) rather than on its own. Wider and further research is needed to establish which superficial heating modality would provide the maximum benefits and for which conditions.

REFERENCES

Abramson, D. I. (1967). Comparison of wet and dry heat in raising temperature of tissue. *Archives of Physical Medicine and Rehabilitation, 48*, 654.

Abramson, D. I., Chu, L. S. W., & Tuck, S. (1965). Indirect vasodilation in thermotherapy. *Archives of Physical Medicine and Rehabilitation, 46*, 412.

Abramson, D. I., Tuck, S., & Chu, L. (1964). Effect of paraffin bath and hot fomentations on local tissue temperature. *Archives of Physical Medicine and Rehabilitation, 45*, 87–94.

Alptekin, H. K., Aydin, T., Iflazoglu, E. S., & Alkan, M. (2016). Evaluating the effectiveness of frozen shoulder treatment on the right and left sides. *Journal of Physical Therapy Science, 28*(1), 207–212.

Ayling, J., Marks, R. (2000). Efficacy of paraffin wax baths for rheumatoid arthritic hands. *Physiotherapy, 86*(4), 190–201.

Aytar, A., Baltaci, G., Uhl, T. L., Tuzun, H., Oztop, P., & Karatas, M. (2015). The effects of scapular mobilization in patients with subacromial impingement syndrome: A randomized, double-blind, placebo-controlled clinical trial. *Journal of Sport Rehabilitation, 24*(2), 116–129.

Bagdatli, A. O., Donmez, A., Eroksuz, R., et al. (2015). Does addition of 'mud-pack and hot pool treatment' to patient education make a difference in fibromyalgia patients? A randomized controlled single blind study. *International Journal of Biometeorology, 59*(12), 1905–1911.

Bahadir, C., Dayan, V. Y., Ocak, F., & Yiğit, S. (2010). Efficacy of immediate rewarming with moist heat after conventional vapocoolant spray therapy in myofascial pain syndrome. *Journal of Musculoskeletal Pain, 18*(2), 147–152.

Behmanesh, F., Pasha, H., & Zeinalzadeh, M. (2009). The effect of heat therapy on labor pain severity and delivery outcome in parturient women. *Iranian Red Crescent Medical Journal, 11*(2), 188–192.

Benjaboonyanupap, D., Paungmali, A., & Pirunsan, U. (2015). Effect of therapeutic sequence of hot pack and ultrasound on physiological response over trigger point of upper trapezius. *Asian Journal of Sports Medicine, 6*(3), e23806.

Binzoni, T., Tchernin, D., Richiardi, J., Van De Ville, D., & Hyacinthe, J. N. (2012). Haemodynamic responses to temperature changes of human skeletal muscle studied by laser-Doppler flowmetry. *Physiological Measurement, 33*(7), 1181–1197.

Bleakley, C. M., & Costello, J. T. (2013). Do thermal agents affect range of movement and mechanical properties in soft tissues? A systematic review. *Archives of Physical Medicine and Rehabilitation, 94*(1), 149–163.

Borell, P. M., Parker, R., & Henley, E. J. (1980). Comparison of in vivo temperatures produced by hydrotherapy, paraffin wax treatment and fluidotherapy. *Physical Therapy, 60*, 1273–1276.

Brink, H., & Werner, J. (1994). Efficiency function: Improvement of classical bioheat approach. *Journal of Applied Physiology, 77*, 1617–1622.

Brosseau, L., Robinson, V., Léonard, G., et al. (2002). Efficacy of balneotherapy for rheumatoid arthritis: A meta-analysis. *Physical Therapy Reviews, 7*(2), 67–87.

Brunt, V. E., Eymann, T. M., Francisco, M. A., Howard, M. J., & Minson, C. T. (2016). Passive heat therapy improves cutaneous microvascular function in sedentary humans via improved nitric oxide-dependent dilation. *Journal of Applied Physiology, 121*(3), 716–723.

Burns, S. P., & Conin, T. A. (1987). The use of paraffin wax in the treatment of burns. *Physiotherapy Canada, 39*, 258.

Cetin, N., Aytar, A., Atalay, A., & Akman, M. N. (2008). Comparing hot pack, short-wave diathermy, ultrasound, and tens on isokinetic strength, Pain, and Functional status of women with osteoarthritic knees: A single-blind, randomized, controlled trial. *American Journal of Physical Medicine and Rehabilitation, 87*(6), 443–451.

Chang, Y. W., Hsieh, S. F., Horng, Y. S., et al. (2014). Comparative effectiveness of ultrasound and paraffin therapy in patients with carpal tunnel syndrome: A randomized trial. *BMC Musculoskeletal Disorders, 15*(1).

Charkoudian, N., Eisenach, J., Atkinson, J., Fealey, R., & Joynder, M. (2002). Effects of chronic sympathectomy on locally mediated cutaneous vasodilation in humans. *Journal of Applied Physiology, 92*, 685–690.

Chou, R., & Huffman, L. H. (2007). Nonpharmacologic therapies for acute and chronic low back pain: A review of the evidence for an American Pain Society/American College of Physicians clinical practice guideline. *Annals of Internal Medicine, 147*(7), 492–504.

Clijsen, R., Taeymans, J., Duquet, W., Barel, A., & Clarys, P. (2008). Changes of skin characteristics during and after local parafango therapy as used in physiotherapy. *Skin Research and Technology : Official Journal of International Society for Bioengineering and the Skin (ISBS) [and] International Society for Digital Imaging of Skin (ISDIS) [and] International Society for Skin Imaging (ISSI), 14*(2), 237–242.

Crockford, G. W., & Hellon, R. F. (1959). Vascular responses of human skin to infrared radiation. *The Journal of Physiology, 149*, 424–432.

Del Pozzi, A. T., Miller, J. T., & Hodges, G. J. (2016). The effect of heating rate on the cutaneous vasomotion responses of forearm and leg skin in humans. *Microvascular Research, 105*, 77–84.

Dellhag, B., Wollersjo, I., & Bjelle, A. (1992). Effect of active hand exercise and wax bath treatment in rheumatoid arthritis patients. *Arthritis Care and Research: The Official Journal of the Arthritis Health Professions Association, 5*(2), 87–92.

Denton, A. L., Hough, A. D., Freeman, J. A., & Marsden, J. F. (2018). Effects of superficial heating and insulation on walking speed in people with hereditary and spontaneous spastic paraparesis: A randomised crossover study. *Annals of Physical and Rehabilitation Medicine, 61*(2), 72–77.

Dilek, B., Gözüm, M., Şahin, E., et al. (2013). Efficacy of paraffin bath therapy in hand osteoarthritis: A single-blinded randomized controlled trial. *Archives of Physical Medicine and Rehabilitation, 94*(4), 642–649.

Ducharme, M. B., VanHelder, W. P., & Radomski, M. W. (1991). Tissue temperature profile in the human forearm during thermal stress at thermal stability. *Journal of Applied Physiology, 71*, 1973–1978.

Evcik, D., Kavuncu, V., Yeter, A., & Yigit, I. (2007). The efficacy of balneotherapy and mud-pack therapy in patients with knee osteoarthritis. Joint, bone, spine. *Revue du Rhumatisme, 74*(1), 60–65.

Freiwald, J., Hoppe, M. W., Beermann, W., Krajewski, J., & Baumgart, C. (2018). Effects of supplemental heat therapy in multimodal treated chronic low back pain patients on strength and flexibility. *Clinical Biomechanics, 57*, 107–113.

French, S. D., Cameron, M., Walker, B. F., Reggars, J. W., & Esterman, A. J. (2006). Superficial heat or cold for low back pain. *Cochrane Database of Systematic Reviews* (1), CD004750.

Ganji, Z., Shirvani, M. A., Rezaei-Abhari, F., & Danesh, M. (2013). The effect of intermittent local heat and cold on labor pain and child birth outcome. *Iranian Journal of Nursing and Midwifery Research, 18*(4), 298–303.

Garcia, L. M., Soares, A. B., Simieli, C., Boratino, A. V. P., & de Jesus Guirro, R. R. (2014). On the effect of thermal agents in the response of the brachial biceps at different contraction levels. *Journal of Electromyography and Kinesiology, 24*(6), 881–887.

Gu, J. Y., Choi, H. S., Lee, D. Y., et al. (2016). Effect of heat treatments for hand in Raynaud's phenomenon. *Indian Journal of Science and Technology, 9*(25).

Gunay Ucurum, S., Kaya, D. O., Kayali, Y., Askin, A., & Tekindal, M. A. (2018). Comparison of different electrotherapy methods and exercise therapy in shoulder impingement syndrome: A prospective randomized controlled trial. *Acta Orthopaedica et Traumatologica Turcica.*

Gungen, G., Ardic, F., Findikoglu, G., & Rota, S. (2012). The effect of mud pack therapy on serum YKL-40 and hsCRP levels in patients with knee osteoarthritis. *Rheumatology International, 32*(5), 1235–1244.

Hardy, J. D. (1956). Spectral transmittance and reflectance of excised human skin. *Journal of Applied Physiology, 9*, 257–264.

Harlen, F. (1980). Infrared irradiation. In M. F. Docker (Ed.), *Physics in physiotherapy, conference report* series – 35 (p. 180). London: Hospital Physicists Association.

Head, M. D., & Helms, P. S. (1977). Paraffin and sustained stretching in the treatment of burns contracture. *Burns, 4*, 136.

Heinonen, I., Brothers, R. M., Kemppainen, J., et al. (2011). Local heating, but not indirect whole body heating, increases human skeletal muscle blood flow. *Journal of Applied Physiology, 111*(3), 818–824.

Henricson, A. S., Fredriksson, K., Persson, I., et al. (1984). The effect of heat and stretching on the range of hip motion. *Journal of Orthopaedic & Sports Physical Therapy, 6*(2), 110–115.

Holwatz, L. A., Houghton, B. L., Wong, B. J., et al. (2003). Nitric oxide and attenuated reflex cutaneous vasodilation in aged skin. *American Journal of Physiology Heart Circulation Physiology, 284*, H1662–H1667.

Homayouni, K., Zeynali, L., & Mianehsaz, E. (2013). Comparison between Kinesio taping and physiotherapy in the treatment of de Quervain's disease. *Journal of Musculoskeletal Research, 16*(4), 1350019.

Horng, Y. S., Hsieh, S. F., Tu, Y. K., et al. (2011). The comparative effectiveness of tendon and nerve gliding exercises in patients with carpal tunnel syndrome: A randomized trial. *American Journal of Physical Medicine & Rehabilitation, 90*(6), 435–442.

Igaki, M., Higashi, T., Hamamoto, S., et al. (2014). A study of the behavior and mechanism of thermal conduction in the skin under moist and dry heat conditions. *Skin Research and Technology: Official Journal of International Society for Bioengineering and the Skin (ISBS) [and] International Society for Digital Imaging of Skin (ISDIS) [and] International Society for Skin Imaging (ISSI), 20*(1), 43–49.

Jarosch, R. (2008). Large-scale models reveal the two-component mechanics of striated muscle. *International Journal of Molecular Sciences, 9*(12), 2658–2723.

Jarosch, R. (2011). The different muscle-energetics during shortening and stretch. *International Journal of Molecular Sciences, 12*(5), 2891–2900.

Kasapoğlu Aksoy M., Altan L. (2018). Short-term efficacy of paraffin therapy and home-based exercise programs in the treatment of symptomatic hand osteoarthritis. *Turkish Journal of Physical Medicine and Rehabilitation, 64*(2), 108–113.

Kenney, W. L., & Hodgson, J. L. (1987). Heat tolerance, thermoregulation and ageing. *Sports Medicine, 4*, 446–456.

Köroğlu, F., Çolak, T. K., & Polat, M. G. (2017). The effect of Kinesio® taping on pain, functionality, mobility and endurance in the treatment of chronic low back pain: A randomized controlled study. *Journal of Back and Musculoskeletal Rehabilitation, 30*(5), 1087–1093.

Kubo, K., Yajima, H., Takayama, M., et al. (2011). Changes in blood circulation of the contralateral Achilles tendon during and after acupuncture and heating. *International Journal of Sports Medicine, 32*(10), 807–813.

Lehmann, J., & de Lateur, B. (1990). Therapeutic heat. In J. Lehmann (Ed.), *Therapeutic heat and cold* (4th ed.) (pp. 470–474). Baltimore: Williams & Wilkins.

Lehmann, J. F., Silverman, D. R., Baum, B. A., Kirk, N. L., & Johnston, V. C. (1966). Temperature distributions in the human thigh, produced by infrared, hot pack and microwave applications. *Archives of Physical Medicine and Rehabilitation, 47*(5), 291–299.

Lentell, G., Hetherington, T., Eagan, J., & Morgan, M. (1992). The use of thermal agents to influence the effectiveness of a low-load prolonged stretch. *Journal of Orthopaedic & Sports Physical Therapy, 16*(5), 200–207.

Leung, M. S. F., & Cheing, G. L. Y. (2008). Effects of deep and superficial heating in the management of frozen shoulder. *Journal of Rehabilitation Medicine, 40*(2), 145–150.

Lewis, S. E., Holmes, P. S., Woby, S. R., Hindle, J., & Fowler, N. E. (2012). Short-term effect of superficial heat treatment on paraspinal muscle activity, stature recovery, and psychological factors in patients with chronic low back pain. *Archives of Physical Medicine and Rehabilitation, 93*(2), 367–372.

Lin, Y. H. (2003). Effects of thermal therapy in improving the passive range of knee motion: Comparison of cold and superficial heat applications. *Clinical Rehabilitation, 17*(6), 618–623.

Lohman, E. B., 3rd. Bains, G. S., Lohman, T., DeLeon, M., & Petrofsky, J. S. (2011). A comparison of the effect of a variety of thermal and vibratory modalities on skin temperature and blood flow in healthy volunteers. *Medical Science Monitor: International Medical Journal of Experimental and Clinical Research, 17*(9), MT72–MT81.

Lung, C. W., Lin, Y. S., Jan, Y. K., et al. (2019). Effect of far infrared radiation therapy on improving microcirculation of the diabetic foot. *Advances in Intelligent Systems and Computing,* 156–163.

Maeda, T., Yoshida, H., Sasaki, T., & Oda, A. (2017). Does transcutaneous electrical nerve stimulation (TENS) simultaneously combined with local heat and cold applications enhance pain relief compared with TENS alone in patients with knee osteoarthritis? *Journal of Physical Therapy Science, 29*(10), 1860–1864.

Matsumoto, S., Kawahira, K., Etoh, S., Ikeda, S., & Tanaka, N. (2006). Short-term effects of thermotherapy for spasticity on tibial nerve F-waves in post-stroke patients. *International Journal of Biometeorology, 50*(4), 243–250.

Matsumoto, S., Shimodozono, M., Etoh, S., et al. (2010). Beneficial effects of footbaths in controlling spasticity after stroke. *International Journal of Biometeorology, 54*(4), 465–473.

Mayer, J. M., Mooney, V., Matheson, L. N., et al. (2006). Continuous low-level heat wrap therapy for the prevention and early phase treatment of delayed-onset muscle soreness of the low back: A randomized controlled trial. *Archives of Physical Medicine and Rehabilitation, 87*(10), 1310–1317.

McAlindon, T. E., Bannuru, R. R., Sullivan, M. C., et al. (2014). OARSI guidelines for the non-surgical management of knee osteoarthritis. *Osteoarthritis and Cartilage, 22*(3), 363–388.

McLellan, K., Petrofsky, J., Zimmerman, G., et al. (2009a). Multiple stressors and the response of vascular endothelial cells: The effect of aging and diabetes. *Diabetes Technology & Therapeutics, 11,* 73–79.

McLellan, K., Petrofsky, J. S., Bains, G., et al. (2009b). The effects of skin moisture and subcutaneous fat thickness on the ability of the skin to dissipate heat in young and old subjects, with and without diabetes, at three environmental room temperatures. *Medical Engineering & Physics, 31*(2), 165–172.

Minson, C. T., Berry, L. T., & Joyner, M. J. (2001). Nitric oxide and neutrally mediated regulation of skin blood flow during local heating. *Journal of Applied Physiology, 91,* 1619–1626.

Moss, C., Ellis, R., Murray, W., & Parr, W. (1989). *Infrared radiation, nonionising radiation protection.* Copenhagen: WHO Regional Publications.

Myrer, J. W., Johnson, A. W., Mitchell, U. H., Measom, G. J., & Fellingham, G. W. (2011). Topical analgesic added to paraffin enhances paraffin bath treatment of individuals with hand osteoarthritis. *Disability & Rehabilitation, 33*(6), 467–474.

Nakano, J., Yamabayashi, C., Scott, A., & Reid, W. D. (2012). The effect of heat applied with stretch to increase range of motion: A systematic review. *Physical Therapy in Sport, 13*(3), 180–188.

Nuhr, M., Hoerauf, K., Bertalanffy, A., et al. (2004). Active warming during emergency transport relieves acute low back pain. *Spine, 29*(14), 1499–1503.

Ojoawo, A. O., Hassan, M. A., Olaogun, M. B., Johnson, E. O., & Mbada, C. E. (2017). Comparative effectiveness of two stabilization exercise positions on pain and functional disability of patients with low back pain. *Journal of Exercise Rehabilitation, 13*(3), 363–371.

Oosterveld, F. G. J., Rasker, J. J., Floors, M., et al. (2008). Infrared sauna in patients with rheumatoid arthritis and ankylosing spondylitis. *Clinical Rheumatology, 28*(1), 29.

Ordahan, B., & Karahan, A. Y. (2017). Efficacy of paraffin wax bath for carpal tunnel syndrome: A randomized comparative study. *International Journal of Biometeorology, 61*(12), 2175–2181.

Ozkurt, S., Donmez, A., Zeki Karagulle, M., et al. (2012). Balneotherapy in fibromyalgia: A single blind randomized controlled clinical study. *Rheumatology International, 32*(7), 1949–1954.

Pennes, H. (1948). Analysis of tissue and arterial blood temperature in the resting human forearm. *Journal of Applied Physiology, 1,* 93–122.

Petrofsky, J., Bains, G., Prowse, M., et al. (2009a). Does skin moisture influence the blood flow response to local heat? A re-evaluation of the Pennes model. *Journal of Medical Engineering & Technology, 33*(7), 532–537.

Petrofsky, J., Bains, G., Prowse, M., et al. (2009b). Dry heat, moist heat and body fat: Are heating modalities really effective in people who are overweight? *Journal of Medical Engineering & Technology, 33*(5), 361–369.

Petrofsky, J., Berk, L., Alshammari, F., et al. (2012a). The effect of moist air on skin blood flow and temperature in subjects with and without diabetes. *Diabetes Technology & Therapeutics, 14*(2), 105–116.

Petrofsky, J. S., Berk, L., Alshammari, F., et al. (2012b). The interrelationship between air temperature and humidity as applied locally to the skin: The resultant response on skin temperature and blood flow with age differences. *Medical Science Monitor: International Medical Journal of Experimental and Clinical Research, 18*(4), CR201–C208.

Petrofsky, J., Goraksh, N., Alshammari, F., et al. (2011). The ability of the skin to absorb heat; the effect of repeated exposure and age. *Medical Science Monitor, 17*(1), CR1–CR8.

Petrofsky, J., Gunda, S., Raju, C., et al. (2010). Impact of hydrotherapy on skin blood flow: How much is due to moisture and how much is due to heat? *Physiotherapy Theory and Practice*, 26(2), 107–112.

Petrofsky, J. S., Laymon, M., & Lee, H. (2013). Effect of heat and cold on tendon flexibility and force to flex the human knee. *Medical Science Monitor: International Medical Journal of Experimental and Clinical Research*, 19, 661–667.

Petrofsky, J., & Lind, A. R. (1975a). The insulative power of body fat on deep muscle temperature and isometric endurance. *Journal of Applied Physiology*, 39, 639–642.

Petrofsky, J., & Lind, A. R. (1975b). The relationship of body fat content to deep muscle temperature and isometric endurance in man. *Clinical Science & Molecular Medicine*, 48, 405–412.

Rashid, S., Salick, K., Kashif, M., Ahmad, A., & Sarwar, K. (2013). To evaluate the efficacy of mobilization techniques in post-traumatic stiff ankle with and without paraffin wax bath. *Pakistan Journal of Medical Sciences*, 29(6).

Robertson, V. J., Ward, A. R., & Jung, P. (2005). The effect of heat on tissue extensibility: A comparison of deep and superficial heating. *Archives of Physical Medicine and Rehabilitation*, 86(4), 819–825.

Robinson, V., Brosseau, L., Casimiro, L., et al. (2002). Thermotherapy for treating rheumatoid arthritis. *Cochrane Database of Systematic Reviews* (2), CD002826.

Sarsan, A., Akkaya, N., Özgen, M., et al. (2012). Comparing the efficacy of mature mud pack and hot pack treatments for knee osteoarthritis. *Journal of Back and Musculoskeletal Rehabilitation*, 25(3), 193–199.

Satpute, K. H., Bhandari, P., & Hall, T. (2015). Efficacy of hand behind back mobilization with movement for acute shoulder pain and movement impairment: A randomized controlled trial. *Journal of Manipulative and Physiological Therapeutics*, 38(5), 324–334.

Selkins, K. M., & Emery, A. F. (1990). Thermal science for physical medicine. In J. Lehmann (Ed.), *Therapeutic heat and cold* (4th ed.) (pp. 62–112). Baltimore: Williams & Wilkins.

Singer, D. (2007). Why 37 degrees C? Evolutionary fundamentals of thermoregulation. *Anaesthetist*, 56, 899–902, 904–906.

Slivka, D., Tucker, T., Cuddy, J., Hailes, W., & Ruby, B. (2012). Local heat application enhances glycogenesis. *Applied Physiology Nutrition and Metabolism*, 37(2), 247–251.

Smith, C. A., Levett, K. M., Collins, C. T., et al. (2018). Massage, reflexology and other manual methods for pain management in labour. *Cochrane Database of Systematic Reviews*, (3), CD009290.

Song, G. S. (2008). Effect of floor surface temperature on blood flow and skin temperature in the foot. *Indoor Air*, 18(6), 511–520.

Szekeres, M., MacDermid, J. C., Birmingham, T., Grewal, R., & Lalone, E. (2017a). The effect of therapeutic whirlpool and hot packs on hand volume during rehabilitation after distal radius fracture: A blinded randomized controlled trial. *Hand (New York, NY)*, 12(3), 265–271.

Szekeres, M., MacDermid, J. C., Grewal, R., & Birmingham, T. (2017b). The short-term effects of hot packs vs therapeutic whirlpool on active wrist range of motion for patients with distal radius fracture: A randomized controlled trial. *Journal of Hand Therapy: Official Journal of the American Society of Hand Therapists*, 31(3), 276-281.

Taavoni, S., Abdolahian, S., & Haghani, H. (2013). Effect of sacrum-perineum heat therapy on active phase labor pain and client satisfaction: A randomized, controlled trial study. *Pain Medicine*, 14(9), 1301–1306.

Tüzün, E. H., Gıldır, S., Angin, E., et al. (2017). Effectiveness of dry needling versus a classical physiotherapy program in patients with chronic low-back pain: A single-blind, randomized, controlled trial. *Journal of Physical Therapy Science*, 29(9), 1502–1509.

Vaht, M., Birkenfeldt, R., & Übner, M. (2008). An evaluation of the effect of differing lengths of spa therapy upon patients with osteoarthritis (OA). *Complementary Therapies in Clinical Practice*, 14(1), 60–64.

Warner, B., Kim, K. M., Hart, J. M., & Saliba, S. (2013). Lack of effect of superficial heat to the knee on quadriceps function in individuals with quadriceps inhibition. *Journal of Sport Rehabilitation*, 22(2), 93–99.

Yurtkuran, M., Yurtkuran, M., Alp, A., et al. (2006). Balneotherapy and tap water therapy in the treatment of knee osteoarthritis. *Rheumatology International*, 27(1), 19–27.

7

Pulsed and Continuous Shortwave and Radiofrequency Therapies

Maryam M. Al-Mandeel, Tim Watson

CHAPTER OUTLINE

INTRODUCTION AND HISTORY

Radiofrequencies are part of the electromagnetic (EM) spectrum that fall in the range of 3 kHz–300 GHz. This frequency band contains short, medium and long radio waves (see Chapter 2, Fig. 2.20). High frequency radio waves (HFRW) have been used for many purposes, including therapy to heat tissues and treat pathologies. Shortwave therapy (SWT) involves the coupling of non-ionizing HFRW to tissues and can be delivered as continuous shortwave therapy (CSWT) or in an interrupted mode as pulsed shortwave therapy (PSWT). The therapeutic use of radiofrequency (RF) is not limited to SWT. Low range radiofrequency was historically used in therapy (longwave diathermy), though was largely discontinued given the difficulties in its clinical application. This chapter focuses on SWT in both continuous and pulsed modes of delivery and discusses other RF frequencies used in therapy. The term 'diathermy', although historically popular, is largely omitted and the term 'shortwave therapy' (SWT) used in preference.

In the 19th century, the French physiologist d'Arsonval passed a current of 1 ampere through his body and the body of his assistant. Despite the belief that a current of such strength would be deadly, they only experienced gentle warmth. Experimentation by d'Arsonval, Tesla and Hertz continued. The term diathermy was first used by the German physician Nagelschidt in 1907 to mean heating through the tissues (Reif- Acherman 2017).

Three modes of diathermy have been developed: shortwave, longwave and microwave (Belanger 2015). Many trade names for shortwave devices are encountered, such as Diapulse, Curapuls and Megapulse. These are device names rather than a modality or treatment per se. Shortwave therapy (SWT) will be employed as an overarching term in this chapter repetitious.

Diathermy has undergone several fashionable shifts in clinical utilization. Microwave devices have almost disappeared from the majority of clinics (Kumaran & Watson 2015a; Shah & Farrow 2013), and clinicians have largely turned to PSWT, replacing their use of CSWT in the belief that the use of lower levels of energy can achieve therapeutic outcomes with minimal thermal effects (Al-Mandeel & Watson 2006; Shah & Farrow 2013; Watson 2000).

In general, the use of SWT has declined over recent years when compared with other electrophysical agents (EPAs). This is underpinned by several factors, such as equipment

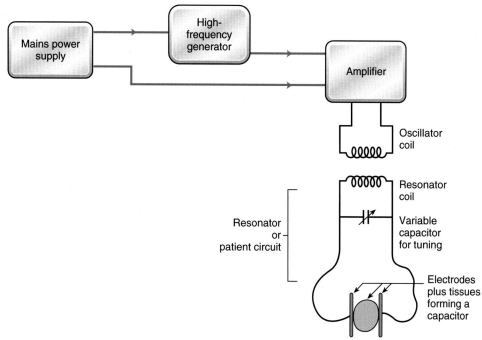

Fig. 7.1 Electrical circuits with SWT generators. (From Low & Reed 2000).

size, cost, growing concerns about the potential hazards to both patients and therapists, and interference with other electrical equipment in the vicinity (Cameron 2013).

SWT remains an under-explored modality compared with other EPAs, with limited research exploring its biological mechanisms (Shields et al 2004) and associated dosage (Fukuda et al 2011). This has changed in the last 5 years with renewed clinical use (Prentice et al 2018) and the move towards researching the effectiveness of SWT and other RF applications with better quality research.

PHYSICAL PRINCIPLES

Shortwave equipment is one of several medical devices that utilizes high RF. The Federal Communication Commission (1947) assigned three frequencies at the short end of the RF band for the medical use of shortwave (Belanger 2015). These are: 40.68 MHz ± 20k Hz and a wavelength of 7.5 m; 13.56 MHz ± 6.25 kHz at a wavelength of 22 m; and 27.12 MHz ± 160 kHz and a wavelength of 11 m (Prentice et al 2018). The frequencies employed relate to international regulation rather than known efficacy. The majority of the research reported in this chapter relates to the use of the 27.12 MHz frequency, which is the most widely employed in current clinical practice, though recent reviews (Kumaran & Watson 2015a, 2016) have included all employed frequencies.

SWT generators produce high frequency electromagnetic fields (EMFs) incorporating two electrical circuits. The machine (or oscillator) circuit is composed of a high frequency generator, amplifier (to raise the output to therapeutic levels) and a power supply (Fig. 7.1). The second circuit is the patient (or resonator) circuit, which includes a variable capacitor (to account for the type of tissue treated) and a method of transferring energy to the tissues without direct link to the main power circuit; this is achieved by either capacitive or inductive electrodes. The same circuit can operate in pulsed or continuous modes.

In CSWT, the energy is delivered to the patient continuously during the treatment time and is primarily associated with higher energy delivery and thermal effects. With PSWT, the output is delivered to the tissues in a train of pulses of varying durations and variable repetition rate, allowing a higher peak amplitude of energy to be delivered to the tissues with either primarily thermal or non-thermal effects (Watson 2006). Depending on the specific machine, the operator can vary the pulse repetition rate (PRR; pulses per second), pulse duration (PD; µs) and pulse peak power (PP; Watts). Mean power (MP; also Watts) can be controlled by changing PRR, PD and PP according to Eq. (7.1) (and illustrated in Fig. 7.2). Table 7.1 illustrates the typical ranges of pulse parameters available on modern PSWT devices.

Mean power = Pulse duration (µs)
(Watts)   × Pulse repetition rate (pps)
              × Peak pulse power(Watts)   **[7.1]**

For example, using a machine with a MP of 200 W, a PRR of 400 pps and a PD of 200 µs, the MP applied to the patient would be 16 W, whereas using the same machine (PP 200 W) with a low PRR (35 pps) and a short duration pulse (65 µs), the MP delivery would be 0.46 W. A modern PSWT device would typically be capable of delivering mean powers in the range of 0.1–48 W.

BIOPHYSICAL EFFECTS, INTERACTIONS AND RESPONSES

Shortwave RF energy has two basic fields: the electric (E) and magnetic (H) fields (see Chapter 2). The application of these fields and the subsequent currents that arise in the tissues are responsible for the physiological effects, such as the rise in tissue temperature and changes in blood flow as well as non-thermal changes affecting cellular activity and tissue repair.

The interaction between the E and H fields and the tissues is affected by the 'complex permittivity', which in turn is related to the dielectric constant. The dielectric constant represents the ease of polarization of tissue molecules of a tissue and is primarily dependent upon the water content. Complex permittivity is also a function of the field frequency, and thus, the propagation and attenuation of the electromagnetic waves are dependent upon frequency (Gabriel & Peyman 2018).

Although SWT units produce both an E and an H field in the tissue, their ratio will differ according to the mode of application, the type of electrode in use and the operating frequency. Differences in the carrying frequency will also result in further variance of the ratio of H and E fields (Markov & Colbert 2000).

The energy distribution in the tissues varies with application system: capacitive versus inductive, and is briefly considered here as it will influence the biophysical effects. The use of different electrode systems is further considered in the Application section.

Capacitive electrodes (Fig 7.3) produce a higher proportion of E than H field in the tissues, the field being stronger in the centre of the treated area. The strength of the field is governed by the electrode placement in relation to the tissue (there is a stronger field with the electrodes situated closer to the skin), the size of the electrodes (small electrodes have less penetration than larger electrodes) and spacing (uniform field in the tissues is achieved by using electrodes slightly larger than the treated area; unequal electrode pairs generate a distorted or unevenly concentrated field distribution) (Prentice et al 2018). The heat produced using the capacitive method is the result of the movement of three components: charged ions/molecules, dipolar molecules and non-polar molecules, and is governed by the strength of the E field and the conductivity of the tissues. A capacitive application is expected to concentrate the field in the superficial tissues, such as the skin

TABLE 7.1 Typical Ranges of Pulse Parameters in Modern Pulsed Shortwave Therapy Devices

Pulse parameter	Units	Typical range
Pulse repetition rate (frequency)	Pulses per second (pps) or Hz	26–800
Pulse duration	Microseconds (µs)	20–400
Pulse peak power	Watts	150–200
Applied mean power	Watts	0.1–30+

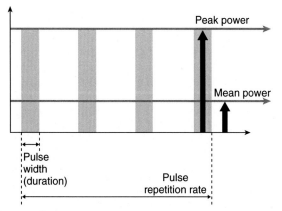

Fig. 7.2 The essential relationship between pulse repetition rate, pulse duration, peak and mean power.

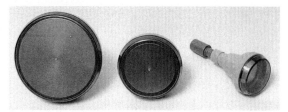

Fig. 7.3 Air spaced electrodes of different sizes in clinical use.

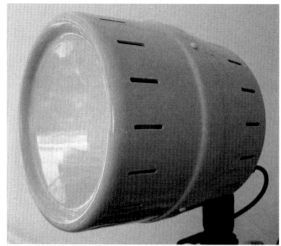

Fig. 7.4 Monode (drum) type applicator for use with continuous or pulsed shortwave modes.

and fat layers, rather than the deep tissues (He et al 2005; William & Roshini 2009). This energy delivery mode is possibly best suited for treating superficial areas of low subcutaneous fat (Prentice et al 2018).

The inductive energy delivery systems predominantly produce an H field via a cable that is either wrapped around the extremity or a conducting wire coiled inside an electrode housing (monode or drum applicator). The use of the monode (Fig. 7.4) has become the clinical norm in current practice, and the wraparound cable application is rarely employed. The drum electrode is placed perpendicular to the part to be treated. The alternating current in the coils produces an H field, which is directed into the tissue, and is set up at right-angles to the direction of current flow. The E field emission from monode-type electrodes is usually limited by a Faradic screen built into the drum. The strength of the H field is determined by the rate at which the current alternates and by the number of wire coils contained within a conductor (Belanger 2015).

The H field induces secondary currents in the tissues known as eddy currents. The eddy currents are alternating in nature, and it is this induced alternating current that is responsible for the increase in molecular vibration and thus, heat generation. This form of heating is not associated with strong sensory stimulation as there is less superficial (skin and fat) heating and the heat will be less obvious to the patient compared with the capacitive application (Prentice et al 2018).

The inductive application is believed to result in selective energy absorption and heating. Tissues with a high electrolyte content and low impedance, such as muscle and blood, will be heated to a greater extent, with the superficial layers, such as skin and fat, being minimally affected (Watson 2006). Draper et al (1999) were able to demonstrate an increase in intramuscular temperature of up to 4°C using inductive electrodes. The inductive application can be employed with continuous or pulsed shortwave modes, although the most common combination in current practice is to use the drum applicator in pulsed mode.

Shortwave therapy can be employed in either thermal or 'non-thermal' modes. The use of CSWT is usually considered to be thermal, whereas PSWT can bring about thermal or non-thermal effects. In theory it is possible to deliver CSWT at a very low dose and achieve a non-thermal effect, though in practice, this option is not utilized following the advent of PSWT devices. The rise in tissue temperature during the application of SWT depends on the specific absorption rate (SAR), which is the rate at which energy is absorbed by a known mass of tissue and is calculated in units of Watts per kilogram (W/kg). SAR is a function of tissue conductivity and the electromagnetic field magnitude. Tissue conductivity reflects the ease with which an electric field can be set up in the tissue. The SAR, and the heating produced by SWT, is dependent upon the electrical properties of tissue within the EM field (Nagaoka et al 2003; Okabe et al 2018).

The physical effects of heat are considered in Chapter 2 and the physiological effects in Chapter 5. If SWT is employed at sufficient energy levels to achieve a tissue heating effect, the biophysical changes would be as described in these chapters.

PSWT can be employed in a 'thermal' or 'non-thermal' fashion with the applied MP being the main determinant (Bricknell & Watson 1995). The thermal mode of PSWT can be achieved by using longer pulse durations and high repetition rates. The non-thermal mode is achieved when short pulses are interposed by long interpulse periods. This is not strictly a 'non-thermal' mode, but there is no perceived increase in temperature ($\triangle$T) as the heat gained during the 'on phase' is dissipated by the circulating blood during the interpulse period (Scott 2002; Watson 2006). When long-duration treatments are applied with these parameters, it is possible that an accumulative heating effect may still be achieved. The differences between thermal and non-thermal effects of therapy are further considered in Chapter 5.

Heat generated in the tissues is the product of tissue resistance and current density as explained in Eq. (7.2) (Prentice et al 2018):

$$\text{Heating} = \text{Current density}^2 \times \text{Resistance} \qquad [7.2]$$

Tissues contain ions, polar molecules and non-charged molecules. Heat can be produced as a result of the oscillation of charged ions and molecules, such as proteins, about a mean position along the lines of the forces that are created by the energy field. The oscillation and friction converts the molecular kinetic energy to heat.

The second type of molecule (water and some proteins) possesses permanent electric dipoles (e.g. water and some proteins). These dipoles are normally randomly arranged. Under the influence of an E field, these dipolar molecules undergo polarization and align themselves to the opposite charged pole. The alternating nature of the field causes the dipoles to rotate and collide (so called 'dipole rotation'), and the friction between these dipoles generates heat. Additionally, each of these polar molecules possesses a weak field of its own, extending from the positive to the negative pole and, when the substance is under the influence of the E field, the net result of these fields governs the electric properties of the matter. Dipolar molecules produce a mixture of real and displacement currents. Real current refers to the current that develops in the tissues and determines the electrical properties and heat production in a matter, as opposed to the displacement current, which does not play a great role in the electrical properties of a matter (Prentice et al 2018; Gabriel & Peynman 2018).

The third type of molecule is the non-charged molecule. The E field affects non-charged molecules by polarizing and distorting their electron cloud fields. Movement of the non-charged molecules in response to the E field results in displacement currents and contributes the least to heat production in the tissues (Durney & Christensen 2000).

The changes in the field distribution in response to implanted metal in the tissues have been considered in detail by Virtanen et al (2006), and the clinical use of PSWT with metal implants is discussed by Draper (2014, 2017) and Seiger and Draper (2006) and is further considered in Chapter 22.

The response of biological systems to EM energy can be the result of either thermal or non-thermal mechanisms. The heat developing in the tissues after 20 minutes of application of SWT was found to peak at 15 minutes, after which it plateaued for 5 minutes and then started to decline slowly at a rate of around 1°C per 5 minutes (Draper et al 1999). Similar findings were achieved by Sousa et al (2017) where the temperature peaked after 10 minutes, plateaued between minute 10 and minute 20, and tissue retained the heat till minute 40 post treatment. Therapeutically, a temperature increase of around 1°C is useful for mild inflammation and an increase between 2 and 3°C is helpful in reducing pain and muscle spasm, whereas an increase of 3–4°C is necessary to cause changes in tissue extensibility (Prentice et al 2018). Based on the work of Sousa et al (2017) using SWT for 10 minutes in a continuous mode is

capable of raising the temperature of the tissues an average of 6° C.

The mechanism of response to EM energy is thought to occur at several sites within the cell: one of the main interactions is thought to be the cell membrane selectivity to ions. It is suggested that EM energy changes the rate of opening and the formation of ion channels across the protein bilayer found in the cell membrane. Cations such as Na^+ and K^+ leak from inside the cell to the extracellular fluid under the influence of the energy, altering the intracellular and extracellular environments and possibly restoring haemostasis (Pall 2013).

Whereas the response of the nucleus to exogenous EM energy is governed by the presence of ions such as Ca^{2+}, the magnitude of the response was seen to correlate with the amount of energy delivered to the cell. For example, using PSWT, the reaction was higher with PD 400 μs, PRR 400 pps, intensity 1, for 10 minutes than with PD 400 μs, PRR 80 pps, intensity 4, and the same duration utilising a Diapulse PSWT device (Pop 1989).

The delivery of SWT energy stimulates the release of various cytokines, which appear to be primarily responsible for the vasodilatation response. Mediators such as NO (nitric oxide) bring about vasodilatation by reducing the tone in blood vessel smooth muscle (Minson et al 2001) and would be consistent with various other therapies (Watson 2016). The axon reflex, much discussed historically, has a short-term vasodilatation effect but the mediator mechanisms dominate.

With vasodilatation, there may be a decrease in blood viscosity to ease blood flow (Jan et al 2006). These proposals were validated by Sousa et al (2017). They report that the application of SWT for 20 minutes is capable of increasing skin temperature and changing blood flow velocity in the treated area. The heat generated and change in blood flow velocity are dependent on the size of the treated area. The pattern of heating is not confined to the area under the electrodes but extends to neighbouring tissues. It is thought that the increase in velocity is proportional to the increase in thermal energy, which was found to be related to the cessation of neural activity responsible for vasoconstriction. Tissues were found to be able to retain temperature increase for up to 40 minutes post treatment.

The increased volume and velocity of blood flow and the accompanying thermal changes in and around the cell were considered to be effective in speeding the recovery of open wounds, increasing tissue extensibility, decreasing oedema and haematoma, and relieving inflammation, joint stiffness and pain (Cameron 2013).

Reducing pain is one of the most common reasons for employing SWT (Al Mandeel and Watson 2006). Pain reduction could occur as a result of the inhibition of sensory impulse transmission, which may lead to a sedative effect. Inflammatory pain is expected to reduce as a result of the vasodilatation and absorption of the exudates accumulating in the tissues (Ward 1980). The pain resulting from muscle spasm could decrease as a consequence of vasodilatation and the removal of excess lactic acid and other metabolic products in the muscle that cause muscle soreness (Cameron 2013). PSWT was shown to be effective when used to treat persistent pain that had failed to respond to medication, immobilization and other forms of physical therapy (Cortes et al 2013).

CLINICAL EVIDENCE

A reasonable amount of research has been published relating to the use of both continuous and pulsed SWT in various clinical areas. It is interesting to note that very little was published during the 1990s, but recently the publication rate appears to have increased and improved in quality. There is a degree of ambiguity in the literature concerning the differences between pulsed electromagnetic fields (PEMFs) and pulsed shortwave therapy (PSWT), and the extensive literature concerning PEMFs is not reviewed here (see Chapter 12). It remains to be seen whether there is, or is not, a direct correlation between these two different forms of intervention. Treatment investigations involving SWT are divided up into several clinical topic areas in this section.

Osteoarthritis

Numerous systematic and narrative reviews have either focused on shortwave or have included shortwave in their interventions.

In a systematic review and meta-analysis conducted by Wang et al (2017), 8 trials involving 542 patients were compiled to evaluate the effects of SWT on osteoarthritis (OA) symptoms. Patients were from an age range of 42 to 85 and were female dominant. Trial quality was evaluated with both the Cochrane Collaboration and PEDro tools. Fifty percent of the trials utilized CSWT and 50% PSWT. Pain was an outcome common to all trials, some using a visual analogue scale (VAS) and some a numerical rating scale (NRS). Function was also a common outcome, though various tools were employed, including Western Ontario and McMaster Universities Osteoarthritis Index (WOMAC) and Knee Osteoarthritis Outcome Score (KOOS).

SWT was shown to be effective in reducing pain with PSWT providing a greater benefit. Function was also shown to have improved but failed to reach a statistically significant level. Wang et al (2017) noted that an increase in knee extensor strength was demonstrated. It is unlikely that the SWT was directly responsible for the

muscle strength changes, but that greater force generation was a likely result of the decreased pain experienced by the patients. The review recommended the use of PSWT as it was associated with better results.

Amongst the reviewed studies, there was a range of treatment sessions (from 6 to 24) covering a timeframe of 2 to 8 weeks – so these may not have been directly comparable programmes, since demonstrating considerable heterogeneity. The methodology of the reported trials varied considerably with regard to sham treatment, blinding and group allocation and therefore the associated risk of bias.

Cacolice et al (2013) reviewed 43 articles ranging in level of evidence between I and V but this review was concerned with SWT across several indications, not only OA. Six papers (Level I/II) were concerned with knee OA. Positive results included pain reduction, reduction of synovial thickness and improved function. Results were found to be related to age, as younger patients demonstrated better outcomes. SWT was found to result in short-term benefit, which may support the notion that EPAs are not best used as a sole modality and improvement gained should be maintained with other interventions, such as exercise. The authors do not clearly differentiate between SWT in continuous or pulsed mode in their discussions, though the tables describing the individual trials do make this clear. Longer-term benefits were not reported in this review.

Laufer and Dar (2012) reviewed the effectiveness of SWT in OA treatment. The authors commented on the difficulty in drawing conclusions due to extensive variation in treatment protocols in terms of the energy delivered, number of sessions and treatment duration. This notwithstanding, the review concludes that there was significant effect on pain and muscle performance if using CSWT. The review also discussed that some of the insignificant results may be attributed to the low power doses employed.

In two recent narrative reviews (Kumaran & Watson 2015a, 2016), the effect of RF applications, predominantly SWT, across a wide range of acute and chronic clinical conditions, was presented. The 2016 paper considered chronic conditions. Of the 59 papers employing classic shortwave treatments, 28 studies evaluated the use of SWT on OA, predominantly of the knee. Many of the studies published before the 1990s were methodologically compromised, of low power and low quality. More recent studies, employing active treatment, placebo and control groups, failed to consistently demonstrate clinically significant benefits of the active treatment; however, the studies are heterogeneous with wide variations in treatment parameters, number and frequency of sessions. The most recent, robust clinical studies have provided support for the use of SWT in OA with the pulsed application mode providing stronger benefit. The authors concluded that PSWT with a mean power at or above 14.5 W with 8–12 sessions over 4–6 weeks treating for 15–20 minutes per session is supported by the best quality evidence.

There are numerous examples of original SWT clinical trials (as evidenced in the reviews cited above). Teslim et al (2013) compared the use of CSWT with PSWT in treating 24 patients complaining of grade III OA. Patients were randomly allocated to CSWT or PSWT groups. Treatment was delivered twice weekly for 20 minutes over a 4-week period. A contraplanar technique with electrodes medially and laterally was employed. Comparing outcomes (10 point pain scale, active and passive joint ranges) between baseline and the end of the treatment period revealed a statistically and clinically significant decrease in pain, with an increase in both passive and active range of motion (ROM). In this trial, CSWT was shown to be more effective than in pulsed mode in contrast to some other trials noted in this section. There was no follow up beyond the treatment period, thus any longer-term effects are not known. The lack of a control group and no information with regard to any concurrent exercise programme potentially weaken this investigation, though the patients made a clear and significant improvement in clinical status.

Atamaz et al (2012) compared the effectiveness of CSWT, transcutaneous nerve stimulation and interferential current, each compared with a sham delivery of the same modality in treating knee OA. The study was a double-blind, randomized controlled, multicentre trial. All groups received education and exercise. Two hundred and three patients, ranging in age between 50 and 80 years, were enrolled in the study against a range of inclusion/exclusion criteria. This sample size was determined to provide adequate power for the multi-arm trial. All groups received exercise. Treatments were delivered five times weekly for 3 weeks. Response to treatment was measured using a VAS for pain, time to walk 15 metres, the WOMAC, Nottingham Health Profile, and paracetamol intake. Patients were followed up at 1 month, 3 months and 6 months post treatment. Active groups demonstrated better outcomes than sham groups, though these differences were not significant for any of the interventions. While the study has shown no significant difference in the reported pain between CSWT and sham group, the active group showed a significant decrease in analgesic use, which could reflect a clinical response to the application of SWT. Absence of a no treatment (i.e. control) group may have decreased significance. A capacitive application of CSWT with a mean power of 3.2 W was employed, though the shortwave delivery was not well reported.

In a study conducted by Fukuda et al (2011) the effectiveness of high and low dose PSWT was investigated in 121 women, mean age 60 ±9 years, complaining of grade II and III knee OA. The study was a multicentre, randomized,

placebo-controlled clinical trial with follow-up through to 12 months. Treatment was given 3 times per week for a total of 9 sessions. Low dose was delivered for 19 minutes with 17 kJ of energy, while high dose was given for 38 minutes and a total of 33 kJ of energy; PRR was 145 Hz and MP was 14.5 W. A control and a sham group were included for comparison. A numerical pain rating scale and the KOOS were used as outcome measures. There was statistically significant and clinically meaningful reduction in pain levels and improvement in function with both low and high dose PSWT treatment when compared with placebo and control groups. There was no statistically significant difference in outcomes between the two PSWT groups, though the low dose group appear to have achieved better results in the longer term based on an intention-to-treat analysis. This was a robust trial.

In general, the findings of the various OA studies are in favour of SWT, with the majority reporting significant improvement in function and reduction in pain especially in the short term. Both CSWT and PSWT appear to be effective in managing pain, improving muscle strength, increasing joint range, enhancing function, reducing stiffness and supporting activities of daily life in individuals with different levels of OA. There is support for SWT in both CSWT in thermal (Jorge et al 2017) and PSWT in non-thermal mode (Kumaran & Watson 2016).

Musculoskeletal Disorders

SWT in both continuous and pulsed modes has been evaluated across a wide range of musculoskeletal presentations.

The effectiveness of SWT for subacromial impingement syndrome was explored by Yilmaz et al (2018). Fifty-seven patients aged 35–65 years were randomized to either night pain group or no night pain group. The two groups were further subdivided into active or sham SWT. Responsiveness to treatment was measured using VAS, Constant Murley scale and shoulder disability questionnaire. There was modest improvement in outcomes, more obvious at 1 month, in the group without night pain. The small improvement may have been influenced by the small number (n=14) of patients in each group.

Incebiyik et al (2015) examined the effect of superficial heat versus deep heat on mild and moderate idiopathic carpal tunnel syndrome (CTS). Thirty-one patients with either single or bilateral wrist involvement were included in the study. Patients were either enrolled in a hot pack, SWT and nerve and tendon gliding exercises group or in a hot pack, placebo SWT and nerve and tendon gliding exercises group. Treatment was delivered over 15 sessions, 5 times per week. The outcome was evaluated using the Tinel test, Phalen test, carpal compression using the reverse Phalen test, Boston Carpal Tunnel Questionnaire (BCTQ),

Symptom Severity Scale (SSS), Functional Status Scale and VAS pre and post treatment. Significant improvements in pain level and hand function were detected (p<0.001) in the active SWT group. The improvements identified in the sham group failed to reach a significant level. SWT was therefore demonstrated to be of clinical value.

Boyaci et al (2014) compared the effect of PSWT and CSWT to placebo in treating CTS. The study was a double blind, controlled, randomized trial. Thirty subjects complaining of mild or moderate symptoms were included in the study. Treatment was administered 5 times a week for a total of 15 sessions each of 20 minutes. Tinel's test, Phalen's and reverse Phalen's manoeuvres, carpal compression test, the BCTQ (symptom severity scale and functional status scale), VAS, median nerve motor distal latency, sensory distal latency, and nerve conduction velocity were used as outcome measures. Outcomes were evaluated at the beginning and end of the therapy but lacked longer-term follow-up. Multiple outcomes (pain, function, electrophysiological measures) were improved with both active groups when compared with placebo intervention. On balance, although those in receipt of CSWT were advantaged for pain, those in the PSWT group fared better.

Draper (2014) examined the effects of thermal SWT in reducing chronic stiffness of what? the condition being treated has got lost and regaining ROM in 6 patients complaining of stiffness as a result of surgery or trauma. The patients received 20 minutes of SWT with MP ranging between 40–48 W (800 Hz, 400 µsec). Treatment was followed with mobilization. Interestingly, all these patients had a metal implant and did not report adverse effects, and 4 out of the 6 patients achieved full ROM within the first 4 days of treatment.

Several studies have evaluated the effect of SWT already indicates therapy in patients with low back pain (LBP). Nine studies were included in the Kumaran and Watson (2016) review. There is supportive evidence for SWT in both CWST and PSWT amongst this group.

For example, Kerem and Yigiter (2002) investigated the effects of PSWT in 60 patients with LBP. Patients were either assigned to CSWT or one of two PSWT groups (200 Hz or 46 Hz); all groups followed an exercise programme. Ten sessions, each of 20 minutes, were delivered. Patients were evaluated for their pain level, muscle strength and ROM. Findings showed significant improvements in outcomes measured in all groups, with PSWT showing significantly better outcomes than CSWT.

Three studies (Ahmed et al 2009; Shakoor et al 2008; Shakoor et al 2010) have all evaluated the effects of CSWT in LBP, typically delivering 18 sessions in 6 weeks, each of 15 minutes duration. Significant benefits were reported in terms of both pain and functional outcomes.

On balance, there are more papers that have evaluated CSWT than PSWT. There is stronger overall support for CSWT especially when the LBP is chronic. The SWT parameters and treatment details are lacking in several of these studies, making strong treatment recommendations problematic.

SWT use in chronic neck pain is not as prevalent as for LBP, but there is sufficient material to warrant inclusion. In the Kumaran and Watson (2016) review, three quality RCTs were considered. Foley-Nolan et al (1990) compared the use of PSWT against a placebo intervention, considering pain and neck movement. The therapy was not, however, classical PSWT in that the applicator was embedded in a soft collar and the treatment was delivered for 6–8 hours a day. The dose (power) was extremely low, but the cumulative effect over many hours approximates that which is delivered in a single clinic session. Patient numbers were small (n=20) and there was no follow-up period in this trial and thus, the longer-term benefits remain unevaluated.

A larger (n=350) and more recent trial (Dziedzic et al 2005) compared manual therapy, PSWT and a control condition in a three-group RCT. The PSWT was delivered for 15–20 minutes with 8 sessions over 6 weeks. All groups received advice and exercise, but neither the PSWT nor the manual therapy added significant value to the outcomes. This trial, whilst involving large patient numbers, was pragmatic in design, and over 50 different therapists were involved in treatment delivery. There were no set parameters for the PSWT, so the treatment was certainly not consistent, which weakens the results. A further publication related to the same trial (Lewis et al 2007) carried out an economic evaluation and, as might be predicted, concluded that advice and exercise was the more economic intervention.

Several studies have evaluated the effect of SWT for tissue stiffness in various clinical conditions. Leung and Cheing (2008) reported a significantly better outcome when treating 30 subjects complaining of stiffness (frozen shoulder) with thermal SWT and stretching. Treatment was compared to superficial heat (hot pack) and stretching or stretching alone. All groups demonstrated improvement. The addition of CSWT resulted in greater effect (p=0.046) than stretch alone. Treatments were delivered for 20 minutes, 3 times weekly over 4 weeks, at a comfortable thermal level using a contraplanar capacitive electrode application.

Draper and colleagues have evaluated the effect of SWT as a means to enhance the effect of stretching and mobilization in various clinical circumstances. Draper and Patten 2010 combined stretching with thermal SWT when treating post-surgical patients who had decreased knee ROM. Findings were positive, and in one case the patient was able to regain full ROM following 4 sessions of thermal SWT. Seiger and Draper (2006) employed PSWT in 4 patients with restricted ankle range with metal present in the tissue. PSWT was delivered at 800 PPS; 400 µs PD and a mean power of 48W over a 20-minute period combined with mobilization. A good result was achieved with all patients and no untoward or adverse effects were noted, despite the presence of metal in the tissue. Draper (2011) also presented a case series of 7 patients with restricted elbow range of motion. PSWT (at 48 W MP) was employed with mobilization to good effect. This is replicated by Draper (2014) in a further case series. Whilst these case series do not achieve the robust evidence level of an RCT, the results provide useful insight that PSWT applied at thermal levels and combined with mobilization can achieve significant benefit in terms of restricted joint range.

Useful studies are published with patients experiencing plantar fasciitis (Brook et al 2012; Michel 2012). A small portable device (along the lines of the Foley Nolan et al (1990) study) was utilized, evaluating effectiveness for morning pain and stiffness. Forty patients were allocated to treatment or sham groups in the Brook et al study, wearing the device overnight for 7 days. The Michel research was based on a case series of 6 patients. Positive outcomes were achieved in both studies though a lack of statistical power detracts from the Brook et al results.

Studies in a range of musculoskeletal conditions are reported in the literature including temporomandibular disorder (TMD). Gray et al (1994) evaluated the effects of four different modalities, including both CSWT and PSWT, in addition to laser, ultrasound and placebo groups. All four active treatments were significantly effective in terms of the success rate when compared against the placebo condition (success rates ranged between 70 and 78%), though there was no significant difference between the four tested modalities.

More recently, Adley et al (2017) examined SWT in a single-blind trial with 32 patients presenting with temporomandibular joint pain. Patients were randomly allocated to SWT or placebo groups. Treatment was given for 3 sessions per week over 4 weeks. Patients were followed up at 1 week and 6 weeks post intervention. Pain was evaluated using VAS and joint clicking was evaluated with a stethoscope. Results showed that SWT is a significantly effective treatment in reducing pain and clicking associated with TMD, both during and after treatment. Whilst not a large trial, SWT may provide an effective intervention for TMD alongside other EPAs recently reviewed (Gil-Martinez et al 2018).

In acute clinical presentations, PSWT dominates the literature – almost certainly on the basis that heat can be clinically disadvantageous in these circumstances, and PSWT offers the opportunity to deliver effective treatment without gross temperature changes in the tissue.

In the Kumaran and Watson (2015a) review considering only the acute clinical situation, 30 trials were identified, most of which employed PSWT, and 22 of the 30 related to clinical pain and inflammatory lesions.

Postoperative pain dominated the reviewed studies (n=9) followed by acute ankle injuries (n=6), then smaller numbers for fracture pain, hand injury, acute LBP and whiplash. Only the post-operative pain and ankle study groups are considered in this section.

Kaplan and Weinstock (1968) employed twice daily PSWT following foot surgery in a group of 100 patients divided into treatment and sham groups. Like several studies of this era, the PSWT was delivered not only to the operated foot, but also to the epigastrium. Patients in the treatment group experienced significant reduction in pain and oedema, though it is not possible to disaggregate the PSWT effects that can be ascribed to the foot treatment or the epigastric exposure.

Several recent studies have tested the effect of small, portable, wearable PSWT devices (akin to that used in the Foley-Nolan et al (1990) trial) used in the acute postoperative period (Heden and Pilla 2008; Rawe 2012; Rohde et al 2010). Treatment was typically delivered for 30 minutes between 3 and 6 times daily over the first post-operative days (usually 5–6 days). The Rawe et al study (2012) treated with a continuous application over a 7-day period. Compared with placebo intervention, significant pain reduction was experienced by patients in the treatment group.

Whilst there are several studies in the acute postoperative group, which have methodological limitations and small sample numbers, the weight of the evidence falls in favour of treatment over sham exposure. Delivering sufficient treatment sessions can be potentially problematic, but utilizing portable 'wearable' devices makes that a more realistic intervention.

The final acute group of studies considered in this chapter are those relating to acute ankle injury. An oft-cited study by Wilson (1972), though now somewhat dated, used PSWT delivered 60 minutes a day for the first 3 days post injury, comparing treatment and sham groups (20 in each). The treatment group experienced reduction of pain and 'disability' when compared with those in the sham group. A similar study by the same author with the same clinical condition (Wilson 1974) compared the outcomes for n=40 patients with acute ankle injury, divided (matched pairs) into CSWT and PSWT groups. Inductive CSWT (using an inductothermy cable application) was delivered to the ankle, twice daily for 3 days. The PSWT was similarly delivered over two 15 minute sessions daily over the 3-day period. The results (pain, swelling, disability) clearly favoured those in the PSWT group with a reported 82% improvement in the PSWT group compared with 44% in the CSWT group. The PSWT improvements were greater given an equivalent amount of treatment.

A more recent (though still dated) study involving patients with acute ankle injury (McGill 1988) involved a larger sample (n=37) in treatment and placebo groups – though no clear control group. Patients received 3 sessions of PSWT of 15 minutes duration with a MP delivery of 19.6 W using a monode applicator. The author concluded that the PSWT failed to generate a measurable benefit for this patient group in terms of pain, swelling or time to full weight bearing, though in the light of more recent studies, the applied power would now be considered high for an acute lesion. Lastly in the acute ankle group was the study by Pennington et al (1993). Fifty patients participated in the trial which was randomized and double blind – giving an advantage over earlier study protocols. The application of PSWT in a single session achieved a significant (p<0.01) reduction in post injury ankle swelling (Grade I/II ankle sprain in a military group). The device employed was a Diapulse PSWT unit through precise dose information is not provided.

The use of SWT was recommended for treating chronic sinusitis in historical EPA books with little supportive evidence beyond the anecdotal. A recent study investigated the use of deep heat on 30 patients, aged 18 to 50 years, to treat headache, pain and discharge associated with acute sinusitis. Patients were randomly allocated to 20 minutes of CSWT (using a crossfire technique) or a placebo treatment of similar duration. Both groups were given medications for 5 days. Outcome was measured using SNOT-22 (Sinonasal Outcome Test -22) questionnaire. SWT was significantly effective (p=0.0001), with the percentage of change in SNOT-22 scores in placebo group being 23.36% compared to 46.54% in the active SWT group. The between group differences at the end of the treatment period was highly significant (p=0.00002) (Heggannavar et al 2017).

Almost all the studies reported in these sections have included pain as a primary outcome. An example of a pain focused study is presented by Lamina et al (2011) in which 32 patients were treated for pain resulting from chronic pelvic inflammatory disease. This was a double blind, randomised study with three groups: SWT, analgesia and control. SWT treatment was 20 minutes duration using CSWT (crossfire technique) for an average of 15 sessions. There was significant (p<0.05) difference between groups. VAS pain level decreased from 5.09 ±0.83 to 0.55 ±0.52 in the SWT group, compared to 6.00 ±0.63 to 2.27 ±1.35 in the analgesic group. This magnitude of pain reduction is clinically as well as statistically significant.

In summary, the use of SWT in both continuous and pulsed modes is supported by a range of clinical trial evidence, though this support is by no means universal. In the musculoskeletal and orthopaedic specialities, there is strong support. In other areas, some not detailed here, there are fewer studies and the support is mixed. As a general trend, continuous mode applications with overtly thermal effects dominate in the more chronic conditions, whilst pulsed mode, mainly at non-thermal levels are more strongly supported in the acute conditions.

THERAPEUTIC EFFECTS AND USES

As indicated in the Clinical Evidence section, there is a range of application areas for the use of both continuous and pulsed shortwave, dominated by musculoskeletal and orthopaedic speciality areas.

Pain

Many clinical trials have reported changes in pain perception as a primary outcome, and a high percentage of those trials report significant beneficial effects. The modes of action whereby SWT achieves pain relief are almost certainly multiple. In chronic pain states, increased tissue temperature is known to bring about reduction in pain (see Chapter 5). Increasing local blood flow will have a 'flushing' effect on local metabolites in addition to a direct effect on local nerve endings – possibly having the long cited 'sedative effect' though more likely causing stimulation of peripheral sensory fibres and thereby stimulating gating mechanisms at spinal cord level. This would be consistent with all other heating modalities and with known pain modulation pathways (see Chapter 3).

In pulsed mode, the observed reduction in perceived pain is clearly not tied to a thermal response. In trials where no gross tissue heating is observed, clinically meaningful pain relief has been demonstrated. Increased local blood flow is a strong contender, influencing the local inflammatory response, reducing local metabolites, cytokine and mediator concentrations.

Reduction in oedema, as demonstrated in several clinical trials including Barclay et al (1983) and Pennington et al (1993), will also serve to reduce local tissue pressure, with a secondary effect of reduction in pain

Facilitated Tissue Healing and Repair

A range of clinical applications relate to the demonstrated capacity for SWT to facilitate the tissue repair response after injury, trauma or surgery (see Chapter 3). This tissue response is consistent with the responses observed with ultrasound and laser-based therapies. The primary difference with SWT – in continuous, or particularly in pulsed mode, is that the effect is dominant in the tissue which absorbs the delivered energy (Watson 2006, 2016).

If the monode applicator is employed to deliver PSWT, the energy absorption will be dominantly in the low impedance tissues (e.g. muscle, tissue with high fluid content, such as oedema, haematoma, effusion). Whereas ultrasound has a dominant tissue repair effect in the dense collagenous tissue, PSWT enhanced repair is predominant in these highly ionic (wet) tissues – thereby making SWT applications optimal following injury and where oedema, effusion and haematoma are present.

In addition to musculoskeletal lesions, SW based therapies have demonstrated clinical benefit after fracture, though PEMF-based therapies (see Chapter 12) dominate this field. Enhanced repair in peripheral nerves has been demonstrated – at least in animal model studies (e.g. Raji 1984; Wilson & Jagadeesh 1976). Post-surgical repair can be enhanced with the application of SWT, predominantly PSWT. In addition to the recent work cited in the clinical evidence section, there is a long history of using PSWT in chronic wounds – skin ulcers (e.g. Comorosan et al 1993; Itoh et al 1991) and pressure ulcers (e.g. Seaborne et al 1996).

Much of the work with wounds and skin lesions was conducted in the 1980s and 90s. Whilst these SWT applications are still delivered, more therapists opt for laser (photobiomodulation) based treatments (see Chapter 10) ultraviolet therapy (see Chapter 11) or various electrical stimulation options (see Chapter 19) in modern practice.

With the recent developments in alternative RF application (see later sections) there is currently something of a resurgence of research in these applications and practice may change again taking SWT and RF from backstage to a more prominent status.

APPLICATION

There are two methods of transferring energy to the tissues when using SWT: the capacitive and the inductive methods.

Capacitive Method

The capacitive application utilizes electrodes in pairs, generating an alternating electrostatic field in the tissue located between them. There is no necessity for tissue contact as the radiofrequency energy travels across an air gap. Capacitive electrodes are illustrated in Figs 7.3 (air spaced) and 7.5 (flexible) with a typical clinical arrangement illustrated in Fig. 7.6.

Air Spaced Electrodes

Air spaced electrodes are composed of two metal plates (ranging in diameter from 7.5 to 17.5 cm) enclosed in a plastic or glass guard (Fig. 7.3). Two electrodes are needed for

this application and the patient is part of the electrical circuit effectively acting as a dielectric. The distance between the skin and the electrodes can be adjusted by changing either the skin/electrode distance or by adjusting the metal plate position within the electrode housing (this normally having a 2–3 cm adjustment). Technically, given the capacity to adjust the electrode position within the housing, there is no need to leave a space between the skin and the electrode, though this is commonly practised. No consensus exists in the literature on the ideal skin–electrode distance, with some suggesting 2.5 cm (Wadsworth and Chanmugam 1983), others recommending 2–4 cm (Low 2000, Scott 2002), 2–10 cm (Cameron 2013), or 2.5–7.5 cm (Prentice et al 2018). Whilst no justification is given for the choice of these values, it should be remembered that the greater the distance between the metal electrode and the skin surface, the more circulating air is allowed between electrode and treated part, which may influence heat build-up in the tissues.

Pad (Rubber) Electrodes

These electrodes are composed of a metal plate encased in rubber (Fig. 7.5). They are placed on the treated part with the electrode in a more uniform and even contact with the tissues which can be useful over uneven tissue surfaces. The treatment effect with the Pad (Rubber) electrodes is

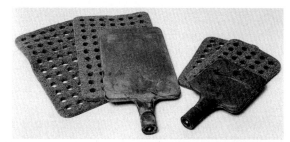

Fig. 7.5 Flexible (rubber-encased metal) electrodes and felt spacers.

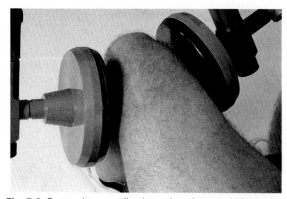

Fig. 7.6 Contraplanar application using air-spaced electrodes.

equivalent to that achieved with the Air Spaced electrodes. Spacing between the skin and the electrodes is controlled with layers of towelling or felt spacers. The amount of heating generated in the tissue is dependent on the spacing between skin and electrodes (more distance between the pads is thought to provide deeper penetration) (Prentice et al 2018). The use of one air spaced and one pad electrode is possible and at times provides an advantageous arrangement. Flexible electrode use has diminished in recent years.

Electrode Arrangement

With capacitive techniques, electrodes can be positioned in a contraplanar, coplanar, longitudinal or crossfire arrangement. In contraplanar, the electrodes are placed opposite to each other on either side of the treated area (Fig. 7.6). The distance between the skin and the electrodes can be symmetrical if an even field is desirable, or the electrodes can be positioned with uneven distances if the aim is to concentrate the field on one side of the treated area (the closer electrode) (Balenger 2015). The same applies for electrode size. The size of the applicators is considered an important factor in determining the strength of the field in the tissues. The use of two electrodes of similar size results in uniform distribution of the field in the tissues. Using electrodes of different sizes results in the concentration of the field under the smaller electrode. To achieve optimal heating, it is considered important that the electrodes are centred over the treatment area (Prentice et al 2018; He et al 2005).

Electrodes can also be positioned in a coplanar arrangement (Fig. 7.7), where both electrodes are placed on the same aspect of the treated area. For safety reasons, the distance between the two electrodes needs to be more than the sum of skin–electrode distance in order to result in an effective field distribution. Although this technique generally produces a more superficial treatment effect, the depth of the field can be increased by increasing the distance between the two electrodes and/or increasing the skin–electrode distance (Prentice et al 2018).

Other electrode arrangements include the longitudinal application, when the electrodes are placed at either end of a limb parallel to the alignment of the tissues. In the crossfire technique the electrodes are placed diagonally over the treated tissue for half the time and are then changed to the other diagonal for the rest of the time. Historically, this latter technique was used to treat cavities containing air, such as sinuses and the uterus (Heggannavar et al 2017); though clinical experience has revealed this technique to be effective, it lacks robust research evidence.

Inductive Method

Inductive SWT can be applied to the tissues by means of either a drum or a cable electrode (Prentice et al 2018; Watson 2006). The inductive method produces predominantly an H field via a cable that is either wrapped around the extremity or coiled inside an electrode housing. The use of the monode or drum applicator has become the clinical norm in current practice, and the cable application is rarely employed. Unlike the conductive technique, the patient is not part of the circuit. A modern monode applicator is illustrated in Fig. 7.4.

Monode (Drum) Electrode

The drum is composed of one or more monoplanar coils (sometimes referred to as a 'pancake' arrangement) encased inside a plastic housing (Fig. 7.4). The applicator has the advantage of being very straightforward to set up, although the disadvantage with this technique is that the drum electrode is minimally compliant with the skin contour. Maximum penetration with this technique is believed to be 3–5 cm, given that the subcutaneous fat layer does not exceed 2 cm. The face of the monode can be placed in contact with the skin, though most practitioners leave a small air gap or place the monode face in contact with a dry towel on the skin surface. There is no demonstrated difference in the treatment effect when using these different application methods.

Cable Electrode

The cable is a thick, insulated wire with plugs on either end. It can be wrapped in a pancake arrangement and placed over the treated area or it can be wrapped around the extremity. It has the advantage of fitting the contour of the body, unlike air-space or drum electrodes. A distance

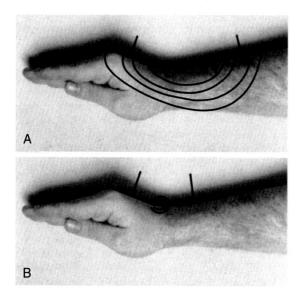

Fig. 7.7 Coplanar electrode placement illustrating (A) correct and (B) incorrect electrode spacing.

of at least 1 cm should be kept between the skin and the electrode (by wrapping the limb in a few layers of towelling), and a distance of about 5cm should be kept between the turns of the cable to prevent overheating (Al-Mandeel and Watson 2008). The cable application method is rarely employed in current clinical practice, the drum or monode applicator being considered more efficient to set up and thus more (cost) effective.

Treatment Time

Historically a 20-minute application was considered to be normal for SWT treatments. With the advent of PSWT applications, treatment durations as short as 10 minutes have been shown to be effective, and numerous studies (reviewed in the clinical evidence section) have employed 15-minute applications. In general, the more chronic the clinical condition, the longer the optimal treatment time (15–20 minutes). In acute and sub-acute conditions, 10–15 minute treatments would appear to be sufficient.

It is of interest to know that most of the theories explaining the field distribution under the various types of electrodes, their depth of penetration, and the possible approaches for arrangements remain theoretical, with little directly supportive researched evidence. Although these beliefs are widely accepted, further research is warranted, especially with regard to the actual penetration depths achieved with these various fields and applicators.

NON-TRADITIONAL RADIOFREQUENCY IN THERAPY

As identified in recent reviews regarding the use of radiofrequency applications in practice, several devices operate at frequencies other than the 'classic' 27.12 MHz (Kumaran and Watson 2015a, 2016). Given that the use of different frequencies relates to issues of regulation (FCC) rather than efficacy, these alternative RF frequency generators may be equally effective when compared with those classically employed, or indeed, may transpire to be more or less effective. Whilst there is some research on the individual RF applications, there is currently a smaller volume of published research when compared with classic SWT applications.

ReBound Diathermy Units

ReBound diathermy is one of the newer additions to the shortwave family. The unit operates in a continuous mode and utilizes a permitted frequency of 13.56 MHz. This device was first designed and developed by ReGear Life Sciences Inc. with the intention of using it in the military. Later it was introduced to the medical field as a possible replacement to the older generations of SWT with the advantage of being more portable, easily manageable and capable of providing homogeneous heating and energy distribution.

The ReBound electrodes are essentially cylindrical garment sleeves that contain a coil wrapped in fabric. The unit works on the same principle as the pancake coil (above), and has the advantage of fitting the contour of the area treated whether it is an extremity or flat area, like the trunk. The energy delivery is most like inductive shortwave as explained in the main part of this chapter.

Draper et al (2013) compared the heating pattern developed by both PSWT (using Megapulse II) and ReBound devices on 12 subjects. Temperature was measured at a depth of 3 cm in the triceps surae. The muscle was irradiated using the highest settings on both machines for a period of 30 minutes. The Megapulse II increased muscle temperatures by 4.32°C ±1.79°C and ReBound increased temperatures by 2.31°C ±0.87°C. Though Megapulse was capable of generating more heat in the tissues, the ReBound had a slower rate of dissipation in regard to temperature decay.

Hawkes et al (2013) examined the superficial heating with the ReBound device, comparing its effects with those achieved using a hot pack in a group of 12 healthy college students. Measurements were taken from triceps surae at a depth of 1 cm. The hot pack was capable of increasing superficial heating in the range of 3.69°C ±1.50°C with the ReBound unit resulting in 2.82°C ±0.90°C.

The ReBound units operate at a lower frequency than classic shortwave, and whilst they appear to generate smaller changes in tissue temperature, there may be differences that are advantageous in the clinical environment (such as a slower rate of thermal dissipation), which have yet to be fully explored.

Radiofrequency Electric Current (RFEC) Applications

The use of radiofrequency electric currents (RFEC) has gained traction in recent years with several manufacturers making devices available that typically operate at frequencies between 0.3 MHz (300 kHz) and 1 MHz, though some operate at frequencies up to 10 MHz or higher. Whilst these devices operate in the RF range, the energy application to the tissues involves direct contact (i.e. the electrodes are in contact with the tissues). Whilst nominally falling into the radiofrequency application group, the delivery of energy to the tissues is therefore different from that employed with classic shortwave devices.

Several different terms have been employed to describe this mode of therapy including: Capacitive Resistive Electric Transfer (CRET), Capacitive Resistive Monopolar Radiofrequency Therapy (CRMRT) and Transferencia Electrica

Capacitiva Resistiva (TECAR). Whilst TECAR has been used in the past as an abbreviation for this energy delivery mode, it has since been adopted as a specific device name and is therefore avoided in this text except when referring to these specific devices. Given that the therapy involves the delivery of electric currents to the tissue and that these currents are delivered in the radiofrequency range, the general term 'radiofrequency electric currents' (RFEC) is adopted in this section as an overarching term.

Devices which deliver RFEC energy and are available in the therapy arena would include the Indiba family of devices and TECAR therapy devices. There are many others which are used in the aesthetics field including physio-aesthetics, though this topic area is also generally excluded from this text.

RFEC therapy is primarily used to activate the tissue repair and recovery system, though its effects in terms of pain relief are also evident. Much as in classic shortwave the energy can be delivered in two modes: capacitive and resistive. RFEC devices utilize the long wave radiofrequency, typically in the range of 300 kHz to 2.0 MHz and a power output that does not normally exceed 300 W (though the energy delivery is reported differently in the capacitive and resistive modes). The frequencies delivered by RFEC systems are lower than traditional shortwave and higher than those causing muscle contraction. Unlike conventional SWT a conductive cream must be employed as a coupling medium between the electrode and the skin surface to facilitate the passage of the RF energy. It is proposed that these units can facilitate polarization of the cell membrane, encouraging intra and extracellular fluid exchange, reducing pain, inducing inflammatory modulation effects and increasing lymphatic mobility. The therapy is promoted to manage both acute and chronic musculoskeletal conditions (reviewed in Kumaran & Watson 2015a, 2016). The energy delivery can be employed at lower levels, producing a non-thermal application, whilst at higher energy levels, the treatment effects are overtly thermal in nature.

Spottorno et al (2017) provide a useful analysis of the different current pathways through the tissues and compare the capacitive and resistive modes of application using a finite element analysis (based on the Indiba device). An extensive range of cell studies (e.g. Hernandez-Bule et al 2014a, b; 2017) have demonstrated both safety and effectiveness with interesting and established stem cell differentiation and cancer cell related effects.

Whilst there is less published evidence for the RFEC application than for classic shortwave, there is sufficient material beyond that provided by the manufacturers to justify their inclusion in evidence-based reviews provided by Kumaran and Watson 2015a, 2016.

Healthy Human Participants

The thermal characteristics and physiological responses of RFEC were studied in 15 healthy subjects by Kumaran and Watson (2015b) using the Indiba Activ device. The unit has a peak power of 200 W and operates at a frequency of 448 kHz. It was noted that resistive and capacitive application modes generated dissimilar patterns of heating. The capacitive achieved faster build-up of temperature and a more rapid decay post treatment whilst the resistive mode application resulted in a slower rate of thermal change, which was retained for a longer period post application. Forty-five minutes after the termination of the treatment, 60% of capacitance heat was lost as opposed to only 15% with the resistive application. These changes did not alter core temperature and there was no cross talk to the neighbouring untreated areas, possibly because of lower levels of scattering of RF waves. The energy application resulted in significant changes in tissue temperature and both superficial and deep blood flow, which were sustained for a prolonged period following cessation of the treatment. These results are consistent with those obtained by Tashiro et al (2017) evaluating temperature and haemoglobin saturation in the tissues, demonstrating not only significant change, but stronger effects when compared with a heat (hot pack) based intervention. In a further study (Kumaran et al 2017) the effect of the RFEC (Indiba) application was compared with a PSWT application at the nearest equivalent energy level. The RFEC treatment generated a more pronounced change in temperature and blood flow, the effects of which lasted for a significantly longer period post intervention. Deep blood flow increased by 79% over the treatment period compared with 4% for the control condition and a reduction of 14% following PSWT application. The application of RFEC energy, therefore, appears to generate significant physiological change in temperature and blood flow in healthy participants. The resistive mode of delivery generates a longer-lasting effect and when compared with other interventions (hot pack, pulsed shortwave) these changes are significantly more pronounced. If temperature and vascular change are a treatment aim (such as to facilitate repair post injury), the magnitude and duration of these tissue responses could have clinical value.

Clinical Studies

In a study by Ganzit (2000), 327 patients aged between 18 and 60 years were divided into two groups; acute and chronic. The device used was composed of a generator that distributes signals at a frequency of 0.5 MHz and a peak power of 300W. The sessions were started with a resistive treatment, the electrode was positioned on the area to be treated for 10 minutes, followed by another 10 minutes with a capacitive electrode applied on the same area. Outcome measures were Steinbroker Index modified for athletic activity and VAS. Results showed a reduction in pain and improved function. Improvement was seen in both (acute and chronic) groups.

Osti et al (2015) employed a combination of RFEC (Pharon, Italy) with laser in managing low back pain. Sixty-six patients complaining of back pain, with or without leg pain, were treated using both laser (I-Triax) and Pharon-based TECAR therapy. Treatment was provided three times weekly on alternate days, for a total of 10 sessions. Outcome was evaluated with VAS and the Oswestry Disability Scale. Results indicated a significant reduction in pain and a significant improvement in their Oswestry score. Best results were seen with patients having leg pain. It is not possible to disaggregate the contribution made by the laser and the RFEC components of this treatment package.

Notarnicola et al (2017) compared the efficacy of RFEC (Doctor TECAR Therapy) with laser therapy, each group receiving 10 (daily) treatment sessions over 2 weeks. Sixty patients complaining of back pain were enrolled. VAS, Oswestry and Roland Morris scores were employed as outcome measures. Significant improvement was evident with both modalities in the short term. However, the RFEC treatment group results were superior when the follow-up results were compared.

In a randomized controlled clinical trial, a similar comparison was carried out (Kumaran & Watson 2019) recruiting patients with chronic osteoarthritis of the knee. Forty-five patients were randomized into an active treatment group, placebo intervention group and a control group. The control group only received best current standard care (exercise and advice) which was common to all three groups. The RFEC was delivered using an Indiba Activ device, with 8 sessions over a 4-week period with a 15 minute treatment time (5 minutes in capacitive mode, 10 minutes in resistive mode) at a comfortable thermal level. The active treatment group demonstrated significantly greater pain relief post treatment when compared with both the placebo and control groups, sustained at follow-up. Function was evaluated using the WOMAC scale and also demonstrated significant improvement over the treatment period compared with the control. Benefits were not claimed for the treatment as a replacement for existing best care but as an adjunct to its use.

The results obtained from both healthy participants and in clinical trials are interesting and indicate that RFEC is a potentially useful tool in the treatment of musculoskeletal pathologies. Given that there is still a relatively small evidence base regarding the interaction between RFECs and biological systems, more evidence is required to substantiate its apparent efficacy.

REFERENCES

Adly, M., Alzamzami, M., Altukroni, A., et al. (2017). Evaluating the effectiveness of shortwave diathermy on temporomandibular joint disorder. *International Journal of Healthcare sciences, 4*(2), 2064–2067.

Ahmed, M. S., Shakoor, M. A., & Khan, A. A. (2009). Evaluation of the effects of shortwave diathermy in patients with chronic low back pain. *Bangladesh Medical Research Council Bulletin, 35*(1), 18–20.

Al-Mandeel, M., & Watson, T. (2006). An evaluative audit of patient records in electrotherapy with specific reference to pulsed shortwave therapy. *International Journal of Therapy and Rehabilitation, 13*(9), 414–419.

Al-Mandeel, M., & Watson, T. (2008). Shortwave and pulsed shortwave therapies. In T. Watson (Ed.), *Electrotherapy: Evidence-based practice* (12th ed.). London: Elsevier.

Atamaz, F., Durmaz, B., Baydar, M., et al. (2012). Comparison of the efficacy of transcutaneous electrical nerve stimulation, interferential currents, and shortwave diathermy in knee osteoarthritis: A double-blind, randomized, controlled multicenter study. *Archives of Physical Medicine and Rehabilitation, 93*(5), 748–756.

Barclay, V., Collier, R. J., & Jones, A. (1983). Treatment of various hand injuries by pulsed electromagnetic energy (Diapulse). *Physiotherapy, 69*(6), 186–188.

Belanger AY. (2015) *Therapeutic electrophysical agents: Evidence behind practice* (3rd ed.). Lippincott Williams & Wilkins, Philadelphia.

Boyaci, A., Tutoglu, A., Koca, I., Kocaturk, O., & Celen, E. (2014). Comparison of the short-term effectiveness of short-wave diathermy treatment in patients with carpal tunnel syndrome: A randomized controlled trial. *Archives of Rheumatology, 29*(4), 298–304.

Bricknell, R., & Watson, T. (1995). The thermal effects of pulsed shortwave therapy. *British Journal of Therapy and Rehabilitation, 2*(8), 430–434.

Brook, J., Dauphinee, D. M., Korpinen, J., & Rawe, I. M. (2012). Pulsed radiofrequency electromagnetic field therapy: A potential novel treatment of plantar fasciitis. *The Journal of Foot and Ankle Surgery, 51*(3), 312–316.

Cacolice, P., Scibek, J., & Martin, R. (2013). Diathermy: A literature review of current research and practices. *Orthopedics Practice, 25*, 3–13.

Cameron, M. (2013). *Physical agents in rehabilitation: From research to practice* (4th ed.). Philadelphia: Saunders.

Comorosan, S., Vasilco, R., Arghiropol, M., Paslaru, L., Jieanu, V., & Stelea, S. (1993). The effect of diapulse therapy on the healing of decubitus ulcer. *Romanian Journal of Physiology, 30*(1–2), 41–45.

Cortes, J., Kubat, N., & Japour, C. (2013). Pulsed radio frequency energy therapy use for pain relief following surgery for tendinopathy-associated chronic pain: Two case reports. *Military Medicine, 178*, e125–e129.

Draper, D. O. (2011). Injuries restored to ROM using PSWD and mobilizations. *International Journal of Sports Medicine, 32*(4), 281–286.

Draper, D. O. (2014). Pulsed shortwave diathermy and joint mobilizations for achieving normal elbow range of motion after injury or surgery with implanted metal: A case series. *Journal of Athletic Training*, 49(6), 851–855.

Draper, D. (2017). Can pulsed shortwave diathermy be used over surgically implanted metal? *Human Kinetics journal*, 22(6), 23–27.

Draper, D., Hawkes, A., Johnson, A., et al. (2013). Muscle heating with Megapulse II shortwave diathermy and ReBound diathermy. *Journal of Athletic Training*, 48(4), 477–482.

Draper, D., Knight, K., Fujiwara, T. & Castel, J. (1999). Temperature change in human muscle during and after pulsed short-wave diathermy. *J Orthop Sports Phys Ther*, 29(1): 13–22.

Draper, D., & Patten, J. (2010). Shortwave diathermy and joint mobilisation for post-surgical restoration of knee motion. *Human Kinetics Journal*, 15(1), 39–41.

Durney, C., & Christensen, D. (2000). *Basic introduction to electromagnetics*. Boca Raton: CRC Press.

Dziedzic, K., Hill, J., Lewis, M., Sim, J., Daniels, J., & Hay, E. M. (2005). Effectiveness of manual therapy or pulsed shortwave diathermy in addition to advice and exercise for neck disorders: A pragmatic randomized controlled trial in physical therapy clinics. *Arthritis & Rheumatism*, 53(2), 214–222.

Foley-Nolan, D., Barry, C., Coughlan, R. J., O'Connor, P., & Roden, D. (1990). Pulsed high frequency (27MHz) electromagnetic therapy for persistent neck pain. A double blind, placebo-controlled study of 20 patients. *Orthopedics*, 13(4), 445–451.

Fukuda, T., Cunha, A., Fukuda, V., et al. (2011). Pulsed shortwave treatment in women with knee osteoarthritis: A multicenter, randomized, placebo-controlled clinical trial. *Physical Therapy*, 91(7), 1009–1017.

Gabriel, C., & Peyman, A. (2018). Dielectric properties of biological tissues; variation with age. In J. Ram & M. Conn (Eds.), *Conn's handbook of models for human aging* (2nd ed.). (pp. 939–952) Cambridge: Academic Press.

Ganzit, G. (2000). New methods in the treatment of joint-muscular pathologies in athletes. The TECAR therapy. *Medicina Dello Sport*, 53(4), 361–367.

Gil-Martinez, A., Paris-Alemany, A., Lopez-de-Uralde-Villanueva, I., & La Touche, R. (2018). Management of pain in patients with temporomandibular disorder (TMD): Challenges and solutions. *Journal of Pain Research*, 11, 571–587.

Gray, R., Quayle, A., Hall, C., et al. (1994). Physiotherapy in the treatment of temporomandibular joint disorders: a comparative study of four treatment methods. *British Dental Journal*, 176(7), 257–261.

Hawkes, A., Draper, D., Johnson, W., et al. (2013). Heating capacity of ReBound shortwave diathermy and moist hot packs at superficial depths. *Journal of Athletic Training*, 48(4), 471–476.

He, X. X., Weng, Y., Ye, B., Shu, Y., Chen, J., Zhu & Mao G. (2005). "Study on Thermal Map Distribution in Phantom by Short Wave Capacitance Coupled Heating." *Chinese Journal of Biomedical Engineering* 24(5), 560–565.

Heden, P., & Pilla, A. A. (2008). Effects of pulsed electromagnetic fields on postoperative pain: A double-blind randomized

pilot study in breast augmentation patients. *Aesthetic Plastic Surgery*, 32(4), 660–666.

Heggannavar, A., Harugop, A., Madhale, D., et al. (2017). Randomised controlled study to evaluate the effectiveness of shortwave diathermy in acute sinusitis. *International Journal of Physiotherapy and Research*, 5(3), 2066–2072.

Hernández-Bule, M. L., Paíno, C. L., Trillo, M. Á., & Úbeda, A. (2014a). Electric stimulation at 448 kHz promotes proliferation of human mesenchymal stem cells. *Cellular Physiology and Biochemistry*, 34(5), 1741–1755.

Hernandez-Bule, M. L., Trillo, M. A., & Ubeda, A. (2014b). Molecular mechanisms underlying antiproliferative and differentiating responses of hepatocarcinoma cells to subthermal electric stimulation. *PLoS One*, 9(1), e84636.

Hernandez Bule, M. L., Angeles Trillo, M., Martinez Garcia, M. A., Abilahoud, & Ubeda, A. (2017). Chondrogenic differentiation of adipose-derived stem cells by radiofrequency electric stimulation. *Journal of Stem Cell Research & Therapy*, 7(12), 7–12.

He, X., Weng, X., Ye, Y., et al. (2005). Study on thermal map distribution in phantom by shortwave capacitance coupled heating. *Chinese Journal of Biomedical Engineering*, 24(5), 560–565.

Incebiyik, S., Boyaci, A., & Tulogu, A. (2015). Short term effectiveness of shortwave diathermy treatment on pain, clinical symptoms, and hand function in patients with mild or moderate idiopathic carpal tunnel syndrome. *Journal of Back and Musculoskeletal Rehabilitation*, 28(2), 221–228.

Itoh, M., Montemayor, J. S., Jr., Matsumoto, E., Eason, A., Lee, M. H. M., & Folk, F. S. (1991). Accelerated wound healing of pressure ulcers by pulsed high peak power electromagnetic energy (Diapulse). *Decubitus*, 4(1), 24–25.

Jan, M., Ming, H., Chung, L., et al. (2006). Effects of repetitive shortwave diathermy for reducing synovitis in patients with knee osteoarthritis: An ultrasonographic study. *Physical Therapy*, 86, 236–244.

Jorge, M. S. G., Zanin, C., Knob, B., & Wibelinger, L. M. (2017). Effects of deep heating to treat osteoarthritis pain: Systematic review. *Revista Dor*, 18(1), 79–84.

Kaplan, E. G., & Weinstock, R. E. (1968). Clinical evaluation of diapulse as adjunctive therapy following foot surgery. *Journal of the American Podiatry Association*, 58(5), 218–221.

Kerem, M., & Yigiter, K. (2002). Effects of continuous and pulsed shortwave diathermy in low back pain. *The Pain Clinic*, 14(1), 55–59.

Kumaran, B., Herbland, A., & Watson, T. (2017). Continuous-mode 448 kHz capacitive resistive monopolar radiofrequency induces greater deep blood flow changes compared to pulsed mode shortwave: A crossover study in healthy adults. *European Journal of Physiotherapy*, 19(3), 137–146.

Kumaran, B., & Watson, T. (2015a). Radiofrequency based treatment in therapy related clinical practice – a narrative review. Part: I Acute conditions. *Physical Therapy Reviews*, 20(4), 241–254.

Kumaran, B., & Watson, T. (2015b). Thermal build-up, decay and retention responses to local therapeutic application of 448 kHz capacitive resistive monopolar radiofrequency: A prospective randomised crossover study in healthy adults. *International Journal of Hyperthermia, 31*(8), 883–895.

Kumaran, B., & Watson, T. (2016). Radiofrequency based treatment in therapy related clinical practice – a narrative review. Part II: Chronic conditions. *Physical Therapy Reviews, 20*(5–6), 325–343.

Kumaran, B., & Watson, T. (2018). Skin thermophysiological effects of 448 kHz capacitive resistive monopolar radiofrequency in healthy adults: A randomised crossover study and comparison with pulsed shortwave therapy. *Electromagnetic Biology and Medicine, 37*(1), 1–12.

Kumaran, B., & Watson, T. (2019). Treatment using 448kHz capacitive resistive monopolar radiofrequency improves pain and function in patients with osteoarthritis of the knee joint: a randomised controlled trial. *Physiotherapy, 105*(1), 98–107.

Lamina, S., Hanif, S., & Gagarawa, Y. (2011). Shortwave diathermy in symptomatic management of chronic pelvic inflammatory disease pain. A randomized controlled trial. *Physiotherapy Research International, 16*, 50–56.

Laufer, Y., & Dar, G. (2012). Effectiveness of thermal and athermal short-wave diathermy for the management of knee osteoarthritis: A systematic review and meta-analysis. *Osteoarthritis and Cartilage, 20*(9), 957–966.

Leung, M. S., & Cheing, G. L. (2008). Effects of deep and superficial heating in the management of frozen shoulder. *Journal of Rehabilitation Medicine, 40*(2), 145–150.

Lewis, M., James, M., Stokes, E., Hill, J., Sim, J., Hay, E., et al. (2007). An economic evaluation of three physiotherapy treatments for non-specific neck disorders alongside a randomized trial. *Rheumatology, 46*(11), 1701–1708.

Low, J., & Reed, A. (2000). *Electrotherapy explained: Principles and practice* (3rd ed.). Oxford: Butterworth–Heinemann.

Markov, M., & Colbert, A. (2000). Magnetic and electromagnetic field therapy. *Journal of Back and Musculoskeletal Rehabilitation, 15*(1), 17–29.

McGill, S. N. (1988). The effects of pulsed shortwave therapy on lateral ligament sprain of the ankle. *New Zealand Journal of Physiotherapy, 16*(3), 21–24.

Michel, R. (2012). Use of pulsed radio frequency energy in the effective treatment of recalcitrant plantar fasciitis: Six case histories. *The Foot, 22*(1), 48–52.

Minson, C. T., Berry, L. T., & Joyner, M. J. (2001). Nitric oxide and neurally mediated regulation of skin blood flow during local heating. *Journal of Applied Physiology, 91*(4), 1619–1626.

Nagaoka, T., Watanabe, S., Sakurai, K., et al. (2003). Development of realistic high resolution whole body voxel models of Japanese adult males and females of average height and weight and application of models to radiofrequency electromagnetic field dosimetry. *Physics in Medicine and Biology, 49*(1), 1–16.

Notarnicola, A., Maccagnano, G., Gallone, M., et al. (2017). Short term efficacy of capacitive-resistive diathermy therapy in patients with low back pain: A prospective randomized controlled trial. *Journal of Biological Regulators & Homeostatic Agents, 31*(2), 509–515.

Okabe, T., Fujimuta, Okajima, J., et al. (2018). Non invasive measurement of effective thermal conductivity of human skin with a guard heated thermister probe. *International Journal of Heat Transfer, 126 part B*, 625–635.

Osti, R., Paris, C., Salvatori, G., et al. (2015). Tri-length laser therapy associated to TECAR therapy in the treatment of low back pain in adults: A preliminary report of prospective case scenario. *Laser in Medical Science, 30*(1), 407–412.

Pall, M. (2013). Electromagnetic fields act via activation of voltage gated calcium channels to produce beneficial or adverse effects. *Journal of Cellular and Molecular Medicine, 17*(8), 958–965.

Pennington, G. M., Danley, D. L., Sumko, M. H., Bucknell, A., & Nelson, J. H. (1993). Pulsed, non-thermal, high-frequency electromagnetic energy (Diapulse) in the treatment of grade I and grade II ankle sprains. *Military Medicine, 158*(2), 101–104.

Pop, L., Muresan, M., Comorosan, S., & Paslaru, L. (1989). The effects of pulsed, high frequency radio waves on rat liver (ultrastructural and biomedical observations). *Physiological Chemistry and Physics and Medical NMR, 21*(1), 45–55.

Prentice, W., & Draper, D. (2018). Shortwave and microwave diathermy. In W. E. Prentice (Ed.), *Therapeutic modalities in rehabilitation*. New York: McGraw-Hill Medical.

Raji, A. M. (1984). An experimental study of the effects of pulsed electromagnetic field (Diapulse) on nerve repair. *Journal of Hand Surgery, 9B*(2), 105–112.

Rawe, I. M., Lowenstein, A., Barcelo, C. R., & Genecov, D. G. (2012). Control of postoperative pain with a wearable continuously operating pulsed radiofrequency energy device: A preliminary study. *Aesthetic Plastic Surgery, 36*(2), 458–463.

Reif-Acherman, S. (2017). Jacques Arsene d'Arsonval: His life and contributions to electrical instrumentation in physics and medicine. Part III: High-frequency experiences and the beginnings of diathermy. *Proceedings of the IEEE, 105*(2), 394–404.

Rohde, C., Chiang, A., Adipoju, O., Casper, D., & Pilla, A. A. (2010). Effects of pulsed electromagnetic fields on interleukin-1b and postoperative pain: A double-blind, placebo-controlled, pilot study in breast reduction patients. *Plastic and Reconstructive Surgery, 125*(6), 1620–1629.

Scott, S. (2002). Diathermy. In S. Kitchen (Ed.), *Electrotherapy: Evidence-based practice* (pp. 145–165). Edinburgh: Churchill Livingstone.

Seaborne, D., Quirion DeGirardi, C., Rousseau, M., Rivest, M., & Lambert, J. (1996). The treatment of pressure sores using pulsed electromagnetic energy (PEME). *Physiotherapy Canada, 48*(2), 131–137.

Seiger, C., & Draper, D. O. (2006). Use of pulsed shortwave diathermy and joint mobilization to increase ankle range of motion in the presence of surgical implanted metal: A case series. *Journal of Orthopaedic and Sports Physical Therapy, 36*(9), 669–677.

Shah, S., & Farrow, A. (2013). Assessment of physiotherapists' occupational exposure to radiofrequency electromagnetic fields from shortwave and microwave diathermy devices: A literature review. *Journal of Occupational and Environmental Hygiene, 10*(6), 312–327.

Shakoor, M. A., Al Hasan, S., Moyeenuzzaman, M., & Deb, A. K. (2010). Treatment with short wave diathermy on chronic low back pain. *Journal of Chittagong Medical College Teachers' Association, 21*(1), 40–44.

Shakoor, M. A., Rahman, M. S., & Moyeenuzzaman, M. (2008). Effects of deep heat therapy on the patients with chronic low back pain. *Mymensingh Medical Journal, 17*(2 Suppl. l), S32–S38.

Shields, N., O'Hare, N., & Gormley, J. (2004). Contra-indications to shortwave diathermy: Survey of Irish physiotherapists. *Physiotherapy, 90*, 42–53.

Sousa, N., Guirro, E., Calio, J., et al. (2017). Application of shortwave diathermy to the lower limb increases arterial blood flow velocity and skin temperature in women: Randomized controlled trial. *Brazilian Journal of Physical Therapy, 21*(2), 127–137.

Spottorno, J., Gonzalez de Vega, C., Buenaventura, M., & Hernando, A. (2017). Influence of electrodes on the 448 kHz electric currents created by radiofrequency: A finite element study. *Electromagnetic Biology and Medicine, 36*(3), 306–314.

Tashiro, Y., Hasegawa, S., Yokota, Y., Nishiguchi, S., Fukutani, N., Shirooka, H., et al. (2017). Effect of capacitive and resistive electric transfer on haemoglobin saturation and tissue temperature. *International Journal of Hyperthermia, 33*(6), 696–702.

Teslim, O., Adebowale, A., Ojoawo, A., et al. (2013). Comparative effects of pulsed and continuous short wave diathermy on pain and selected physiological parameters among subjects with chronic knee osteoarthritis. *Technical Health Care, 21*(5), 433–440.

Virtanen, H., Keshvari, J., & Lappalainen, R. (2006). Interaction of radio frequency electromagnetic fields and passive metallic implants – a brief review. *Bioelectromagnetics, 27*(6), 431–439.

Wadsworth, H., & Chanmugam, P. (1983). *Electrophysical agents in physiotherapy* (2nd ed.). Marrickville, NSW: Science Press.

Wang, H., Zhang, C., Gao, C., et al. (2017). Effects of short-wave therapy in patients with knee osteoarthritis: A systematic review and meta-analysis. *Clinical Rehabilitation, 31*(5), 660–671.

Ward, A. (1980). *Electricity, fields and waves in therapy.* Marrickville, NSW: Science Press.

Watson, T. (2000). The role of electrotherapy in contemporary physiotherapy practice. *Manual Therapy, 5*(3), 132–141.

Watson, T. (2006). Electrotherapy and tissue repair. *Sport Ex Med, 29*, 7–13.

Watson, T. (2016). *Expanding our understanding of the inflammatory process and its role in pain & tissue healing.* Glasgow: IFOMPT 2016.

William, B. R. J. (2009). *Experimental Study of Heating effects of 27.12 MHz Diathermy unit on clay models for Hyperthermia applications in cancer treatment.* (MSc), California State University: Sacramento. http://hdl.handle.net/10211.9/528.

Wilson, D. H. (1972). Treatment of soft-tissue injuries by pulsed electrical energy. *British Medical Journal, 2*(5808), 269–270.

Wilson, D. H. (1974). Comparison of short-wave diathermy and pulsed electromagnetic energy in treatment of soft tissue injuries. *Physiotherapy, 60*(10), 309–310 1974.

Wilson, D. H., & Jagadeesh, P. (1976). Experimental regeneration in peripheral nerves and the spinal cord in laboratory animals exposed to a pulsed electromagnetic field. *Paraplegia, 14*(1), 12–20.

Yilmaz, M., Akpinar, P., Aktas, I., et al. (2018). Effectiveness of shortwave diathermy for subacromial impingement syndrome and value of night pain for patient selection: A randomized placebo-controlled trial. *American Journal of Physical Medicine and Rehabilitation, 97*(3), 178–186.

Cryotherapy

Chris Bleakley

INTRODUCTION AND HISTORY

Cryotherapy is the use of cold for therapeutic purpose. It is one of the simplest and oldest therapeutic modalities and dates back to 3000 BCE when the Egyptians were reported to use cold compresses to treat inflammation and infection (Korpan 2007). By the early 1800s, the Europeans were using cooling for anaesthesia and even amputation, and later that century, an English physician named James Arnott was the first to use cryotherapy in the treatment of tumours. Today, cryotherapy is one of the most popular treatments for managing acute soft tissue injury and musculoskeletal pain conditions, and is commonly recommended as an adjunct to rehabilitation.

Cryotherapy has traditionally been applied using crushed-ice packs or gel packs. However, newer techniques of cryotherapy have broadened its use for postsurgical patients, and it is a common postoperative intervention. Since the late 1990s, many athletes have been using cold-water immersion (CWI) baths to treat the effects of exercise-induced muscle damage and to expedite recovery post exercise. Most recently, whole-body cryotherapy (WBC), which involves exposure to extremely cold, dry air (below -100°C) for short periods of time, has gained popularity. Although this technique was originally developed to treat chronic medical conditions, such as multiple sclerosis and rheumatoid arthritis, WBC is also increasingly employed by athletes to treat muscle soreness and facilitate recovery after exercise (Costello et al 2015).

PHYSICAL PRINCIPLES

Cryotherapy achieves its clinical effect by extracting heat energy from the body. As topical cooling relies primarily on conduction for heat extraction, temperature reductions at skin level are consistently larger compared with muscle tissue or joints. Overlying adipose tissue also creates a large insulating effect due to its low thermal conductivity and diffusivity. Indeed, it is estimated that a 1-cm increase in adipose thickness reduces the rate of cooling (at 1-cm intramuscular depth) from 0.72 to 0.45°C/min in healthy subjects (Myrer et al 2001). In effect, the potential to induce large or fast changes to deep tissue may be restricted to the lean athletic population, or to body parts with less adipose distribution.

BIOPHYSICAL EFFECTS

Local Cooling

It is proposed that topical cooling after acute injury can facilitate recovery by reducing pain, altering blood flow and reducing inflammation and metabolism, which cumulatively can protect tissue around the injury site.

Hypoalgesia

Hypoalgesia is one of the most fundamental physiological effects associated with cryotherapy. This may be underpinned by a number of mechanisms, but one of the most commonly purported is cold-induced reduction in nerve conduction velocity (NCV). Indeed, a number of early studies confirm the linear relationship between skin temperature and NCV (Greathouse et al 1989). More recent evidence from healthy human models shows that cooling skin temperature to approximately 15°C results in a 33% reduction in NCV, with corresponding localized analgesia (Algafly & George 2007). Other research by Herrera et al (2010) shows that cryotherapy has different effects on motor and sensory nerves, with larger reductions in NCV occurring in sensory compared to motor nerves. Interestingly, these authors also recorded a cold-induced decrease in compound action potential amplitude, and they consequently suggest that the inactivation of some nerve fibres could be a related physiological mechanism underpinning the hypoalgesic effect of cryotherapy. Other purported mechanisms for cold-induced hypoalgesia include: closing of the pain gate, decreased receptor sensitivity, reduced muscle spasm and counter irritant effects that activate inhibitory control mechanisms (Bleakley et al 2012; Ernst & Fialka 1994).

Altered Haemodynamics

Topical cooling results in an immediate constriction of superficial blood vessels. The general consensus is that this is mediated by adrenergic and non-adrenergic pathways. However, larger reductions in tissue temperature will also increase Rho kinase activity and decrease endothelial nitric oxide production, which also culminates into a reduction in blood flow (Bailey et al 2004). There is consistent evidence that various modes of cryotherapy can significantly reduce blood flow in large vessels. For example, a 20-minute ice application on healthy forearms reduces radial artery flow by 25% (Topp et al 2013), and full limb immersion in cold water is associated with reductions in superficial femoral artery blood flow and vessel diameter ranging between 16 and 80% (Mawhinney et al 2017; Menetrier et al 2015). Data on the effect of cryotherapy on the microvasculature show similar patterns. In healthy human tendons (Knobloch et al 2006; Knobloch et al 2008), 10 minutes of cooling decreased capillary flow, with the greatest changes observed in the first 1–3 minutes; and there were also cold-induced decreases in post-capillary filling pressure and an improvement of venous outflow. One of these studies (Knobloch et al 2008) used intermittent applications based on three 10-minute periods of cooling, separated by 10 minutes of recovery at room temperature. Interestingly, removal of the cooling modality was associated with an increase in capillary flow towards baseline levels.

It is logical that topical cooling will have more effect on the superficial vasculature. Indeed, the research of Knobloch et al (2006, 2008) recorded microcirculation at two different tissues depths, with a clear attenuation of cold-induced effects occurring at 8 mm compared to 2 mm. There is little research into the effect that topical cryotherapy can have on the deep vessels. One study (Selkow et al 2012) used contrast enhanced ultrasound (CEU) to quantify microvascular volume in the gastrocnemius muscle of healthy adults, but found no effect of cryotherapy, even though intramuscular temperature reductions of 7°C were achieved.

We must also consider that it is most relevant to ascertain the effects of cryotherapy on the vasculature when applied in the immediate stages after trauma. Indeed, an acute soft-tissue injury causes significant changes to the microvasculature, including increases in vessel diameter, blood vessel permeability and macromolecular leakage, with subsequent decreases in tissue perfusion. While it is proposed that cryotherapy can help to regulate or reverse some of these effects, this hypothesis has not been studied at all in injured human subjects. Furthermore, intravital microscopy studies undertaken on animal models have failed to delineate any marked or consistent effect of cryotherapy on microvascular diameters or blood flow velocities in the early stages post injury (Schaser et al 2006; Schaser et al 2007; Westermann et al 1999).

Anti-inflammatory

Although many clinicians agree that cryotherapy has a protective effect on injured tissue, the biochemical mechanisms have not been extensively investigated in clinical models. However, through basic scientific research in animals, we can estimate the extent to which cryotherapy attenuates inflammation, and determine which cellular pathways may be most affected. Much of this field has examined the effect of cooling on the activation and extravasation of white blood cells (neutrophils, monocytes, eosinophils and macrophages), an event that dominates the early stages of inflammation. Although white blood cells have a critical role in healing through their removal of necrotic debris and release of cytokines, they can also have a negative effect on soft tissue healing after injury. For example, white cell activation results in a series of reactions termed the 'respiratory burst' (Blake et al 1987), which produces reactive oxygen species (ROS), such as superoxide, hydrogen peroxide and hypochlorous acid, which is a powerful antibacterial agent. In certain circumstances, the production of ROS and antibacterial agents are important immune defence mechanisms, but overproduction of ROS in the absence of bacteria or infection may cause unwanted collateral damage to adjacent tissues and surrounding molecules. A number of animal models have used fluorescent intravital microscopy to observe the real-time effect that cryotherapy has on white blood cell activity within the microvasculature, and there is clear consensus that over the first 24 hours after injury, cryotherapy lowers the percentage of both adherent and rolling neutrophils after injury, in comparison to untreated injured tissue (Lee et al 2005; Schaser et al 2006; Schaser et al 2007; Westermann et al 1999). There are concurrent findings from histological analysis on injured animal models. A study by Schaser et al (2006) found that cooling decreased neutrophilic granulocyte muscle infiltration, in comparison to control muscle. In a follow-up study (Schaser et al 2007) using longer periods of cooling (5 hours), tissue analysis at 24 hours post trauma also found lower levels of neutrophilic granulocytes in the cold treated muscle. More recent animal studies (Puntel et al 2013; Singh et al 2017) concur, reporting significantly lower levels of white blood cells in tissue treated with cryotherapy, compared with injured untreated tissue. Of particular interest was that one of these studies by Puntel et al (2013) used an ischaemia and reperfusion (I/R) model of injury. I/R is a crucial factor in the generation of oxidative damage following soft tissue trauma, particularly those involving skeletal muscle. Interestingly, Puntel et al's 2013 study concluded that cryotherapy successfully reduced oxidative damage, a finding that corresponds with previous research by Carvalho et al (2010) and Siqueira et al (2017).

A number of injured animal models have also examined the effect of local cryotherapy on gene expression patterns for inflammatory cytokines; these are small proteins that play a key role in cell signalling in the early stages of inflammation. There is evidence that cooling is associated with a down regulation of gene expression levels for key cytokines in the first 48 hours post injury including IL-6, IL-17A and IL-1β (Guillot et al 2017), and TNF-α, with similar patterns in other important enzymes such as MMP-9 (Vieira Ramos et al 2016). Although these molecules can be involved in a wide variety of biological functions, these data provide further evidence that cryotherapy attenuates key aspects of the inflammatory response to injury.

It is more difficult to replicate this type of research in injured human subjects. A number of studies have used exercise induced muscle damage models to try to quantify the effects of cryotherapy on a number of important biomarkers of inflammation (IL-1β; IL-6; IL-10; CRP) and muscle damage (creatine kinase (CK); lactate dehydrogenase (LDH); myoglobin), but there are few clear patterns (Bleakley et al 2012). One novel study (Stalman et al 2008) used a microdialysis technique to examine levels of prostaglandin E2 (PGE2) in human subjects after knee surgery (PGE2 is a principle mediator of inflammation). The authors found reductions in PGE2 levels associated with cryotherapy and compression; however, their methods were limited to a case control design, with confounding due to surgery type and the concomitant use of morphine.

Attenuation of Tissue Damage

The patho-physiological events associated with acute inflammation can lead to collateral damage to cells peripheral to the primary injury. This may be due to enzymatic and/or hypoxic mechanisms, but the corollary can be an increase in injury site size. This phenomenon is often referred to as secondary cell death (or secondary hypoxic death). The pragmatic use of cryotherapy can reduce cellular metabolism at and around the injury site, helping surrounding cells to better tolerate the ischaemic conditions, and ultimately decrease the risk of secondary cell injury. This theory is supported by early studies of limb preservation whereby muscle cells survived better at lower muscle temperatures (Sapega et al 1988). There is also some evidence from animal studies supporting the 'secondary injury theory', whereby 5 hours of continuous cooling in animal models inhibited the loss of mitochondrial oxidative function after experimental injury (Merrick et al 1999).

Related animal work further highlights the protective potential of cryotherapy. Schaser et al (2007) found that 6 hours of consecutive cryotherapy reduced the extent of myonecrosis (desmin ratio) in injured animal muscle. Using a shorter intermittent cryotherapy protocol, Oliveira et al (2006) also found cooling was associated with a 25% reduction in injury site size compared to untreated injured muscle tissue. Interestingly this study also found that compression on its own had little effect on injury size, potentially suggesting that the observed protective effect of cryotherapy is more likely due to cold induced reductions in metabolism than circulatory change. There is related evidence that cryotherapy can attenuate apoptosis after a chemically induced inflammation (Westermann et al 1999). Although apoptosis is the normal mechanism for cells to end their life span, there is often a large increase in apoptosis in the early stages after an acute injury.

The underpinning mechanism for the observed cold-induced reductions in tissue damage and apoptosis post injury is unclear. Indeed there is likely to be a combination of factors including an attenuation of inflammation, metabolism and secondary free radical production (Bleakley & Davison 2010a). Others suggest that cryotherapy could optimize muscle regulation after injury through regulation of gene expression. Indeed, it has been proposed that prolonged cooling could upregulate 'cold shock' genes. As these genes are also upregulated during skeletal muscle hypertrophy, it is logical that they could play a role in protecting myoblasts in the immediate stages of muscle injury (Ferry et al 2011). This has not been validated, however, and a recent study by Sarver et al (2017), which examined muscle biopsies from eight healthy humans in the immediate hours after cryotherapy, concluded that tissue cooling had no effect on cold shock gene expression, or on signal transduction pathways that are known to be important in muscle growth and metabolism.

Paradoxically, there remains a concern that since cold therapy can suppress key inflammatory pathways, this could negatively impact on proliferation, culminating in an impaired healing response. This may be particularly relevant when extreme or prolonged applications of cryotherapy are applied. Data from rat muscle injury models highlight that cryotherapy, undertaken every other day for 2 weeks post injury, results in excessive fibrosis (Shibaguchi et al 2016). Crush injury models in rat muscle have also found that icing is associated with excessive collagen deposition with additional delays and impairments to muscle regeneration at 28 days post injury (Takagi et al 1985). The authors speculate that the observed detriments were mediated by a cold-induced reduction in macrophages at the injury site, which subsequently attenuated the expression of growth factors (IGF-I and TGF-1) associated with optimal muscle regeneration and regulation through the activation, proliferation and differentiation of satellite cells.

Partial and Full Body Cooling

It is increasingly popular to either partially or fully expose the body to cryotherapy, in order to achieve various therapeutic outcomes. This is typically undertaken using immersion in cold water (CWI) (at temperatures of <15°C) or whole-body cryotherapy (WBC) which entails brief exposures to extremely cold, dry air (usually between −100°C and −140°C). CWI and WBC are used primarily as a post-exercise recovery strategy and as a method of treating acute soft tissue injuries. It is also purported that full or even partial body exposure to cold temperature will also incur a number of systemic effects. This is sometimes referred to as therapeutic 'cryostimulation' based on its potential to enhance the body's anti inflammatory and oxidant barriers, to counteract harmful stimuli and improve overall health.

CWI remains one of the most popular post-exercise recovery strategies. Despite positive anecdotal reports, the exact physiological rationale for CWI has not been elucidated. Furthermore, a 2010 review (Bleakley & Davison 2010b) outlined the broad biochemical and physiological effects associated with acute immersion in cold water, and questioned whether some may even be deleterious for sports recovery. For example, undertaking a sudden immersion in very cold water (<5°C) causes an extreme cutaneous stimulation, a cold shock response, and an increase in sympathetic nervous activity, norepinephrine levels, oxidative stress and a possible increase in free radical-species formation. Although the mechanisms associated with free radical production following CWI may be multifold and difficult to determine, both shivering and non-shivering thermoregulation may be influencing factors (Bleakley & Davison 2010b). An important caveat is that most of these effects are extenuated in the following scenarios: when an individual has little experience of cryotherapy exposure; during acute exposure to extreme temperatures; or when prolonged durations of immersion are employed.

Paradoxically, other physiological effects associated with CWI align well with the broader objectives of post-exercise recovery. Ice water immersion (<3°C) induces core temperature cooling rates of 0.35°C per minute and is a primary strategy for reducing thermal strain after exercise (McDermott et al 2009). Even more moderate exercise can place a thermal strain on the body, which can culminate in central nervous system fatigue. This often manifests as a decrement in neural drive to the muscle, reduced force production and an increased perception of exertion (Ihsan et al 2016). A number of studies have demonstrated reduced ratings of perceived exertion (RPE) during exercise following CWI. The mechanism for this is unclear, but it may be due to an increase in cerebral perfusion, which is ultimately mediated by increased central blood volume following CWI (Ihsan et al 2016). Reducing thermal strain can have additional benefits on the cardiovascular system; indeed, it negates the need to dissipate heat from the body via the cutaneous circulation, leaving more blood retained within the active musculature, maximizing oxygen (O_2) delivery. Other evidence from laboratory studies in humans is contradictory, whereby a single bout of CWI post exercise is associated with positive effects, such as enhanced muscle oxidative adaptations, but also deleterious effects, such as obstructions in hypertrophic/strength adaptations after resistance training (Roberts et al 2015). Others have shown that cold-water immersions can help to optimize parasympathetic reactivation post exercise (Buchheit et al 2009), which is regarded as an important marker of post-exercise recovery.

Whole-body cryotherapy (WBC) represents an alternative method of body cooling. Many of the acute effects are purported to be similar to CWI. In a series of reviews Banfi et al (2010) and Lombardi et al (2017) highlight that WBC exposure is associated with a possible mobilization of leukocytes (especially neutrophils), a dose-dependent improvement on lipid profile, decreases in proinflammatory cytokines, adaptive changes in antioxidant status, and positive effects on muscular enzymes associated with muscle damage (creatine kinase and lactate dehydrogenase). They also concluded that exposure to WBC is safe and does not deleteriously affect cardiac or immunological function.

A key consideration is that an individual's response to either CWI or WBC will depend on their previous exposure. A number of studies have profiled the status of winter swimmers (individuals who regularly undertake short CWIs or swimming in cold temperatures) and there is some evidence that these individuals adapt to oxidative stress associated with CWI with resultant improvements in antioxidant protection (Bleakley & Davison 2010b). This may explain some of the perceived benefits reported by athletes during recovery from exercise, particularly those at an elite level, undertaking regular CWI.

CLINICAL EVIDENCE

The majority of studies examining the clinical effects of cryotherapy have been undertaken in a postsurgical population (ACL reconstruction, knee arthroplasty, knee arthroscopy). Such orthopaedic procedures are associated with significant pain, swelling and loss of function during the immediate stages of recovery, and evidence in this field has some applicability to closed soft tissue injuries such as sprains and strains.

In clinical practice, ice is commonly combined with compression and elevation, making it difficult to determine the value of cryotherapy alone. Therefore, the aim of many surgical studies has been to compare the effectiveness of various combinations of ice and compression in a bid to try and disentangle their individual effects. A review by Bleakley et al (2004) included 12 studies comparing the effectiveness of concomitant ice and compression to compression alone. Unfortunately, four of these studies were of little value as they failed to standardize the mode of compression between comparison groups. In the remaining studies, six found that ice and compression was no more effective than compression alone, and two recorded significantly larger decreases in pain with ice and compression. More recently, Song et al (2016) undertook a meta-analysis based on n=10 randomized controlled trials (RCTs), comparing the effectiveness of cryotherapy and compression versus cryotherapy alone after common knee surgeries (ACL reconstruction, arthroplasty, arthroscopy). They recorded lower levels of pain and oedema in the early stages post-surgery (days 1–3) in groups using a combination of cryotherapy and compression; but there was little difference between groups after this time point. A systematic review by Gatewood et al (2017) found further evidence that combined application of cryotherapy and compression is more effective than traditional icing for reducing pain and narcotic consumption after knee arthroscopic surgery.

Since 2005, there have been two systematic reviews evaluating the effectiveness of cryotherapy after ACL reconstruction. The first by Raynor et al (2005) included seven randomized clinical trials with comparisons made to control interventions. There were no between-group differences for postoperative drainage or range of motion; however, cryotherapy was associated with significantly lower postoperative pain. An updated review by Martimbianco et al

(2014), which included ten RCTs (a total of 573 patients), again concluded that the use of cold compression devices was associated with a reduction in postoperative pain compared to no cryotherapy. However, there was not strong evidence that cryotherapy had a positive effect on any of the following postoperative outcomes: oedema, knee function, analgesic medication use, range of motion, blood loss, hospital stay, quality of life and patient satisfaction. A Cochrane Review (Adie et al 2012) also found little evidence to support the use of cryotherapy after total knee arthroplasty (TKA). Although patients using cryotherapy in the immediate stages after TKA had higher knee range of motion (ROM), and lower levels of pain and postoperative blood loss compared to control groups, the between-group differences were consistently small.

Few studies in this field have recruited participants with closed soft tissue injury, such as ligament tears or injuries to the musculo-tendinous unit. For example, Bleakley et al's (2004) systematic review was limited to just five studies assessing the effectiveness of cryotherapy on closed soft tissue injuries, all of which focused on patients with acute lateral ankle sprains. Of note, effect sizes were consistently small and the consensus was that single applications using ice and compression were no more effective than no treatment. We are aware of two other randomized controlled studies that have recruited participants with injuries other than ankle sprain. A randomized controlled study (Prins et al 2011) investigated the effects of cryotherapy versus control on acute gastrocnemius tear. Although this was a feasibility study based on n=19 participants, a novel part of the design was that interventions were initiated within 6 hours after the injury. In spite of this, they found little to no effects when 20-minute ice treatments (repeated every 3 hours over a 36-hour period) were compared to no ice control in the acute stages of strain. Using a different method of cryotherapy, Airaksinen et al (2003) found that four daily applications of a topical cooling gel, initiated within 48 hours of injury, reduced pain in comparison to placebo gel. These results were based on general minor soft tissue injuries to the extremities and cannot be generalized to more moderate or severe injuries.

Cryokinetics is the use of cooling as an adjunct to therapeutic exercise, and there is some evidence that this combination of treatments can have positive short-term effect. One randomized controlled study (Lessard et al 1997) compared the effect of an intermittent icing protocol combined with knee exercises to exercises alone, after minor arthroscopic knee surgery. Moderate effects sizes were reported in favour of the ice and exercise group for both pain and weight-bearing status at 1 week post-surgery, but there were no between-group differences for knee girth and knee ROM. Bleakley et al (2010) also found similar patterns in subjects with acute ankle sprain, whereby a combination of intermittent icing and exercise resulted in lower pain levels and higher function at weeks 1 and 2, compared to ice alone. However, groups were similar at weeks 3 and 4, and there were no between-group differences in re-injury rate at 4-month follow-up. Finally, an RCT (Sefiddashti et al 2018) that included elite athletes with an acute grade I or II hamstring strain compared cryotherapy and exercise to cryotherapy alone. Their findings also suggest that the combination (cryostretching) was of most clinical benefit based on improvements in function and passive knee extension.

Limitations in the Clinical Evidence Base

A perennial concern is that many clinical studies to date did not employ appropriate doses of cryotherapy, which could have attenuated clinical effectiveness, and therefore increased the risk of type II error (i.e. rejection of an effective intervention as ineffective because the observed effect size was neither statistically nor clinically significant). A related concern is that the majority of clinical research examining the effects of cryotherapy on injury is derived from postsurgical models. Whilst such a setting facilitates early initiation of treatment, other limitations have been noted (Bleakley et al 2004). Of particular concern is that postsurgical patients require the use of postsurgical dressing or socks, which risks mitigating the cooling effect and diminishing the clinical effectiveness. Finally, much of the evidence is of limited quality, underpowered with consistent limitations due to selection and retention biases. Furthermore, as cryotherapy is a popular and accessible treatment modality, there is often a risk of contamination of control participants. In one example, 60% of subjects randomized to the no ice group had actually applied ice as a self-treatment prior to recruitment (Bleakley et al 2004). Such contamination can reduce the point estimate of an intervention's effectiveness creating additional risk of a type II error.

CWI and WBC

The clinical evidence base to support the use of CWI after exercise is equivocal. A Cochrane Review published in 2012 (Bleakley et al 2012) included 17 small RCTs involving a total of 366 participants. Muscle soreness data was pooled from 14 studies with moderate effects in favour of CWI over passive interventions. However, the clinical relevance of these effects is questionable, and there was no evidence to suggest that CWI enhanced other important correlates of recovery (strength, ROM, function, swelling). A 2016 meta-analysis (Machado et al 2016) also found evidence that CWI is superior to passive recovery in terms of managing post exercise muscle soreness. Most recently, a 2017 systematic review and meta-analysis (Higgins et al 2017) exclusively examined the effect of CWI on recovery after team sports. Interestingly, they found no effect of CWI perceptions of muscle soreness, but they did find a positive effect for some components of neuromuscular recovery after team sports. In general, there is little evidence that CWI is more effective than other popular recovery interventions, such as contrast water therapy, active recovery or soft tissue massage.

The clinical evidence supporting the use of WBC is also limited. In an initial review, Bleakley et al (2014) found evidence from a number of small randomized studies showing that WBC offered improvements in subjective recovery and muscle soreness following metabolic or mechanical overload, but was of little benefit for other objective markers of recovery. In 2015 a Cochrane Review (Costello et al 2015) was published examining the clinical effectiveness of WBC on pain, function and other markers of recovery. The review included just four studies comparing WBC versus control (no WBC or passive rest), three of which were laboratory-based studies based on an exercise induced muscle damage model. Although there were trends towards lower levels of post exercise soreness in the WBC group at short-term follow ups, the effect sizes were small. There were also no significant differences between groups in relation to other outcomes. A more recent review (Rose et al 2017) that included 16 laboratory-based studies concluded that WBC may improve recovery from muscle damage, with multiple exposures more likely to be associated with improvements in recovery from pain, loss of muscle function, and markers of inflammation and damage. Of note, much of the research in this field includes younger male athletic volunteers. A further limitation is that although no complications or side effects are reported within any of the individual studies, it is generally unclear whether any study actively monitored specific adverse effects. This is an important area for further research and there is evidence from case reports of frostbite and even transient global amnesia (Carrard et al 2017) associated with WBC exposure.

Finally, there are very few studies examining the effectiveness of WBC on recovery from a musculoskeletal injury. In one trial (Ma et al 2013) participants with adhesive capsulitis were randomized to receive either physiotherapy alone or physiotherapy in addition to WBC. After 4 weeks of treatment, both groups improved in terms of pain, shoulder function and ROM. Between-group comparisons were significantly in favour of the WBC for ROM, pain, and shoulder function. Of note, this study did not continue outcome assessment beyond the 4 weeks of treatment, therefore any long-term effectiveness is unclear.

THERAPEUTIC EFFECTS

The consensus from the current clinical evidence base is that applying local cryotherapy after soft tissue injury or post-surgery is an effective treatment for managing pain symptoms. Cooling should also be regarded as an important adjunctive therapy for therapeutic exercise. The primary limitation is that there is little evidence of any long-term clinical effect associated with cryotherapy after common acute soft tissue injures, such as muscle strains or ligament injury.

A key consideration is that all of the physiological effects discussed are mediated by the magnitude of temperature reduction attained during treatment. Pain relief is a fundamental therapeutic effect associated with cryotherapy as hypoalgesia can be readily achieved with only moderate changes in skin temperature. This is substantiated with the consensus from clinical research, where reductions in pain have been reported after using cryotherapy. Furthermore, these effects are consistent across a number of conditions including post-surgery, after soft-tissue injury, and for exercise induced muscle soreness. A number of studies have reported reductions of 20–30% compared to non-cryotherapy controls. The clinical relevance of these effect sizes is debatable and will ultimately depend on the nature of the conditions, concomitant symptoms and patient expectations. Notwithstanding this, it is clear that cryotherapy application has a drug dose sparing potential and should therefore be considered as a core therapy for common pain conditions involving the musculoskeletal system. This is particularly relevant today, given the high risks associated with prescription medication and opioid use disorders.

Muscle weakness is a common clinical problem presenting after acute injury but is also seen in more chronic conditions, such as osteoarthritis. Such strength deficits are often difficult to address without first considering underlying neurophysiological impairments. Indeed, a significant component of strength loss observed after injury may be due to arthrogenic muscle inhibition. This is an acute protective response which seems to be driven by reflexive inhibition of musculature surrounding an injured joint, coupled with changes in cortical excitability. The current clinical evidence base highlights the potential for cryotherapy to act as a disinhibitory intervention, which may ultimately help to address neurophysiological impairments after injury. Much of the supporting research in this area is based on patients with acute ankle injury or recovering after knee surgery. The primary mechanism is that cooling stimulates receptors around the joint, which alters the afferent signal propagated to the central nervous system; the net effect is that this allows therapeutic exercises to be performed in a state of diminished neuromuscular inhibition, thereby maximizing strength gains during rehabilitation (Harkey et al 2014). The magnitude of this therapeutic effect may be high, with evidence that decreasing neuromuscular inhibition in people with knee osteoarthritis predicts 47% of the variance strength improvement (Pietrosimone et al 2012). It is also proposed that using cryotherapy to address underlying neurophysiological impairments not only expedites strength gains, but can also have a cumulative effect on restoration of motor patterns, gait and functional capacity (Pietrosimone et al 2015).

There is consistent evidence from animal models that cooling can result in attenuation of inflammation, with subsequent reductions in secondary cell death and oxidative stress. This creates a clinical paradox, as whilst controlling inflammation could protect the injury site (through reductions in secondary cell death and oxidative stress), complete attenuation of key inflammatory cells could negatively impact on healing response. This has led some clinicians to question the relevance of using cryotherapy in the therapeutic setting. We would suggest that this is unfounded based on current evidence. Fundamentally, it is very difficult for topical cooling to induce clinically meaningful changes in metabolism and inflammation within an injured human. Although animal models suggest that cooling can attenuate muscle regeneration after injury, this is associated with very large intramuscular (IM) temperature reductions, many of which could not be reproduced within an injured human. For example, a 20-minute ice application on an average person might reduce superficial muscle temperature by as little as 3°C. This contrasts starkly with the large reductions in intramuscular temperature reported within the animal literature, some of which are in excess of 30°C. Furthermore, even if small attenuations in inflammation did result, any deleterious effects must be placed in context with cryotherapy's positive therapeutic effects due to hypoalgesia and disinhibition.

Local cooling also has potential to produce concomitant effects on many other physiological systems. The importance of these effects may depend on the clinical context. For example, changes in temperature can influence the mechanical properties of soft tissue, with cold induced increases in terminal stiffness at the knee joint (Muraoka et al 2008) and ankle (Kubo et al 2005) reported. A related concern is that undertaking short periods of cryotherapy can deleteriously affect proprioceptive acuity, muscle strength and sports performance. Although initial data in this area were conflicting (Dover & Powers 2004; Torres et al 2017; Uchio et al 2003; Wassinger et al 2007) a more recent systematic review (Bleakley et al 2012) concluded that athletes may be at a performance disadvantage if they return to activity immediately after longer periods of cooling (>15 minutes).

CWI remains as a useful intervention for controlling the symptoms of exercise-induced muscle soreness, reducing thermal strain, and therefore ameliorating the level of perceived exertion post exercise. These effects may be more valuable for athletes participating in multiple training bouts (in hot conditions) within 24 hours, leaving little time for recovery between exercise sessions. Notwithstanding this, there is conflicting evidence around whether CWI can also impact on objective clinical markers of recovery, such as joint ROM, swelling, strength, and even sports performance. We must also consider that the perception of both CWI and WBC may be changing from a conventionally intended symptomatic therapy to a stimulating treatment that aims to enhance the anti-inflammatory and oxidant barriers through multiple exposure. An interesting finding is the preliminary association between WBC and the expression of certain myokines. As these are normally produced during muscular contraction, it is proposed that WBC in some ways mimics exercise, which could introduce a range of new therapeutic strategies for obesity and type 2 diabetes.

GENERAL PRINCIPLES OF APPLICATION

There are now many different types of cooling modalities available, but often these have different thermal qualities. In recent years, commercially developed cryotherapy devices that incorporate ice and compression have become more popular. Early versions were essentially gravity-fed devices, manually filled with iced water; however, many now include a motorized unit that both cools and circulates the chilled water or another cooling medium. These units also offer options to alter the temperature of the cooling interphase and set specific treatment durations. These are significantly more expensive than traditional forms of cryotherapy (ice bags, ice packs) and whilst they may be more user friendly, it is important to determine if they offer greater clinical effectiveness.

A recent systematic review (Chughtai et al 2017) included six studies examining the effectiveness of continuous cold flow devices versus ice packs after knee arthroplasty. Results found that three studies favoured the use of continuous flow devices, with no differences reported in the others. We did note that in spite of these studies assessing a number of similar outcomes, there was little consistency in the magnitude and direction of effect. Furthermore, in two of these studies, the effects in favour of continuous cold flow were generally small based on between-group differences (e.g. 1 unit on a pain scale, or 6 degrees of knee flexion) which may not be clinically relevant.

There is a supposition that because of its extreme temperatures (-110°C), WBC offers an enhanced cooling effect over traditional forms of cryotherapy. Whilst exposure to -110°C creates a large thermal gradient, heat transfer depends on a number of additional factors. For example, ice cubes have a much higher heat transfer coefficient (the ability of a material to transfer heat) compared to both water and air, meaning that it is a more efficient material for extracting heat energy from the body. A 2014 review (Bleakley et al 2014) illustrated that larger reductions in skin temperature were associated with a 10-minute ice pack application in comparison to a 5-minute CWI or 2.5–3-minute WBC exposure (-110 to -195°C). Ice also has more potential to extract heat energy from the skin based on its ability to undergo phase change. The results of this review also confirmed negligible intramuscular temperature variation regardless of the cooling modality.

Some confusion exists within clinical practice and published literature over the most effective cryotherapy duration. Indeed, textbooks, clinical guidelines and surveys of practice show wide discrepancies in its application. In general, it is important that treatment protocols strike a balance between safety and efficacy. Whilst mild cooling may not be of any physiological benefit to the patient, excessive temperature reduction is harmful and adverse effects have been reported. A survey of practitioners' experiences of adverse events estimated that cryotherapy accounted for a larger number of complications than heat, electrical stimulation and therapeutic exercise (Nadler et al 2003) with the majority involving skin burns, frostbite, intolerance or allergy. There have been a number of cases reporting the iatrogenic adverse events associated with various modes of cryotherapy. Many are serious and have involved frostbite requiring surgical decompression (Rivlin et al 2014), necrosis and eventual skin loss (Dundon et al 2013) and neuropathy (Babwah 2011). Other reported side effects include cold urticaria (wheal formation and skin discoloration), which occurred during an experimental study (Dover et al 2004), but symptoms had fully resolved within 48 hours.

There is perhaps an erroneous supposition that a panacea dosage exists, i.e. a treatment dose that is equally effective regardless of the time since injury, pathological condition or body tissue affected. Although empirical guidance from injured humans is lacking, it is pragmatic to suggest that cooling dose should be broadly tailored according to the patient (levels of adiposity at the injury site) and the desired physiological effect. For example, in some clinical situations, e.g. a deep muscle injury with high levels of overlying adipose tissue, the therapeutic effects of cryotherapy are essentially limited to hypoalgesia. Indeed, for certain injuries/patients/body parts, even if treatment application is extended beyond 60 minutes, changes in tissue temperature at the injury site will still be negligible. In contrast, applying 20 minutes of crushed ice to a superficial muscle injury with low adiposity could significantly reduce injury site temperatures; and we speculate greater potential for reducing metabolism and attenuation of inflammation.

There is a dearth of studies comparing the relative effectiveness of different cryotherapy doses. A previous review of the evidence base proposed that short intermittent applications of cryotherapy are most effective for relieving pain and dysfunction after injury (MacAuley 2001). An RCT by Bleakley et al (2006) found some trends that intermittent icing (10 minutes on, 10 minutes off, 10 minutes on) was preferable to a standard 20-minute protocol after acute ankle sprain. In general, shorter intermittent use of cryotherapy seems to strike a balance between safety and efficacy. Indeed 10 minutes of cooling is highly likely to provide hypoalgesia in the presence of most pain conditions, whilst avoiding excessive tissue temperature reductions. Cell death occurs when tissue temperature reaches approximately -10°C (Gage 1979); such extreme reductions would not be expected in a clinical setting when a short intermittent application is stringently applied. Indeed, many of the case reports of adverse events cite patient or practitioner error as key risk factor, and the corollary is prolonged application times and/or excessive concomitant compression. Although it is purported that using a barrier between the cooling surface and the skin minimizes the risk of adverse effects, a pragmatic approach is required and excessively thick dressings or barriers will create excessive insulation, with little to no reduction in skin temperature.

Shorter intermittent durations are also appropriate when the goal is to exploit the disinhibitory effects of ice prior to exercise. Others have recommended that cryotherapy should be applied during exercise, which may be facilitated through CWI. Logistically, traditional cryotherapy treatments, such as ice packs, may be cumbersome and it would be difficult to perform active exercises while these are actively applied. However, as the disinhibitory effects of cryotherapy can last for a period of time following cryotherapy removal, clinicians may be able to implement cryotherapy prior to therapeutic exercise, with similar therapeutic effects. Note that other interventions, such as electrical stimulation or manual therapy, will also induce a disinhibitory effect and when combined with exercise can have a similar therapeutic effect on strength. But these interventions are sometimes less accessible (in relation to cost and/or expertise) when compared to cryotherapy.

It is difficult to determine an optimal dose for CWI or WBC. A subgroup analysis from a recent systematic review (Machado et al 2016) reported effects favouring moderate water temperatures of 11–15°C (compared to severe: 5–10°C) and longer immersion times of 11–15 minutes (compared to <10 minutes). However, findings from subgroup analyses should be interpreted with caution, particularly if they do not concur with evidence from individual studies. Indeed, recent RCTs (Bleakley et al 2004; Gatewood et al 2017; Lombardi et al 2017; Song et al 2016), making direct comparisons between different cooling doses, failed to find strong evidence to suggest dose-response relationship for CWI.

WBC involves exposing individuals to extremely cold dry air (achieved through liquid nitrogen or refrigerated cold air). Individuals wear minimal clothing during the exposure, but to reduce the risk of cold-related injury, they typically wear gloves, a woollen headband covering the ears, and a nose and mouth mask, in addition to dry shoes and socks. Air temperature ranges between -180 and -100°C, and treatment duration from 2 to 4 minutes. Choice of temperature and duration are largely anecdotal. The vast majority of evidence in this area is derived from studies using trained individuals. Given the extreme nature of these treatments, the magnitude and even the direction effects may be moderated by an individual's past exposure to WBC. Recreational athletes have started to emulate elite athletes in using these treatments after exercise, but we should be cognizant that their responses to either acute or chronic cryostimulation may not concur with the patterns presented in the current evidence base.

SUMMARY

There is consistent clinical evidence that topical cooling reduces pain across a range of conditions including ankle sprain, exercise-induced muscle soreness and post-surgery. Cryotherapy should also be considered as a key adjunct for therapeutic exercise, particularly when addressing neurophysiological impairments associated with joint injury (e.g. arthrogenic muscle inhibition). There remains a dearth of clinical studies investigating the effectiveness of cryotherapy on acute muscle tears and tendinopathies. The effects of cryotherapy on inflammation and tissue damage remain equivocal. Animal models suggest that tissue cooling modulates components of the inflammatory process; however, these effects are attenuated in human subjects due to the insulating effects of overlying body fat and potentially greater injury depths. Current trends involving partial or full body exposure to extreme cold (e.g. WBC) after musculoskeletal injury are not substantiated in the evidence base. Similarly, further research is required to determine the potential use of WBC or CWI for therapeutic 'cryostimulation'. However there is preliminary evidence that this can enhance the body's anti-inflammatory and oxidant barriers.

REFERENCES

Adie, S., et al. (2012). Cryotherapy following total knee replacement. *Cochrane Database of Systematic Reviews* (9), CD007911.

Airaksinen, O. V., et al. (2003). Efficacy of cold gel for soft tissue injuries: A prospective randomized double-blinded trial. *The American Journal of Sports Medicine*, 31(5), 680–684.

Algafly, A. A., & George, K. P. (2007). The effect of cryotherapy on nerve conduction velocity, pain threshold and pain tolerance. *British Journal of Sports Medicine*, 41(6), 365–369; discussion 369.

Babwah, T. (2011). Common peroneal neuropathy related to cryotherapy and compression in a footballer. *Research in Sports Medicine*, 19(1), 66–71.

Bailey, S. R., et al. (2004). Rho kinase mediates cold-induced constriction of cutaneous arteries: Role of alpha2C-adrenoceptor translocation. *Circulation Research*, 94(10), 1367–1374.

Banfi, G., et al. (2010). Whole-body cryotherapy in athletes. *Clinics in Sports Medicine*, 40(6), 509–517.

Blake, D. R., Allen, R. E., & Lunec, J. (1987). Free radicals in biological systems--a review orientated to inflammatory processes. *British Medical Bulletin*, 43(2), 371–385.

Bleakley, C. M., Costello, J. T., & Glasgow, P. D. (2012). Should athletes return to sport after applying ice? A systematic review of the effect of local cooling on functional performance. *Clinics in Sports Medicine*, 42(1), 69–87.

Bleakley, C., & Davison, G. W. (2010a). Cryotherapy and inflammation: Evidence beyond the cardinal signs. *Physical Therapy Reviews*, 15(6), 430–435.

Bleakley, C. M., & Davison, G. W. (2010b). What is the biochemical and physiological rationale for using cold-water immersion in sports recovery? A systematic review. *British Journal of Sports Medicine*, 44(3), 179–187.

Bleakley, C. M., et al. (2006). Cryotherapy for acute ankle sprains: a randomised controlled study of two different icing protocols. *British Journal of Sports Medicine*, 40(8), 700–705; discussion 705.

Bleakley, C. M., et al. (2010). Effect of accelerated rehabilitation on function after ankle sprain: randomised controlled trial. *BMJ (Clinical research ed.)*, 340, c1964.

Bleakley, C., et al. (2012). Cold-water immersion (cryotherapy) for preventing and treating muscle soreness after exercise. *Cochrane Database of Systematic Reviews* (2), CD008262.

Bleakley, C. M., et al. (2014). Whole-body cryotherapy: Empirical evidence and theoretical perspectives. *Open Access Journal of Sports Medicine*, 5, 25–36.

Bleakley, C., McDonough, S., & MacAuley, D. (2004). The use of ice in the treatment of acute soft-tissue injury: A systematic review of randomized controlled trials. *The American Journal of Sports Medicine*, 32(1), 251–261.

Buchheit, M., et al. (2009). Effect of cold water immersion on postexercise parasympathetic reactivation. *American Journal of Physiology. Heart and Circulatory Physiology*, 296(2), H421–H427.

Carrard, J., Lambert, A. C., & Genne, D. (2017). Transient global amnesia following a whole-body cryotherapy session. *BMJ Case Reports, 2017.*

Carvalho, N., et al. (2010). Protective effects of therapeutic cold and heat against the oxidative damage induced by a muscle strain injury in rats. *Journal of Sports Sciences*, 28(9), 923–935.

Chughtai, M., et al. (2017). Cryotherapy treatment after unicompartmental and total knee arthroplasty: A review. *The Journal of Arthroplasty*, 32(12), 3822–3832.

Costello, J. T., et al. (2015). Whole-body cryotherapy (extreme cold air exposure) for preventing and treating muscle soreness after exercise in adults. *Cochrane Database of Systematic Reviews* (9), CD010789.

Dover, G., Borsa, P. A., & McDonald, D. J. (2004). Cold urticaria following an ice application: A case study. *Clinical Journal of Sport Medicine: Official Journal of the Canadian Academy of Sport Medicine*, 14(6), 362–364.

Dover, G., & Powers, M. E. (2004). Cryotherapy does not impair shoulder joint position sense. *Archives of Physical Medicine and Rehabilitation*, 85(8), 1241–1246.

Dundon, J. M., Rymer, M. C., & Johnson, R. M. (2013). Total patellar skin loss from cryotherapy after total knee arthroplasty. *The Journal of Arthroplasty*, 28(2), 376 e5–7.

Ernst, E., & Fialka, V. (1994). Ice freezes pain? A review of the clinical effectiveness of analgesic cold therapy. *Journal of Pain and Symptom Management*, 9(1), 56–59.

Ferry, A. L., Vanderklish, P. W., & Dupont-Versteegden, E. E. (2011). Enhanced survival of skeletal muscle myoblasts in response to overexpression of cold shock protein RBM3. *American Journal of Physiology. Cell Physiology*, 301(2), C392–C402.

Gage, A. A. (1979). What temperature is lethal for cells? *The Journal of Dermatologic Surgery and Oncology*, 5(6), 459–460 464.

Gatewood, C. T., Tran, A. A., & Dragoo, J. L. (2017). The efficacy of post-operative devices following knee arthroscopic surgery: a systematic review. *Knee Surgery, Sports Traumatology, Arthroscopy: Official Journal of the ESSKA*, 25(2), 501–516.

Greathouse, D. G., et al. (1989). Electrophysiologic responses of human sural nerve to temperature. *Pediatric Physical Therapy: The Official Publication of the Section on Pediatrics of the American Physical Therapy Association*, 69(11), 914 922.

Guillot, X., et al. (2017). Local cryotherapy improves adjuvant-induced arthritis through down-regulation of IL-6 / IL-17 pathway but independently of TNFα. *PLoS One*, 12(7), e0178668.

Harkey, M. S., Gribble, P. A., & Pietrosimone, B. G. (2014). Disinhibitory interventions and voluntary quadriceps activation: A systematic review. *Journal of Athletic Training*, 49(3), 411–421.

Herrera, E., et al. (2010). Motor and sensory nerve conduction are affected differently by ice pack, ice massage, and cold water immersion. *Journal of Geriatric Physical Therapy*, 90(4), 581–591.

Higgins, T. R., Greene, D. A., & Baker, M. K. (2017). Effects of cold water immersion and contrast water therapy for recovery from team sport: A systematic review and meta-analysis. *Journal of Strength and Conditioning Research*, 31(5), 1443–1460.

Ihsan, M., Watson, G., & Abbiss, C. R. (2016). What are the physiological mechanisms for post-exercise cold water immersion in the recovery from prolonged endurance and intermittent exercise? *Journal of Science and Medicine in Sport*, 46(8), 1095–1109.

Knobloch, K., et al. (2006). Microcirculation of the ankle after Cryo/Cuff application in healthy volunteers. *International Journal of Sports Medicine, 27*(3), 250–255.

Knobloch, K., et al. (2008). Midportion Achilles tendon microcirculation after intermittent combined cryotherapy and compression compared with cryotherapy alone: A randomized trial. *The American Journal of Sports Medicine, 36*(11), 2128–2138.

Korpan, N. N. (2007). A history of cryosurgery: Its development and future. *Journal of the American College of Surgeons, 204*(2), 314–324.

Kubo, K., Kanehisa, H., & Fukunaga, T. (2005). Effects of cold and hot water immersion on the mechanical properties of human muscle and tendon in vivo. *Clinical Biomechanics (Bristol, Avon), 20*(3), 291–300.

Lee, H., et al. (2005). Effects of cryotherapy after contusion using real-time intravital microscopy. *Medicine and Science in Sports and Exercise, 37*(7), 1093–1098.

Lessard, L. A., et al. (1997). The efficacy of cryotherapy following arthroscopic knee surgery. *The Journal of Orthopaedic and Sports Physical Therapy, 26*(1), 14–22.

Lombardi, G., Ziemann, E., & Banfi, G. (2017). Whole-body cryotherapy in athletes: from therapy to stimulation. An updated review of the literature. *Frontiers in Physiology, 8*, 258.

Ma, S. Y., et al. (2013). Effects of whole-body cryotherapy in the management of adhesive capsulitis of the shoulder. *Archives of Physical Medicine and Rehabilitation, 94*(1), 9–16.

MacAuley, D. (2001). Do textbooks agree on their advice on ice? *Clinical Journal of Sport Medicine: Official Journal of the Canadian Academy of Sport Medicine, 11*(2), 67–72.

Machado, A. F., et al. (2016). Can water temperature and immersion time influence the effect of cold water immersion on muscle soreness? A systematic review and meta-analysis. *Clinics in Sports Medicine, 46*(4), 503–514.

Martimbianco, A. L., et al. (2014). Effectiveness and safety of cryotherapy after arthroscopic anterior cruciate ligament reconstruction. A systematic review of the literature. *Physical Therapy in Sport, 15*(4), 261–268.

Mawhinney, C., et al. (2017). Cold water mediates greater reductions in limb blood flow than whole body cryotherapy. *Medicine and Science in Sports and Exercise, 49*(6), 1252–1260.

McDermott, B. P., et al. (2009). Acute whole-body cooling for exercise-induced hyperthermia: A systematic review. *Journal of Athletic Training, 44*(1), 84–93.

Menetrier, A., et al. (2015). Changes in femoral artery blood flow during thermoneutral, cold, and contrast-water therapy. *The Journal of Sports Medicine and Physical Fitness, 55*(7-8), 768–775.

Merrick, M. A., et al. (1999). A preliminary examination of cryotherapy and secondary injury in skeletal muscle. *Medicine and Science in Sports and Exercise, 31*(11), 1516–1521.

Muraoka, T., et al. (2008). Effects of muscle cooling on the stiffness of the human gastrocnemius muscle in vivo. *Cells Tissues Organs, 187*(2), 152–160.

Myrer, W. J., et al. (2001). Muscle temperature is affected by overlying adipose when cryotherapy is administered. *Journal of Athletic Training, 36*(1), 32–36.

Nadler, S. F., et al. (2003). Complications from therapeutic modalities: Results of a national survey of athletic trainers. *Archives of Physical Medicine and Rehabilitation, 84*(6), 849–853.

Oliveira, N. M., Rainero, E. P., & Salvini, T. F. (2006). Three intermittent sessions of cryotherapy reduce the secondary muscle injury in skeletal muscle of rat. *Journal of Sports Science and Medicine, 5*(2), 228–234.

Pietrosimone, B., et al. (2015). Clinical strategies for addressing muscle weakness following knee injury. *Clinics in Sports Medicine, 34*(2), 285–300.

Pietrosimone, B. G., & Saliba, S. A. (2012). Changes in voluntary quadriceps activation predict changes in quadriceps strength after therapeutic exercise in patients with knee osteoarthritis. *The Journal of Knee Surgery, 19*(6), 939–943.

Prins, J. C., et al. (2011). Feasibility and preliminary effectiveness of ice therapy in patients with an acute tear in the gastrocnemius muscle: A pilot randomized controlled trial. *Clinical Rehabilitation, 25*(5), 433–441.

Puntel, G. O., et al. (2013). Cryotherapy reduces skeletal muscle damage after ischemia/reperfusion in rats. *Journal of Anatomy, 222*(2), 223–230.

Raynor, M. C., et al. (2005). Cryotherapy after ACL reconstruction: A meta-analysis. *The Journal of Knee Surgery, 18*(2), 123–129.

Rivlin, M., et al. (2014). Frostbite in an adolescent football player: A case report. *Journal of Athletic Training, 49*(1), 97–101.

Roberts, L. A., et al. (2015). Post-exercise cold water immersion attenuates acute anabolic signalling and long-term adaptations in muscle to strength training. *The Journal of Physiology, 593*(18), 4285–4301.

Rose, C., et al. (2017). Whole-body cryotherapy as a recovery technique after exercise: A review of the literature. *International Journal of Sports Medicine, 38*(14), 1049–1060.

Sapega, A. A., et al. (1988). The bioenergetics of preservation of limbs before replantation. The rationale for intermediate hypothermia. *The Journal of Bone and Joint Surgery. American Volume, 70*(10), 1500–1513.

Sarver, D. C., et al. (2017). Local cryotherapy minimally impacts the metabolome and transcriptome of human skeletal muscle. *Bioscience Reports, 7*(1), 2423.

Schaser, K. D., et al. (2006). Local cooling restores microcirculatory hemodynamics after closed soft-tissue trauma in rats. *The Journal of Trauma, 61*(3), 642–649.

Schaser, K. D., et al. (2007). Prolonged superficial local cryotherapy attenuates microcirculatory impairment, regional inflammation, and muscle necrosis after closed soft tissue injury in rats. *American Journal of Speech-Language Pathology / American Speech-Language-Hearing Association, 35*(1), 93–102.

Sefiddashti, L., et al. (2018). The effects of cryotherapy versus cryostretching on clinical and functional outcomes in athletes with acute hamstring strain. *Journal of Bodywork and Movement Therapies, 22*(3), 805–809.

Selkow, N. M., et al. (2012). Microvascular perfusion and intramuscular temperature of the calf during cooling. *Medicine and Science in Sports and Exercise, 44*(5), 850–856.

Shibaguchi, T., et al. (2016). Effects of icing or heat stress on the induction of fibrosis and/or regeneration of injured rat soleus muscle. *The Journal of Physiological Sciences, 66*(4), 345–357.

Singh, D. P., et al. (2017). Effects of topical icing on inflammation, angiogenesis, revascularization, and myofiber regeneration in skeletal muscle following contusion injury. *Frontiers in Physiology, 8*, 93.

Siqueira, A. F., et al. (2017). Multiple cryotherapy applications attenuate oxidative stress following skeletal muscle injury. *Redox Report: Communications in Free Radical Research, 22*(6), 323–329.

Song, M., et al. (2016). Compressive cryotherapy versus cryotherapy alone in patients undergoing knee surgery: A meta-analysis. *Springerplus, 5*(1), 1074.

Stalman, A., et al. (2008). Local inflammatory and metabolic response in the knee synovium after arthroscopy or arthroscopic anterior cruciate ligament reconstruction. *Arthroscopy, 24*(5), 579–584.

Takagi, R., et al. (1985). Influence of icing on muscle regeneration after crush injury to skeletal muscles in rats. *Journal of Applied Physiology, 110*(2), 382–388 2011.

Topp, R., Ledford, E. R., & Jacks, D. E. (2013). Topical menthol, ice, peripheral blood flow, and perceived discomfort. *Journal of Athletic Training, 48*(2), 220–225.

Torres, R., et al. (2017). The acute effect of cryotherapy on muscle strength and shoulder proprioception. *Journal of Sport Rehabilitation, 26*(6), 497–506.

Uchio, Y., et al. (2003). Cryotherapy influences joint laxity and position sense of the healthy knee joint. *Archives of Physical Medicine and Rehabilitation, 84*(1), 131–135.

Vieira Ramos, G., et al. (2016). Cryotherapy reduces inflammatory response without altering muscle regeneration process and extracellular matrix remodeling of rat muscle. *Bioscience Reports, 6*, 18525.

Wassinger, C. A., et al. (2007). Proprioception and throwing accuracy in the dominant shoulder after cryotherapy. *Journal of Athletic Training, 42*(1), 84–89.

Westermann, S., et al. (1999). Surface cooling inhibits tumor necrosis factor-alpha-induced microvascular perfusion failure, leukocyte adhesion, and apoptosis in the striated muscle. *Surgery, 126*(5), 881–889.

Non-Thermal, Microthermal and Light Energies

9

Ultrasound

Tim Watson

CHAPTER OUTLINE

INTRODUCTION

Ultrasound is almost certainly the most widely used of the electrophysical modalities in current clinical practice. Ultrasound is a form of mechanical energy (Chapter 2), and the more recently adopted overarching term 'electrophysical modality or agent' encompasses the modality comfortably.

Although therapeutic ultrasound has been widely used for over 50 years, its current use in the clinical environment

has changed significantly over this period, and whereas in the past it was used primarily for its thermal effect, it is now equally widely employed for its non-thermal effects, especially in relation to tissue repair and wound healing.

A variety of surveys have been conducted over the decades (e.g. Pope et al 1995; ter Haar et al 1985) illustrating the high availability and use of therapeutic ultrasound in practice. Ultrasound remained the most widely available electrophysical agent (EPA) modality in various surveys

(Chipchase et al 2009 (Australia); Shah et al 2007 (UK)) while the 2013 international survey of EPA use based on reviewed literature (Shah & Farrow 2013) demonstrated increased ultrasound usage in several countries, despite a general trend of decreased EPA availability and use across multiple modalities.

Ultrasound can be delivered from a multimodal machine (Fig. 9.1A), a standalone ultrasound only device (Fig. 9.1B) or portable handheld devices (Fig. 9.1C).

PHYSICAL PRINCIPLES

The essential physics of therapeutic ultrasound is covered in Chapter 2 and is not repeated in this section; however, it is important to consider some behavioural characteristics before considering therapeutic effects, evidence and clinical use.

Ultrasound Transmission

All materials present an impedance to the passage of sound waves. The specific impedance of a tissue will be determined by its density and elasticity. For maximal transmission of energy from one medium to another, the two media need to have the same impedance, in which case reflection at the interface will be minimized. Clearly, in the case of ultrasound passing from the generator to the body and then through the different tissue types, this cannot be achieved. The greater the difference in impedance between boundary tissues, the greater the reflection that will occur, and hence the smaller the amount of energy that will be transferred.

The difference in impedance is greatest for the metal–air interface at the face of the applicator. To minimize this difference, a suitable coupling medium should be used. If an air gap exists between the transducer and the skin, the proportion of ultrasound that will be reflected approaches 99.998%, which means that there will be no effective transmission.

The coupling media used in this context include water, various oils, creams and gels. Ideally, the coupling medium should be sufficiently fluid to fill all available spaces; relatively viscous, so that it stays in place; have an impedance appropriate to the media with which it connects; and should allow transmission of ultrasound with minimal absorption, attenuation or disturbance (for more extensive reading, see Casarotto et al 2004; Klucinec et al 2000). The gel-based media are preferable to the oil- and cream-based media. Water is an effective and useful alternative, but it fails to

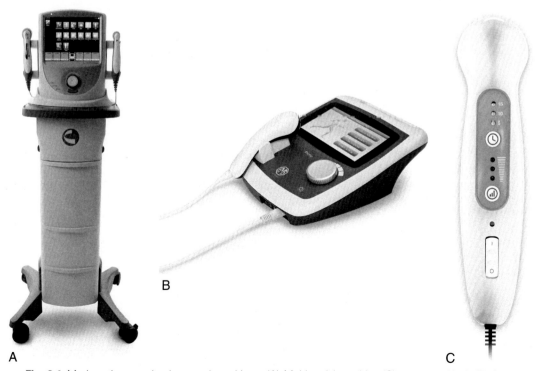

Fig. 9.1 Modern therapeutic ultrasound machines. (A) Multimodal machine (Chattanooga Neo). (B) Stand-alone ultrasound device (Primo Therasonic (EMS Physio)). (C) Handheld ultrasound device (Revitive).

meet the above criteria in terms of its viscosity. A detailed study considering the effect of different coupling gels on ultrasound transmission demonstrated differences in transmission characteristics and absorption levels of commonly employed gels, but there was no clinically significant difference between them (Poltawski & Watson 2007a).

In addition to the reflection that occurs at a boundary due to differences in impedance, there will also be some refraction if the wave does not strike the boundary surface at 90°. Essentially, the ultrasound beam angles away from the original pathway as it crosses the boundary between adjacent tissue layers. The critical angle for ultrasound at the skin interface appears to be approximately 15°.

Penetration and Absorption of Ultrasound Energy

The absorption of ultrasound energy follows an exponential pattern, i.e. more energy is absorbed in the superficial tissues than in the deep tissues. For energy to have an effect, it must be absorbed. Transmission and attenuation of ultrasound energy are considered in detail in Chapter 2.

Because the absorption (penetration) of ultrasound energy is exponential, there is (in theory) no point at which all the energy has been absorbed, but there is certainly a point at which the energy levels are not sufficient to produce a therapeutic effect.

The 'half value depth' is often quoted in relation to ultrasound. It represents the depth in the tissues at which half the surface energy remains. This will be different for each tissue and also depends on ultrasound frequencies (detailed in Chapter 2). As the thickness of different tissue layers (subcutaneous fat, muscle, etc.) is patient specific, average half value depths are employed for each frequency:
3 MHz 2.0 cm
1 MHz 4.0 cm.

These values are not universally accepted (see Ward 1986) and ongoing research suggests that in the clinical environment they may be significantly lower. To achieve a particular ultrasound intensity at depth, account must be taken of the proportion of energy that has been absorbed by the superficial tissue layers (Watson 2002).

Absorption and Attenuation

Ultrasound is not absorbed equally in different tissue types; tissues with a higher protein content will absorb ultrasound to a greater extent. Consequently, tissues such as blood and fat, which have a high water content and a low protein content, absorb little of the ultrasound energy, whereas those with a lower water content and a higher protein content will absorb ultrasound far more efficiently. The best-absorbing tissues in terms of clinical practice are those with high collagen content: ligament, tendon, fascia, joint capsule and scar tissue (Nussbaum 1998; ter Haar 1999;

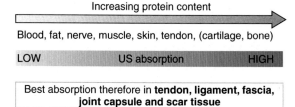

Fig. 9.2 Ranking of musculoskeletal tissues according to their relative absorption of ultrasound energy. *US,* Ultrasound.

Watson 2000, 2002). It has been suggested that tissues can therefore be ranked according to their relative absorption (Fig. 9.2). Although cartilage and bone are at the upper end of this scale, the problems associated with wave reflection at the tissue surface mean that a significant proportion of ultrasound energy striking the surface of either of these tissues is likely to be reflected.

The application of therapeutic ultrasound to tissues with a low energy-absorption capacity will be less effective than the application to a highly absorbing material.

EFFECTS OF ULTRASOUND

Ultrasound exerts an effect on the cells and tissues through both thermal and non-thermal mechanisms.

Thermal Effects

Absorption of ultrasound manifests in a rise in tissue temperature. A biologically significant thermal effect can be achieved if the temperature of the tissue is raised to between 40 and 45°C for at least 5 minutes. Controlled heating can produce desirable effects (Lehmann & deLateur 1982; Dalecki 2004), which include pain relief, decrease in joint stiffness and increased local blood flow. The therapeutic benefits of tissue heating are well established (see Chapter 5), but ultrasound is relatively inefficient at generating sufficient thermal change in large tissue volumes in order to achieve temperature changes at this level.

Thermal ultrasound dominated early applications, became less prevalent compared with non-thermal applications in 1980's and 1990's (Watson 2000, 2006a, 2010), but has started to re-emerge as a viable treatment option (e.g. Aydin et al 2016; Jorge et al 2017).

Gallo et al (2004) demonstrated that both continuous and pulsed ultrasound generated measurable thermal changes in muscle tissue, but that considering the temperature changes achieved, they would be of minimal therapeutic value. Garrett et al (2000) compared the heating effect of a pulsed shortwave treatment with an ultrasound treatment; the shortwave intervention was clearly more effective at achieving the required thermal change for therapeutic benefit. A patient treated with ultrasound in continuous mode at a relatively high dose will feel a temperature change (mainly in the skin, which is where thermal receptors are predominantly located) but this is not the same as achieving a clinically significant thermal change in deeper tissues. There is some evidence (Lehmann et al 1967a,b; Draper & Ricard 1995) that if the ultrasound is delivered to soft tissue overlying bone, significant heating at depth can be achieved.

A possible complication can occur when an ultrasound beam strikes bone or a metal prosthesis. Because of the great acoustic impedance difference between these structures and the surrounding soft tissues at least 30% of the incident energy will be reflected back through the soft tissue. This means that further energy is deposited as heat during the beam's return journey. Therefore, heat rise in soft tissue could be higher when it is situated in front of a reflector. To complicate matters further, an interaction termed 'mode conversion' occurs at the interface of the soft tissue and the reflector (e.g. bone or metal prosthesis). During mode conversion, a percentage of the reflected incident energy is converted from a longitudinal waveform into a transverse or shear waveform, which cannot propagate on the soft tissue side of the interface and is therefore absorbed rapidly, causing heat rise (and sometimes pain) at the bone–soft-tissue interface (periosteum).

Non-Thermal Effects

There are many situations where ultrasound produces bioeffects and yet significant temperature change is not involved, e.g. low spatial-average temporal-average (SATA) intensity (see Chapter 2). It is not strictly true to talk about 'non-thermal' mechanisms, in that absorption of energy in the tissues will result in a temperature rise. The term 'non-thermal' in this context relates to the fact that there is no apparent thermal accumulation in the tissues (see Chapter 5), which is sometimes referred to as a 'microthermal' effect.

There is evidence indicating that non-thermal mechanisms play a primary role in producing therapeutic effects: stimulation of tissue regeneration (Dyson et al 1968), soft-tissue repair (Dyson et al 1976; Watson 2006a), blood flow in tendon (Chang et al 2015), protein synthesis (Webster et al 1978) and bone repair (Malizos et al 2006; Padilla et al 2016). The essential ultrasound biophysics of non-thermal effects is reviewed in Izadifar et al (2017).

The physical mechanisms thought to be involved in producing these non-thermal effects are one or more of the following: cavitation, acoustic streaming and standing waves (Baker et al 2001; Izadifar et al 2017; ter Haar 1999).

Cavitation

Ultrasound can cause the formation of micrometre-sized bubbles or cavities in gas-containing fluids. Depending on the pressure amplitude of the energy, the resultant bubbles can be either useful or potentially dangerous. Low-pressure amplitudes result in the formation of bubbles that vibrate (stable cavitation) leading to reversible permeability changes in cell membranes near to the cavitational event (Mortimer & Dyson 1988; Speed 2001). Changes in cell permeability to various ions such as calcium can have a profound effect upon the activity of the cell (Sutherland & Rall 1968).

High-pressure amplitudes can result in a more violent cavitational event (unstable, transient, inertial, or collapse cavitation). During this event, the bubbles collapse during the positive pressure part of the cycle, resulting in very high local pressures (>1000 MPa) and temperatures (>10000 K) (Donikov & Bouakaz 2010). Unstable cavitation can lead to the formation of highly reactive free radicals. Although free radicals are produced by cells naturally, they are removed by free-radical scavengers. Production in excess of the natural scavenger system capacity could be damaging. Avoidance of a standing-wave field and use of low intensities during therapy make it unlikely that transient cavitation will occur and there is no evidence of these effects when using therapeutic ultrasound appropriately (Koulakis et al 2018). Some applications of ultrasound deliberately employ the unstable cavitation effect (reviewed in Izadifar et al 2017), e.g. high-intensity focused ultrasound (HIFU), but it is beyond the remit of this chapter (see Maloney & Hwang 2015; Singal et al 2016; Wu 2006).

Acoustic Streaming

This refers to the unidirectional movement of a fluid in an ultrasound field. High-velocity gradients develop in boundary fluids adjacent to structures such as cells, bubbles and tissue fibres. Acoustic streaming can stimulate cell activity if it occurs at the boundary of the cell membrane and the surrounding fluid (El Ghamrawy et al 2019). The resultant viscous stress on the membrane, providing it is not too severe, can alter the membrane's permeability and second-messenger activity (Dyson 1982, 1985). This could result in therapeutically advantageous changes, such as increased protein synthesis (Webster et al 1978), increased secretion from mast cells (Fyfe & Chahl 1982), fibroblast mobility changes (Mummery 1978), increased uptake of the second-messenger calcium (Mortimer & Dyson 1988; Mummery 1978), and increased production of growth factors by macrophages (Padilla et al 2016; Watson, 2016; Young & Dyson 1990a). Such effects could account for the acceleration of repair following ultrasound therapy, and interaction at the cell membrane level is considered to be the primary mechanism (Hanson 2010).

Standing Waves

When an ultrasound wave encounters the interface between two tissues of different acoustic impedances (e.g. bone and muscle), a percentage of the wave energy is reflected. The reflected waves can interact with oncoming incident waves to form a standing-wave field in which the peaks of intensity (antinodes; see Chapter 2) of the waves are stationary and are separated by half a wavelength. Because the standing wave consists of two superimposed waves in addition to a travelling component, the peak intensities and pressures are higher than the normal incident wave. Between the antinodes, which are points of maximum and minimum pressure, are nodes, which are points of fixed pressure. Gas bubbles collect at the antinodes and suspended cells collect at the nodes (National Council on Radiation Protection (NCRP) 1983; Padilla et al 2014). Fixed cells that are situated at the antinodes, such as endothelial cells, can be damaged by microstreaming forces around bubbles. Erythrocytes can be lysed if they are swept through the arrays of bubbles situated at the pressure antinodes. Reversible blood cell stasis has been demonstrated, the cells forming bands half a wavelength apart centred on the pressure nodes (Dyson et al 1974). The increased pressure produced in standing-wave fields can cause transient cavitation and consequently the formation of free radicals (Nyborg 1977). It is therefore important to move the applicator continuously throughout treatment, and also use the lowest intensity required to cause an effect, to minimize possible hazards of standing-wave field production (Dyson et al 1974; ter Haar et al 1979).

The combination of stable cavitation and acoustic streaming is thought to be responsible for the cellular 'upregulation' that occurs during an ultrasound treatment (Izadifar et al 2017). The therapeutic effects (see following sections) of this type of intervention arise as a consequence of this stimulated cellular activity; in reality, the 'effects' of ultrasound are primarily at a cell membrane level (Fig. 9.3).

BIOPHYSICAL EFFECTS AND TISSUE RESPONSES

The Effect of Ultrasound on the Inflammatory Phase of Repair

During the inflammatory phase, ultrasound has a stimulating effect on the mast cells, platelets, phagocytic white cells and macrophages (Li et al 2003; Nussbaum 1997; ter Haar 1999; Watson 2008). For example, ultrasound induces the degranulation of mast cells, causing the release of arachidonic acid, which itself is a precursor for the synthesis of prostaglandins and leukotriene – which act as inflammatory mediators (Leung et al 2004a; Mortimer & Dyson 1988; Nakamura et al 2010; Palidda et al 2014; Watson 2016; Wilson et al 2014). By increasing the activity of these cells, the overall influence of therapeutic ultrasound is certainly pro-inflammatory rather than anti-inflammatory. The benefit is not through increasing the inflammatory response as such (though if applied with too great intensity at this stage, it is a possible outcome) (Ciccone et al 1991), but rather by acting as an 'inflammatory optimiser' (Watson 2007, 2008, 2016). The inflammatory response is essential to the effective repair of tissue, and the more efficiently the process can complete, the more effectively the tissue can progress to the proliferative phase.

Further confirmation of this has been shown experimentally in acute surgical wounds (Young & Dyson 1990b). In this study, full-thickness excised skin lesions in rats were exposed to therapeutic ultrasound (0.1 W/cm^2 SATA, 0.75 MHz or 3.0 MHz) daily for 7 days (5 minutes per day per wound). By 5 days after injury, the ultrasound-treated groups had significantly fewer inflammatory cells in the wound bed and more extensive granulation tissue than the sham-irradiated controls. Also, the alignment of the fibroblasts – parallel to the wound surface – in the wound beds of the ultrasound-treated groups was indicative of a more advanced stage of tissue organization than the random

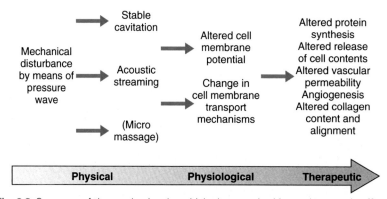

Fig. 9.3 Summary of the mechanism by which ultrasound achieves therapeutic effects.

alignment of fibroblasts seen in the control wounds. The results obtained suggest that there had been an acceleration of the wounds through the inflammatory phase repair in response to ultrasound therapy. It was also noted that no abnormalities were seen, such as hypertrophy of the wound tissue in response to ultrasound therapy.

Studies that attempted to demonstrate an anti-inflammatory effect of ultrasound in fact failed to do so (e.g. El Hag et al 1985; Hashish 1986, 1988), and suggested that ultrasound is ineffective. Anti-inflammatory effects are not the mechanism by which ultrasound achieves beneficial outcome. Ultrasound promotes the normality of the inflammatory events and, as such, has therapeutic value in promoting overall tissue repair (ter Haar 1999; Watson 2008). A further benefit is that chemically mediated events during the inflammatory phase are associated with stimulation of the ensuing proliferative phase of repair (Chapter 3).

Employed at an appropriate treatment dose, with optimal treatment parameters (intensity, pulsing and time), the benefit of ultrasound is to make the inflammatory phase as efficient as possible, and thus have a promotional effect on the whole healing cascade. For tissues in which there is an inflammatory reaction, but in which there is no 'repair' to be achieved, the benefit of ultrasound is to promote the normal resolution of the inflammatory events, and hence resolve the 'problem'. This will, of course, be most effectively achieved in the tissues that preferentially absorb ultrasound – i.e. the dense collagenous tissues.

The Effect of Ultrasound on the Proliferative Phase of Repair

During the proliferative phase (scar production) ultrasound also has a stimulative effect (cellular up regulation), though the primary active targets are now the fibroblasts, endothelial cells and myofibroblasts (Dyson & Smalley 1983; Maxwell 1992; Mortimer & Dyson 1988; Ng 2011; Ramirez et al 1997; Watson 2007, 2008; Watson & Young 2008; Young & Dyson 1990a,b). These are all cells that are normally active during scar production and ultrasound is therefore pro-proliferative in the same way that it is pro-inflammatory – it does not change the normal proliferative phase, but optimizes its efficiency. Harvey et al (1975) demonstrated that low-dose pulsed ultrasound increases protein synthesis, and several research groups have demonstrated enhanced fibroplasia and collagen synthesis (Enwemeka et al 1989, 1990; Huys et al 1993; Ramirez et al 1997; Turner et al 1989; Warden et al 2006; Zhang et al 2004). Recent work has identified the critical role of numerous growth factors in relation to tissue repair, and some accumulating evidence has identified that therapeutic ultrasound has a positive role to play in this context (e.g. Leung et al 2006; Li et al 2002; Lovric et al 2013;

McBrier et al 2007; Reher et al 1999; Tsai et al 2006) and also with heat shock proteins (Nussbaum & Locke 2007).

The Effect of Ultrasound on the Remodelling Phase of Repair

During the remodelling phase of repair, the somewhat generic scar that is produced in the initial stages is refined such that it adopts functional characteristics of the tissue that it is repairing. A scar in ligament will not 'become' ligament, but will partly perform the functions of ligamentous tissue. This is achieved by a number of processes, but mainly related to the orientation of the collagen fibres in the developing scar (Aiyegbusi et al 2012; Culav et al 1999; Gomez et al 1991; Watson 2003) and also to the change in collagen type, from predominantly type III collagen to a more dominant type I collagen, which is more functional. The remodelling process is not a short duration phase – research has shown that it can last for a year or more – yet it is an essential component of quality repair (El Batouty et al 1986; ter Haar 1987).

The application of therapeutic ultrasound can influence the remodelling of the scar tissue in that it appears to enhance the maturing process related to collagen type and orientation thus increasing tensile strength and enhancing scar mobility (Nussbaum 1998; Wang 1998) and thus the functional capacity of the scar tissues (Huys et al 1993; Nussbaum 1998; Tsai et al 2006, 2011; Yeung et al 2006). The influence of ultrasound on collagen fibres has been demonstrated in an elegant study by Byl et al (1996), though their conclusions were, quite reasonably, somewhat tentative.

The effects of ultrasound on the properties of the scar depend very much upon the time at which the therapy was first instigated. The most effective regimens appear to be those that are started soon after injury (i.e. during the inflammatory phase of repair). Webster (1980) found that when wounds were treated three times per week for 2 weeks after injury ($0.1 \ W \ cm^{-2}$ SATA) the resulting tensile strength and elasticity of the scar were significantly higher than those of the control group. Byl et al (1992, 1993) demonstrated an increase in tensile strength and collagen content in incised lesions whose treatment was commenced during the inflammatory phase. They also compared different ultrasound intensities and found that the lower intensity (1 MHz, pulsed, $0.5 \ W \ cm^{-2}$ SATA) was the most effective. Treatment with ultrasound during the inflammatory phase of repair not only increases the amount of collagen deposited in the wound, but also encourages the deposition of that collagen in a pattern whose three-dimensional architecture more resembles that of uninjured skin than the untreated controls (Dyson 1981). Jackson et al (1991) showed that the mechanical properties of injured tendon can be improved with ultrasound if treatment starts early enough; however, the levels used were relatively high, at 1.5 W cm^{-2}. Enwemeka et al (1990) reported that increased tensile strength and elasticity can be achieved in injured tendons using much lower intensities (0.5 W/cm^2 SA).

The application of ultrasound during the inflammatory, proliferative and repair phases is of value not because it changes the normal sequence of events, but because it has the capacity to enhance the normal events and thus increase the efficiency of the repair phases (ter Haar 1999; Watson 2007, 2008; Watson & Young 2008). The effective application of ultrasound to achieve these aims appears to be dose dependent.

CLINICAL EVIDENCE

There is a large body of evidence covering cell, animal and lab studies. The clinical evidence covers a wide range of presentations, which are grouped together in the following sections that dominate the published literature:

- Wound healing
- Osteoarthritis
- Soft-tissue injury
- Pain management.

Some additional indications are included in the Therapeutic Effects section and the use of ultrasound to facilitate fracture repair is included in the section on low-intensity pulsed ultrasound (LIPUS) below.

Ultrasound and Wound Healing

Numerous EPAs have been employed as a means to enhance wound healing in the clinical environment. Ultrasound has a long history of this dating back to at least the 1960s.

A meta-analysis of the early work that employed ultrasound in chronic leg ulceration (Johannsen et al 1998) included 6 studies and 265 patients. The analysis demonstrated a significant effect size of 16.9% (p=0.011) mean difference in healing over a 4-week period when compared with controls (6 studies) and a 14.5% effect size (p=0.005) after 8 weeks of treatment (5 studies). The analysis based on the number of closed ulcers (as opposed to the change in ulcer size) just failed to reach a significant difference (p=0.06) at 8 weeks. The authors conclude that ultrasound has its best effect being delivered in low doses around the ulcer margins.

Accelerated wound closure has also been recorded in other chronic wounds, such as pressure sores (McDiarmid et al 1985; Paul et al 1960). McDiarmid et al also reported an interesting finding that infected ulcers (wound swab results) were more responsive to ultrasound therapy than uninfected sores. It is likely that the low-grade infection had in some way primed or further activated the healing

system (e.g. recruiting more macrophages to the area), which in turn would produce an amplified signal to herald an early start to the other phases of repair.

A Cochrane Review in 2000 (Flemming & Cullum 2000) considered the effectiveness of ultrasound in relation to the treatment of pressure sores (pressure ulcers in current terminology). Randomized controlled trials (RCTs) were included if the ultrasound treatment was compared with a sham treatment or against a treatment without ultrasound. Three studies met the criteria (two of which compared the ultrasound with sham; one of which compared a combination of ultrasound plus ultraviolet against a laser-based intervention). The two studies that compared ultrasound against sham involved a total of 128 patients. The primary outcome was the number of ulcers closed in the trial period. The results indicate no significant advantage using ultrasound. The trial that used combined treatments involved 20 patients, though only 16 (with 18 wounds) completed. In the combined (ultrasound + ultraviolet) group, 100% of the wounds healed; 66% healed in the laser group and 83% in the standard care group. (The results were not significant, though this might be attributed to the small sample.) The review authors conclude that there is no apparent evidence of a benefit with ultrasound in this clinical presentation, though they acknowledge that there may be a real effect which is not (statistically) demonstrated with a low number of RCTs and small sample sizes. There was an update of this Cochrane Review (Baba-Akbari et al 2006) with no substantive change in the papers considered nor the conclusion reached.

It appears that taking complete wound closure as the primary outcome fails to provide results that are as strong as those that take the percentage of wound closure as their primary measure.

A number of more recent studies have provided mixed evidence with regard to the effectiveness of ultrasound as part of the management of chronic wounds (predominantly venous leg ulcers and, to a lesser extent, pressure ulcers). Trials with positive outcomes include those by Ennis et al (2005), Franek et al (2004, 2006) and Polak et al (2014); trials with no demonstrated advantage for ultrasound include that by Selkowitz et al (2002) and Watson et al (2011).

While the results of ultrasound use in wound healing are mixed, it would appear that the variable results may be attributed to a dose dependency (see Chapter 1; Uhlemann et al 2003; Uhlemann & Wollina 2003) and, with continuing research in this field, it is possible that the optimal treatment parameters will be identified. Furthermore, comparison of different EPAs is clearly needed. Ultrasound is only one of several modalities (e.g. laser (see Chapter 10), electrical stimulation (see Chapter 19), ultraviolet (see Chapter 11), shockwave (see Chapter 13) that have been demonstrated to have an effect on wound healing, and few studies have directly compared their effectiveness. Demir et al (2004) compared the effectiveness of laser therapy and ultrasound, identifying both as better than control intervention but stating that laser therapy was advantageous over ultrasound. Franek et al (2006) made a similar comparison between electrical stimulation, laser therapy and ultrasound. The electrical stimulation and ultrasound were found to be significantly effective; laser therapy was not. This ambiguous evidence generates some confusion, but it is hoped that, with further comparative research, clarification can be achieved.

Ultrasound and Osteoarthritis

There have been numerous trials (over 150) in which ultrasound (alone or as a care package component) has been employed in the management of osteoarthritis. Whilst this therapy is not currently capable of resolving the underlying disease process, it appears to be capable of reducing pain, reducing stiffness, improving function and significantly influencing the patient's quality of life (QoL) when comparing pre- to post-treatment outcomes. Interesting studies are evaluating the potential capacity for ultrasound to influence chondrogenesis and thereby directly affect the pathophysiology of this complaint (reviewed in Rothenberg et al 2017). The future use of ultrasound in this condition may therefore be very different from the current applications considered further on.

Robinson et al (2005) published a Cochrane Review covering this topic with an update of the 2001 review. Three papers (294 patients) were included in the review. The authors conclude that ultrasound appears to have no benefit over placebo or over shortwave diathermy for patients with osteoarthritis (OA) of the hip or knee. One trial compared ultrasound with sham (74 patients) demonstrating no significant difference between groups for pain, movement or gait velocity. The other trials compared ultrasound with other therapies (220 patients) demonstrating no significant difference between the treatments (ultrasound, galvanic stimulation, shortwave). The results of this review are somewhat misleading in that ultrasound achieved significantly greater pain relief when compared with galvanic stimulation, but the physician global assessment failed to achieve a difference. The salient point is that patients in all three groups (ultrasound, galvanic stimulation and shortwave) all achieved a significant reduction in pain. That there was no significant difference between the modalities does not negate the pain reduction achieved with ultrasound (86% of patients reporting an excellent or good therapy effect in the ultrasound group, and no patients were worsened). Concluding that there was no

effect is not a valid reflection of the evidence provided in the trials reviewed.

A recent umbrella review (Ferreira et al 2018) evaluated multiple modalities (non-surgical, non-pharmacological) for patient management in osteoarthritis based on existing systematic review evidence. Ultrasound was deemed to provide silver level of evidence for pain reduction and improved function. Three systematic reviews reported on ultrasound benefits and the authors conclude that 1 MHz; 2.5 W cm^{-2} for 15 minutes, 3 times weekly may be an optimal dose for these patients.

More recent trials include a combined therapy study in which ultrasound and laser were used in combination, either with or without exercise and compared with a sham group. Forty-two patients with OA knee were included, and the results support the combined therapy as having a significant benefit over the placebo group. Combining ultrasound, laser and exercise gave the greatest improvement in pressure pain threshold and sit-to-stand activity (Paoillo et al 2018).

Zeng et al (2014) evaluated both continuous and pulsed modes of ultrasound in the management of OA knee, taking a systematic review and meta-analysis approach. Twelve papers were included in the analysis, and the authors concluded that pulsed mode ultrasound provided significant pain relief and functional improvement, whereas continuous ultrasound provided significant benefit only in terms of pain relief. There was no significant difference between the pulsed and continuous ultrasound in terms of the magnitude of the pain relief achieved.

Briani et al (2018) considered interventions that could improve QoL or psychological factors for patients with knee OA, taking a systematic review and meta-analysis approach. Whilst acknowledging that the available evidence was limited, ultrasound-based therapy was supported.

Examples of modern ultrasound studies include Yegin et al (2017) who conducted an RCT with 62 patients presenting with OA knee. Ultrasound treatment (1 MHz; 1 W cm^{-2} in continuous mode) was compared with sham. Treatment benefits for pain and function and activity demonstrated significant improvement in the ultrasound group over the short term, though these benefits were not maintained in the longer term follow-up.

Rodriguez-Grande et al (2017) set out to evaluate the effect of ultrasound (1 MHz, 20% duty cycle, 0.44 W cm^{-2}, 4 minutes, 10 sessions) on pain, mobility, strength, function and QoL in 17 patients with knee OA. Significant reductions in pain (p=0.03), improved function (p=0.008), strength (p=0.04) and QoL (p=0.0001) were demonstrated in this single arm pre-post study.

A large number of studies have evaluated the effects of ultrasound in this patient group. Many have demonstrated highly significant improvements in multiple outcomes, most notably pain, function and QoL. The systematic reviews covering the topic provide mixed levels of support, largely depending on their inclusion criteria and the publication age – that is, the trials that were included. On balance, patients with OA knee exposed to an appropriate ultrasound treatment protocol would reasonably expect to experience significantly less pain, improved function and improved QoL by the end of the treatment period.

Ultrasound and Soft-Tissue Injury

Ultrasound is a widely employed therapy modality in soft-tissue injury and is one of the more widely cited (empirical) uses for the modality. Despite the popularity of this intervention, there are relatively few quality clinical trials that evaluate the effect of ultrasound against a placebo treatment or against a no treatment control.

Page et al (2016) published a Cochrane Review concerning electrotherapy (EPA) interventions for rotator cuff disease, evaluating 47 research papers. In relation to the use of ultrasound, the authors conclude that there is some support for its use in calcific tendinitis around the shoulder. There was high heterogeneity in the ultrasound trials – some comparing with placebo and some against other treatments. Much of the published research was of low quality and at high risk of bias based on the authors' analysis. There was no strong support for the addition of ultrasound to other treatment options involving rotator cuff pathologies. As is typical with this type of review, the conclusion was that more high-quality research with larger numbers is needed in order to reach a more definitive conclusion.

Page et al (2014) also compiled a Cochrane Review looking at EPA interventions for adhesive capsulitis (frozen shoulder) including 19 trials and 1249 patients in their analysis (four trials involved the use of ultrasound). In one study (Dogru et al 2008), ultrasound (3 MHz; 1.5 W cm^{-2}) was delivered in conjunction with hot pack and exercise (compared with sham ultrasound, hot pack and exercise). Both groups significantly improved, but there were no significant between-group differences indicating that the use of ultrasound provided no additional benefit to the patients. The trial was at high risk of bias (review author comment) though ironically, they do not comment about the dose of ultrasound – at 3 MHz being unlikely to even reach the target tissue in the shoulder. The review authors conclude that they could not be certain of a beneficial effect for ultrasound (along with several other modalities) in the treatment of adhesive capsulitis.

Several recent papers have evaluated the use of ultrasound in various shoulder pathologies. Yu et al (2015) reviewed several 'passive' modalities for shoulder pain (including subacromial impingement, non-specific shoulder pain and calcific tendinitis), with 22 papers included for consideration. Ultrasound was not supported in their conclusions based on the inclusion of three published trials.

Yavuz et al (2014) compared the effectiveness of laser and ultrasound (1 MHz, 2.0 W cm^{-2}, continuous, 5 minutes) treatments in subacromial impingement. Thirty-one patients each received 10 treatments over 2 weeks and were followed up for 3 months. Both treatments were significantly (all $p<0.05$) effective in terms of pain relief, function and sleep improvements. There was no significant difference between the laser and ultrasound group changes.

Analan et al (2015) evaluated the effect of continuous mode ultrasound plus exercise on pain, function and muscle strength in 22 patients with rotator cuff disease. All patients received hot pack, transcutaneous electrical nerve stimulation (TENS) and exercise together with verum (1.1 MHz, 1.5 W cm^{-2}, continuous, 5 minutes) or sham ultrasound. The treatment programme was shown to be effective, but the addition of ultrasound made no significant difference to the outcome and therefore was not supported. The additional use of TENS (20 minutes) and hot pack (20 minutes) then exercise (30 minutes) is likely to have confounded the results. That notwithstanding, the lack of difference between ultrasound and sham additions to this treatment package implies that ultrasound may not have value at these parameters with a rotator cuff disease patient group.

In a broad review for the use of ultrasound in relation to soft-tissue injury (Watson 2014) a range of clinical improvements are identified following soft-tissue injury. This was not a systematic review and took a narrative approach to the topic – making it possibly less robust than others.

Ultrasound and Pain Relief

Whilst not primarily employed as a pain relief modality, some clinical trial evidence would support the contention that patients in receipt of ultrasound therapy do report a reduction in pain. It is most commonly ascribed a second order effect (i.e. that the ultrasound has an effect on the underlying injury/problem and that as a result, there is a subsequent reduction in pain).

Gam and Johannsen (1995) present a meta-analysis based on 22 papers in which ultrasound was employed as a treatment for musculoskeletal pain. The authors conclude that the evidence to support its use in this context is lacking, but further identify that poor reporting, low trial quality and missing essential treatment parameters confound the issue. Some trials included in their analysis date back to the 1960s, so to some extent this is inevitable. The Gam and Johannsen analysis was primarily concerned with pain as an outcome rather than recovery from injury per se.

Several trials have been published in which ultrasound is employed as part of a comparison group either alone or as one of several interventions. This group is sometimes the 'EPA' group of the 'passive intervention' group. For example, Murtezani et al (2015) compared McKenzie therapy with an electrophysical agents group in back pain. The EPA group received interferential therapy, heat and ultrasound. Similarly, Ulug et al (2017) set out to compare various exercise programmes (Pilates, yoga and isometric) in chronic neck pain. All groups were in receipt of ultrasound alongside hot pack and TENS as part of a standard care package. It is not possible to disaggregate the relative contribution that the ultrasound component makes to this improvement (or lack of change) and contributes little to the ultrasound research literature.

Jorge et al (2017) evaluated the effectiveness of a variety of heating modalities, including ultrasound, in terms of their capacity to manage OA knee pain, following a systematic review format. The authors conclude that ultrasound has demonstrable benefits for OA knee pain, though along with other modalities, this effect is improved when combined with exercise.

Ultrasound has been evaluated against a control group in myofascial pain syndrome (Ilter et al 2015). Continuous mode (3 MHz; $1.0 \, W \, cm^{-2}$) was compared with pulsed mode (3 MHz; $1.0 \, W \, cm^{-2}$ pulsed 50%) and a control (sham) group (each with 20 patients). Pain was a primary outcome, but function, QoL and depression were also evaluated. All groups improved on several outcomes, but in terms of pain, the patients in the continuous ultrasound group achieved the greatest pain relief, the differences between groups being significant ($p < 0.05$).

Ruiz-Molinero et al (2014) compared ultrasound against a placebo ultrasound in 54 patients post whiplash injury. There was a statistically significant ($p < 0.05$) reduction in pain after the treatment programme was completed, though at the end of ten sessions, the differences were not apparent. The results are confounded by the simultaneous use of microwave diathermy therapy and massage in both groups – the only substantive difference being in the real versus sham ultrasound component. Both the microwave and the massage therapies could have achieved real treatment benefit. That notwithstanding, those in the ultrasound group did demonstrate a better outcome at follow up.

Ultrasound has been used by clinicians for the treatment of carpal tunnel syndrome (e.g. Ebenbichler et al 1998) and in a recent systematic review of RCTs, Huissstede et al (2018) clearly identified that ultrasound has a significant effect on carpal tunnel pain when tested as a standalone therapy, when compared with placebo intervention and

when compared with other therapies, such as steroid injection. In the Page et al (2013) Cochrane Review covering the same topic area, the reviewers conclude that ultrasound can have a short-term benefit in carpal tunnel syndrome, but that the evidence they considered was of a low quality.

Armagan et al (2014) conducted an RCT in which placebo ultrasound was compared with continuous or pulsed ultrasound (at 1 MHz; $1.0 \, W \, cm^{-2}$ either continuous mode or pulsed at 20% duty cycle) with 15 sessions over 3 weeks. All patients were provided with a night splint. Pain was significantly reduced in all groups ($p < 0.006$) but there was not significant difference between groups. Those in the continuous ultrasound group achieved the strongest pain relief, the magnitude of which was sufficient to claim a clinically significant change. Function and symptom scores were similarly improved across all groups. Those in the ultrasound groups demonstrated significant nerve conduction changes, which were not identified in the placebo group. This would suggest that if ultrasound has a real effect on pain relief over and above a placebo intervention, it may be attributed to nerve conduction changes.

Sharma et al (2015) compared ultrasound with laser therapy in the treatment of de Quervain's tenosynovitis pain. The ultrasound was delivered at 3 MHz; pulsed 1:1; $0.8 \, W \, cm^{-2}$ for 3 minutes). Both therapies were effective, significantly reducing pain and other symptoms, but there was no advantage of one therapy over the other.

Whilst ultrasound is not routinely employed as a pain management modality, there is evidence that it can result in reduced pain perception, certainly in the short term. The biophysics evidence would suggest that this is most likely a second order rather than a primary effect and other modalities are likely to be more effective if pain relief is a primary treatment objective. Patients being treated with ultrasound for an underlying musculoskeletal problem are likely to experience a reduced pain perception.

Phonophoresis/Sonophoresis

Phonophoresis is defined as the migration of drug molecules through the skin under the influence of ultrasound. The term sonophoresis is sometimes employed for the same application.

Theoretically, phonophoresis is possible using the acoustic streaming forces that exist in the ultrasound field. However, it is debatable whether these forces are strong enough to produce a net forward movement capable of pushing all drugs through the skin to their target tissue. In addition, it is often difficult to determine whether a biological effect of a topically applied drug is a result of its direct action on the underlying target tissue or of a systemic effect, or indeed, the ultrasound energy which is being used to achieve drug transmission. This complexity may partly explain why the results of phonophoresis research are somewhat mixed. It is likely that phonophoresis will be dependent not only on the frequency, intensity, duty cycle and treatment duration of the ultrasound (Mitragotri et al 2000), but also on the nature of the drug molecule itself. A further complexity is added with the sequential use of ultrasound and drug-based therapy – for example, Rosim et al (2005) evaluated the effect of using ultrasound prior to the drug application on the skin rather than using the ultrasound to 'drive' the agent into the tissues. The outcome was positive and provides an interesting avenue for further work.

There is a wide range of phonophoresis research studies relating to musculoskeletal clinical issues.

Takla et al (2018) compared ultrasound phonophoresis with TENS on active trigger points using four treatment groups (diclofenac phonophoresis with TENS; diclofenac phonophoresis; ultrasound with standard gel and sham ultrasound). There were statistically significant improvements in post intervention pressure pain threshold and range of motion values in treatment groups (p < 0.0001). The sham group demonstrated no significant change. The detailed analysis demonstrated that there were significant differences between the three treatment group outcomes for pain (p<0.0001) with the combined TENS and phonophoresis giving the strongest effect followed by phonophoresis and then standard ultrasound. The trial involved 100 patients, and whilst all three active treatments provided significant benefits, the use of phonophoresis, especially when combined with electrical stimulation, appears to provide an advantage to the patient.

Perez-Marino et al (2016) evaluated three different treatments in subacromial impingement syndrome (SIS) with a group of 96 patients. The groups received either ultrasound, phonophoresis with dexketoprofen or iontophoresis using dexketoprofen. Whilst there were some differences at the end of the treatment period (the ultrasound group doing better than the drug-based groups), by 1 month post intervention, group results were not significantly different.

Similarly, Garcia et al (2016) compared phonophoresis and iontophoresis in shoulder impingement syndrome with 88 patients divided into three groups: a standard treatment group (cryotherapy plus exercise plus placebo phonophoresis plus placebo iontophoresis); standard treatment plus iontophoresis plus placebo phonophoresis; and standard treatment plus phonophoresis plus placebo iontophoresis. Patients in the phonophoresis group demonstrated significant benefits over the standard care group whilst those receiving iontophoresis were no better than standard care. It appears therefore, based on a randomized and reasonably large sample trial, that the addition of phonophoresis

(1 MHz continuous; 0.7 W cm^{-2} plus sodium diclofenac) to a standard care programme confers an advantage to this patient group.

Ojoawo et al (2015) evaluated the effect of phonophoresis in comparison with a standard treatment (exercise) in 70 patients with chronic low back pain. Patients in both groups received the exercise programme and ultrasound (1 MHz; 1.5 W cm^{-2}; continuous mode; 10 minutes; 12 sessions over 6 weeks). In the control group, the ultrasound was delivered with standard gel. Those in the phonophoresis group received ultrasound through Lofnac gel (diclofenac diethylamine plus methyl salicylate). Patients in both groups significantly improved in terms of pain (p<0.001) and disability (p<0.001), but statistically, those receiving phonophoresis were advantaged.

Many similar reports involving patients with chronic rhinosinusitis (Ansari et al 2013); OA knee (Boonhong et al 2018); tennis elbow (Baktir et al 2018) and medial tibial stress syndrome (Winters et al 2013) have been published. The results are mixed with some demonstrating significant benefit, some showing equivalence with other treatments and some demonstrating the phonophoresis is less effective than others.

One significant issue appears to be the sheer number of potentially confounding variables – the condition, the ultrasound parameters, the drug, its dose and application. Clearly further research may serve to identify optimal parameters. In the current state of the evidence, there is sufficient evidence to support the use of phonophoresis in some, but not all, clinical presentations.

Alternative Ultrasound Application and Devices

There are two main alternatives to classic MHz clinical ultrasound, which are both evidenced and employed clinically: (i) Ultrasound generated in the kilohertz frequency range (kHz or 'longwave' ultrasound) and (ii) MHz ultrasound delivered at a very much lower intensity – so called low-intensity pulsed ultrasound – or LIPUS.

Low-Frequency (kHz) Ultrasound

Since the early 1990s there has been an interest in the use of low-frequency (longwave) therapeutic ultrasound for the treatment of a variety of tissue injuries (Bradnock et al 1996) (Fig. 9.4). Typically, this modality operates at a frequency of around 44–48 kHz, which is significantly lower than the usual therapy range of 1–3 MHz. It is suggested that one benefit of using such a low frequency is that the depth of penetration is greatly enhanced and the risks of standing waves are minimized. There is considerable debate whether this 'greater penetration' benefit is of clinical relevance given, for example, the arguments made by Robertson and Ward (1997) illustrating the important

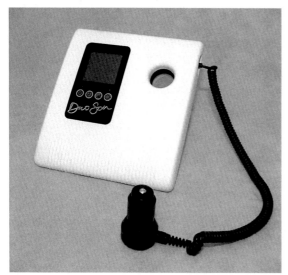

Fig. 9.4 Low-frequency (longwave) ultrasound equipment (Orthosonics).

relationship between the penetration depth and the relative proportion of longwave ultrasound energy that is absorbed in the superficial tissues. It is suggested that because the majority of the energy is absorbed in the superficial tissues, the immediate pain relief and extensibility changes are more akin to those seen as a result of thermal treatments. A recent study (Meakins & Watson 2006) compared the effect of longwave ultrasound and superficial contact heating on tissue extensibility: both were effective but, although there was no statistically significant difference in their outcomes, there was a trend for the heat treatment to be more effective.

Apart from the Bradnock et al (1996) study, there have been few published clinical trials and one of these (Basso & Pike 1998) demonstrated no benefit when low-frequency ultrasound was employed post wrist fracture in terms of mobility gains. Several studies have considered the effect of this intervention with regard to chronic wound management, wound infection and associated problems. Although not numerous, these studies do suggest that there may be a significant benefit of using the modality in these areas (Pavlov 2002; Sedov et al 1998).

The application for wound care typically employs an ultrasound frequency of 20–25 kHz and can be delivered with a contact or non-contact application mode, the latter employing a saline 'mist' in order to achieve energy transmission to the tissue (Keltie et al 2013). Voigt et al (2011) provide a review of this application, though several developments and numerous trials have been published since this time, so it does not fully reflect current evidence.

Zhang et al (2017) included this intervention in their review of ultrasound, expanding on potential mechanisms of actions. Liu et al (2016) evaluated kHz ultrasound effects in terms of antimicrobial activity with supportive data presented, as do Harris et al (2014).

Samuels et al (2013) evaluated the effect of kHz ultrasound at varying doses in a group of 20 patients with chronic venous stasis ulcers. Ultrasound at 20 kHz delivered over a 15-minute time frame achieved the best results with 100% of wounds closed by the fourth treatment. This was a small-scale study and the results should be considered in that context. Olyaie et al (2013) compared the more traditional ultrasound with a contactless application of low-frequency (20 kHz) ultrasound on a group of patients with venous leg ulcers. Both interventions were significantly effective compared with standard wound care, but there was no difference between the ultrasound groups.

There is a lack of clinical or laboratory research in this field compared with 'traditional' ultrasound, and there is a need for large controlled trials to establish where this relatively new modality can be used most effectively. It may be that there are circumstances or clinical conditions for which the low-frequency (kHz; longwave) ultrasound has 'better' effects than traditional (MHz) ultrasound, and the anecdotal evidence would support this contention to some extent. However, without quality published research it is a difficult contention to support from the evidence to date.

Low-Intensity Pulsed Ultrasound (LIPUS)

LIPUS is a relatively recent development in ultrasound therapy, most work having been completed in the last 20 years. LIPUS devices typically operate at 1.5 MHz, 0.03 W cm^{-2} (often described as 30 mW cm^{-2}) and using pulse regimens of 1000 Hz delivered at a 1:4 regimen (20% duty cycle).

These parameters cannot normally be delivered with a traditional ultrasound therapy machine, and dedicated LIPUS devices are available for this application (Fig. 9.5). The Exogen device (used in many of the reported studies) was first available in 1994. Warden et al (1999, 2006) provide an interesting analysis and review of the early work in this field, whilst Pounder and Harrison (2008) provide a useful update which includes mechanism of action considerations. Given the effectiveness of LIPUS in fracture management (below), several groups have considered its potential benefit in other musculoskeletal presentations (e.g. Khanna et al 2009).

Over 200 papers (laboratory, animal and clinical studies) have been published to date which consider the use of LIPUS in fracture management. LIPUS is considered for its effects in fresh fractures, and for enhanced repair in both delayed and non-union clinical presentations. These are briefly outlined below. Its use in distraction osteogenesis is also briefly considered.

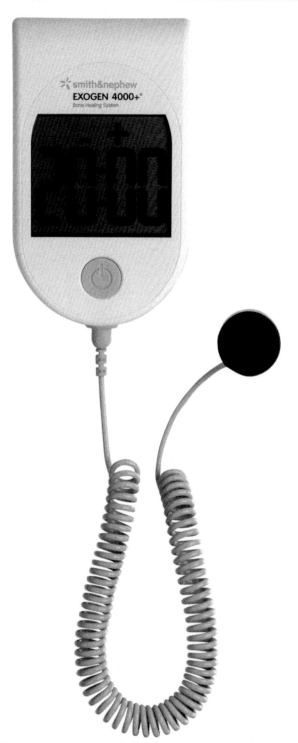

Fig. 9.5 Low-intensity pulsed ultrasound (Exogen) device used to enhance fracture healing.

Early work with traditional ultrasound (e.g. Dyson & Brookes 1983) showed that it was possible to accelerate the repair of fibular fractures using therapeutic levels of ultrasound (1.5 or 3 MHz, pulsed, 0.5 W cm^{-2} SATA). The treatments were for 5 minutes, four times per week. The most effective treatments were found to be those which were carried out during the first 2 weeks of repair. Of the two frequencies used, 1.5 MHz was the more effective. Pilla et al (1990) and Tsai et al (1992a,b) extended this work and further identified PGE2 as a strong contender for the mechanism of effect and also identified that the fracture healing response was dose dependent (high doses were detrimental).

Over 35 papers have reviewed the LIPUS evidence – with mixed conclusions. Schandelmaier et al (2017) reviewed 26 trials considering patient-related factors (such as return to work) as being of importance. They observe that the highest quality trials do not provide convincing evidence of benefit whilst acknowledging multiple publications with reports of significant benefit. Padilla et al (2016) provide an extensive consideration of the potential mechanisms through which LIPUS can exert its influence (dominated by chemical mediator stimulation in response to mechanotransduction effects). Their consideration of the clinical effects is supportive for the use of LIPUS, certainly in the non-union state. Harrison et al (2016) also consider the mechanism of benefit, reaching the same basic conclusions as Padilla et al (2016).

Zura et al (2015) present an extensive cohort study (over 4000 patients) treated with LIPUS, with particular emphasis on age-related effects. Their analysis suggests that older patients with fractures would normally have a significantly reduced healing rate. In their cohort treated with LIPUS, the healing rate in the elderly was brought to the same level as for the younger population.

Hannemann et al (2014) review data from 735 patients reported in 13 trials (pulsed electromagnetic fields (PEMF) and LIPUS applications) and conclude that PEMF or LIPUS can be beneficial in the treatment of acute fractures regarding time to radiological and clinical union. PEMF and LIPUS significantly shorten time to radiological union for acute fractures undergoing non-operative treatment and acute fractures of the upper limb. Furthermore, PEMF or LIPUS bone growth stimulation accelerates the time to clinical union for acute diaphyseal fractures.

Mehta et al (2015) provide a detailed economic evaluation of this therapy comparing the intervention costs with surgery. They conclude that surgery patients used significantly and substantially more healthcare resources in non-union fracture treatment, and that the use of LIPUS as a conservative measure could potentially result in cost savings approaching $1 billion. Additional supportive reviews are provided by Busse et al (2002), Busse and Bhandari (2004), Malizos et al (2006), Rubin et al (2001), Stein et al (2005) and Warden (2003).

In addition to the demonstrated benefits of ultrasound in terms of 'normal' fracture healing, additional experimental and review material considers its effective application for delayed and non-unions (Gebauer et al 2005; Lerner et al 2004; Leung et al 2004b; Mayr et al 2000; Nolte et al 2001). Furthermore, a range of recent publications demonstrates the application of LIPUS in the management of distraction osteogenesis (Dudda et al 2005; El-Mowafi & Mohsen 2005; Fujishiro et al 2005; Gebauer & Correll 2005) though the recent systematic review from Lou et al (2018) casts some doubt on the value of LIPUS in distraction osteogenesis.

On balance, there is both original research and review support for the use of LIPUS in fresh fractures, delayed and non-unions. The quality of this research is mixed and some of the strongest (supportive) data is derived from trials which have been criticized for their potential risk of bias and low patient numbers. On balance, it is difficult to dismiss this therapy as being without evidence, and with increasing patient numbers being exposed to this intervention, it is anticipated that its real clinical value will become clearer with time.

THERAPEUTIC EFFECTS

The evidence considered in the previous section on clinical evidence considered the application of ultrasound in wound healing, osteoarthritis, soft-tissue injury, and as a pain management tool. These applications were broadly supported by the reviewed evidence. Some additional supported ultrasound applications are identified below:

Ultrasound in Neck and Low Back Pain

Ultrasound has been included in comparative treatment packages which aim to evaluate intervention effects in neck and back pain. For example, Ulug et al (2017) set out to compare various exercise programmes – Pilates, yoga and isometrics – in chronic neck pain. All groups were in receipt of ultrasound alongside hot pack and TENS as part of a standard care package. There was a significant improvement in pain, disability, depression and QoL in all groups ($p < 0.05$) though it is not possible to disaggregate the relative contribution that the ultrasound component made to this improvement.

In the Cochrane Review (Ebadi et al 2014) 7 trials with a total of 362 patients were included for analysis. The authors conclude that there was no high-quality evidence to support the use of ultrasound for improving pain or QoL in patients with non-specific chronic low back pain (LBP). There is some evidence that therapeutic ultrasound has a small effect on improving low-back function in the short term, but this benefit is unlikely to be clinically important.

Louw et al (2016) conducted insightful research involving the use of ultrasound in chronic LBP. They employed a 3-group design each of 20 patients where all received the same ultrasound treatment (1 MHz; 1.5 W cm^{-2}; 20% duty cycle; 10 minutes) based on previously successful research outcomes. What was different between the groups in this study was the education about the applied ultrasound – the control group receiving the standard education, one group receiving an inflated explanation and the third group an extra-inflated explanation. Multiple outcomes were evaluated and the straight leg raise distance increased significantly in both the inflated education groups compared with the control ($p < 0.0001$). Those receiving the extra education were on average 4.4 times more likely to make a clinically significant improvement. There was no significant difference in pain (back or leg) or flexion range between groups, though in each instance, those in the extra education group fared best.

The single blind trial of continuous ultrasound in chronic low back pain reported by Ebadi et al (2012) employed a two-group design: ultrasound (1 MHz; 1.5 W cm^{-2}) plus exercise or a sham ultrasound plus exercise with 50 patients recruited. Ten ultrasound sessions were delivered over 4 weeks and followed up for a month thereafter. Across a range of outcome measures, both groups were determined to have significantly improved. There were significant differences between groups for movement and function ($p < 0.05$) but not for pain.

The same lead author provides a further ultrasound study in chronic, non-specific, LBP (Ebadi et al 2013) demonstrating significant changes in muscle endurance, an increase in function (by 17%) and a reduction in pain (by 24%) in a group of 22 patients. This was not an RCT nor was there any kind of control, thus the positive results should be considered in that light.

Overall in spinal (neck and back) pain presentations, there is a mixed body of evidence including systematic reviews, RCT and cohort studies. There appears to be sufficient support for the use of ultrasound, but the dose required appears to be relatively high and numerous treatment sessions are needed. The primary benefits do not actually appear to be pain focused but rather related to function.

The use of ultrasound at trigger points has been used clinically for some time and is well supported from the anecdotal evidence. A study by Srbely et al (2007) raises some interesting points and demonstrates a measurable benefit. Other studies in this area include Aguilera et al (2009), Draper et al (2010), Majlesi and Unalan (2004), Manca et al (2014), Sarrafzadeh et al (2012) and Unalan et al (2011). More recently, Morishita et al (2014) have demonstrated some interesting effects of ultrasound (to trapezius muscle), stretch and pain effects, which may link to trigger point applications.

Ultrasound in Sinusitis and Rhinosinusitis

There is an increasing body of evidence which supports the use of ultrasound in chronic sinusitis and rhinosinusitis. This has been usefully reviewed in Bartley et al (2014) and detailed clinical trials can be found in Ansari et al (2007, 2014), Naghdi et al (2008) and Young et al (2010). Doses applied in these trials were typically at 1 MHz; 0.5-1.0 W cm^{-2}, pulsed mode, 15–18 minutes, 3 × weekly, 10 sessions with significant clinical benefit.

Temporomandibular Disorder (TMD)

Anecdotal support abounds for the use of ultrasound for patients with various TMD presentations. Early papers (e.g. Mohl et al 1990) do not report positive outcomes when ultrasound is employed for patients with TMD, and in a broad scoping review Shaffer et al (2014) also suggest that ultrasound has limited value, as do Butts et al (2017). Grey et al (1994, 1995) compared several different treatment options for TM pain, ultrasound being one of them (also shortwave – continuous and pulsed, and laser). All interventions were demonstrated to have a significant benefit compared with placebo, though no significant differences were identified between treatments.

There is a paucity of quality original research, and whilst numerous treatment reviews generally lack support, their conclusions are reached on the basis of a weak evidence base. For example, Oh et al (2002) evaluated the effect of a physiotherapy treatment package in post TMJ surgery patients. Ultrasound was one of the included components. Twenty-two patients received the therapy package while 22 others did not. The patients in the treatment group were significantly advantaged, but given that ultrasound was one component of several, it is not possible to disaggregate the results and identify the contribution it made to recovery.

Therapy Ultrasound as a Diagnostic Tool for Stress Fractures

The use of ultrasound therapy to 'detect' a stress fracture is a technique that has been employed sporadically for many years. Some claim (anecdotally) that it is very effective whilst others dismiss the technique. Essentially, a 'strong' ultrasound application (typically 1 MHz; 1.0 W cm^{-2}; continuous) is applied over the suspect area. If there is a stress fracture (or other significant bony injury) it is common for a sharp pain to be felt by the patient. It can be a useful technique when working without immediate access to x-ray, MRI or other higher-level imaging technology. The research reports covering this technique are mixed. The more recent papers include Papalada et al (2012) who suggest that the technique is reproducible and reliable whilst Khatri et al (2008) suggest that the technique is not as accurate as MRI. Other papers include Devereaux et al (1984) and Delacerda (1981).

ULTRASOUND APPLICATION

A number of factors should be considered when using therapeutic ultrasound:

- choice of ultrasound machine
- calibration
- choice of coupling medium
- frequency
- intensity
- pulsed or continuous mode
- treatment intervals
- duration of treatment.

Choice of Ultrasound Machine

Most ultrasound machines have the same basic design, consisting of an ultrasound generator, which may be mains or battery powered (or both) (see Fig. 9.1). The applicator houses the transducer, which produces ultrasound when stimulated by the oscillating voltage from the generator. Machines may operate at single or multiple frequencies, most commonly 1 and 3 MHz. The intensity can be varied, as can the choice of output: from pulsed mode (a range of pulses is usually available) to continuous mode. Typically, 'large' (approximately 5 cm^2) and 'small' (approximately 1 cm^2) treatment applicators are available (Fig. 9.6). The beam non-uniformity ratio (BNR) represents the difference between the peak and the mean power output across the transducer face, and the lower this value, the better for clinical applications. Typically, the values for modern machines range between 4 and 6.

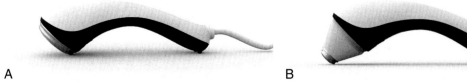

A   B

Fig. 9.6 Ultrasound transducers. (A) Large applicator. (B) Small applicator (EMS Physio).

Calibration

The machine should be calibrated on a regular basis (at least annually) and the output checked at more frequent intervals (ideally once a week). It is important to note that the reading on the machine power-output meter is not an accurate guide to what is actually emitted by the treatment head: the machine must be calibrated against a dedicated calibration device. It has been suggested that the effective calibration of therapy machines is currently inadequate (Artho et al 2002; Guirro et al 1997; Pye & Milford 1994; Sutton et al 2006), and although full technical calibration may not be realistic more than every 6 months, a regular check of power output using a water balance is advised.

Choice of Coupling Medium

A coupling medium must be employed as ultrasound will not travel through air. The most efficient coupling agent in terms of acoustic properties is water. The difference in acoustic impedance between water and soft tissue is small, which means that there is only approximately 0.2% reflection at the interface between the two. Alternatively, aqueous gels are almost as effective as water in terms of absolute transmission, but with the added advantage of higher viscosity, which means that they meet more of the 'essential requirements' for a clinical coupling medium (Dyson 1990).

As identified in an earlier section of this chapter, and also in Chapter 2, there is no clinically relevant difference between currently available coupling gels (Poltakski & Watson 2007a). Water is an effective medium for treating small areas and body parts with significant bony protuberances, although with the advent of the 'small' treatment head this is now less of a clinical problem.

Treatment 'under water' has other advantages in that the treatment head need not actually touch the skin; this may be considered beneficial for patients with significant tenderness.

For the treatment of open wounds, it is important to use a transmission system that will enable the ultrasound energy to reach the wound surface while not compromising the sterility of the area. Being able to treat through an existing wound dressing is considered to be advantageous in that there is less compromise to the wound environment and also less risk of introducing infective agents (Poltawski & Watson 2007b).

Some wound dressings demonstrate very good ultrasound transmission characteristics whereas others transmit very little, and still others absolutely no ultrasound energy at all. A recent review of 48 different wound dressings identified the characteristics and qualities of each. This is an important and necessary consideration for any therapist working in this field (Poltawski & Watson 2007b).

Frequency

Having control over the frequency of the ultrasound output gives the therapist control over the depth of transmission. The basic principle is that the higher the frequency, the more superficial the energy absorption (related to the half value depth). Lower frequency ultrasound energy has a lower absorption rate and thus a greater proportion of the energy reaches the deeper tissues. It is generally considered advantageous to have access to a dual-frequency device, and hence the capacity to be effective in both deep and superficial lesions. The average half value depths (noted previously in this chapter and in Chapter 2) will assist in determining the effective penetration of the energy in the clinical setting.

Intensity

There is no quantitative scientific or clinical information that indicates that 'high' levels of ultrasound (greater than 1 W cm^{-2} (SATA)) need to be used to cause a significant biological effect in injured tissues. On the contrary, the data presented earlier in this chapter support the use of intensities of 0.5 W cm^{-2} (SATA), and less, to achieve maximum healing rates in damaged tissues. The use of higher intensities in the more acute lesions is potentially detrimental, though in chronic lesions, high-intensity applications are strongly evidenced.

There has been a trend over recent years towards the use of lower-intensity treatments. The advice is to always use the lowest intensity that produces the required therapeutic effect, as higher intensities may be damaging (Dyson 1990). Generally, with acute conditions the intensity used should be between 0.1 and 0.3 W cm^{-2} and should not usually be higher than 0.5 W cm^{-2} (SATA). For more chronic conditions, the levels would typically be between 0.3 and 0.8 W cm^{-2}, and should be no higher than 2.5 W cm^{-2} (SATA). Although detailed information as regards treatment dose selection is beyond the remit of this section, the important point to consider is that these intensity values are those that are needed at the target, which clearly may not be the same as those delivered at the skin surface. Details of clinically effective intensities are available from numerous sources, including Watson (2002) and http://www.electrotherapy.org.

Pulsed or Continuous Mode?

Pulsing ultrasound has a major effect on reducing the amount of heat generated in the tissues. A controversy exists as to what the major mechanisms are by which ultrasound stimulates injured tissue to heal. It is unlikely that a specific bioeffect occurs as a result of the exclusive action of either thermal or non-thermal mechanisms; it is more likely to be an effect of both. Therefore, the area is rather a grey one. However, based on the literature available, the more acute the presentation, the lower the duty cycle should be (start at around 1:4 or 20% duty cycle). With less acute (or more chronic) lesions, a lower pulse ratio (1:3, 1:2, duty cycles of 25% or 33%) is more effective. With truly chronic lesions, still lower pulse ratios (1:1 or continuous, duty cycles of 50% and 100%) appear to be most efficacious.

Treatment Intervals

The interval between successive treatments depends upon the nature of the injury. In general terms, the more acute the lesion, the better result will be achieved with low-dose treatments applied relatively frequently – daily in the ideal setting. Treatment more than once a day is a practice employed in some clinical areas (most commonly sports medicine, but also some acute orthopaedic units). There is no absolute evidence to demonstrate that treatment more than once a day is any more effective, and it is advised that if this practice is followed, then a gap of at least 6 hours is maintained between ultrasound interventions. With the less acute lesions, a higher but less frequent treatment dose seems to be effective and, as a general rule of thumb, three times a week for subacute and twice a week for chronic lesions appears to be effective. These are 'ideal' treatment frequencies and it is accepted that it might not be possible to achieve them in the clinical environment. It is also suggested that any level of intervention, with a treatment at the 'right' dose, will have a measurable benefit, although it may not be as effective as the ideal.

Duration of Treatment

The duration of treatment depends upon the area of the injury. Typically, the area should be divided into zones that are approximately the same size as the treatment head, and then each zone should be treated for 1 minute (Oakley 1978; Watson 2002, 2006a). Hoogland (1986) recommends a total maximal treatment time of 15 minutes, and that at least 1 minute should be spent in treating an area of 1 cm^2. If the intention is to raise tissue temperature to above 40°C, then a minimum of 10 minutes treatment will be required.

Compiling the Treatment Dose

Whilst recipe-based treatment settings are not appropriate in an evidenced based viewpoint, it is possible to employ the available evidence in order to construct the combined ultrasound treatment dose that is most likely to be effective – based on the best available evidence. The detail of this dose 'calculation' is beyond the remit of this chapter, but is published (Watson, 2002) and is freely available at http://www.electrotherapy.org for those who wish to consult this resource.

ULTRASOUND APPLICATION GUIDE

Much like any other EPA application, the basic principles are reasonably straightforward and are covered in Chapter 22; some guidelines specific to ultrasound treatment follow:
- Clean the treatment head with an alcohol wipe (or equivalent) for infection control.
- Sufficient coupling medium gel is required to ensure air-free contact. There is no advantage in using large quantities.
- The gel needs to be bubble free – avoid shaking the bottle – the more air in the gel, the less effective the treatment becomes.
- Set the machine (parameters) – it is easiest to set all parameters except for the intensity – do this last once the treatment head is in contact with the skin.
- Apply the treatment. The treatment head should move throughout the treatment. You should never use a stationary transducer application unless applying LIPUS.
- The direction of movement is not a critical issue, nor is speed, but it is normal to move at around 2–4 cm/second and most commonly to use an overlapping circles technique – but that is not a rule.
- Keep the treatment applicator as flat as possible on the skin surface. The critical angle is approximately 15 degrees, therefore tilting the applicator to 15 degrees or more from the perpendicular position will significantly reduce ultrasound penetration into the tissue.
- Ensure that you only treat the area that you plan to – avoid spreading out the treatment as the session proceeds – 'chasing the gel'.
- The patient should not feel anything with low-dose applications, other than the treatment head moving on the skin. If they report any tingling, pain, irritation or similar issues, then stop, check the applied dose, and if all was set up as planned, try at a lower dose (intensity). If the patient still reports adverse sensations, then discontinue. With higher dose treatments, some gentle warming of the skin is considered normal – but should not be uncomfortably warm.
- Terminate the application and remove the applicator.
- Clean the applicator. Clean and check the skin.

TREATMENT APPLICATOR CONTAMINATION AND MICROBIAL SPREAD

The potential for the transmission of infective agents by means of ultrasound treatment devices has been considered by Schabrun et al (2006). It was demonstrated that a high proportion of ultrasound devices in clinical use showed significant levels of nosocomial infective organisms (as did a high proportion of ultrasound gel containers). Importantly, the microbiological agents identified were those normally found on the skin rather than treatment-resistant varieties. Furthermore, the use of a 70% alcohol wipe on the treatment head significantly reduced the microorganism count. It is suggested, therefore, that the treatment head is wiped with a 70% alcohol wipe prior to each and every treatment. This finding was broadly replicated by Spratt et al (2014) and an additional consideration of MRSA was included. The use of an antibacterial agent was shown to be effective for cleaning the ultrasound applicator between treatments.

SUMMARY

Therapeutic ultrasound has the capacity to positively influence the normal processes of tissue repair following injury. Although the effects appear to be strongest during the inflammatory phase, they are certainly evident throughout all the other repair phases. Ultrasound has clinical effects on a range of conditions other than tissue damage, including osteoarthritis and various musculoskeletal syndromes such as carpal tunnel syndrome and the management of trigger points. The developing use of ultrasound (LIPUS) to assist fracture healing and the application of kHz ultrasound in wound management provides new treatment options.

The published evidence for cell, animal and laboratory studies is ironically stronger than the clinical research. Some systematic reviews note the low quality and high risk of bias for ultrasound clinical studies, though this is not unique to this modality. There is sufficient original trial evidence to support its application in therapy based on the material reviewed in this chapter. It is important however to apply the energy at the optimal parameters in order to gain maximal benefit.

REFERENCES

Aguilera, F. J., Martin, D. P., Masanet, R. A., Botella, A. C., Soler, L. B., & Morell, F. B. (2009). Immediate effect of ultrasound and ischemic compression techniques for the treatment of trapezius latent myofascial trigger points in healthy subjects: A randomized controlled study. *Journal of Manipulative and Physiological Therapeutics*, 32(7), 515–520.

Aiyegbusi, A. I., Duru, F. I., & Akinbo, S. R. (2012). The morphology of the healing tendon: A comparison of the effects of intrasound therapy and therapeutic pulsed ultrasound. *Connective Tissue Research*, 53(6), 478–484.

Analan, P. D., Leblebici, B., & Adam, M. (2015). Effects of therapeutic ultrasound and exercise on pain, function, and isokinetic shoulder rotator strength of patients with rotator cuff disease. *Journal of Physical Therapy Science*, 27(10), 3113–3117.

Ansari, N. N., Fathali, M., Naghdi, S., Bartley, J., & Rastak, M. S. (2013). Treatment of chronic rhinosinusitis using erythromycin phonophoresis. *Physiotherapy Theory and Practice*, 29(2), 159–165.

Ansari, N. N., Naghdi, S., & Farhadi, M. (2007). Physiotherapy for chronic rhinosinusitis: The use of continuous ultrasound. *International Journal of Therapy and Rehabilitation*, 14(7), 306–310.

Artho, P. A., Thyne, J. G., Warring, B. P., et al. (2002). A calibration study of therapeutic ultrasound units. *Physical Therapy*, 82(3), 257–263.

Aydin, E., Tastaban, E., Omurlu, I. K., Turan, Y., & Sendur, O. F. (2016). Effects of deep heating provided by therapeutic ultrasound on demyelinating nerves. *Journal of Physical Therapy Science*, 28(4), 1278–1283.

Baba-Akbari, S. A., Flemming, K., Cullum, N. A., et al. (2006). Therapeutic ultrasound for pressure ulcers. *Cochrane Database of Systematic Reviews* (3), CD001275.

Baker, K. G., Robertson, V. J., & Duck, F. A. (2001). A review of therapeutic ultrasound: Biophysical effects. *Physical Therapy*, 81(7), 1351–1358.

Baktir, S., Razak Ozdincler, A., Kaya Mutlu, E., & Bilsel, K. (2018). The short-term effectiveness of low-level laser, phonophoresis, and iontophoresis in patients with lateral epicondylosis. *Journal of Hand Therapy*.

Bartley, J., Ansari, N. N., & Naghdi, S. (2014). Therapeutic ultrasound as a treatment modality for chronic rhinosinusitis. *Current Infectious Disease Reports*, 16(3), 398.

Basso, O., & Pike, J. M. (1998). The effect of low frequency, longwave ultrasound therapy on joint mobility and rehabilitation after wrist fracture. *The Journal of Hand Surgery (Br)*, 23(1), 136–139.

Boonhong, J., Suntornpiyapan, P., & Piriyajarukul, A. (2018). Ultrasound combined transcutaneous electrical nerve stimulation (UltraTENS) versus phonophoresis of piroxicam (PhP) in symptomatic knee osteoarthritis: A randomized double-blind, controlled trial. *Journal of Back and Musculoskeletal Rehabilitation*, 31(3), 507–513.

Bradnock, B., Law, H. T., & Roscoe, K. A. (1996). A quantitative comparative assessment of the immediate response to high frequency ultrasound and low frequency ultrasound (longwave therapy) in the treatment of acute ankle sprains. *Physiotherapy*, 82, 78–84.

Briani, R. V., Ferreira, A. S., Pazzinatto, M. F., Pappas, E., De Oliveira Silva, D., & Azevedo, F. M. (2018). What interventions can improve quality of life or psychosocial factors of individuals with knee osteoarthritis? A systematic review with meta-analysis of primary outcomes from randomised controlled trials. *British Journal of Sports Medicine*, 52(16), 1031–1038.

Busse, J. W., & Bhandari, M. (2004). Therapeutic ultrasound and fracture healing: A survey of beliefs and practices. *Archives of Physical Medicine and Rehabilitation*, 85(10), 1653–1656.

Busse, J. W., Bhandari, M., Kulkarni, A. V., et al. (2002). The effect of low-intensity pulsed ultrasound therapy on time to fracture healing: A meta-analysis. *Canadian Medical Association Journal*, 166(4), 437–441.

Butts, R., Dunning, J., Pavkovich, R., Mettille, J., & Mourad, F. (2017). Conservative management of temporomandibular dysfunction: A literature review with implications for clinical practice guidelines (narrative review part 2). *Journal of Bodywork and Movement Therapies*, 21(3), 541–548.

Byl, N. N., Hill Toulouse, L., Sitton, P., Hall, J., & Stern, R. (1996). Effects of ultrasound on the orientation of fibroblasts: An in-vitro study. *European Journal of Physical Medicine and Rehabilitation*, 6(6), 180–184.

Byl, N. N., McKenzie, A. L., West, J. M., et al. (1992). Low-dose ultrasound effects on wound healing: A controlled study with Yucatan pigs. *Archives of Physical Medicine and Rehabilitation*, 73, 656–664.

Byl, N. N., McKenzie, A. L., Wong, T., et al. (1993). Incisional wound healing: A controlled study of low and high dose ultrasound. *The Journal of Orthopaedic and Sports Physical Therapy*, 18, 619–628.

Casarotto, R. A., Adamowski, J. C., Fallopa, F., et al. (2004). Coupling agents in therapeutic ultrasound: Acoustic and thermal behavior. *Archives of Physical Medicine and Rehabilitation*, 85(1), 162–165.

Chang, Y. P., Chiang, H., Shih, K. S., Ma, H. L., Lin, L. C., Hsu, W. L., et al. (2015). Effects of therapeutic physical agents on Achilles tendon microcirculation. *The Journal of Orthopaedic and Sports Physical Therapy*, 45(7), 563–569.

Chipchase, L. S., Williams, M. T., & Robertson, V. J. (2009). A national study of the availability and use of electrophysical agents by Australian physiotherapists. *Physiotherapy Theory and Practice*, 25(4), 279–296.

Ciccone, C., Leggin, B., & Callamaro, J. (1991). Effects of ultrasound and trolamine salicylate phonophoresis on delayed-onset muscle soreness. *Physical Therapy*, 71, 666.

Culav, E. M., Clark, C. H., & Merrilees, M. J. (1999). Connective tissues: Matrix composition and its relevance to physical therapy. *Physical Therapy*, 79(3), 308–319.

Dalecki, D. (2004). Mechanical bioeffects of ultrasound. *Annual Review of Biomedical Engineering*, 6, 229–248.

Delacerda, F. G. (1981). A case study: Application of ultrasound to determine a stress fracture of the fibula. *The Journal of Orthopaedic and Sports Physical Therapy*, 2(3), 134–136.

Demir, H., Yarray, S., Kirnap, M., et al. (2004). Comparison of the effects of laser and ultrasound treatments on experimental wound healing in rats. *The Journal of Rehabilitation Research and Development*, 41(5), 721–728.

Devereaux, M. D., Parr, G. R., Lachmann, S. M., Page-Thomas, P., & Hazleman, B. L. (1984). The diagnosis of stress fractures in athletes. *JAMA*, 252(4), 531–533.

Dogru, H., Basaran, S., & Sarpel, T. (2008). Effectiveness of therapeutic ultrasound in adhesive capsulitis. *Joint Bone Spine*, 75(4), 445–450.

Doinikov, A. A., & Bouakaz, A. (2010). Acoustic microstreaming around an encapsulated particle. *Journal of the Acoustical Society of America*, 127(3), 1218–1227.

Draper, D. O., Mahaffey, C., Kaiser, D., Eggett, D., & Jarmin, J. (2010). Thermal ultrasound decreases tissue stiffness of trigger points in upper trapezius muscles. *Physiotherapy Theory and Practice*, 26(3), 167–172.

Draper, D. O., & Ricard, M. D. (1995). Rate of temperature decay in human muscle following 3 MHz ultrasound: The stretching window revealed. *Journal of Athletic Training*, 30(4), 304–307.

Dudda, M., Pommer, A., Muhr, G., et al. (2005). Application of low intensity, pulsed ultrasound on distraction osteogenesis of the humerus. Case report. *Unfallchirurg*, 108(1), 69–74.

Dyson, M. (1981). The effect of ultrasound on the rate of wound healing and the quality of scar tissue. In A. J. Mortimer & N. Lee (Eds.), *Proceedings of the International Symposium on Therapeutic Ultrasound, Manitoba* (pp. 110–123). Winnipeg: Canadian Physiotherapy Association.

Dyson, M. (1982). Nonthermal cellular effects of ultrasound. *British Journal of Cancer*, 45(Suppl. V), 165–171.

Dyson, M. (1985). Therapeutic applications of ultrasound. In W. L. Nyborg & M. C. Ziskin (Eds.), *Biological effects of ultrasound. Clinics in diagnostic ultrasound* (pp. 121–133). New York: Churchill Livingstone.

Dyson, M. (1990). Role of ultrasound in wound healing. In L. C. Kloth, J. M. McCulloch & J. A. Feedar (Eds.), *Wound healing: Alternatives in management* (pp. 259–285). Philadelphia: FA Davis.

Dyson, M., & Brookes, M. (1983). Stimulation of bone repair by ultrasound. In R. A. Lerski & P. Morley (Eds.), *Ultrasound '82. Proceedings of the third meeting of the World Federation for Ultrasound in Medicine and Biology* (pp. 232–236). Oxford: Pergamon Press.

Dyson, M., Franks, C., & Suckling, J. (1976). Stimulation of healing varicose ulcers by ultrasound. *Ultrasonics*, 14, 232–236.

Dyson, M., Pond, J. B., Joseph, J., & Warwick, R. (1968). Stimulation of tissue repair by pulsed wave ultrasound. *IEEE Trans Sonics Ultrasonics SU*, 17, 133–140.

Dyson, M., Pond, J. B., Woodward, J., & Broadbent, J. (1974). The production of blood cell stasis and endothelial cell damage in the blood vessels of chick embryos treated with ultrasound in a stationary wave field. *Ultrasound in Medicine and Biology*, 1, 133–148.

Dyson, M., & Smalley, D. S. (1983). Effects of ultrasound on wound contraction. In R. Millner, E. Rosenfeld & U. Cobet (Eds.), *Ultrasound interactions in biology and medicine* (p. 151). New York: Plenum Press.

Ebadi, S., Ansari, N. N., Naghdi, S., Fallah, E., Barzi, D. M., Jalaei, S., et al. (2013). A study of therapeutic ultrasound and exercise treatment for muscle fatigue in patients with chronic non specific low back pain: A preliminary report. *Journal of Back and Musculoskeletal Rehabilitation*, 26(2), 221–226.

Ebadi, S., Ansari, N. N., Naghdi, S., Jalaei, S., Sadat, M., Bagheri, H., et al. (2012). The effect of continuous ultrasound on chronic non-specific low back pain: A single blind placebo-controlled randomized trial. *BMC Musculoskeletal Disorders*, 13, 192.

Ebadi, S., Henschke, N., Nakhostin Ansari, N., Fallah, E., & van Tulder, M. W. (2014). Therapeutic ultrasound for chronic low-back pain. *Cochrane Database of Systematic Reviews* (3), CD009169.

Ebenbichler, G. R., Resch, K. L., Nicolakis, P., et al. (1998). Ultrasound treatment for treating the carpel tunnel syndrome: Randomised 'sham' controlled trial. *British Medical Journal*, 316(7133), 731–735.

El Ghamrawy, A., de Comtes, F., Koruk, H., Mohammed, A., Jones, J. R., & Choi, J. J. (2019). Acoustic streaming in a soft tissue microenvironment. *Ultrasound in Medicine and Biology*, 45(1), 208–217.

El Hag, M., Coghlan, K., Christmas, P., et al. (1985). The anti-inflammatory effects of dexamethasone and therapeutic ultrasound in oral surgery. *British Journal of Oral and Maxillofacial Surgery*, 23, 17–23.

El-Batouty, M. F., El-Gindy, M., El-Shawaf, I., Bassioni, N., El-Ghaweet, A., & El-Emam, A. (1986). Comparative evaluation of the effects of ultrasonic and ultraviolet irradiation on tissue regeneration. *Scandinavian Journal of Rheumatology*, 15, 381–386.

El-Mowafi, H., & Mohsen, M. (2005). The effect of low-intensity pulsed ultrasound on callus maturation in tibial distraction osteogenesis. *International Orthopaedics*, 29(2), 121–124.

Ennis, W. J., Foremann, P., Mozen, N., et al. (2005). Ultrasound therapy for recalcitrant diabetic foot ulcers: Results of a randomized, double-blind, controlled, multicenter study. *Ostomy Wound Managementment*, 51(8), 24–39.

Enwemeka, C. S. (1989). The effects of therapeutic ultrasound on tendon healing. *American Journal of Physical Medicine and Rehabilitation*, 68(6), 283–287.

Enwemeka, C. S., Rodriguez, O., & Mendosa, S. (1990). The bio-mechanical effects of low-intensity ultrasound on healing tendons. *Ultrasound in Medicine and Biology*, 16, 801–807.

Ferreira, R. M., Duarte, J. A., & Goncalves, R. S. (2018). Non-pharmacological and non-surgical interventions to manage patients with knee osteoarthritis: An umbrella review. *Acta Reumatologica Portuguesa*, 43(3), 182–200.

Flemming, K., & Cullum, N. (2000). Therapeutic ultrasound for pressure sores (Cochrane Review). *Cochrane Database of Systematic Reviews* (4).

Franek, A., Chmielewska, D., Brzezinska-Wcislo, L., et al. (2004). Application of various power densities of ultrasound in the treatment of leg ulcers. *Journal of Dermatological Treatment*, 15(6), 379–386.

Franek, A., Krol, P., Chmielewska, D., et al. (2006). The venous ulcer therapy in use of the selected physical methods (part 2) – the comparison analysis. *Polski Merkuriusz Lekarski*, 20(120), 691–695.

Fujishiro, T., Matsui, N., Yoshiya, S., et al. (2005). Treatment of a bone defect in the femoral shaft after osteomyelitis using low-intensity pulsed ultrasound. *European Journal of Orthopaedic Surgery and Traumatology*, 15, 244–246.

Fyfe, M. C., & Chahl, L. A. (1982). Mast cell degranulation: A possible mechanism of action of therapeutic ultrasound. *Ultrasound in Medicine and Biology*, 8(Suppl. 1), 62.

Gallo, J. A., Draper, D. O., Brody, L. T., et al. (2004). A comparison of human muscle temperature increases during 3-MHz continuous and pulsed ultrasound with equivalent temporal average intensities. *The Journal of Orthopaedic and Sports Physical Therapy*, 34(7), 395–401.

Gam, A. N., & Johannsen, F. (1995). Ultrasound therapy in musculoskeletal disorders: A meta-analysis. *Pain*, 63, 85–91.

Garcia, I., Lobo, C., Lopez, E., Servan, J. L., & Tenias, J. M. (2016). Comparative effectiveness of ultrasonophoresis and iontophoresis in impingement syndrome: A double-blind, randomized, placebo controlled trial. *Clinical Rehabilitation*, 30(4), 347–358.

Garrett, C. L., Draper, D. O., & Knight, K. L. (2000). Heat distribution in the lower leg from pulsed short-wave diathermy and ultrasound treatments. *The Journal of Athletic Training*, 35(1), 50–55.

Gebauer, D., & Correll, J. (2005). Pulsed low-intensity ultrasound: A new salvage procedure for delayed unions and nonunions after leg lengthening in children. *Journal of Pediatric Orthopaedics*, 25(6), 750–754.

Gebauer, D., Mayr, E., Orthner, E., et al. (2005). Low-intensity pulsed ultrasound: Effects on nonunions. *Ultrasound in Medicine and Biology*, 31(10), 1391–1402.

Gomez, M. A., Woo, S. L., Amiel, D., Harwood, F., Kitabayashi, L., & Matyas, J. R. (1991). The effects of increased tension on healing medical collateral ligaments. *The American Journal of Sports Medicine*, 19(4), 347–354.

Gray, R. J., Quayle, A. A., Hall, C. A., & Schofield, M. A. (1994). Physiotherapy in the treatment of temporomandibular joint disorders: A comparative study of four treatment methods. *British Dental Journal*, 176(7), 257–261.

Gray, R. J. M., Quayle, A. A., Hall, C. A., & Schofield, M. A. (1995). Temporomandibular pain dysfunction: Can electrotherapy help? *Physiotherapy*, 81(1), 47–51.

Guirro, R., Serrao, F., Elias, D., et al. (1997). Calibration of therapeutic ultrasound equipment. *Physiotherapy*, 83, 419–422.

ter Haar, G. (1987). *Recent advances in therapeutic ultrasound. Ultrasound: Method applications, biological effects and hazard potential.* In M. Repacholi, M. Grandolfo & A. Rindi (Eds.). New York: Plenum Press.

ter Haar, G. (1999). Therapeutic ultrasound. *European Journal of Ultrasound*, 9, 3–9.

ter Haar, G., Dyson, M., & Oakley, E. M. (1985). The use of ultrasound by physiotherapists in Britain, 1985. *Ultrasound in Medicine and Biology*, 13, 659–663.

ter Haar, G., Dyson, M., & Smith, S. P. (1979). Ultrastructural changes in the mouse uterus brought about by ultrasonic irradiation at therapeutic intensities in standing wave fields. *Ultrasound in Medicine and Biology*, 5(2), 167–179.

Hannemann, P. F., Mommers, E. H., Schots, J. P., Brink, P. R., & Poeze, M. (2014). The effects of low-intensity pulsed ultrasound and pulsed electromagnetic fields bone growth stimulation in acute fractures: A systematic review and meta-analysis of randomized controlled trials. *Archives of Orthopaedic and Trauma Surgery*, 134(8), 1093–1106.

Hanson, M. A. (2010). *Health effects of exposure to ultrasound and infrasound: Report of the independent advisory group on non-ionising radiation.* Health Protection Agency.

Harris, F., Dennison, S. R., & Phoenix, D. A. (2014). Sounding the death knell for microbes? *Trends in Molecular Medicine*, 20(7), 363–367.

Harrison, A., Lin, S., Pounder, N., & Mikuni-Takagaki, Y. (2016). Mode & mechanism of low intensity pulsed ultrasound (LIPUS) in fracture repair. *Ultrasonics*, 70, 45–52.

Harvey, W., Dyson, M., Pond, J. B., & Grahame, R. (1975). The stimulation of protein synthesis in human fibroblasts by therapeutic ultrasound. *Rheumatology Rehabilitation, 14,* 237.

Hashish, I. (1986). *The effects of ultrasound therapy on post operative inflammation.* PhD Thesis. University of London.

Hoogland, R. (1986). *Ultrasound therapy.* Delft, the Netherlands: Enraf Nonius.

Huisstede, B. M., Hoogvliet, P., Franke, T. P., Randsdorp, M. S., & Koes, B. W. (2018). Carpal tunnel syndrome: Effectiveness of physical therapy and electrophysical modalities. An updated systematic review of randomized controlled trials. *Archives of Physical Medicine and Rehabilitation, 99*(8), 1623–1634.

Huys, S., Gan, B. S., & Sherebrin, M. (1993). Comparison of effects of early and late ultrasound treatment on tendon healing in the chicken limb. *Journal of Hand Therapy, 6,* 58–59.

Ilter, L., Dilek, B., Batmaz, I., Ulu, M. A., Sariyildiz, M. A., Nas, K., et al. (2015). Efficacy of pulsed and continuous therapeutic ultrasound in myofascial pain syndrome: A randomized controlled study. *American Journal of Physical Medicine & Rehabilitation, 94*(7), 547–554.

Izadifar, Z., Babyn, P., & Chapman, D. (2017). Mechanical and biological effects of ultrasound: A review of present knowledge. *Ultrasound in Medicine and Biology, 43*(6), 1085–1104.

Jackson, B. A., Schwane, J. A., & Starcher, B. C. (1991). Effect of ultrasound therapy on the repair of Achilles tendon injuries in rats. *Medicine and Science in Sports and Exercise, 23,* 171–176.

Johannsen, F., Gam, A. N., & Karlsmark, T. (1998). Ultrasound therapy in chronic leg ulceration: A meta-analysis. *Wound Repair and Regeneration, 6*(2), 121–126.

Jorge, M. S. G., Zanin, C., Knob, B., & Wibelinger, L. M. (2017). Effects of deep heating to treat osteoarthritis pain: Systematic review. *Revista Dor, 18*(1), 79–84.

Keltie, K., Reay, C. A., Bousfield, D. R., Cole, H., Ward, B., Oates, C. P., et al. (2013). Characterization of the ultrasound beam produced by the MIST therapy, wound healing system. *Ultrasound in Medicine and Biology, 39*(7), 1233–1240.

Khanna, A., Nelmes, R. T., Gougoulias, N., Maffulli, N., & Gray, J. (2009). The effects of LIPUS on soft-tissue healing: A review of literature. *British Medical Bulletin, 89,* 169–182.

Khatri, S., Sandhu, J., & Kishor, V. (2008). Effectiveness of therapeutic ultrasound in identification of tibial stress fractures. *Indian Journal of Physiotherapy and Occupational Therapy-An International Journal, 2*(1), 51–53.

Klucinec, B., Scheidler, M., Denegar, C., et al. (2000). Effectiveness of wound care products in the transmission of acoustic energy. *Physical Therapy, 80*(5), 469–476.

Koulakis, J. P., Rouch, J., Huynh, N., Dubrovsky, G., Dunn, J. C. Y., & Putterman, S. (2018). Interstitial matrix prevents therapeutic ultrasound from causing inertial cavitation in tumescent subcutaneous tissue. *Ultrasound in Medicine and Biology, 44*(1), 177–186.

Lehmann, J. F., & deLateur, B. J. (1982). Therapeutic heat. In J. F. Lehmann (Ed.), *Therapeutic heat and cold* (3rd ed.) (p. 404). Baltimore, MD: Williams and Wilkins.

Lehmann, J. F., deLateur, B. J., Stonebridge, J. B., & Warren, C. G. (1967a). Therapeutic temperature distribution produced by ultrasound as modified by dosage and volume of tissue exposed. *Archives of Physical Medicine and Rehabilitation, 48*(12), 662–666.

Lehmann, J. F., deLateur, B. J., Warren, C. G., & Stonebridge, J. S. (1967b). Heating produced by ultrasound in bone and soft tissue. *Archives of Physical Medicine and Rehabilitation, 48*(8), 397–401.

Lerner, A., Stein, H., & Soudry, M. (2004). Compound high-energy limb fractures with delayed union: Our experience with adjuvant ultrasound stimulation (exogen). *Ultrasonics, 42*(1–9), 915–917.

Leung, K. S., Lee, W. S., Tsui, H. F., et al. (2004b). Complex tibial fracture outcomes following treatment with low-intensity pulsed ultrasound. *Ultrasound in Medicine and Biology, 30*(3), 389–395.

Leung, M. C., Ng, G. Y., & Yip, K. K. (2004a). Effect of ultrasound on acute inflammation of transected medial collateral ligaments. *Archives of Physical Medicine and Rehabilitation, 85,* 963–966.

Leung, M. C., Ng, G. Y., & Yip, K. K. (2006). Therapeutic ultrasound enhances medial collateral ligament repair in rats. *Ultrasound in Medicine and Biology, 32*(3), 449–452.

Li, J. K., Chang, W. H., Lin, J. C., Ruaan, R. C., Liu, H. C., & Sun, J. S. (2003). Cytokine release from osteoblasts in response to ultrasound stimulation. *Biomaterials, 24*(13), 2379–2385.

Li, J. G., Chang, W. H., Lin, J. C., & Sun, J. S. (2002). Optimum intensities of ultrasound for PGE(2) secretion and growth of osteoblasts. *Ultrasound in Medicine and Biology, 28*(5), 683–690.

Lou, S., Lv, H., Li, Z., Tang, P., & Wang, Y. (2018). Effect of low-intensity pulsed ultrasound on distraction osteogenesis: A systematic review and meta-analysis of randomized controlled trials. *Journal of Orthopaedic Surgery and Research, 13*(1), 205.

Louw, A., Zimney, K., Landers, M. R., Luttrell, M., Clair, B., & Mills, J. (2016). A randomised controlled trial of 'clockwise' ultrasound for low back pain. *South African Journal of Physiotherapy, 72*(1), 306.

Lovric, V., Ledger, M., Goldberg, J., Harper, W., Bertollo, N., Pelletier, M. H., et al. (2013). The effects of low-intensity pulsed ultrasound on tendon-bone healing in a transosseous-equivalent sheep rotator cuff model. *Knee Surgery, Sports Traumatology, Arthroscopy, 21*(2), 466–475.

Majlesi, J., & Unalan, H. (2004). High-power pain threshold ultrasound technique in the treatment of active myofascial trigger points: A randomized, double-blind, case-control study. *Archives of Physical Medicine and Rehabilitation, 85*(5), 833–836.

Malizos, K. N., Hantes, M. E., Protopappas, V., et al. (2006). Low-intensity pulsed ultrasound for bone healing: An overview. *Injury, 37*(Suppl. 1), S56–S62.

Maloney, E., & Hwang, J. H. (2015). Emerging HIFU applications in cancer therapy. *International Journal of Hyperthermia, 31*(3), 302–309.

Manca, A., Limonta, E., Pilurzi, G., Ginatempo, F., De Natale, E. R., Mercante, B., et al. (2014). Ultrasound and laser as stand-alone therapies for myofascial trigger points: A randomized, double-blind, placebo-controlled study. *Physiotherapy Research International, 19*(3), 166–175.

Maxwell, L. (1992). Therapeutic ultrasound: Its effects on the cellular and molecular mechanisms of inflammation and repair. *Physiotherapy, 78*(6), 421–426.

Mayr, E., Frankel, V., & Ruter, A. (2000). Ultrasound – an alternative healing method for nonunions? *Archives of Orthopaedic and Trauma Surgery, 120*(1–2), 1–8.

McBrier, N. M., Lekan, J. M., Druhan, L. J., Devor, S. T., & Merrick, M. A. (2007). Therapeutic ultrasound decreases mechano-growth factor messenger ribonucleic acid expression after muscle contusion injury. *Archives of Physical Medicine and Rehabilitation, 88*(7), 936–940.

McDiarmid, T., Burns, P. N., Lewith, G. T., & Machin, D. (1985). Ultrasound and the treatment of pressure sores. *Physiotherapy, 71*, 66–70.

Meakins, A., & Watson, T. (2006). Longwave ultrasound and conductive heating increase functional ankle mobility in asymptomatic subjects. *Physical Therapy in Sport, 7*, 74–80.

Mehta, S., Long, K., DeKoven, M., Smith, E., & Steen, R. G. (2015). Low-intensity pulsed ultrasound (LIPUS) can decrease the economic burden of fracture non-union. *Journal of Medical Economics, 18*(7), 542–549.

Mitragotri, S., Farrell, J., Tang, H., et al. (2000). Determination of threshold energy dose for ultrasound-induced transdermal drug transport. *The Journal of Controlled Release, 63*, 41–52.

Mohl, N. D., Ohrbach, R. K., Crow, H. C., & Gross, A. J. (1990). Devices for the diagnosis and treatment of temporomandibular disorders. Part III: Thermography, ultrasound, electrical stimulation, and electromyographic biofeedback [published erratum appears in J Prosthet Dent 1990 May;63(5):13A]. *The Journal of Prosthetic Dentistry, 63*(4), 472–477.

Morishita, K., Karasuno, H., Yokoi, Y., Morozumi, K., Ogihara, H., Ito, T., et al. (2014). Effects of therapeutic ultrasound on range of motion and stretch pain. *Journal of Physical Therapy Science, 26*(5), 711–715.

Mortimer, A. J., & Dyson, M. (1988). The effect of therapeutic ultrasound on calcium uptake in fibroblasts. *Ultrasound in Medicine and Biology, 14*, 499–506.

Mummery, C. L. (1978). *The effect of ultrasound on fibroblasts in vitro.* PhD Thesis. University of London.

Murtezani, A., Govori, V., Meka, V. S., Ibraimi, Z., Rrecaj, S., & Gashi, S. (2015). A comparison of McKenzie therapy with electrophysical agents for the treatment of work related low back pain: A randomized controlled trial. *Journal of Back and Musculoskeletal Rehabilitation, 28*(2), 247–253.

Naghdi, S., Ansari, N. N., & Farhadi, M. (2008). A clinical trial on the treatment of chronic rhinosinusitis with continuous ultrasound. *Journal of Physical Therapy Science, 20*(4), 233–238.

Nakamura, T., Fujihara, S., Katsura, T., Yamamoto, K., Inubushi, T., Tanimoto, K., et al. (2010). Effects of low-intensity pulsed ultrasound on the expression and activity of hyaluronan synthase and hyaluronidase in IL-1beta-stimulated synovial cells. *Annals of Biomedical Engineering, 38*(11), 3363–3370.

National Council on Radiation Protection (NCRP). (1983). Biological effects of ultrasound: Mechanisms and implications. *Report No. 74*, 82.

Ng, G. Y. (2011). Comparing therapeutic ultrasound with micro-amperage stimulation therapy for improving the strength of Achilles tendon repair. *Connective Tissue Research, 52*(3), 178–182.

Nolte, P. A., van der Krans, A., Patka, P., et al. (2001). Low-intensity pulsed ultrasound in the treatment of nonunions. *The Journal of Trauma, 51*(4), 693–702, discussion 702–703.

Nussbaum, E. L. (1997). Ultrasound: To heat or not to heat – that is the question. *Physical Therapy Reviews, 2*, 59–72.

Nussbaum, E. L. (1998). The influence of ultrasound on healing tissues. *Journal of Hand Therapy, 11*(2), 140–147.

Nussbaum, E. L., & Locke, M. (2007). Heat shock protein expression in rat skeletal muscle after repeated applications of pulsed and continuous ultrasound. *Archives of Physical Medicine and Rehabilitation, 88*(6), 785–790.

Nyborg, W. L. (1977). *Physical mechanisms for biological effects of ultrasound. DHEW 78-8062.* Washington, DC: US Government Printing Office.

Oakley, E. M. (1978). Applications of continuous beam ultrasound at therapeutic levels. *Physiotherapy, 64*, 169–172.

Oh, D. W., Kim, K. S., & Lee, G. W. (2002). The effect of physiotherapy on post-temporomandibular joint surgery patients. *Journal of Oral Rehabilitation, 29*(5), 441–446.

Ojoawo, A. O., Odewole, O., Odejide, S. A., Arilewola, B. O., & Badru, A. G. (2015). Therapeutic efficacy of Lofnac gel via phonophoresis in the management of chronic nonspecific low back pain: A randomised controlled trial. *Hong Kong Physiotherapy Journal, 33*, 89–94.

Olyaie, M., Rad, F. S., Elahifar, M. A., Garkaz, A., & Mahsa, G. (2013). High-frequency and noncontact low-frequency ultrasound therapy for venous leg ulcer treatment: A randomized, controlled study. *Ostomy Wound Management, 59*(8), 14–20.

Padilla, F., Puts, R., Vico, L., Guignandon, A., & Raum, K. (2016). Stimulation of bone repair with ultrasound. *Advances in Experimental Medicine & Biology, 880*, 385–427.

Padilla, F., Puts, R., Vico, L., & Raum, K. (2014). Stimulation of bone repair with ultrasound: A review of the possible mechanic effects. *Ultrasonics, 54*(5), 1125–1145.

Page, M.J., Green, S., Kramer, S., Johnston Renea, V., McBain, B., & Buchbinder, R. (2014). Electrotherapy modalities for adhesive capsulitis (frozen shoulder). *Cochrane Database of Systematic Reviews*, C 24. https://doi.org/10.1002/14651858.

Page, M. J., Green, S., Mrocki, M. A., Surace, S. J., Deitch, J., McBain, B., et al. (2016). Electrotherapy modalities for rotator cuff disease. *Cochrane Database of Systematic Reviews* (6), CD012225.

Page, M. J., O'Connor, D., Pitt, V., & Massy-Westropp, N. (2013). Therapeutic ultrasound for carpal tunnel syndrome. *Cochrane Database of Systematic Reviews* (3), CD009601.

Paolillo, F. R., Paolillo, A. R., Joao, J. P., Frasca, D., Duchene, M., Joao, H. A., et al. (2018). Ultrasound plus low-level laser therapy for knee osteoarthritis rehabilitation: A randomized, placebo-controlled trial. *Rheumatology International.*

Papalada, A., Malliaropoulos, N., Tsitas, K., Kiritsi, O., Padhiar, N., Del Buono, A., et al. (2012). Ultrasound as a primary evaluation tool of bone stress injuries in elite track and field athletes. *The American Journal of Sports Medicine, 40*(4), 915–919.

Paul, B. J., Lafratta, C. W., Dawson, A. R., et al. (1960). Use of ultrasound in the treatment of pressure sores in patients with spinal cord injuries. *Archives of Physical Medicine and Rehabilitation, 41*, 438–440.

Pavlov, I. V. (2002). Use of low frequency ultrasonic technology in preventing and treating purulent wounds of the lung and pleura. *Khirurgiia, 5*, 64–67.

Perez-Merino, L., Casajuana, M. C., Bernal, G., Faba, J., Astilleros, A. E., Gonzalez, R., et al. (2016). Evaluation of the effectiveness of three physiotherapeutic treatments for subacromial impingement syndrome: A randomised clinical trial. *Physiotherapy, 102*(1), 57–63.

Pilla, A. A., Mont, M. A., Nasser, P. R., et al. (1990). Non-invasive low-intensity pulsed ultrasound accelerates bone healing in the rabbit. *Journal of Orthopaedic Trauma, 4*, 246–253.

Polak, A., Franek, A., Blaszczak, E., Nawrat-Szoltysik, A., Taradaj, J., Wiercigroch, L., et al. (2014). A prospective, randomized, controlled, clinical study to evaluate the efficacy of high-frequency ultrasound in the treatment of Stage II and Stage III pressure ulcers in geriatric patients. *Ostomy Wound Management, 60*(8), 16–28.

Poltawski, L., & Watson, T. (2007a). Relative transmissivity of ultrasound coupling agents commonly used by therapists in the UK. *Ultrasound in Medicine and Biology, 33*(1), 120–128.

Poltawski, L., & Watson, T. (2007b). Transmission of therapeutic ultrasound by wound dressings. *Wounds, 19*(1), 1–12.

Pope, G. D., Mockett, S. P., & Wright, J. P. (1995). A survey of electrotherapeutic modalities: Ownership and use in the NHS in England. *Physiotherapy, 81*(2), 82–91.

Pounder, N. M., & Harrison, A. J. (2008). Low intensity pulsed ultrasound for fracture healing: A review of the clinical evidence and the associated biological mechanism of action. *Ultrasonics, 48*(4), 330–338.

Pye, S., & Milford, C. (1994). The performance of ultrasound physiotherapy machines in Lothian Region. *Ultrasound in Medicine and Biology, 4*, 347–359.

Ramirez, A., Schwane, J. A., McFarland, C., et al. (1997). The effect of ultrasound on collagen synthesis and fibroblast proliferation in vitro. *Medicine and Science in Sports and Exercise, 29*, 326–332.

Reher, P., Doan, N., Bradnock, B., et al. (1999). Effect of ultrasound on the production of IL-8, basic FGF and VEGF. *Cytokine, 11*(6), 416–423.

Robertson, V., & Ward, A. (1997). Longwave ultrasound reviewed and reconsidered. *Physiotherapy, 83*(3), 123–130.

Robinson, V. A., Brosseau, L., Peterson, J., Shea, B. J., Tugwell, P., & Wells, G. (2005). Therapeutic ultrasound for osteoarthritis of the knee. *The Cochrane Database of Systematic Reviews Issue, 1*.

Rodriguez-Grande, E. I., Osma-Rueda, J. L., Serrano-Villar, Y., & Ramirez, C. (2017). Effects of pulsed therapeutic ultrasound on the treatment of people with knee osteoarthritis. *Journal of Physical Therapy Science, 29*(9), 1637–1643.

Rosim, G. C., Barbieri, C. H., Lancas, F. M., & Mazzer, N. (2005). Diclofenac phonophoresis in human volunteers. *Ultrasound in Medicine and Biology, 31*(3), 337–343.

Rothenberg, J. B., Jayaram, P., Naqvi, U., Gober, J., & Malanga, G. A. (2017). The role of low-intensity pulsed ultrasound on cartilage healing in knee osteoarthritis: A review. *Pharmacy Management R, 9*(12), 1268–1277.

Rubin, C., Bolander, M., Ryaby, J. P., et al. (2001). The use of low-intensity ultrasound to accelerate the healing of fractures. *The Journal of Bone and Joint Surgery (American), 83-A*(2), 259–270.

Ruiz-Molinero, C., Jimenez-Rejano, J. J., Chillon-Martinez, R., Suarez-Serrano, C., Rebollo-Roldan, J., & Perez-Cabezas, V. (2014). Efficacy of therapeutic ultrasound in pain and joint mobility in whiplash traumatic acute and subacute phases. *Ultrasound in Medicine and Biology, 40*(9), 2089–2095.

Samuels, J. A., Weingarten, M. S., Margolis, D. J., Zubkov, L., Sunny, Y., Bawiec, C. R., et al. (2013). Low-frequency (< 100 kHz), low-intensity (< 100 mW/cm[sup 2]) ultrasound to treat venous ulcers: A human study and in vitro experiments. *Journal of the Acoustical Society of America, 134*(2), 1541–1547.

Sarrafzadeh, J., Ahmadi, A., & Yassin, M. (2012). The effects of pressure release, phonophoresis of hydrocortisone, and ultrasound on upper trapezius latent myofascial trigger point. *Archives of Physical Medicine and Rehabilitation, 93*(1), 72–77.

Schabrun, S., Chipchase, L., & Rickard, H. (2006). Are therapeutic ultrasound units a potential vector for nosocomial infection? *Physiotherapy Research International, 11*(2), 61–71.

Schandelmaier, S., Kaushal, A., Lytvyn, L., Heels-Ansdell, D., Siemieniuk, R. A., Agoritsas, T., et al. (2017). Low intensity pulsed ultrasound for bone healing: Systematic review of randomized controlled trials. *BMJ, 356*, j656.

Sedov, V. M., Gordeev, N. A., Krivtsova, G. B., et al. (1998). Management of infected wounds and trophic ulcers by low frequency ultrasound. *Khirurgiia Mosk, 4*, 39–41.

Selkowitz, D. M., Cameron, M. H., Mainzer, A., et al. (2002). Efficacy of pulsed low-intensity ultrasound in wound healing: A single-case design. *Ostomy Wound Management, 48*(4), 40–44 46–50.

Shaffer, S. M., Brismee, J. M., Sizer, P. S., & Courtney, C. A. (2014). Temporomandibular disorders. Part 2: Conservative management. *Journal of Manual & Manipulative Therapy, 22*(1), 13–23.

Shah, S. G. S., & Farrow, A. (2013). Trends in the availability and usage of electrophysical agents in physiotherapy practices from 1990 to 2010: A review. *Physical Therapy Reviews, 17*(4), 207–226.

Shah, S., Farrow, A., & Esnouf, A. (2007). Availability and use of electrotherapy devices: A survey. *International Journal of Therapy and Rehabilitation, 14*(6), 260–264.

Sharma, R., Aggarwal, A. N., Bhatt, S., Kumar, S., & Bhargava, S. K. (2015). Outcome of low level lasers versus ultrasonic therapy in de Quervain's tenosynovitis. *Indian Journal of Orthopaedics, 49*(5), 542–548.

Singal, A., Ballard, J. R., Rudie, E. N., Cressman, E. N. K., & Iaizzo, P. A. (2016). A review of therapeutic ablation modalities. *Journal of Medical Devices, 10*(4), 040801-040801-040811.

Speed, C. A. (2001). Therapeutic ultrasound in soft tissue lesions. *Rheumatology, 40*(12), 1331–1336.

Spratt, H. G., Jr., Levine, D., & Tillman, L. (2014). Physical therapy clinic therapeutic ultrasound equipment as a source for bacterial contamination. *Physiotherapy Theory and Practice, 30*(7), 507–511.

Srbely, J. Z., & Dickey, J. P. (2007). Randomized controlled study of the antinociceptive effect of ultrasound on trigger point sensitivity: Novel applications in myofascial therapy? *Clinical Rehabilitation, 21*(5), 411–417.

Stein, H., & Lerner, A. (2005). How does pulsed low-intensity ultrasound enhance fracture healing? *Orthopedics, 28*(10), 1161–1163.

Sutherland, E. W., & Rall, E. W. (1968). Formation of cyclic adenine ribonucleotide by tissue particles. *Journal of Biological Chemistry, 232*, 1065–1076.

Sutton, Y., McBride, K., & Pye, S. (2006). An ultrasound mini-balance for measurement of therapy level ultrasound. *Physics in Medicine and Biology, 51*(14), 3397–3404.

Takla, M. K. N., & Rezk-Allah, S. S. (2018). Immediate effects of simultaneous application of transcutaneous electrical nerve stimulation and ultrasound phonophoresis on active myofascial trigger points: A randomized controlled trial. *American Journal of Physical Medicine & Rehabilitation, 97*(5), 332–338.

Tsai, C. L., Chang, W. H., & Liu, T. K. (1992a). Preliminary studies of duration and intensity of ultrasonic treatments on fracture repair. *The Chinese Journal of Physiology, 35*, 21–26.

Tsai, C. L., Chang, W. H., & Liu, T. K. (1992b). Ultrasonic effect on fracture repair and prostaglandin E2 production. *The Chinese Journal of Physiology, 35*, 168.

Tsai, W. C., Pang, J. H., Hsu, C. C., Chu, N. K., Lin, M. S., & Hu, C. F. (2006). Ultrasound stimulation of types I and III collagen expression of tendon cell and upregulation of transforming growth factor beta. *Journal of Orthopaedic Research, 24*(6), 1310–1316.

Tsai, W. C., Tang, S. T., & Liang, F. C. (2011). Effect of therapeutic ultrasound on tendons. *American Journal of Physical Medicine & Rehabilitation, 90*(12), 1068–1073.

Turner, S., Powell, E., & Ng, C. (1989). The effect of ultrasound on the healing of repaired cockerel tendon: Is collagen cross-linkage a factor? *The Journal of Hand Surgery, 14B*, 428–433.

Uhlemann, C., Heinig, B., & Wollina, U. (2003). Therapeutic ultrasound in lower extremity wound management. *The International Journal of Lower Extremity Wounds, 2*(3), 152–157.

Uhlemann, C., & Wollina, U. (2003). Physiological aspects of therapeutic ultrasound in wound- healing. *Phlebologie, 32*(4), 81–86.

Ulug, N., Yilmaz, O. T., Kara, M., & Ozcakar, L. (2017). Effects of Pilates and yoga in patients with chronic neck pain: A sonographic study. *Journal of Rehabilitation Medicine, 50*(1), 80–85.

Unalan, H., Majlesi, J., Aydin, F. Y., & Palamar, D. (2011). Comparison of high-power pain threshold ultrasound therapy with local injection in the treatment of active myofascial trigger points of the upper trapezius muscle. *Archives of Physical Medicine and Rehabilitation, 92*(4), 657–662.

Voigt, J., Wendelken, M., Driver, V. R., & Alvarez, O. M. (2011). Low-frequency ultrasound (20-40 khz) as an adjunctive therapy for chronic wound healing a systematic review of the literature and meta-analysis of eight randomized controlled trials. *The International Journal of Lower Extremity Wounds, 10*(4), 190–199.

Wang, E. D. (1998). Tendon repair. *Journal of Hand Therapy, 11*(2), 105–110.

Ward, A. R. (1986). *Electricity, fields and waves in therapy.* Marrickville, Australia: Science Press.

Warden, S. (2003). A new direction for ultrasound therapy in sports medicine. *Sports Medicine, 33*(2), 95–107.

Warden, S., Bennell, K., McMeeken, J. M., et al. (1999). Can conventional therapeutic ultrasound units be used to accelerate fracture repair? *Physical Therapy Reviews, 4*, 117–126.

Warden, S. J., Fuchs, R. K., Kessler, C. K., et al. (2006). Ultrasound produced by a conventional therapeutic ultrasound unit accelerates fracture repair. *Physical Therapy, 86*(8), 1118–1127.

Watson, T. (2000). The role of electrotherapy in contemporary physiotherapy practice. *Manual Therapy, 5*(3), 132–141.

Watson, T. (2002). Ultrasound dose calculations. *Touch, 101*, 14–17.

Watson, T. (2003). Soft tissue healing. *Touch, 104*, 2–9.

Watson, T. (2006a). Electrotherapy and tissue repair. *Sportex Medicine, 29*, 7–13.

Watson, T. (2007). *Modality and dose dependency in electrotherapy. 15th International WCPT Congress.* Vancouver, Canada: WCPT.

Watson, T. (2008). Ultrasound in contemporary physiotherapy practice. *Ultrasonics, 48*, 321–329.

Watson, T. (2010). Narrative review: Key concepts with electrophysical agents. *Physical Therapy Reviews, 15*(4), 351–359.

Watson, T. (2014). Crest of a wave: Effectiveness of therapeutic ultrasound in musculoskeletal injury. *International Therapist* (110), 18–20.

Watson, T. (2016). *Expanding our understanding of the inflammatory process and its role in pain & tissue healing.* Glasgow: IFOMPT 2016.

Watson, J. M., Kang'ombe, A. R., Soares, M. O., Chuang, L. H., Worthy, G., Bland, J. M., et al. (2011). Use of weekly, low dose, high frequency ultrasound for hard to heal venous leg ulcers: The VenUS III randomised controlled trial. *BMJ, 342*, d1092.

Watson, T., & Young, S. (2008). Therapeutic ultrasound. In T. Watson (Ed.), *Electrotherapy: Evidence based practice* (12th ed.). Edinburgh: Churchill Livingstone - Elsevier.

Webster, D. F. (1980). *The effect of ultrasound on wound healing.* PhD Thesis. University of London.

Webster, D. F., Pond, J. B., Dyson, M., & Harvey, W. (1978). The role of cavitation in the in vitro stimulation of protein synthesis in human fibroblasts by ultrasound. *Ultrasound in Medicine and Biology, 4*, 343–351.

Wilson, C. G., Martin-Saavedra, F. M., Padilla, F., Fabiilli, M. L., Zhang, M., Baez, A. M., et al. (2014). Patterning expression of regenerative growth factors using high intensity focused ultrasound. *Tissue Engineering Part C: Methods, 20*(10), 769–779.

Winters, M., Eskes, M., Weir, A., Moen, M. H., Backx, F. J., & Bakker, E. W. (2013). Treatment of medial tibial stress syndrome: A systematic review. *Sports Medicine, 43*(12), 1315–1333.

Wu, F. (2006). Extracorporeal high intensity focused ultrasound in the treatment of patients with solid malignancy. *Minimally Invasive Therapy and Allied Technologies, 15*(1), 26–35.

Yavuz, F., Duman, I., Taskaynatan, M. A., & Tan, A. K. (2014). Low-level laser therapy versus ultrasound therapy in the treatment of subacromial impingement syndrome: A randomized clinical trial. *Journal of Back and Musculoskeletal Rehabilitation, 27*(3), 315–320.

Yegin, T., Altan, L., & Kasapoglu Aksoy, M. (2017). The effect of therapeutic ultrasound on pain and physical function in patients with knee osteoarthritis. *Ultrasound in Medicine and Biology, 43*(1), 187–194.

Yeung, C. K., Guo, X., & Ng, Y. F. (2006). Pulsed ultrasound treatment accelerates the repair of Achilles tendon rupture in rats. *Journal of Orthopaedic Research, 24*(2), 193–201.

Young, S. R., & Dyson, M. (1990a). Macrophage responsiveness to therapeutic ultrasound. *Ultrasound in Medicine and Biology, 16*, 809–816.

Young, S. R., & Dyson, M. (1990b). The effect of therapeutic ultrasound on the healing of full-thickness excised skin lesions. *Ultrasonics, 28*, 175–180.

Young, D., Morton, R., & Bartley, J. (2010). Therapeutic ultrasound as treatment for chronic rhinosinusitis: Preliminary observations. *Journal of Laryngology & Otology, 124*(5), 495–499.

Yu, H., Cote, P., Shearer, H. M., Wong, J. J., Sutton, D. A., Randhawa, K. A., et al. (2015). Effectiveness of passive physical modalities for shoulder pain: Systematic review by the Ontario protocol for traffic injury management collaboration. *Physical Therapy, 95*(3), 306–318.

Zeng, C., Li, H., Yang, T., Deng, Z. H., Yang, Y., Zhang, Y., et al. (2014). Effectiveness of continuous and pulsed ultrasound for the management of knee osteoarthritis: A systematic review and network meta-analysis. *Osteoarthritis and Cartilage, 22*(8), 1090–1099.

Zhang, N., Chow, S. K., Leung, K. S., & Cheung, W. H. (2017). Ultrasound as a stimulus for musculoskeletal disorders. *The Journal of Orthopaedic Translation, 9*, 52–59.

Zura, R., Mehta, S., Della Rocca, G. J., Jones, J., & Steen, R. G. (2015). A cohort study of 4,190 patients treated with low-intensity pulsed ultrasound (LIPUS): Findings in the elderly versus all patients. *BMC Musculoskeletal Disorders, 16*(1), 45.

10

Laser/Photobiomodulation

G. David Baxter, Ethne L. Nussbaum

CHAPTER OUTLINE

BRIEF HISTORY

'Laser' is an acronym for Light Amplification by Stimulated Emission of Radiation. Theodore Maiman produced the first burst of ruby laser light at Hughes Laboratories in the United States in 1960. In subsequent decades, various devices based on Maiman's original prototype have found applications ranging from laser pointers and bar-code readers to military range-finders and target acquisition systems.

Lasers have wide application in medicine and surgery: ophthalmic surgeons were the first to use lasers successfully for treatment of detached retina in humans. Most medical applications to date have relied upon photothermal (heating) and photoablative ('explosive') interactions of laser with tissue. The use of lasers as alternatives to metal scalpels, as well as for tumour ablation and tattoo removal, are all based upon these tissue reactions. Early interest also focused on potential clinical applications of non-thermal interactions of laser light with tissue, based upon initial work by Professor Endre Mester's group in Budapest during the late 1960s and early 1970s. Results of this work indicated that relatively low-intensity laser irradiation applied directly to tissue could modulate biological processes – in particular could *photobiostimulate* wound-healing processes (Mester 1985). The ensuing decade saw the promotion of irradiation using He-Ne lasers as an effective treatment for a variety of conditions throughout the countries of the former Soviet Union and in Asia. However, it was not until the introduction of small, compact, laser-emitting photodiodes that the use of this therapy, known as low level laser therapy (LLLT) or photobiomodulation (PBM), started to gain popularity in the West. The modality has found application by physiotherapists (for human and animal use), dentists, acupuncturists, podiatrists and some physicians, for the treatment of open wounds, soft-tissue injuries, arthritic conditions, and various types of pain (Baxter 1991). Subsequent approvals by the Food and Drug Administration (FDA) led to increasing usage in the United States.

DEFINITIONS AND NOMENCLATURE

Photobiomodulation therapy (Anders et al 2015), or low (reactive)-level laser therapy (Ohshiro & Calderhead 1988), are the widely accepted terms to describe the therapeutic application of relatively low-output lasers (typically <500 mW for a single source) and monochromatic light emitting diodes at dosages generally considered to be too low to cause any detectable tissue heating (usually <35 Jcm-2). Photobiomodulation is an accurate term because it encompasses the range of low-level laser effects, from acceleration to inhibition of cellular processes as well as its modulating effects, for example on pain.

Alternative terms are misleading and their use is discouraged: this includes (photo)biostimulation or low intensity laser therapy (LILT), which derive from an early focus of treatment on wound and soft-tissue repair, and 'soft' or 'cold' laser which were supposed to distinguish

therapeutic devices from high-power sources of the type used in surgical, medical and dental applications.

It should be noted that there is an increasing number of higher power lasers (>1 W) becoming available on the market for PBM treatments, which reinforces the importance of defining the therapy in terms of intended biological and clinical effects, rather than the technology used. Similarly, use of the term LED (light emitting diode) therapy, i.e. to attempt to distinguish these devices from laser therapy, is misleading.

PHYSICAL PRINCIPLES

Fuller accounts of the biophysical principles underpinning the therapeutic applications of lasers in PBM are available elsewhere (Nussbaum et al 2003a).

Light Emission, Absorption and the Production of Laser Radiation

The basis of production of stimulated emission is illustrated in Fig. 10.1. In non-laser sources, light is typically produced by spontaneous emission of radiation (Fig. 10.1A). In such circumstances and devices, the atoms and molecules comprising the central emitter (e.g. the element/ filament in a typical household light bulb) are stimulated with (electrical) energy so that the electrons shift to higher energy orbits. Once in such orbits, the electrons are inherently unstable and fall spontaneously within a short period of time to lower energy levels. In so doing they release their extra energy as photons of light. The properties of the

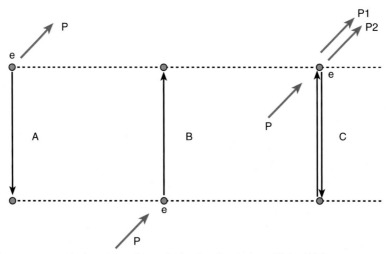

Fig. 10.1 Spontaneous emission, absorption and stimulated emission of light. (A) Spontaneous emission: excited electron (e) drops to lower (resting) level, emitting a single photon (P). (B) Absorption: incident photon is absorbed by resting electron, which moves to higher level. (C) Stimulated emission: incident photon interacts with already excited electron to produce two identical photons (P1, P2).

emitted photons are determined by the difference in energy levels (or valence bands) through which an excited electron 'dropped', as the difference in energy will be exactly the same as the quantal energy of the photon produced. As, for a given photon of light, the quantal energy (specified in electron-volts) is inversely related to the wavelength (in nm), the wavelength is effectively determined by the difference in valence bands; and in turn, molecules produce typical ranges of wavelengths or emission spectra when appropriately stimulated.

Absorption of Radiation

Absorption occurs when a photon of light interacts with an atom or molecule in which the difference in energy of the valence bands exactly equals the energy carried by the photon (Fig. 10.1B). This has two consequences: for a photon of a given quantal energy (and thus wavelength) only certain molecules will be capable of absorbing the light radiation; conversely, for a given molecule, only certain quantal energies (and thus wavelengths) can be absorbed (this is termed the absorption spectrum for the molecule). Thus absorption is said to be wavelength specific. This is an important concept in LLLT/PBM applications, as this wavelength specificity of absorption effectively determines which types of tissue will preferentially absorb incident radiation, and (in turn) the depth of penetration of light produced by a particular treatment unit.

Stimulated Emission of Radiation

Stimulated emission is a unique event that occurs when an incident photon interacts with an atom that is already excited (i.e. where the electron(s) are already in a higher energy orbit). Additionally, the quantal energy of the incident photon must exactly equal the difference in energy levels between the electron's excited and resting states (Fig. 10.1C). Under these exceptional circumstances, the electron, in returning to its original orbit, gives off its excess energy as a photon of light with exactly the same properties (e.g. wavelength) as the incident photon, and completely in phase. In laser devices, the unique circumstances that give rise to stimulated emission of radiation are produced through the selection of an appropriate material or substance (the lasing medium), which, when electrically stimulated, will produce large numbers of identical photons through the rapid excitation of the medium. In order to produce such stimulated emission of radiation, laser treatment devices rely upon three essential components: the lasing medium, the resonating cavity, and the power source.

Lasing Medium

A lasing medium is capable of being 'pumped' with energy to produce stimulated emission. For therapeutic systems,

the energy source is invariably electrical and is delivered to the medium from the electrical mains, or from a battery (see following section). The media most commonly used in LLLT/PBM applications are gallium arsenide (Ga-As), or gallium–aluminium–arsenide (GaAIAs) semiconductors, which typically produce radiation at single wavelengths between 630–950 nm (i.e. visible red to the near infrared). Lasers based on the gaseous mixture of helium and neon (He-Ne) operating at a wavelength of 632.8 nm (i.e. red light) were once commonly used for research and clinical applications; these are now rarely seen in routine clinical practice.

Resonating Cavity

A resonating cavity or chamber consists of a structure to contain the lasing medium and incorporates a pair of parallel reflecting surfaces or mirrors. Within this chamber, photons of light produced by the medium are reflected back and forth between the 'mirrors' to ultimately produce an intense photon resonance. As one of the reflecting surfaces (also termed the output coupler) is not a 'pure' mirror, and so does not reflect 100% of the light striking its surface, some of the radiation is allowed to pass through as the output of the device. The resonating cavity for diode-based units is essentially the lasing medium itself (i.e. the semiconductor diode), the ends of which are carefully polished to form reflecting surfaces. This has important implications for the routine use of these units in clinical practice, as the treatment 'head' or 'probe' is usually not much larger than the size of a pen; this represents another reason why diode-based units (which may be regarded as 'second-generation' laser therapy systems) are so popular with clinicians (Fig. 10.2). Furthermore, most manufacturers now offer multisource 'cluster' arrays, incorporating a number of diodes (e.g. up to 180) to allow simultaneous treatment of larger lesions and (in some cases) to allow several wavelengths of radiation to be used simultaneously (Fig. 10.2B). Such multisource cluster units may be regarded as the 'third generation' of development for therapeutic lasers. Several manufacturers have also introduced 'fourth-generation' flexible multisource arrays, initially developed for the equine market, to allow more efficient delivery of light to tissue surfaces with 'hands-free' application.

Power Source

A power source is required to 'pump' the lasing medium to produce stimulated emission. In most cases, therapeutic devices tend to be electrical mains supplied and incorporate a base unit to contain the transformer and control unit. Alternatively, some devices incorporate rechargeable and battery-powered units to enhance their portability (e.g. for sports injury applications).

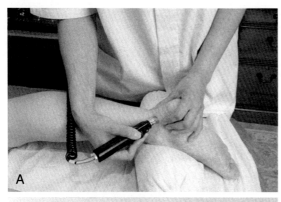

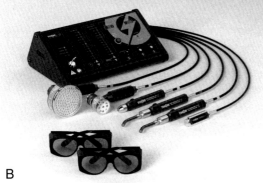

Fig. 10.2 Modern laser treatment units. (A) Single-diode treatment pen and (B) multisource cluster array. (Photographs courtesy of Thor Laser Systems).

Characteristics of Laser Radiation

The radiation generated by therapeutic laser devices differs from that produced by other similar sources (e.g. infrared heat lamps) in the following three respects:

1. Monochromaticity: the light produced by a laser is 'single coloured', most of the radiation emitted by the treatment device being clustered around a single wavelength with a very narrow bandwidth. In contrast, light generated by other sources comprises a wide variety of wavelengths, sometimes ranging from the ultraviolet to the infrared, which results in the sensation of the colour white when the light strikes the retina of a human observer. Wavelength is a critical factor in determining the biological effects produced by laser treatments, as this parameter determines which biomolecules will absorb the incident radiation, and thus the basic photobiological interaction underlying any treatment effect.

2. Collimation: in laser light, the rays of light or photons produced by the laser device are for all practical purposes parallel, with almost no divergence of the emitted radiation over distance; this property keeps the optical power of the device 'bundled' on to a relatively small area over considerable distances. However, highly collimated courses are also inherently more dangerous to the unprotected eye.

3. Coherence: the light emitted by laser devices is also in phase, so in conjunction with the two unique properties already outlined above, the troughs and peaks of the emitted light waves match perfectly in time (temporal coherence) and in space (spatial coherence). The biological and clinical relevance of this property has been debated since the inception of the therapy (e.g. Heiskanen 2018), not least because of the widespread use of so-called 'superluminous diodes', or simply light emitting diodes (LEDs), which possess all the qualities of a 'true' laser diode, less the coherence, but which are a fraction of the cost.

LASER–TISSUE INTERACTION

As already indicated, laser–tissue interaction in medical applications has typically been seen in terms of the potentially destructive effects of irradiation at relatively high power and energy levels; in these circumstances, high intensities of laser light from highly collimated or focused sources with output in the watt range can easily produce photothermal reactions in tissues, including ablative or explosive effects. However, in photobiomodulation, the emphasis is upon the non-thermal (or athermal) reactions of light with tissue.

When applying light from a laser or monochromatic light therapy treatment device to the skin, approximately 4–7% of the incident light is reflected from the stratum corneum surface due to differences in refractive indices at the air-tissue interface. Light transmitted through the stratum corneum can interact with irradiated tissue in two ways:

1. Scattering of incident light: this is essentially a change in the direction of propagation of the light as it passes through tissues, and is due to variability in the refractive indices of tissue components relative to water. Such scattering will cause a 'widening' of the beam as it passes through irradiated tissue, and result in the rapid loss of coherence. Scattering also occurs in a backward direction thereby reducing the amount of energy available for forward transmission but adding to the energy available for absorption in the more superficial tissue layers.

2. Absorption of incident light by a chromophore: a chromophore is a biomolecule that is capable, through its electronic or atomic configuration, of absorbing incident photon(s). Light at the wavelengths typically employed in LLLT/PBM are readily absorbed by a variety of biomolecules, including melanin and haemoglobin; as a consequence, the penetration depth associated

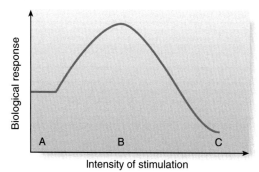

Fig. 10.3 The Arndt–Schultz law (A) Prethreshold: no biological activation (resting); (B) biostimulation: activation of biological processes; (C) bioinhibition: inhibition of biological processes.

with treatment devices is usually considered to be no more than several millimetres. It should be noted that, as the absorption is dependent upon the wavelength of incident light, the depth of penetration is similarly wavelength dependent.

Of these two modes of interaction, absorption may be regarded as the most important in terms of the photobiological basis of laser therapy, as without absorption, no photobiological (nor thus clinical) effects would be possible (this represents the first law of photochemistry).

Conceptual Basis of Laser Photobiomodulation: the Arndt–Schultz Law

The photobiological effects of laser or monochromatic light upon tissue are many and complex, particularly in terms of the variable stimulative/inhibitory reactions that can be effected by such irradiation. In providing a theoretical basis for the observed biological and clinical effects of this modality, the Arndt–Schultz law has been proposed as a suitable model; the main tenets of this law are illustrated in Fig. 10.3. It should be stressed, however, that although this model can account for such phenomena as the 'inverse' dosage dependency reported in some papers (e.g. Lowe et al 1994), it essentially applies to radiant exposure (or energy density – see further sections); the putative relevance of manipulation of other irradiation parameters, such as pulse repetition rate or power output remains, at least for the time being, a matter of debate (Nussbaum et al 2003b).

Biological and Physiological Effects

Investigations of the biological and physiological effects of PBM can usefully be considered under three main areas: cellular studies involving the use of well-established cell lines and explanted cells, studies in various species of animals (in vivo and in vitro), and research in healthy human volunteers.

Although the following provides an overview of the findings to date in these areas, a full and comprehensive review of the literature on the biological and physiological effects of low-level laser radiation is beyond the scope of this chapter; for further detail the reader is directed to the reviews of Baxter (1994), Karu (1998), Tuner and Hode (1999), Peplow et al (2010a) and Anders et al (2017).

Cellular Research

A large number of studies have examined the biological basis of PBM using a variety of bacteria, as well as cell lines and explanted cells, especially fibroblasts and macrophages (Peplow et al 2010b). In these studies, a number of possible indicators have been used to assess the photobiomodulatory effects of laser irradiation, including cell proliferation (Bolton et al 1995; Hawkins & Abrahamse 2006; Stein et al 2005), collagen production (Medrado et al 2003) and gene expression (Byrnes et al 2005). However, it should be stressed that although results from such studies are generally positive, findings in some areas are equivocal (Posten et al 2005).

Cellular studies are important in two respects. In the first instance they provide a scientific basis for the clinical application of low-level lasers for the management of wounds, through demonstration of the photobiological mechanisms underlying such treatments (Karu 1998; Posten et al 2005). Second, by using such well-controlled laboratory research techniques, systematic investigations by some groups have demonstrated the importance of laser irradiation parameters, such as wavelength and dosage, to the observed effects (Peplow et al 2010a, 2010b).

This notwithstanding, the precise relevance of the reported observations to clinical treatments is not always entirely clear. For example, where photobiostimulatory effects might be reported utilizing a radiant exposure of 1.5 Jcm^{-2} in a laboratory study involving the direct irradiation of artificially maintained murine macrophage-like cell lines, what direct relevance has this for dosage selection in the laser treatment of a venous ulcer in a 67-year-old patient? Given such problems, e.g. the differences between the cell lines and the highly complex microenvironment of the clinical wound, a number of groups have employed animal studies and experimental studies on healthy human volunteers to further assess the biological and physiological effects of this modality in the laboratory.

Animal Studies

To date, animal studies have concentrated on two main areas of research: the photobiostimulatory effects of laser irradiation on wound healing in experimentally induced lesions, and the neurophysiological and antinociceptive ('pain-blocking') effects of irradiation. For the former studies, small, loose-skinned animals, such as rats and mice, have been traditionally, and most commonly, used (e.g. Mester et al 1985; Rabelo et al 2006). A range of experimental wounds have been employed in these species, including bone defects (Khadra et al 2004), burns (Bayat et al 2006), tendon and ligamentous injuries (Bayat et al 2005) and open skin wounds based upon models of compromised wound healing (Mester et al 1985; Rabelo et al 2006; Walker 2000). Although such studies have typically reported positive effects of laser irradiation (in terms of increased rates of healing, wound closure, enhanced granulation tissue formation, etc.) (see Peplow et al 2010c; Woodruff et al 2004) experimental lesions in these animals have long been considered to represent a poor model for wounds in humans because of the differences in species integument compared with humans (King 1990).

Perhaps the most interesting aspect of this type of animal work has been reports of the potential of laser irradiation to accelerate regeneration of damaged nerves, together with associated electrophysiological and functional recovery, after various types of experimental lesions (Anders et al 2004). If such effects are also possible in humans, the implications for future applications of this modality would be enormous (Gigo-Benato et al 2005).

The effects of laser irradiation have been studied in various animal models of pain to investigate its mechanism of action and dependence upon irradiation parameters (Ferreira et al 2005; Ponnudurai et al 1987; Wedlock & Shephard 1996a, 1996b). These studies have generally demonstrated a significant hypoalgesic effect of laser irradiation, which seems to be dependent upon the irradiation parameters used (pulse repetition rate: Ponnudurai et al 1987; dosage: Wedlock & Shephard 1996b). Furthermore, the observed hypoalgesia has been found to be naloxone reversible in some studies (Wedlock & Shephard 1996a), but not in others (Ponnudurai et al 1987), suggesting that the pain relief obtained with laser irradiation may be underpinned by a variety of different mechanisms, and in some circumstances may be opiate mediated.

Notwithstanding the utility of such animal work, some of the problems in extrapolating the findings to humans remain. As a consequence, several groups have used controlled studies in healthy human volunteers as a useful means of investigation without recourse to patients and the problems inherent in undertaking controlled clinical research.

Controlled Studies in Humans

One area of study in humans that might have immediate relevance for clinicians relates to the effects of skin colour on reflection, absorption and transmission of laser and LED light (Liebert et al 2012; Nussbaum et al 2007; Souza-Barros et al 2018). The melanin concentrated in highly pigmented skin reduces the amount of light transmitted to subcutaneous tissue and deeper tissue layers, particularly in the red wavebands, indicating that energy dose should be increased when irradiating patients with dark skin compared with fair-skinned patients. When treating deep-seated lesions, for example tendinopathy, the presence of significant adipose tissue also reduces light transmission, particularly in NIR wavebands (Liebert et al 2012; Nussbaum et al 2007). Energy density might need to be doubled when using red light on dark skin in normal weight individuals; additional increase is indicated for overweight and obese individuals (BMI >25). Readers are directed to the research for more precise calculations.

Whereas studies in healthy humans have focused principally on the physiological and hypoalgesic effects of laser radiation, controlled studies on experimental lesions have also been completed and have shown benefits of laser irradiation (Hopkins et al 2004). Nerve conduction studies have long been used to study the effects of laser on peripheral nerves; such studies have typically demonstrated significant effects on peripheral nerve conduction in peripheral nerves, which would appear to depend upon the dosage and pulse repetition rate of the laser source (Basford et al 1993; Baxter et al 1994; Lowe et al 1994; Safavi-Farokhi & Bakhtiary 2005). However, the precise relevance of such observations to the clinical applications of this modality is debatable. Of more direct relevance to clinical practice, a number of studies have assessed the effects of laser upon various types of experimentally induced pain in humans; however, these have produced variable findings (Brockhaus & Elger 1990; Douris 2006; Lowe et al 1997; Vinck et al 2006).

CLINICAL EVIDENCE

Although a large number of clinical studies have been completed and published in this area, generally with positive results, prevalent issues with the literature include:

- Studies reported in the literature are often poorly controlled with only very limited blinding; indeed, a significant proportion of available studies are anecdotal in nature.
- Irradiation parameters and treatment protocols used are frequently inadequately specified, thus limiting comparison of results and rendering replication and application in the clinical setting impossible. Even where irradiation parameters are specified, the bewildering number of possible permutations and combinations of wavelength, irradiance, pulse repetition rate, etc. will often mean that precise replication is problematic. Guidance on better reporting is available to address this issue (Jenkins & Carroll 2011).

- A large proportion of the available studies have been published in foreign-language journals, often without English abstracts, making the work inaccessible to anglophone researchers and clinicians.

It should be noted that these issues are certainly not unique to the field of laser therapy. This notwithstanding, it is important to stress that the published database of clinical studies on LLLT/PBM represents a significant body of evidence in favour of the modality; although the constraints of this text preclude an exhaustive review of this literature, the following provides an overview of some of the most relevant recent reviews in the area.

Wound Healing

The enduring popularity of using laser therapy for the treatment of various types of wounds is evidenced by the results of an early large-scale survey of physiotherapy practice in Northern Ireland (Baxter et al 1991). More recently, the growing number of publications on the topic emanating from South America, Asia, China, Africa and beyond suggest worldwide interest in using PBM for wound management. Treatment of various types of chronic wounds was the first low-level laser application to be trialled in humans during the late 1960s (Mester & Mester 1989); success was noted in terms of enhanced rates of wound healing and pain reduction, using He-Ne sources with dosages of up to 4 Jcm^{-2}.

In recent decades standard wound care (SWC) has been compared with SWC combined with laser therapy in a variety of chronic wounds, however, the strength of the evidence is compromised because of the low quality of many studies due to small numbers, questionable randomization of subjects, lack of blinding of clinicians or absence of a placebo group. Systematic reviews covering the efficacy of laser therapy for venous leg ulcers (Flemming & Cullum 2014), diabetic foot ulcers (Li et al 2018) and pressure ulcers (Chen et al 2014; Machado et al 2017) provide clinicians with some guidance; however, the picture is incomplete due to the restrictive inclusion criteria elected by some review authors.

Chen et al (2014) included seven randomized controlled trials (RCTs) involving 403 subjects with pressure ulcers; six trials compared SWC plus laser therapy with SWC alone. The authors concluded that there was insufficient evidence to determine efficacy. The most common dosage for pressure ulcer treatment appears to be 4 Jcm^{-2} and negative studies might be explained by using lower energy density. The most uncertain parameter for planning treatment, however, appears to be laser wavelength; two studies that delivered four or more wavelengths simultaneously to the ulcers using a multidiode-cluster probe produced negative results. A study by Taradaj et al (2013) that was not included in the Chen et al (2014) review is of particular interest: this double-blind, randomized trial, with concealed allocation

of subjects, compared the effects on pressure ulcer healing of 658 nm, 808 nm, 940 nm or placebo laser therapy at 4 Jcm^{-2} applied for 4 weeks. The protocol in terms of energy density, treatment repetition and study duration was quite similar to studies included in the Chen et al (2014) review. The interesting finding was that 658 nm was significantly beneficial when compared with the other wavelengths and placebo laser. A more recent review by Machado et al (2017) included four trials involving 210 subjects; these authors concluded that using 658 nm lasers was beneficial in treating pressure ulcers.

The efficacy of laser therapy in the treatment of venous leg ulcers is currently undergoing review by the Cochrane Wounds Group (Illescas-Montes et al 2018). The previous 2014 review by the Cochrane Group included four RCTs; however, variation among trial protocols prevented pooling of results. The reviewers concluded that lasers using single wavelengths, 904 nm or He-Ne light, did not improve wound-healing rate; whereas a combination of 904 nm plus He-Ne laser seemed to be beneficial. The quality of the evidence was considered weak. Recent literature includes additional studies, some of which show benefit of PBM for venous ulcers; however, some of these studies still score low on quality assessment. Therapy using a single wavelength of red light, 625–660 nm, or 660 nm combined with infrared light around 880 nm, at 4 Jcm^{-2}, applied for 10 or more weeks has produced benefit, although notably, not when used for a much shorter period (Kopera et al 2005). Infrared light alone at 810 nm or 904 nm has not produced benefit. These findings from individual studies should be viewed carefully as there are issues with some studies with respect to randomization and blinding.

Li et al (2018) included seven RCTs with 194 patients in a review of laser efficacy in treating diabetic foot ulcers. Results in four trials could be pooled for analysis of wound area reduction and in three trials for closure rate; qualitative analysis was conducted when data could not be pooled. The authors concluded that laser decreased wound surface area, increased closure rate, promoted granulation tissue, and decreased foot ulcer pain compared with controls. Treatment using red light around 660 nm alone or 660 nm combined with infrared light, applied at about 3–4 Jcm^{-2}, 3–6 times per week for at least 3 weeks, improved healing. A 2018 study (Frangez & Frangez 2018), using similar parameters, showed no benefit for laser therapy; however, the placebo group in that study seems to have received a low dose of laser irradiation which likely compromised the results.

There are many articles describing positive experiences using laser of various wavelengths in individual cases, in case series, and in large uncontrolled trials involving chronic or post-surgical wounds (Schindl et al 1999; de Oliveira et al 2018). In contrast, when Barreto and Salgado (2010) treated ulcers in cases of peripheral neuropathy due to leprosy, they found no benefit using 660 nm laser when applying 2 Jcm^{-2} to ulcer surfaces and a much higher dose of 4 J per point to wound margins.

Different problems underly the development of diabetic, venous and pressure-type ulcers. Clinicians treating ulcers should consider whether they are dealing with acute tissue ischemia or long-standing tissue oedema and fibrosis, and whether there is presence of slough, necrotic tissue or infection. Intuitively, there is not likely to be a single laser protocol indicated for these different problems. Accordingly, clinicians might consult the literature based on their patient's presenting type of wound, and, based on available laser wavelength, assess the likelihood of benefit from introducing laser treatment.

Mucositis Associated with Chemoradiotherapy

Laser therapy has been assessed in the management of oral mucositis in patients undergoing chemoradiotherapy or radiation therapy for head and neck cancers. Experts in the field have conducted systematic reviews with meta-analysis and a recent article provides a useful summary of the current recommendations. Based on the literature and their experience in the field, Zecha et al (2016) recommend using laser at wavelengths of 633–685 nm or 780–830 nm at energy density of 2–3 Jcm^{-2}, 2–3 times per week applied to single spots rather than scanned over the entire mucosa. Benefits include decreased prevalence, severity and duration of oral mucositis and decrease in associated pain. Examination of possible adverse effects on treatment and patient outcomes has shown that laser therapy is safe for patients with head and neck cancers: follow-up for up to 41 months (range 0.7–101.9 months) post laser therapy using 660 nm at 4 Jcm^{-2}, 5 days per week for an average of 46 days, showed, in addition to short-term benefits for mucositis severity, significant gain in progression-free survival and a tendency to better overall survival (Antunes et al 2017).

Musculoskeletal Disorders

Treatment of musculoskeletal disorders (including pain and soft-tissue injuries) represents the most common application of PBM in routine physiotherapy practice, given the attractions of combining benefits of promotion of tissue repair with pain relief; this is therefore – not surprisingly – the area that has been studied most extensively. As for other areas of application, confusion over the clinical relevance of irradiation parameters and appropriate application techniques initially confounded a systematic approach to research in musculoskeletal disorders (e.g. low-output powers: Waylonis et al 1988; use of non-contact treatment technique: Siebert et al 1987).

Results from systematic reviews in this area have included inconclusive findings for the treatment of lateral epicondylitis ('tennis elbow') (Stasinopoulos & Johnson 2005), although this review has been criticized for including trials of laser acupuncture alongside 'regular' laser therapy treatments (Chow 2006). Apart from reductions in pain associated with treatment effects in the musculoskeletal conditions already indicated, laser therapy has also been reported as effective in the treatment of various types of pain, including neuropathic and neurogenic pain syndromes. The modality has long been a popular treatment method with physiotherapists for the relief of pain, and is highly rated against alternative electrotherapeutic modalities (Baxter et al 1991).

While early reviews of the field were critical of the quality of work, and typically did not find consistent evidence to support the use of laser therapy, more recent systematic reviews in this area of musculoskeletal management have generally shown benefits of LLLT/PBM. This shift is in part due to better understanding of the biophysical principles and underlying mechanisms of actions, as well as better insight into the relevance of irradiation parameters. In addition, the quality and quantity of the research literature – and of the reviews – has increased markedly. Findings from salient reviews are outlined below.

Laser therapy has been recommended as a potentially effective intervention in sports to promote tissue repair and recovery post exercise. Leal-Junior and colleagues (2015) have published a number of studies assessing the potential of PBM to reduce muscle fatigue and enhance recovery post exercise, and reviewed these studies alongside relevant work from other groups in the area. Findings from 13 controlled studies have reported consistent benefits in a range of outcome measures and markers including peak muscle force or time to fatigue, or levels of creatine kinase or lactic acid. Interestingly, from this synthesis of the work to date, there appears to be a dosage dependency to such effects, as benefits were associated with power and energy dosages of 50–200 mW, and 5–6 J per point respectively.

Low back pain is recognized globally as a prevalent, costly, and frequently intractable condition, which has significant impacts on the individual, families, and communities; for some these impacts are pronounced and long term as the pain may become chronic (e.g. Maher et al 2017). LLLT/PBM, typically used in combination with other therapies, has been recommended as a safe and effective treatment option, although the results from systematic reviews are somewhat mixed. Glazov et al (2016) included laser acupuncture interventions – as well as regular LLLT/PBM – in their meta-analysis of 15 controlled clinical studies on chronic low back pain (n=1039 patients; n=5 laser acupuncture). Primary outcome measures of interest were pain relief and global assessment of improvement in the short term; the team also assessed (through sub-group analysis) the potential relevance to clinical effects of treatment approach, chronicity, and dosage parameters. Findings were positive, at least for effectiveness in the short term/immediately following treatment. Better effects were seen with shorter duration of back pain (noting that the overall focus was on chronic low back pain), and with application of higher energy dosages (>3 J per point). Results from the laser acupuncture trials were more mixed, which might have been as a result of the appropriateness of the intervention parameters applied (dosage and points selected) rather than an inherent failure of laser acupuncture per se (see below). In an earlier meta-analysis which focused solely on laser therapy treatments, Huang et al (2015a) similarly found evidence of effectiveness in terms of pain relief within the short term, but no significant effects upon functional or range of movement measures (n=7 RCTs; n=394 patients). Given the emergence of the use of higher power laser systems for routine use in rehabilitation, it is interesting that a recent randomized trial (Alayat et al 2014) investigated treatment of chronic low back pain utilizing an Nd:YAG laser (peak power 3 W), with a total dosage of 3000 J applied in three phases of treatment. In this three-arm trial (n=72 patients), laser treatment combined with a standardized exercise programme was found to be more effective for pain relief, and for functional improvement, than laser therapy in isolation, or the exercise programme combined with sham laser, at least in the short term.

For the treatment of neck pain, Chow and colleagues (2009) systematically reviewed results from 16 RCT studies (n=820 patients) and found that LLLT reduced pain immediately after treatment, and for up to 22 weeks post treatment. This was a timely and interesting review, given the previous scepticism around the pain-relieving effects of laser therapy, and ongoing controversy around potential mechanisms of action (Devor 1990). In a subsequent review of controlled neurophysiological studies in animals and humans (n=44 studies), Chow et al (2011) found consistent evidence of inhibitory effects peripherally and centrally, providing evidence of a putative mechanism of action for the clinically observed laser-mediated pain relief.

Laser therapy has also been promoted as a safe and effective treatment for temporomandibular disorders (TMD). Chang et al (2014) completed a review of randomized controlled trials of laser therapy for relief of TMD pain: a total of seven RCTs met their inclusion criteria, based upon which there was evidence of a moderate effect of laser in the short term. However, reported laser parameters varied significantly across the included trials (e.g. dosages ranged from ~1 to >100 Jcm^{-2}), which for now precludes definitive recommendations for optimal treatment of this condition.

Carpal tunnel syndrome has proved to be a popular condition for researchers interested in the potential benefits from PBM as a non-pharmacological, non-surgical alternative. Franke et al (2018) completed a systematic review, based upon 17 RCTs, which found evidence of benefit in the short term (<5 weeks) compared to placebo/sham irradiation; evidence of benefit in the medium to longer term was equivocal (moderate at 7 weeks, and conflicting at 12 weeks). The variety of parameters used in studies precluded definitive conclusions concerning the relevance of dosage and power, etc.

Tendinopathy is a disabling condition, which shows increasing prevalence with increasing age. Laser therapy has been promoted for decades as a potentially effective management option for tendinopathy of various aetiologies, with mixed results. Tumilty S. et al (2010) systematically reviewed the literature from randomized controlled trials in this field and found benefits in only 12/25 trials included in their review. However, in assessing potential relevance of dosage of laser therapy to reported benefit, the positive trials all employed dosages within the recommended dosage window (WALT, 2005), highlighting – again – that clinical effectiveness is dosage dependent.

Similarly, in the management of shoulder conditions, a systematic review by Haselrud et al (2015) incorporating 17 RCTs found that benefits for pain and functional outcome measures were dependent upon application of recommended dosages. Better outcomes for functional measures were also associated with use of LLLT as a monotherapy (i.e. not in combination or as an adjunctive treatment).

The potential of laser to improve the signs and symptoms of plantar fasciitis has been examined by several authors and, where pooling was possible, meta-analysis was performed; all studies were at least of moderate quality. Heel pain, tenderness and functional status improved when compared with placebo laser or alternative treatments using 830 nm or 904 nm lasers at about 6–8 J per point (Cinar & Uygur 2018a, 2018b; Kiritsi et al 2010) or 10 J using a scanning technique (Ulusoy et al 2017) applied to numerous points around the medial tubercle of the heel and the medial aspect of the plantar fascia. In addition to symptomatic relief, the use of ultrasonography (Kiritsi et al 2010; Macias 2015) and MRI (Ulusoy et al 2017) demonstrated that laser therapy decreased plantar fascia thickness. Meta-analysis involving two studies favoured laser on visual analogue scale (VAS) pain (Salviolia et al 2017). Treatment using a multidiode laser comprising red and infrared wavelengths was also shown to improve plantar fascia pain, tenderness and functional status when compared with placebo laser; however, shockwave therapy was superior to laser on measures of tenderness and function (Takla & Rezk-Allah 2018). In contrast to the positive outcomes, Basford et al (1998) found no benefit in treating the plantar fascia using an 830 nm laser; the lack of effect might be related to the use of a low treatment dose of 1 J per point and 3 J total per session for a condition characterized by deep-seated fibrous tissue. Macias et al (2015) reported that 635 nm laser applied twice weekly for 3 weeks at about 10 J per point improved pain and reduced plantar fascia thickness on MRI at 8 weeks; function, however, improved equally in laser and placebo groups. Overall PBM using 830 nm or 904 nm lasers appears to be an effective treatment for chronic plantar fasciitis: the key to benefit may be using adequate energy. Additional studies are needed to confirm the benefit shown using 635 nm.

Arthritic Conditions

The role of laser therapy in the management of arthritic conditions, such as rheumatoid arthritis, osteoarthritis and arthrogenic pain has been extensively investigated for decades. Reviews of clinical trials in these conditions have produced mixed conclusions and have been criticized as suffering from systematic biases (Bjordal et al 2005; Stausholm et al 2017). Previous systematic reviews in this area have provided some support for the effectiveness of laser therapy in rheumatoid arthritis (Brosseau et al 2005; Ottawa Panel 2004), particularly for relief of pain and early morning stiffness in the short term (based upon five randomized controlled trials and 222 patients); in contrast, the evidence for its effectiveness in the treatment of osteoarthritis is more equivocal (Brosseau et al 2004; Huang et al 2015b). Huang et al (2015b) reviewed a total of nine randomized controlled trials on knee osteoarthritis, comprising 518 patients, and did not find evidence to support the benefit of laser therapy. Immediate effects (within two weeks) on pain (VAS) were not significantly different between LLLT and control (a total of seven studies); similarly, there were no such differences at 12 weeks (five studies). Furthermore, there was no evidence of effectiveness from any other outcome measures reported, including Western Ontario and McMaster Universities Arthritis Index (WOMAC) pain, stiffness, or function outcomes. Interestingly, no significant differences were identified in those studies (n=4) conforming to the World Association of Laser Therapy (WALT) dosage recommendations (WALT 2005).

A recent cohort study (Ip 2015) on older individuals with bilateral knee osteoarthritis (n=100, aged 60–72 years), who received routine physiotherapy (both knees) and – for a single knee – a standardized laser treatment protocol (820 cm, 20 mW, 3.6 Jcm⁻²) found there were fewer joint replacements required in the laser treated knee. This is a particularly interesting finding given the length of the follow-up period (~6 years).

Although the precise reasons for conflicting research findings are not entirely clear, these may be due in part to the selection of laser parameters in these studies, including the use of relatively low-output powers in some of the earlier studies (Basford et al 1987). Current opinion and evidence favours the use of infrared wavelengths (>700 nm), along with relatively higher power (>30 mW) and dosage (>2–3 J per point) levels for the effective treatment of arthritic conditions. It is also interesting to note that benefits of treatment may persist well beyond the period of treatment: extended follow-ups in one trial (>6 months) showed ongoing benefits following a 3-week course of laser therapy (904 nm, 3 Joules/point), followed by 8 weeks of a strengthening programme (Alfredo et al 2017).

Laser Acupuncture

In China and Japan, the main method of laser application has been as an alternative to needles for acupuncture. Although the comparative effectiveness of this application technique with respect to needles or other non-invasive alternatives (e.g. TENS, acupressure) is still unclear, there are a number of positive reports in the literature of successful application of laser acupuncture for pain relief (Gur et al 2004; Hakguder et al 2003). Taut muscles with associated well-localized areas of pain upon palpation (i.e. trigger points) (Baldry 1993) may also be treated with laser irradiation; reviews by Baxter et al (2008), and (updated) by Law et al (2015) provide evidence of effectiveness in the treatment of myofascial trigger points in the short and medium term. The former review included nine RCTs on myofascial pain, seven of which reported positive outcomes. While a variety of parameters were used in the included studies, better outcomes were typically associated with the use of infrared wavelengths, higher power outputs (at least 10 mW) and dosages above 0.5 J per point. The updated review of Law et al (2015) found 49 studies that met their inclusion criteria, which included musculoskeletal pain as the generic indication of interest (13 specifically investigated effects in myofascial trigger points). The overall conclusions supported the continued use of laser acupuncture as an effective non-pharmacological treatment for myofascial pain, at least when appropriate dosages were employed. Interestingly, the review also highlighted better outcomes in terms of pain in the medium to longer term, compared to immediately after treatment, which is similar to findings in laser therapy treatment of other conditions, such as tendinopathy (see above).

Although there are no definitive recommendations on dosage for laser acupuncture used for trigger-point therapy, these reviews indicate that best results have been achieved with higher power and dosages of at least 0.5 J. Treatment dosages of 1–3 J per point can be routinely used, in line with general recommendations for routine musculoskeletal treatments (WALT 2005). Thus laser therapy used in this way may be regarded as a safe and effective alternative to needles, particularly for the needle-phobic, for children, or where there are risks of cross infection with puncture (e.g. patients with hepatitis).

Breast Cancer-Related Lymphoedema

Breast cancer is one of the most common cancers affecting women, and breast cancer-related lymphedema (BCRL) is a prevalent complication for breast cancer survivors, secondary to breast cancer treatments. A number of studies have evidenced increasing use of PBM for the management of the condition, typically applying laser therapy in combination with other forms of management, such as massage and use of compression garments.

A recent systematic review assessed the literature in this area (Baxter et al 2017), using a best evidence synthesis focusing primarily on limb circumference/volume as well as pain and range of motion as outcome measures. A total of seven RCTs were chosen for analysis, of which the quality was generally high (three were rated as 'high quality'). However, reporting of treatment parameters was limited, which precluded definitive recommendations for practice.

Results indicated strong evidence (three high-quality trials) showing LLLT/PBM to be more effective than sham treatment for the reduction of limb circumference/volume reduction, at least at short-term follow-up, and moderate evidence (one high-quality trial) indicating LLLT/PBM was more effective than sham laser for short-term pain relief, and limited evidence (one low-quality trial) that LLLT/PBM was more effective than no treatment for decreasing limb swelling at short-term follow-up. These findings were in keeping with an earlier systematic review by Smoot et al (2015), which also found some benefit in terms of pain reduction with laser therapy treatment.

Based upon the findings of these reviews, LLLT/PBM may be considered an effective treatment option for women with BCRL, particularly where laser therapy is used in conjunction with other physical interventions. This notwithstanding, the optimal treatment parameters for clinical application have yet to be determined, and there is a clear need for further well-designed high-quality trials in this area.

THERAPEUTIC EFFECTS AND USES

Laser therapy finds a variety of applications in clinical practice; these can be usefully summarized under the following headings:

- Wound management: stimulation of wound-healing processes in various types of open wounds, and particularly chronic ulcers.
- Treatment of soft-tissue injuries.
- Treatment of arthritis: treatment of arthritic conditions.
- Pain relief: relief of pain of various aetiologies.

The treatment of open wounds and ulcers represents the cardinal application for low-level laser devices and combined phototherapy/LLLT units. In the treatment of muscle tears and injuries, laser therapy can be effective in accelerating the repair process and thus the return to normal function. This, coupled with its ability to be applied early in the acute stage – in some cases immediately after injury – makes it a popular modality with sports teams and sports physiotherapists for the treatment of sports injuries.

Classification of Lasers and Ocular Hazard

Under an internationally agreed classification system (revised in 2002), laser devices are classed on a scale from 1 to 4 according to the associated dangers to the unprotected skin and eye: 1, 1M, 2, 2M, 3R, 3B, 4. The units typically used in LLLT/PBM are designated as class 3R or 3B lasers, although higher power class 4 systems are becoming more common, and much lower output class 1 and 2 devices have also been previously used. This essentially means, for the majority of systems used in physiotherapy applications (i.e. class 3R and 3B units), that although the laser's output may be considered harmless when directed on to the unprotected skin, it poses a potential hazard to the eye if viewed along the axis of the beam (i.e. intrabeam viewing) owing to the high degree of collimation of the laser light. For this reason, the use of protective goggles, which must be appropriate for the wavelength(s) used, is recommended for operator and patient. Care is also recommended in ensuring that the beam is never directed towards the unprotected eye; the patient should be specifically warned about the ocular hazard associated with the device and asked not to stare directly at the treatment site during application. Furthermore, the laser treatment unit should ideally be used only in an area specifically designated for this purpose; outside this area, the appropriate laser warning symbols should be clearly displayed. Having outlined these fundamental safety rules, it is important to stress that the ocular hazard associated with therapeutic units of classes 1–3 is practically negligible, especially where the treatment head or probe is used with the recommended 'in-contact' technique (see the following section, Principles of Clinical Application). The increasing use of class 4 devices is associated with higher risk (in terms of unprotected skin and eyes, as well as local tissue heating), and requires commensurately higher regulatory and safety measures; however, this is generally mitigated through use of defocused device settings, and use of standard tests for thermal modalities (i.e. skin testing).

In addition, the output of the treatment unit should be regularly tested to ensure the optimal operation (and thus effectiveness) of the device; this is particularly important as it has been reported that a large proportion of laser units in routine use may not be providing adequate power output to be effective (Nussbaum et al 1999).

Contraindications to LLLT/PBM are covered in Chapter 22.

Special Devices for Treatment

A number of special devices have been produced and marketed to simplify and improve the efficiency and effectiveness of treatments. In the first instance, several manufacturers have produced scanning devices that mechanically direct the output of the device over an area defined by the operator by means of controls on the scanning unit. While these devices have been popular in some circles in offering a 'hands-off' approach to providing standardized treatment, for example across wound areas, particularly in cases of more extensive wounds (e.g. burns), the relatively high cost and potentially greater hazards associated with these units have prevented them becoming popular.

As an alternative to scanners, many manufacturers now provide the option of so-called 'cluster' units, typically incorporating an array of diodes in a single hand-held unit. The number of diodes provided in these clusters can vary between 3 and 200, but it is generally true that the larger units incorporate a mixture of superluminous (monochromatic) diodes (simply referred to as LEDs) as well as (true) laser sources in their arrays, owing to the prohibitive cost of the latter. Such cluster units allow simultaneous treatment of an area of tissue, the extent of which is decided by the number and configuration of the diodes included in the array. Furthermore, some manufacturers have incorporated diodes operating at a variety of wavelengths (i.e. multisource/multiwavelength arrays) in their cluster units, claiming enhanced clinical effects through parallel (and possibly synergistic) wavelength-specific effects. In routine clinical practice, the relative difficulty in treating extensive ulceration with single-diode units underpinned the prevalent use of cluster units (Baxter et al 1991). In treating wound beds, cluster units can be used in isolation or in conjunction with single probes to access deeper or recessed areas, and in either case provide a more time efficient means of treatment than single probes units used in isolation.

PRINCIPLES OF CLINICAL APPLICATION

These are considered in outline below, after an overview of the principles underlying effective laser treatment. As a basis for subsequent sections and to aid the reader in more critical review of the work published in this area, the method of calculating dosage and the importance of other irradiation parameters are presented below.

Dosage and Irradiation Parameters

Apart from wavelength, which is determined by the lasing medium used in the device, the other irradiation parameters that are important to consider in laser treatments are as follows.

Power Output

The power output of a unit is usually expressed in milliwatts (mW), or thousandths of a watt. This is usually fixed and invariable. However, some machines allow operator selection of the percentage of the total power output (e.g. 10%, 25%); in addition, where pulsing of the output is provided as an option for the operator, this can affect the power output of the unit in some devices. The last few decades have seen units with increasingly higher-power output devices (generally 30–200 mW per source) replace the once-popular 1–10 mW devices for routine clinical use, not least because higher-output units can deliver a specified treatment in a much shorter period of time. More recently, higher power units operating in the watt range (i.e. > 1000 mW) have become commercially available for PMB, and found applications in physiotherapy as well as veterinary practice. Treatment with these devices is usually based on defocused outputs (to limit power densities at the site of application); however, such devices can also produce (photo)thermal effects in addition to photobiomodulation. A detailed review of findings in these class 4 units is not provided here, given that these are not currently widely used in routine physiotherapy practice. It is also important to reiterate that therapeutic application is defined with respect to the tissue response, rather than the output parameters of the device used.

Irradiance (Power Density)

The power per unit area (mW/cm^2) is an important irradiation parameter. It is usually kept as high as possible for a given unit by use of the so-called 'in-contact' treatment technique, and by applying a firm pressure through the treatment head during treatment. It should be noted that, even with the small degrees of divergence associated with laser treatment devices, treatment out of contact with the target tissue will significantly reduce the effectiveness of treatment as the irradiance falls owing to the inverse square law and because of increased reflection from the skin or tissue interface. For in-contact treatments for single point/probe devices, the irradiance is simply calculated by dividing the power output (or average power output for a pulsed unit) by the spot size of the treatment head; typical values for the latter are 0.1–0.125 cm^2.

It is important to note that lasers are available with probe areas as small as 0.01 cm², and whilst such lasers have the appearance of delivering very high power per unit area (mW/cm²), light penetration is significantly decreased compared with a laser of the same power output and a large beam diameter, such as 4 mm (0.125 cm²).

It is worth noting that laser beam sizes are typically much smaller than LEDs; thus the resulting reported power density of a laser is typically much greater than an LED of a similar average power.

Energy

This is given in joules (J) and is usually specified per point irradiated, or sometimes for the 'total' treatment where a number of points are treated. It is calculated by multiplying the power output in watts by the time of irradiation or application in seconds. Thus a 30 mW (i.e. 0.03 W) device applied for 1 minute (i.e. 60 seconds) will deliver 1.8 J of energy. For routine clinical practice, dosage can be recorded in joules per point: thus, for treatment of a tendon using a 100 mW laser for 30 seconds per point, dose could be recorded as 3 J per point.

Radiant Exposure (Energy Density)

This can be considered a better means of specifying dosage, at least for research papers, and is given in joules per unit area (i.e. J cm⁻²); typical values for routine treatments may range from 1 to 30 Jcm². Energy density is usually calculated by dividing the energy delivered (in joules) by the spot size of the treatment unit (in cm²). This can lead to some variance in calculated dosage where manufacturers provide different estimates of spot size for their units (e.g.

consider the same dose of 1 J delivered over spot sizes of 0.01 or 0.1 cm²). Energy density can be a useful measure of dosage for treatment of wounds, especially where using 'cluster' units, where the total energy (in J) is divided by the wound area (in cm², established as part of wound assessment). Thus the treatment of a pressure injury (decubitus ulcer) using a multisource array with a total output of 500 mW for a total of 2 minutes (120 seconds) over a wound of 12 cm² would result in an average energy density of 5 Jcm⁻².

Pulse Repetition Rate

Although some of the laser units routinely used in clinical practice are continuous wave (CW) output (i.e. the output power is essentially invariable over time), most units currently available allow for some form of pulsing of their output. For pulsed units, the pulse repetition rate is expressed in hertz (Hz, pulses per second). Typical values for pulse repetition rate can vary from 2 to tens of thousands of Hz (or kHz). Although the potential biological and clinical relevance of pulse repetition rate is still far from being universally accepted, cellular research would suggest that this parameter is critical to at least some of the biological effects of this modality (Nussbaum et al 2002; Rajaratnam et al 1994).

Importance of the Use of Contact Technique

Although the method of application may vary depending on the presenting condition, wherever possible the treatment head or probe should be applied with a firm pressure to the area of tissue to be treated (Fig. 10.4). In the first instance, this makes the laser treatment inherently safer by reducing the potential for accidental intrabeam viewing (and thus the risk of eye injury). However, the

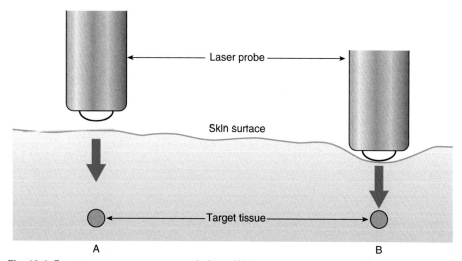

Fig. 10.4 Contact versus non-contact technique. (A) Non-contact technique; (B) contact technique.

primary reason for using so-called contact technique is to maximize the irradiance or power density on the tissue surface, and hence the light flux within the target tissue, which are important in ensuring the effectiveness of laser treatment. Where the treatment head is used out of contact, the light flux within the tissue is reduced owing to several factors; most importantly, the inverse square law applies to such non-contact applications, leading to reduced incident irradiance on the surface of the irradiated tissue.

Apart from producing the highest levels of light flux within the tissue, application of the contact technique will also allow the operator to press the treatment probe into the tissues to treat deeper-seated lesions more effectively. As well as compensating for the relatively limited penetration of therapeutic laser devices by approximating the treatment probe with the target tissue, the deep pressure will drive red blood cells from the area of tissue directly under the probe head and thus reduce the attenuation of light due to absorption by such cells (Nussbaum et al 2007).

Application of the laser treatment probe also affords the opportunity of applying pressure treatments to key points (e.g. trigger or acupoints) and thus effectively combines laser with acupressure-type treatments; indeed, 'laser acupuncture' has long been proposed as a viable alternative (and non-invasive) means of stimulating acupuncture points (Baxter 1989).

Despite the above, there are situations in which laser treatment cannot be applied using contact technique, principally when such application would be too painful or when an aseptic technique is required (e.g. in cases of open wounds). Less commonly, the contours of the tissue to be treated may not allow use of a so-called 'cluster' head in full contact, and so non-contact technique must be used. Where this is the case, the treatment head should not generally be held more than 0.5–1 cm from the surface of the target tissue.

Treatment of Open Wounds and Ulcers

For comprehensive treatment of open wounds, irradiation is applied in two stages: the first using standard contact technique around the edges of the wound; the second, during which the wound bed is treated, using non-contact technique (Fig. 10.5).

Treatment of Wound Margins

For this, a single-diode probe is the ideal unit to apply treatment around the circumference of wound at approximately 1–2 cm from its edges. Points of application should be no more than 2–3 cm apart, and the treatment unit should be applied with a firm pressure to the intact skin, within the patient's tolerances.

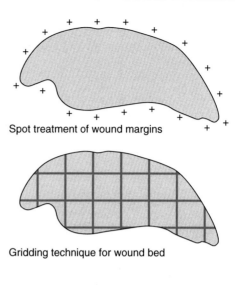

Spot treatment of wound margins

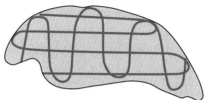

Gridding technique for wound bed

Treatment of wound bed using a scanning technique

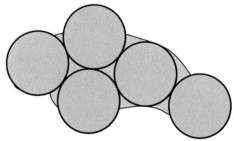

Treatment of wound margins and bed with 'cluster' array

Fig. 10.5 Laser treatment of wounds. Wound margin is treated with single probe using contact technique (1 cm from wound; 2-cm intervals); wound bed is treated using non-contact technique using either gridding or scanning technique (single-diode probe) or multidiode 'cluster' unit.

For such treatments of the wound margins, dosages should be initiated at 0.4 J per point (approximately 4 Jcm^{-2} assuming a 0.1 cm^2 spot size).

Treatment of the Wound Bed

As indicated above, treatment of the wound bed will invariably be completed using non-contact technique. As the wound lacks the usual protective layer of dermis, the dosages applied during treatment will be much lower than during application over intact skin; typically cited radiant exposures are somewhere in the range of 1–10 Jcm^{-2}, with 4 Jcm^{-2} being most commonly recommended as the so-called 'Mester protocol' (i.e. based upon the early work of Professor Endre Mester's group).

However, the problem of applying such a dosage in a standardized fashion across the surface of an open wound is obvious and has led to several means of application being recommended in these conditions. At the simplest level, where only a single probe or fibreoptic applicator is available, the wound may be 'mapped' with a hypothetical grid of equal-sized squares (typically 1–2 cm^2), each of which may be regarded as an individual area of target tissue and treated accordingly at the recommended dosage. Apart from such gridding, some therapists have also employed some variant of scanning technique to treat the wound bed where single-diode or fibreoptic applicators are used. In these cases, the probe is moved slowly over the area of the lesion using a non-contact technique and taking care to deliver a standardized radiant exposure to all areas, while maintaining the head at a distance of no more than 1 cm from the wound bed.

Treatment of Other Conditions

As already indicated, when treatment is applied to intact skin, contact technique is the application method of choice. For treatment of general musculoskeletal conditions, laser therapy can usefully be applied via contact method in a number of ways.

Direct Treatment of the Lesion

In such cases, the laser probe is applied directly to the lesion (area of bruising, site of pain, etc.) using a firm pressure within the patient's tolerance. Where extensive bruising/haematoma is present, an 'in-contact' version of wound treatment (as above) is applied; for these cases, dosages applied are correspondingly higher than those used for the treatment of open wounds, given the presence of the skin as a barrier to laser irradiation.

Irradiation Over Nerve Roots, Trunks, etc.

In the laser treatment of pain syndromes, or in cases where pain represents a major feature of the clinical presentation of the condition to be treated, irradiation may usefully be applied to the skin overlying the appropriate nerve root, plexus, or trunk. For example, in treating upper limb pain, laser therapy might be applied over the relevant cervical nerve roots or the brachial plexus by irradiation over Erb's point, as well as to points where the nerves in the arm are relatively superficial, such as the radial, median, or ulnar nerves at the elbow or wrist.

KEY POINTS ON LASER TREATMENT OF SOME SELECTED CONDITIONS

Soft-Tissue Injuries

Treatment for such injuries should be initiated as early as is practically possible within the acute stage, using relatively low dosages in the region of 1 J per point or 10 Jcm^{-2} applied directly to the site of injury as well as to any areas of palpable pain. Within the first 72–96 hours after injury, treatment may be applied up to three times daily with no risk of overtreatment, provided that dosages are kept low. It is important to reiterate that low-level laser treatment is athermal, and thus eminently suitable for treatment in these situations. As the condition resolves, the frequency of laser treatment may be reduced and dosage correspondingly increased, up to a maximum of 3–4 J per point, or 30–40 Jcm^{-2}. Where pulsed systems are available, early treatments should be initiated with relatively low pulse repetition rates (100 Hz) and increased into the kilohertz range as treatment progresses. Where haematoma or bruising is present, it should be treated using the general principles already outlined for the treatment of open wounds, although in this case a firm contact technique should be used within the patient's tolerance, particularly where the lesion is relatively deep.

Neuropathic and Neurogenic Pain

Where the patient presents with chronic neurogenic pain, laser irradiation is typically applied in a systematic fashion to all relevant nerve roots, plexus and trunks, using a middle-range dosage of 1–2 J per point (10–20 Jcm^{-2}) to initiate treatment. Where trigger or tender points are identified, these are also treated, using the same dose level, which is increased to achieve desensitization of the point upon repalpation (i.e. as is normal practice with treatment of trigger points with other modalities). Irradiation is also applied directly to any areas of referred pain, and to the affected dermatome, etc.

Arthrogenic Pain and Arthritis

Best results in treatment of arthritis and arthralgia of various aetiologies is achieved with laser treatment when it is applied in a comprehensive manner to the affected joints at the appropriate dosages (2–10 J per point; WALT 2005). Care is needed (especially with regard to patient positioning) to ensure that all aspects of the joint are systematically treated.

SUMMARY

Laser technology has evolved remarkably over recent decades: robust, high powered devices have become available for treatment using red or infrared (IR) light, as well as arrays housing up to a hundred or more diodes that are often assembled in combinations of both red and IR light. Systematic reviews find that laser therapy (PBM) is beneficial in a wide variety of clinical conditions, including wound healing, post breast cancer lymphoedema (particularly where used in conjunction with other physical interventions) and mucositis. Early reviews of PBM in the area of soft-tissue injuries and pain were generally inconclusive; however, recent reviews are largely supportive of PBM in this area and that may partly be due to clinicians' better understanding of the biophysical principles and underlying mechanisms of actions, as well as better insight into the relevance of irradiation parameters. Benefit has been found for neck pain, TMD, back pain and carpal tunnel syndrome, at least in the short term. Studies of PBM in rheumatoid and osteoarthritis have produced conflicting findings; however, some older studies used very low dosage. Results appear best using IR wavelengths with dosage >2–3 J per point. Numerous controlled trials support PBM intervention in sports to promote tissue repair and recovery post exercise; results appear to be dependent on dose with 5–6 J per point being the optimal range. Further research is needed to establish optimal treatment protocols in most clinical conditions; investigators should be attentive to using consistent terminology to report their work to allow comparisons and replication by others.

REFERENCES

Alayat, M. S. M., Atya, A. M., Ali, M. M. E., et al. (2014). Long-term effect of high-intensity laser therapy in the treatment of patients with chronic low back pain: A randomized blinded placebo-controlled trial. *Lasers in Medical Science, 29,* 1065–1073.

Alfredo, P. P., Bjordal, J. M., Junior, W. S., et al. (2017). Long-term results of a randomized, controlled, double-blind study of low-level laser therapy before exercises in knee osteoarthritis: Laser and exercises in knee osteoarthritis. *Clinical Rehabilitation, 32,* 173–178.

Anders, J. J., Geuna, S., & Rochkind, S. (2004). Phototherapy promotes regeneration and functional recovery of injured peripheral nerve. *Neurological Research, 26,* 233–239.

Anders, J. J., Ketz, A. K., & Wu, X. (2017). Basic principles of photobiomodulation and its effects at the cellular, tissue, and system levels. In R. J. Reigel & J. C. Godbold (Eds.), *Laser therapy in veterinary medicine: Photobiomodulation* (pp. 36–51). USA: John Wiley & Sons.

Anders, J. J., Lanzafame, R. J., & Arany, P. (2015). Low-level light/laser therapy versus photobiomodulation therapy. *Photomedicine and Laser Surgery, 33,* 183–184.

Antunes, H. S., Herchenhorn, D., Small, I. A., et al. (2017). Long-term survival of a randomized phase III trial of head and neck cancer patients receiving concurrent chemoradiation therapy with or without low-level laser therapy (LLLT) to prevent oral mucositis. *Oral Oncology, 71,* 11–15.

Baldry, P. (1993). *Acupuncture, trigger points and musculoskeletal pain* (2nd ed.). New York: Churchill Livingstone.

Barreto, J. G., & Salgado, C. G. (2010). Clinic-epidemiological evaluation of ulcers in patients with leprosy sequelae and the effect of low level laser therapy on wound healing: A randomized clinical trial. *BMC Infectious Diseases, 10,* 237–244.

Basford, J. R., Hallman, J. O., Matsumoto, J. Y., et al. (1993). Effects of 830 nm laser diode irradiation on median nerve function in normal subjects. *Lasers in Surgery and Medicine, 13,* 597–604.

Basford, J. R., Malanga, G. A., Krause, D. A., & Harmsen, W. S. (1998). A randomised controlled evaluation of low-intensity laser therapy: Plantar fasciitis. *Archives of Physical Medicine and Rehabilitation, 79,* 249–254.

Basford, J. R., Sheffield, C. G., Mair, S. D., et al. (1987). Low energy helium neon laser treatment of thumb osteoarthritis. *Archives of Physical Medicine and Rehabilitation, 68,* 794–797.

Baxter, G. D. (1989). Laser acupuncture analgesia: An overview. *Acupuncture Medicine, 6,* 57–60.

Baxter, G. D. (1994). *Therapeutic lasers: Theory and practice.* New York: Churchill Livingstone.

Baxter, G. D., Bell, A. J., Ravey, J., et al. (1991). Low level laser therapy: Current clinical practice in Northern Ireland. *Physiotherapy, 77,* 171–178.

Baxter, G. D., Bleakley, C., & McDonough, S. (2008). Clinical effectiveness of laser acupuncture: A systematic review. *Journal of Acupuncture and Meridian Studies, 1,* 65–82.

Baxter, G. D., Liu, L., Petrich, S., et al. (2017). Low level laser therapy (photobiomodulation therapy) for breast cancer-related lymphedema: A systematic review. *BMC Cancer, 17,* 833.

Baxter, G. D., Walsh, D. M., Lowe, A. S., et al. (1994). Effects of low intensity infrared laser irradiation upon conduction in the human median nerve *in vivo. Experimental Physiology, 79,* 227–234.

Bayat, M., Delbari, A., Almaseyeh, M. A., et al. (2005). Low-level laser therapy improves early healing of medial collateral ligament injuries in rats. *Photomedicine and Laser Surgery, 23,* 556–560.

Bayat, M., Vasheghani, M. M., & Razavi, N. (2006). Effect of low-level helium-neon laser therapy on the healing of third-degree burns in rats. *Journal of Photochemistry and Photobiology B-Biology, 83,* 87–93.

Bjordal, J. M., Bogen, B., Lopes-Martins, R. A., et al. (2005). Can Cochrane reviews in controversial areas be biased? A sensitivity analysis based on the protocol of a systematic Cochrane review on low-level laser therapy in osteoarthritis. *Photomedicine and Laser Surgery, 23,* 453–458.

Bolton, P., Young, S., & Dyson, M. (1995). The direct effect of 860 nm light on cell proliferation and on succinic dehydrogenase activity of human fibroblasts in vitro. *Laser Therapy, 7,* 55–60.

Brockhaus, A., & Elger, C. E. (1990). Hypoalgesic efficacy of acupuncture on experimental pain in man. Comparison of laser acupuncture and needle acupuncture. *Pain, 43,* 181–186.

Brosseau, L., Robinson, V., Wells, G., et al. (2005). Low level laser therapy (classes I, II and III) for treating rheumatoid arthritis. *Cochrane Database of Systematic Reviews,* CD002049.

Brosseau, L., Welch, V., Wells, G., et al. (2004). Low level laser therapy (classes I, II and III) for treating osteoarthritis. *Cochrane Database of Systematic Reviews*, CD002046.

Byrnes, K. R., Wu, X., Waynant, R. W., et al. (2005). Low power laser irradiation alters gene expression of olfactory ensheathing cells in vitro. *Lasers in Surgery and Medicine, 37*, 161–171.

Chang, W., Lee, C., Lin, H., et al. (2014). A meta-analysis of clinical effects of low-level laser therapy on temporomandibular joint pain. *Journal of Physical Therapy Science, 26*, 1297–1300.

Chen, C., Hou, W. H., Chan, E. S. Y., Yeh, M. L., & Lo, H. L. D. (2014). Phototherapy for treating pressure ulcers. *Cochrane Database of Systematic Reviews* (7), CD009224. https://doi.org/10.1002/14651858.CD009224.pub2.

Chow, R. (2006). Laser acupuncture studies should not be included in systematic reviews of phototherapy. *Photomedicine and Laser Surgery, 24*, 69.

Chow, R., Armati, P., Laakso, E.-L., et al. (2011). Inhibitory effects of laser irradiation on peripheral mammalian nerves and relevance to analgesic effects: A systematic review. *Photomedicine and Laser Surgery, 29*, 365–381.

Chow, R. T., Johnson, M. I., Lopes-Martins, R. A. B., et al. (2009). Efficacy of low-level laser therapy in the management of neck pain: A systematic review and meta-analysis of randomised placebo or active-treatment controlled trials. *Lancet, 374*, 1897–1908.

Cinar, E., Saxena, S., & Uygur, F. (2018a). Combination therapy versus exercise and orthotic support in the management of pain in plantar fasciitis: A randomized controlled trial. *Foot & Ankle International, 39*, 406–414.

Cinar, E., Saxena, S., & Uygur, F. (2018b). Low-level laser therapy in the management of plantar fasciitis: A randomized controlled trial. *Lasers in Medical Science, 33*, 949–958.

Devor, M. (1990). What's in a beam for pain therapy? *Pain, 43*, 139.

Douris, P., Southard, V., Ferrigi, R., et al. (2006). Effect of phototherapy on delayed onset muscle soreness. *Photomedicine and Laser Surgery, 24*, 377–382.

De oliveira, R. A., Boson, L. L. B., Portela, S. M. M., Filho, A. L. M. M., & de Oliveira Santiago, D. (2018). Low-intensity LED therapy (658 nm) on burn healing: A series of cases. *Lasers in Medical Science, 33*, 729–735.

Ferreira, D. M., Zangaro, R. A., Villaverde, A. B., et al. (2005). Analgesic effect of He-Ne (632.8 nm) low-level laser therapy on acute inflammatory pain. *Photomedicine and Laser Surgery, 23*, 177–181.

Flemming, K., & Cullum, N. (2014). Laser therapy for venous leg ulcers. *Cochrane Database of Systematic Reviews 7*, CD001182. https://doi.org/10.1002/14651858. CD001182.pub.

Frangez, I., Nizic-Kos, T., & Frangez, H. B. (2018). Phototherapy with LED shows promising results in healing chronic wounds in diabetes mellitus patients: A prospective randomized double-blind study. *Photomedicine and Laser Surgery, 36*, 377–382.

Franke, T. P., Koes, K. W., Geelen, S. J., et al. (2018). Do patients with carpal tunnel syndrome benefit from low-level laser therapy? A systematic review of randomized controlled trials. *Archives of Physical Medicine and Rehabilitation, 99*, 1650–1659.

Gigo-Benato, D., Geuna, S., & Rochkind, S. (2005). Phototherapy for enhancing peripheral nerve repair: A review of the literature. *Muscle & Nerve, 31*, 694–701.

Glazov, G., Yelland, M., & Emery, J. (2016). Low-level laser therapy for chronic non-specific low back pain: A meta-analysis of randomised controlled trials. *Acupuncture in Medicine, 34*, 328–341.

Gur, A., Sarac, A. J., Cevik, R., et al. (2004). Efficacy of 904 nm gallium arsenide low level laser therapy in the management of chronic myofascial pain in the neck: A double-blind and randomized-controlled trial. *Lasers in Surgery and Medicine, 35*, 229–235.

Hakguder, A., Birtane, M., Gurcan, S., et al. (2003). Efficacy of low level laser therapy in myofascial pain syndrome: An algometric and thermographic evaluation. *Lasers in Surgery and Medicine, 33*, 339–343.

Haselrud, S., Magnussen, L. H., & Joensen, J. (2015). The efficacy of low–level laser therapy for shoulder tendinopathy: A systematic review and meta–analysis of randomized controlled trials. *Physiotherapy Research International, 20*, 108–125.

Hawkins, D. H., & Abrahamse, H. (2006). The role of laser fluence in cell viability, proliferation, and membrane integrity of wounded human skin fibroblasts following helium-neon laser irradiation. *Lasers in Surgery and Medicine, 38*, 74–83.

Heiskanen, V., & Hamblin, M. R. (2018). Photobiomodulation: Lasers vs. light emitting diodes? *Photochemical and Photobiological Sciences, 8*, 1003–1017.

Hopkins, J. T., McLoda, T. A., Seegmiller, J. G., et al. (2004). Low level laser therapy facilitates superficial wound healing in humans: A triple-blind, sham-controlled study. *Photomedicine and Laser Surgery, 39*, 223–229.

Huang, Z., Ma, J., Chen, J., et al. (2015a). The effectiveness of low-level laser therapy for nonspecific chronic low back pain: A systematic review and meta-analysis. *Arthritis Research and Therapy, 17*, 360.

Huang, Z., Chen, J., Ma, J., et al. (2015b). Effectiveness of low-level laser therapy in patients with knee osteoarthritis: A systematic review and meta-analysis. *Osteoarthritis and Cartilage, 23*, 1437–1444.

Illescas-Montes, R., Atkinson, R. A., & Cullum, N. (2018). Low-level light therapy for treating venous leg ulcers. *Cochrane Database of Systematic Reviews 6*, CD013061. https://doi.org/10.1002/14651858.CD013061.

Ip, D. (2015). Does addition of low-level laser therapy (LLLT) in conservative care of knee arthritis successfully postpone the need for joint replacement? *Lasers in Medical Science, 30*, 2335–2339.

Jenkins, P., & Carroll, J. (2011). How to report low-level laser therapy (LLLT)/photomedicine dose and beam parameters in clinical and laboratory studies. *Photomedicine and Laser Surgery, 12*, 785–787.

Karu, T. (1998). *The science of low power laser therapy*. Amsterdam: Gordon & Breach.

Khadra, M., Kasem, N., Haanaes, H. R., et al. (2004). Enhancement of bone formation in rat calvarial bone defects using low-level laser therapy. *Oral Surgery, Oral Medicine, Oral Pathology, and Oral Radiology Endodontics, 97*, 693–700.

King, P. R. (1990). Low level laser therapy: A review. *Physiotherapy Theory and Practice, 6*, 127–138.

Kiritsi, O., Tsitas, K., Malliaropoulos, N., et al. (2010). Ultrasonographic evaluation of plantar fasciitis after low-level laser therapy: Results of a double-blind, randomized, placebo-controlled trial. *Lasers in Medical Science, 25*, 275–281.

Kopera, D., Kokol, R., Berger, C., et al. (2005). Does the use of low-level laser influence wound healing in chronic venous leg ulcers? *Journal of Wound Care, 14*, 391–394.

Law, D., McDonough, S., Bleakley, C., Baxter, G. D., & Tumilty, S. (2015). Laser acupuncture for treating musculoskeletal pain: A systematic review with meta-analysis. *Journal of Acupuncture and Meridian Studies, 8*, 2–16.

Leal-Junior, E. C. P., Vanin, A. A., Miranda, E. F., et al. (2015). Effect of phototherapy (low-level laser therapy and light-emitting diode therapy) on exercise performance and markers of exercise recovery: A systematic review with meta-analysis. *Lasers in Medical Science, 30*, 925–939.

Liebert, A., Waddington, G., Bicknell, B., Chow, R., & Adams, R. (2012). *Quantification of the absorption of low-level 904 nm super pulsed laser light as a function of skin colour. Proceedings of the 9th WALT Congress, September 28-30.* Australia: QT Gold Coast, Surfers Paradise.

Li, S., Wang, C., Wang, B., Liu, L., Tang, L., Liu, D., et al. (2018). Efficacy of low-level light therapy for treatment of diabetic foot ulcer: A systematic review and meta-analysis of randomized controlled trials. *Diabetes Research and Clinical Practice, 143*, 215–224.

Logan, I. D., McKenna, P. G., & Barnett, Y. A. (1995). An investigation of the cytotoxic and mutagenic potential of low intensity laser irradiation in Friend erythroleukaemia cells. *Mutation Research, 347*, 67–71.

Lowe, A. S., Baxter, G. D., Walsh, D. M., et al. (1994). The effect of low intensity laser (830 nm) irradiation upon skin temperature and antidromic conduction latencies in the human median nerve: Relevance of radiant exposure. *Lasers in Surgery and Medicine, 14*, 40–46.

Lowe, A. S., McDowell, B. C., Walsh, D. M., et al. (1997). Failure to demonstrate any hypoalgesic effect of low intensity laser irradiation of Erb's point upon experimental ischaemic pain in humans. *Lasers in Surgery and Medicine, 20*, 69–76.

Machado, R. S., Viana, S., & Sbruzzi, G. (2017). Low-level laser therapy in the treatment of pressure ulcers: Systematic review. *Lasers in Medical Science, 32*, 937–944.

Macias, D. M., Coughlin, M. J., Zang, K., et al. (2015). Low-level laser therapy at 635 nm for treatment of chronic plantar fasciitis: A placebo-controlled, randomized study. *Journal of Foot and Ankle Surgery, 54*, 768–772.

Maher, C., Underwood, M., & Buchbinder, R. (2017). Non specific low back pain. *Lancet, 389*, 736–747.

Medrado, A. R., Pugliese, L. S., Reis, S. R., et al. (2003). Influence of low level laser therapy on wound healing and its biological action upon myofibroblasts. *Lasers in Surgery and Medicine, 32*, 239–244.

Mester, A. F., & Mester, A. (1989). Wound healing. *Laser Therapy, 1*, 7–15.

Mester, E., Mester, A. F., & Mester, A. (1985). The biomedical effects of laser application. *Lasers in Surgery and Medicine, 5*, 31–39.

Nussbaum, E. L., Baxter, G. D., & Lilge, L. (2003a). A review of laser technology and light tissue interactions as a background to therapeutic applications of low intensity lasers and other light sources. *Physical Therapy Reviews, 8*, 31–44.

Nussbaum, E. L., Lilge, L., & Mazzulli, T. (2002). Effects of 630-, 660-, 810-, and 905-nm laser irradiation delivering radiant exposure of 1–50 J/cm^2 on three species of bacteria *in vitro*. *Journal of Clinical Laser Medicine and Surgery, 20*, 325–333.

Nussbaum, E. L., Lilge, L., & Mazzulli, T. (2003b). Effects of low-level laser therapy (LLLT) of 810 nm upon in vitro growth of bacteria: Relevance of irradiance and radiant exposure. *Journal of Clinical Laser Medicine and Surgery, 21*, 283–290.

Nussbaum, E., Van Zuylen, V., & Baxter, G. D. (1999). Specification of treatment dosage in laser therapy: Unreliable equipment and radiant power determination as confounding factors. *Physiotherapy Canada, 51*, 159–167.

Nussbaum, E. L., Van Zuylen, J., & Jing, F. (2007). Transmission of light through human skin folds during phototherapy: Effects of physical characteristics, irradiation wavelength, and skin-diode coupling. *Quantification of the absorption of low-level 904 nm super pulsed laser light as a function of skin colour Canada, 59*(3), 194–207.

Ohshiro, T., & Calderhead, R. G. (1988). *Low level laser therapy: A practical introduction.* Chichester, UK: Wiley.

Ottawa Panel. (2004). Evidence-based clinical practice guidelines for electrotherapy and thermotherapy interventions in the management of rheumatoid arthritis in adults. *Physical Therapy, 84*, 1016–1043.

Peplow, P. V., Chung, T.-Y., & Baxter, G. D. (2010a). Application of low level laser technologies for pain relief and wound healing: Overview of scientific bases. *Physical Therapy Reviews, 15*, 253–285.

Peplow, P. V., Chung, T.-Y., & Baxter, G. D. (2010b). Laser photobiomodulation of proliferation of cells in culture: A review of human and animal studies. *Photomedicine and Laser Surgery, 28*, S3–S40.

Peplow, P. V., Chung, T.-Y., & Baxter, G. D. (2010c). Laser photobiomodulation of wound healing: A review of experimental studies in mouse and rat animal models. *Photomedicine and Laser Surgery, 28*, 291–325.

Pogrel, M. A., Chen, J. W., & Zang, K. (1997). Effects of low-energy gallium-aluminium-arsenide laser irradiation on cultured fibroblasts and keratinocytes. *Lasers in Surgery and Medicine, 20*, 426–432.

Ponnudurai, R. N., Zbuzek, V. K., & Wu, W. (1987). Hypoalgesic effect of laser photobiostimulation shown by rat tail flick test. *Int J Acupuncture Electrother Res, 12*, 93–100.

Posten, W., Wrone, D. A., Dover, J. S., et al. (2005). Low-level laser therapy for wound healing: Mechanism and efficacy. *Dermatologic Surgery, 31*, 334–340.

Rabelo, S. B., Villaverde, A. B., Nicolau, R., et al. (2006). Comparison between wound healing in induced diabetic and nondiabetic rats after low-level laser therapy. *Photomedicine and Laser Surgery, 24*, 474–479.

Rajaratnam, S., Bolton, P., Dyson, M. (1994). Macrophage responsiveness to laser therapy with varying pulsing frequencies. *Laser Therapy*, 6, 107–112.

Safavi-Farokhi, Z., & Bakhtiary, A. H. (2005). The effect of infrared laser on sensory radial nerve electrophysiological parameters. *Electromyography & Clinical Neurophysiology*, 45, 353–356.

Salviolia, S., Guidib, M., & Marcotulli, G. (2017). The effectiveness of conservative, non-pharmacological treatment, of plantar heel pain: A systematic review with meta-analysis. *The Foot*, 33, 57–67.

Schindl, M., Kerschan, K., Schindl, A., et al. (1999). Induction of complete wound healing in recalcitrant ulcers by low level laser irradiation depends on ulcer cause and size. *Photodermatology, Photoimmunology & Photomedicine*, 15, 18–21.

Siebert, W., Siechert, N., Siebert, B., et al. (1987). What is the efficacy of 'soft' and 'mid' lasers in therapy of tendinopathies? *Archives of Orthopaedic and Trauma Surgery*, 106, 358–363.

Smoot, B., Chiavola-Larson, L., Lee, J., et al. (2015). Effect of low-level laser therapy on pain and swelling in women with breast cancer-related lymphedema: A systematic review and meta-analysis. *Journal of Cancer Survivorship*, 9, 287–304.

Souza-Barros, L., Dhaidan, G., Maunula, M., Solomon, V., Gabison, S., Lilge, L., et al. (2018). Skin color and tissue thickness effects on transmittance, reflectance and skin temperature when using 635 nm and 808 nm lasers in low intensity therapeutics. *Lasers in Surgery and Medicine*, 50(4), 291–301.

Stasinopoulos, D. I., & Johnson, M. I. (2005). Effectiveness of low-level laser therapy for lateral elbow tendinopathy. *Photomedicine and Laser Surgery*, 23, 425–430.

Stausholm, M. B., Bjordal, J. M., Lopes-Martins, R. A. B., et al. (2017). Methodological flaws in meta-analysis of low-level laser therapy in knee osteoarthritis: A letter to the editor. *Osteoarthritis and Cartilage*, 25, e9–e10.

Stein, A., Benayahu, D., Maltz, L., et al. (2005). Low-level laser irradiation promotes proliferation and differentiation of human osteoblasts in vitro. *Photomedicine and Laser Surgery*, 23, 161–166.

Takla, M. K. N., & Rezk, S. S. R. (2019). Clinical effectiveness of multi-wavelength photobiomodulation therapy as an adjunct to extracorporeal shock wave therapy in the management of plantar fasciitis: A randomized controlled trial. *Lasers in Medical Science*, 34(3), 583–593.

Taradaj J., Halski T., Kucharzewsi M., Urbanek T., Halska U., Kucio C. (2013) Effect of laser irradiation at different wavelengths (940, 808, and 658 nm) on pressure ulcer healing: Results from a clinical study. *Evidence-based Complementary & Alternative Medicine*, Article Number: 960240.

Tumilty, S. T., Munn, J., McDonough, S., et al. (2010). Low level laser treatment of tendinopathy: A systematic review with meta-analysis. *Photomedicine and Laser Surgery*, 28, 3–16.

Tuner, J., & Hode, L. (1999). *Low level laser therapy. Clinical practice and scientific background. Spjutvägen.* Sweden: Prima Books.

Ulusoy, A., Cerrahoglu, L., & Orguc, S. (2017). Magnetic resonance imaging and clinical outcomes of laser therapy, ultrasound therapy, and extracorporeal shock wave therapy for treatment of plantar fasciitis: A randomized controlled trial. *The Journal of Foot & Ankle Surgery*, 56, 762–767.

Vinck, E., Cagnie, B., Coorevits, P., et al. (2006). Pain reduction by infrared light-emitting diode irradiation: A pilot study on experimentally induced delayed-onset muscle soreness in humans. *Lasers in Medical Science*, 21, 11–18.

Walker, M. D., Rumpf, S., Baxter, G. D., et al. (2000). Effect of low level laser irradiation (660 nm) on a radiation-impaired wound-healing model in murine skin. *Lasers in Surgery and Medicine*, 26, 41–47.

Waylonis, G. W., Wilkie, S., O'Toole, D., et al. (1988). Chronic myofascial pain: Management by low output helium-neon laser therapy. *Archives of Physical Medicine and Rehabilitation*, 69, 1017–1020.

Wedlock, P. M., & Shephard, R. A. (1996a). Cranial irradiation with Gaalas laser leads to naloxone reversible analgesia in rats. *Psychological Reports*, 78, 727–731.

Wedlock, P., Shephard, R. A., Little, C., & McBurney, F. (1996b). Analgesic effects of cranial laser treatment in two rat nociception models. *Physiology & Behavior*, 59, 445–448.

Woodruff, L. D., Bounkeo, J. M., Brannon, W. M., et al. (2004). The efficacy of laser therapy in wound repair: A meta-analysis of the literature. *Photomedicine and Laser Surgery*, 22, 241–247.

World Association for Laser Therapy (WALT). (2005). Recommended *Anti-Inflammatory Dosage for Low Level LaserTherapy.* WALT. Online. Available: http://www.walt.nu.

Zecha JAEM., Raber-Durlacher J. E., Nair R. G., Epstein J. B, Elad S., Hamblin MR., et al. (2016) Low-level laser therapy/photobiomodulation in the management of side effects of chemoradiation therapy in head and neck cancer: part 2: *proposed applications and treatment protocols Support Care Cancer;* 24(6): 2793–2805.

Ultraviolet Therapy

Ethne L. Nussbaum

INTRODUCTION

Ultraviolet radiation (UV) has been used therapeutically for more than a century. Initially UV was used to treat skin conditions, including chronic wounds (Freytes et al 1965), tuberculosis and acne, as a whole-body treatment in conditions such as psoriasis and rickets, and to improve immunity. However, the use of UV declined during the last quarter of the 20th century owing to awareness of the adverse effects of chronic sun exposure, primarily the risks of skin cancer and premature aging, the availability of drugs to treat some of the conditions, and an emphasis on delivering evidence-based healthcare.

PHYSICAL PRINCIPLES

Ultraviolet radiation occupies the non-ionizing, electromagnetic waveband region and is divided into three bands: UVC at 180–280 nm, UVB at >280–315 nm and UVA at >315–400 nm. Absorption by epidermal chromophores initiates photochemical events in the superficial skin layers with effects extending to deeper layers by chemical diffusion. Penetration decreases with wavelength: UVA, UVB and UVC reach the dermis, the epidermal basal layer and the upper epidermis, respectively. It is known that UV-induced cell mutation in the basal layer of the deep epidermis is an important factor in skin cancer development. UVC is relatively ineffective in producing skin cancer: likely because it does not reach the lower skin layers and is absorbed by the non-living epidermal stratum corneum cells, which are regularly sloughed off. Sunlight UVC

is absorbed by the earth's atmosphere and does not reach the earth's surface.

UV is produced artificially by passing a high voltage current across a quartz tube containing an inert gas and a small amount of mercury vapour. Photons transmitted through the quartz tube form the device output. A reflector behind the tube directs the output towards the intended target. The intensity at each wavelength depends on the parent atom, pressure of the gas, properties of the glass tubing, and possible UV filters fitted to the lamp. A small amount of visible blue light is usually emitted together with the invisible UV to alert users when these lamps are in active mode.

There are various types of lamps used in patient care: hand-held, low-pressure and cool-to-the-touch UVC lamps are used for treating skin wounds (Fig. 11.1). The latter lamps have largely replaced medium-pressure water-cooled lamps that emit UV plus infrared (IR) radiation for treating localized conditions. Low-pressure fluorescent tubes mounted in a semicircular reflector and emitting UVA 300–380 nm were used in the past to treat psoriasis; patients were given oral photosensitizers – usually psoralen – giving rise to a treatment known as PUVA. The newer approach for managing psoriasis in cases that have not responded adequately to drug therapy utilizes narrow-band UVB lamps, predominantly at 311–313 nm (Shelk & Morgan 2000). Tanning parlours, promising a quick tan, use UVA sunbeds; survey results revealing the association between parlour tanning and skin melanoma have somewhat diminished this dangerous practice (Veierød et al 2010).

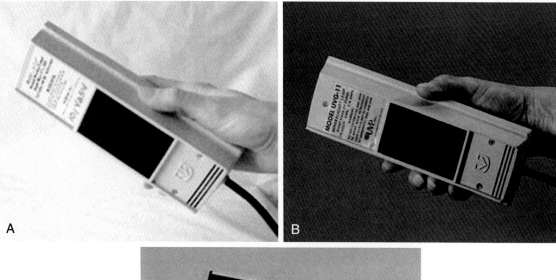

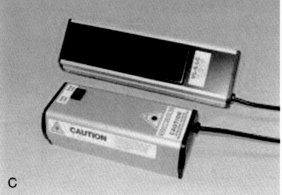

Fig. 11.1 UVC filtered lamps. (A) V-254 lamp (USA), nominal irradiance 14.5 mW/cm². (B) UVP lamp (Cambridge, UK); a stand is available for hands-free operation; output 4 W. (C) Vilber Lourmat lamp (Germany); output 6 W, can be hand-held or operated with a stand.

In recent decades UVA and UVB treatments for psoriasis, other skin diseases and allergic conditions have increasingly been delivered by technicians working under the direction of dermatologists. There are numerous review articles for readers who would like more information on these therapies (Matz 2010; Vangipuram & Feldman 2016). Physiotherapists currently use UV primarily for the treatment of wounds. The remainder of this chapter will be devoted specifically to use of UV for wounds with emphasis on UVC.

BIOPHYSICAL INTERACTIONS

A large variety of cell types absorb UV, including epidermal cells, mast cells, endothelial cells, fibroblasts and melanocytes. The primary effector site is lipid membrane. UV disruption of cytoplasmic membranes and ultrastructural membranes, e.g. cell nuclei, causes release of membrane metabolites, such as arachidonic acid, which trigger a local inflammatory response. Studies have identified UV-induced chemical mediators, such as histamine, prostaglandin E2 and interleukin-1 in the epidermis; these likely diffuse to the dermis and account for the observed capillary dilatation and overall increased blood flow to the skin that is seen to reach a maximum within 24–48 hours (Diffey & Farr 2017), and increased vascular permeability, which leads to increased interstitial fluid and cells. Vasodilatation is rapidly established and may begin several hours before erythema is visible (Diffey & Oakley 1987).

Natural sunlight causes tanning in susceptible individuals (Fitzpatrick skin types III–VI): experimentally, pigmentation may develop after even one erythemogenic exposure of UVA. In contrast, Kaidbey and Klingman (1981) showed that after five consecutive days of erythemogenic doses of

UVC there were no cases of pigmentation among 10 and 11 individuals with skin types I and II respectively, whilst 3 of 11 individuals with skin type III developed pigmentation.

UV offers a non-antibiotic approach to killing pathogenic microorganisms. All open wounds are contaminated to some extent, although healing continues in the presence of a low bacterial load. Healing ceases, however, and the wound may in fact regress, if the host tissue is overwhelmed by bacteria and is no longer able to meet the tissues' oxygen needs (Wysocki 2002). UVC kill rates of 99.9% have been shown in vitro for vancomycin-resistant *Enterococcus* (VRE) (Conner-Kerr et al 1998), Group A *Streptococcus pyogenes* (Rao 2011; Sullivan & Conner-Kerr 2000), MRSA (Conner-Kerr et al 1998; Rao 2011) and *P. aeruginosa* (Sullivan & Conner-Kerr 2000). Fungal killing requires 3–5 times longer exposure than bacterial killing (Sullivan & Conner-Kerr 2000). Studies in vitro suggest that microorganism resistance to UVC does not develop unless exposure is excessive – about 80 treatment cycles (Alcantara-Diaz et al 2004). Furthermore, a prophylactic role has been shown for UVC in a cutaneous wound model in mice (Dai 2012b).

Other important effects of UV include induction and modification of growth factors and their receptors, possibly activated by reactive oxygen species (ROS). Vascular-endothelial growth factor (VEGF), transforming growth factor-α (TGFα) and epidermal growth factor (EGF) receptors have been identified (Huang 1996; Rosette 1996). In turn, these factors might be responsible for the increased keratinocyte and fibroblast activation, increased DNA synthesis and increased cell turnover that have been shown in cell culture studies. Following repeated skin exposures, cell proliferation results in epidermal hyperplasia, which temporarily adds strength to the wound peri skin; hyperplasia subsides when UV is discontinued. Morykwas and Mark (1998) showed UVC-induced collagen lattice contraction in a cell culture model: this finding supports the application of UVC to the wound borders in order to accelerate wound closure.

The intensity needed to induce UV effects is wavelength dependent. For example, effectiveness to produce a minimal erythema is higher at 250 nm than at any other wavelength in the UV spectrum. In contrast, moderate and severe erythema of the skin develop more easily using UVB: this means that there is a low likelihood of producing a harmful sunburn during UVC clinical application (Farr & Diffey 1985). The action spectrum for keratinocyte absorption peaks in the UVC region and UVC is significantly more efficient for bacterial killing than UVB or UVA. However, UVC is the least effective region for melanogenesis (Parrish 1982). The high bactericidal rate and high keratinocyte absorption rate combined with low melanogenesis capacity is the reason why UVC is clinically employed for treating open wounds. It should be noted that UVC is not effective for clearing psoriasis.

THERAPEUTIC EFFECTS AND USES

UVC is widely used for bactericidal effects in settings that do not directly involve patients but are nevertheless relevant to health. For instance, UVC is utilized on a large scale for liquids and especially water purification. It is used to clear airborne pathogens in work spaces, including in surgical operating rooms and food processing facilities, and is also used to sterilize solid surfaces (Lee 2017).

In patient care the main use is in wound management. Specific indications include clearing wounds of necrotic tissue and eschar, managing bacterial load, stimulating granulation and accelerating epithelialization. Treatment dose is different for each of these indications. Dose strength is defined by the skin erythemal response to UV radiation using the levels of subE, through E1 to E4, or at the strongest level 2E4. Alternatively, the energy dose can be used to indicate treatment strength based on the irradiance of the lamp $(W/cm^2) \times$ radiation time in seconds (J/cm^2).

Granulation tissue must fill the wound space as a prerequisite to epithelialization. Low dose UVC is used on clean wound surfaces to stimulate endothelial budding, which is the basis of granulation. Low dose UVC is also applied to the wound perimeter to stimulate epithelial growth across existing granulation tissue and to promote wound contraction. Three to four times higher UVC intensity is required to kill bacteria than to promote tissue growth. High doses are also used to debride yellow fibrous tissue and grey slough. The highest doses are reserved for removing black eschar.

CLINICAL EFFECTIVENESS

There is good evidence in vivo that UVC has bactericidal and fungicidal effects (Chauvin & LaPier 2005). Thai and colleagues (2002) applied 180 seconds of UVC to chronic infected leg ulcers in three patients. *P. aeruginosa*, *S. aureus* and methicillin-resistant *S. aureus* (MRSA) were completely eradicated in two ulcers and MRSA was markedly reduced in a third ulcer. Two ulcers were healed after one week of treatment. The work of Dai and colleagues (2011) counters concerns that bactericidal doses of UVC might damage healthy tissue; they demonstrated that the UVC exposure required to inactivate *P. aeruginosa* and *S. aureus* was much lower than the exposure that would inactivate keratinocytes. Thai et al (2005) in later work examined the effects of a single 180-second UVC exposure on the bioburden in 22 chronic superficial wounds. Effectiveness was measured using semi-quantitative swab tests taken pre-radiation and 5 minutes post-radiation. The results showed partial to complete eradication of some bacteria, including MRSA; however, the lack of effect on MRSA in two wounds suggests that multiple UVC exposures might be needed in some patients.

Multiple exposures were found to be effective for disinfecting catheter exit-sites in patients receiving continuous peritoneal dialysis (Shimomura et al 1995). Among 18 affected patients who applied UVC at home twice daily for 30–60 seconds, 10 sites became negative, three showed decreased microbial growth, and five sites were unchanged. The findings suggest there may be a prophylactic role for UVC. Given the global concerns over drug-resistant bacteria, UVC is attracting attention as an alternative to oral and topical antibiotics (Dai et al 2012a; Yin et al 2013). A further advantage of using UVC is that it eradicates microorganisms in less than 1 hour (2–3-log10 eradication in vivo), while antibiotics usually take several days (Dai et al 2012a).

A number of authors have examined UV effects on wound healing. However, the body of literature has limitations: sample sizes are generally small and investigators have used different study end points, including percentage area reduction, wound closure rate, percentage of wounds closed, etc., which precludes pooling of results for meta-analysis. A 2014 Cochrane Review of phototherapy for treating pressure ulcers found that UV reduced the mean time to complete healing based on the pooled results of two studies (Chen 2014). Studies were excluded from the review if patients had more than one ulcer entered into the trial.

Wills and colleagues (1983) performed one of the earliest randomized, placebo-controlled trials: 18 patients with pressure ulcers were treated with UVB or a placebo lamp. Wound beds were initially exposed to an E4 dose to address infection and thereafter E2 was applied twice weekly to the wound beds and 1 mm of periwound skin. Healing was 33% slower in the placebo group, p<0.02; significance was unaltered when patient age and initial ulcer size were accounted for. Crous and Malherbe (1988) applied UV (lamp emitted UVA, B and C) in three patients with venous ulcers present for as long as 30 years: an E4 or 2E4 dose was applied to necrotic tissue and an E1 to peri skin and clean granulating tissue three times weekly for 4 weeks. At the end of 4 weeks new granulation tissue was prominent in all three ulcers while infected tissue was markedly reduced; area reduction was between 10 and 50%. Onigbinde and colleagues (2010) examined UVB effectiveness on pressure ulcers in 10 patients with bilateral pressure ulcers. Right-sided ulcers were designated as controls and received standard wound care (SWC); left-sided ulcers received SWC plus UVB, beginning with a 45-second exposure at 7.5 cm distance from the wound surface, and increasing to 5 minutes over the first 7 sessions. Treatment was applied two to three times per week for 6 weeks. Benefit was evaluated by amount of exudate, type of exudate, wound appearance and depth using the Pressure Sore Status Tool. UVB was significantly more beneficial than SWC on all outcomes.

UVC has been used in combination with other electrophysical agents. Nussbaum et al (1994) compared effects of SWC alone, SWC plus a UVC-ultrasound combination (US/UVC) and SWC plus laser on pressure ulcers. Eighteen patients with spinal cord injuries were randomized to one of the three treatment groups. Laser was applied three times weekly using a cluster probe (660, 820, 880, 950 nm, 4 J/cm^2). US/UVC was applied five times weekly, alternating the modality each day. The 3 MHz US was applied to wound peri skin at 1 W/cm^2, pulsed 1:4, spatial-average temporal-peak, for 5 minutes per 5 cm^2 of ulcer area. UVC was applied to wound peri skin using an E1 dose and to wound surfaces using an E1 for red granulating surfaces and higher doses according to wound appearance up to an E4 for heavily sloughing or necrotic surfaces. The assessor was blinded to group allocation; however, therapists and patients knew which treatment they were getting. Wound closure ranged from 4–14 weeks in SWC group, 6–20 weeks in the laser group and 2–6 weeks in the US/UVC group. US/UVC was superior to SWC alone and significantly better than SWC plus laser. The study limitations should be noted: power was low with considerable risk of a type 2 error. In addition, there was no intention to treat analysis and results for two SWC group subjects, who were withdrawn by medical physicians because they were not making progress, were ignored in the analysis; their withdrawal had the effect of improving SWC group results.

Chandrasekaran and colleagues (2012) used a UVC and laser combination for managing an extensive, infected and intolerably painful wound following transmetatarsal amputation in a patient with diabetes. The UVC protocol was based on the above Nussbaum study. Laser therapy was applied using an 820 nm, single diode at 2 J/cm^2 in contact around the wound edge and a multiprobe consisting of 4 × 660 nm and 4 × 880 nm diodes at 4 J/cm^2 on the wound bed. Both modalities were applied daily. Wound closure was achieved following 23 sessions over a 5-week period. Follow-up at 3 months showed no wound breakdown in spite of patients' metabolic instability.

Nussbaum et al (2013) conducted a further study on pressure ulcer healing in people with spinal cord injury in order to determine whether UVC was beneficial without adding US. The later study was performed in a double-blind, placebo-controlled fashion. Forty-three subjects with 58 ulcers were assigned to groups by concealed randomization with stratification for ulcer area on the basis that the earlier study showed that lower extremity ulcers were slower healing than pelvic ulcers. UVC or placebo UVC was applied 3 days each week until ulcers were closed, or patients were discharged from the facility. Ulcers were photographed weekly, measured digitally and analysed for percent wound area relative to baseline each week, mean weekly percent wound area change (averaged over weeks of participation for each ulcer) and weeks to closure. During weeks 1 through 8, stage 2 pelvic ulcers had decreased from 76% to 26% of the baseline area using UVC versus from 180% to 111% in the placebo group; achieved significant level (ASL) 0.03–0.08; effect size 0.5–0.8. For all stage 2 ulcers the mean weekly percentage reductions in wound sizes were 36.6% and 5.8% for UVC and placebo groups, respectively (ASL=0.09); the UVC effect greatly exceeded the Minimal Clinically Important Difference. There were no group differences for stage 3 and 4 ulcers. The authors discussed limitations of their study, including the unbalanced distribution of subjects. They advised that further stratification should have been performed to address time since onset, which was significantly longer in the UVC group, ulcer size and patient status with respect to institution-based versus outpatient status. The authors noted the very wide variance associated with the results and suggested that heterogeneity of the sample compromised ability to show significance in some measures. In addition, they recommended that in future studies researchers should consider using wound depth or volume as an outcome measure on the basis that stage 4 ulcers heal from the wound base upwards, therefore wound surface area is a poor measure of short-term response to treatment in the case of deep ulcers.

APPLICATION PRINCIPLES AND TREATMENT PARAMETERS

Dosimetry

UV lamps vary in output and beam area. Irradiance (W/cm^2) is calculated using the lamp output/beam area; energy dose, J/cm^2, is calculated by irradiance × time (seconds). However, introducing a space between the lamp face and the skin surface results in beam expansion which changes the irradiance; this confounds attempts to report the energy dose at the wound surface without use of expensive equipment, such as a radiometer-photometer. It is even more problematic to determine UV dose at the base of a cavity.

TABLE 11.1 Erythema Characteristics of an E1 Dose of UVC	
Latency	Appears in 3–6 hours
Colour at 8 hrs	Patchy pink with no clear borders
Duration	Fades in 24–36 hours
Blister formation	None
Desquamation	None

Past custom among physiotherapists has been to describe dosage in terms of skin response to UV rather than in J/cm^2. The response factor is erythema (E) and the response level (E1–E4) is determined by the following erythema factors: latency (response delay, measured in hours), duration (hours to disappear), colour intensity (at peak presentation), blister formation and desquamation. Table 11.1 shows E1 characteristics for UVC. Dermatologists describe UV intensity using the term MED (Minimal Erythema Development) with levels of sub-MED and MED1–4. An E1 as described in Table 11.1 is approximately equal to a MED1.

Skin colour (e.g. Fitzpatrick type I–VI) significantly affects erythema and pigmentation development when using UVA and UVB due to absorption of these wavelengths by melanin. Thus, when using UVA or UVB, individual skin sensitivity tests must be performed to determine individual E1 exposure times. Generally, fair-skinned people, because they have less melanin, which provides sun protection, have a shorter E1 time than dark-skinned individuals. Importantly, skin colour plays a minimal role in UVC effects because UVC absorption takes place in the keratin layer rather than in epidermal layers that could be rich in melanin. It is sufficient to establish the average time for an E1 dose for a particular UVC lamp and that time functions as the E1 for all patients, regardless of skin colour, when using that specific lamp.

Manufacturers usually rate the output of their UV lamps. UVC lamps of the type shown in Fig. 11.1A have a rated output of about 14–15 mW/cm^2. Exposing skin for 15 seconds with 2.5 cm spacing between the lamp face and the skin surface typically produces an E1 response using these lamps. New lamps should be tested on 6–10 individuals to confirm that on average a 15 second exposure at 2.5 cm spacing produces an E1 dose. Lamps should be re-tested annually to confirm the output has not changed. A quick method of testing lamps is suggested in Box 11.1.

BOX 11.1   Procedure for Establishing Average E1 Dose for a UVC Lamp

Recruit six or more persons with light, medium light or medium dark skin colouring. While UVC also produces erythema in dark skin, the colour change is difficult to see. Using an alcohol swab, clean the lamp face and test area, usually anterior forearm skin.

Prepare a template using strong paper or an index card. Cut out three shapes, each about the size of a thumbnail and spaced about 3 cm apart. Expose the first shape to UVC at 2.5 cm distance from the skin (measured accurately) while shielding the other two shapes from the beam. Repeat for the remaining two shapes, using a graded series of exposures, usually 10, 15 and 20 seconds. The objective is to determine for each recruit which exposure most closely represents the characteristics of an E1 dose when considering latency, colour and duration. All three exposures are in the range of an E1 dose: if the 10-second response is barely visible and has faded by 18 hours, it is closer to a sub-E1 dose; a dark pink patch with clearly defined borders is closer to an E2 dose. The average E1 time for the group is taken as the *lamp* E1 exposure time.

TABLE 11.2   Calculation of Treatment Time as a Function of E1 Dose for UVC Lamps

Erythema Level	Time as Multiple of E1 Dose
E2	3 × E1
E3	6 × E1
E4	12 × E1
2E4	24 × E1

Five levels of erythema, E1–E4 and 2E4, are used in practice. Exposure time for doses in excess of E1 are calculated from the E1 dose, as shown in Table 11.2.

Treatment Technique

The clinician washes hands appropriately and dons gloves: clean but not sterile technique is required. The lamp face, lamp body and supply cord are thoroughly cleaned using 70% alcohol wipes. Supplies as needed are laid out on a clean or sterile paper towel including sterile spatula or cotton-tipped probe, petroleum jelly and a timer.

Wound preparation. The wound is irrigated prior to radiation. The wound is assessed for area and depth, surface appearance, discharge and odour.

Protective goggles are donned by the patient and therapist to prevent conjunctival irritation.

Treatment is delivered in two steps.
1. The *peri skin* is always irradiated with an E1 dose.
2. The *wound bed* is irradiated with an E1 dose when red granulation tissue fills the wound to within 0.5 cm of the surface. Additional exposure may be needed to address increasing wound depth and increasing severity of surface appearance. Different areas within the wound might require different doses.

Periwound skin should be screened from UVC in excess of an E1 dose using petroleum jelly and paper towel (Fig. 11.2A–C). Figs 11.3–11.5 illustrate dose selection and treatment progression based on wound surface appearance, depth and discharge. A further guide for treating the wound bed is provided in Table 11.3.

Completion. After radiation, petroleum jelly is lightly removed using a cotton bud or moist gauze. Petroleum jelly is inert and forms the basis of many popular wound dressing materials: a small residual amount in or around the wound is not harmful. The wound is covered using suitable dressings to keep it moist.

Treatment Tips

- UVC does not penetrate through wound dressings, including transparent membrane-type dressings (Rao et al 2011).
- UVC readily penetrates through 2- or 3-ply facial tissues, such as Kleenex, therefore facial-type tissue should not be used for screening purposes.
- Beam penetration is maximum at perpendicular incidence, which means the lamp face should be held parallel to the tissue surface. Reflectance at the air-tissue interface increases with increasing angle of incidence, which means dosage is reduced.
- Incidence will not be perpendicular when radiating wounds that encircle body parts, for example, the distal lower leg. To compensate for the loss of intensity, the curved surface should be irradiated from two directions, off-set from each other by about 90°. Approximately 2 half doses will be delivered in the area where the beams overlap.
- The established treatment time for an E1 dose of UVC is not increased for repeat exposures. UVC is absorbed in the upper epidermis where it has minimal effects on melanocyte proliferation and migration in the lower epidermis; thus successive exposures do not interfere with absorption in the keratin skin layer. The same rule does not apply to UVA and UVB: for these, treatment time must be increased at succeeding sessions to account for increasing skin pigmentation which screens UVA and UVB from reaching their absorption sites in the lower epidermis and dermis.

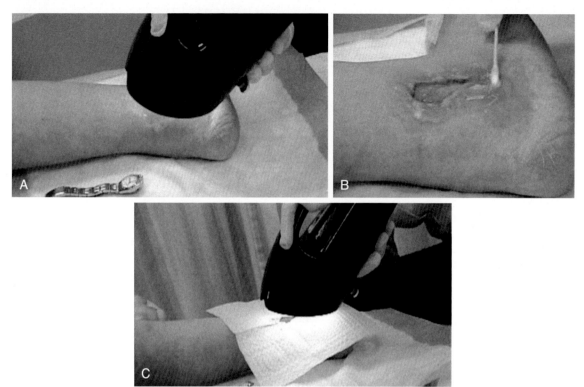

Fig. 11.2 (A) Step 1: An E1 dose to the periwound skin and wound bed. The lamp face is centred over the wound and held parallel to the skin surface. Exposure time is 15 seconds at 2.5 cm skin-lamp distance. (B) Step 2: petroleum jelly and paper towel are applied to screen the periwound skin from any further UVC. (C) Continuing Step 2: During the initial exposure (2A), the wound base received 15 seconds of UVC. The base is about 5 mm deep, is poorly granulating and there are some areas covered in thin yellow fibrous tissue – indication for an E3 exposure. An E3 dose is 90 seconds: thus, an additional 75 seconds is delivered to the wound base.

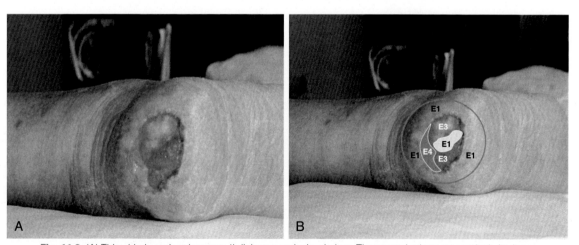

Fig. 11.3 (A) This elderly patient has type II diabetes and a heel ulcer. The wound edges are vertical. At deepest point the wound depth is 5 mm. The wound surface shows healthy granulation over a small area and other areas of either light or heavy fibrous tissue. (B) Suggested UVC exposure for the ulcer areas shown in A: To be efficient, the peri skin and surface are exposed to an E1 dose using multiple exposures, based on the size of the lamp face versus wound size, and curvatures of the heel. Next, the areas designated as E1 are screened from additional dose using petroleum jelly and paper cut-out. The remaining wound surface areas are exposed for an additional 75 seconds to make up to an E3 dose (15 + 75 = 90 s). Next, the areas designated for E3 dose are screened using petroleum jelly and paper cut-out and the remaining area is exposed for 90 seconds to make up to an E4 dose (90 + 90 = 180 s).

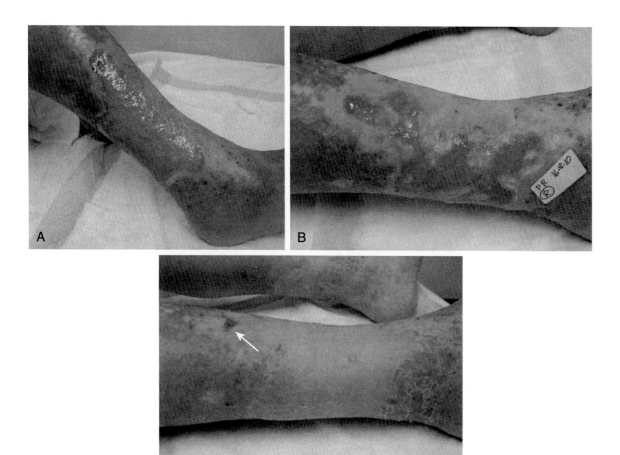

Fig. 11.4 (A) This 60-year-old female patient had a 10-year history of steadily deteriorating bilateral venous ulcers. Her problems included debilitating pain and copious wound drainage. She used high doses of oxycontin and applied absorbent dressings plus abdominal pads around her ankles to manage the discharge. Examination showed ulceration completely encircling both lower legs. Wound surfaces were pale pink, very wet and level with surrounding skin; wound edges were not advancing. Due to transport problems, the patient agreed to attend clinic no more than twice weekly. All ulcerated areas and surrounding peri skin were exposed to an E1 dose. The lateral lower right leg is shown on treatment day 1. (B) The right lower leg after 6 treatments (3 weeks). (C) The right lower leg after 14 weeks. Ulcers are closed bilaterally except for the last remaining area indicated by an arrow.

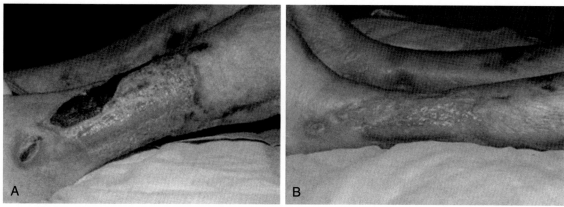

Fig. 11.5 (A) This hospitalized patient had cardiovascular disease and lung cancer. The ischemic ulcer on her lower leg consisted partly of thick, black eschar, partly of yellow fibrous tissue turning brown and some pale granulation. Treatment plan for day 1 was to expose peri skin to E1, the granulating area to E2, the fibrous tissue to E4 and eschar to 2E4. (B) At the end of 3 weeks of 3 times weekly UVC, the wound bed was clear of eschar. A change in treatment plan was indicated at this time: areas of fibrous tissue were exposed to E3 and granulating areas and peri skin to E1 dose 3 times weekly.

TABLE 11.3	Recommended UVC Treatment for the Wound Bed or Part of the Wound Bed	
Erythema Dose	**Surface Features and Depth Factor**	**Treatment Objective**
E1	The surface displays beefy red granulation. There is no slough. The wound edges slope towards the wound base. Depth is 1–5 mm. If these features combine with depth of more than 5 mm, replace with an E2 dose.	Stimulate epithelialization
E2	The surface is pale pink or greyish; depth is 1–5 mm. There is no slough. If these features combine with depth of more than 5 mm, replace with an E3 dose.	Stimulate granulation
E3	The surface shows yellow or grey slough, OR is infected, OR produces purulent or malodorous discharge. OR the wound is deep with vertical edges joining a pale wound base. OR the wound base is red but depth is greater than 1 cm.	Eradicate bacteria; stimulate granulation
E4–2E4	The wound surface displays dense yellow slough and necrotic debris, or brown or black eschar. The wound depth may not be visible because of necrotic fill.	Debridement

SUMMARY

The literature strongly supports the use of UVC as an alternative to oral and topical antibiotics for eradicating bacteria in open wounds; UVC may also have a role in preventing infection. There is evidence that UV accelerates the rate of closure of pressure ulcers. Case studies show the potential of UV to improve healing of other types of wounds, including venous ulcers and diabetic foot ulcers; however, controlled trials are lacking for these wound types. Treatment is formulated based on immediate wound assessment; intact skin is exposed to no more than a mildly stimulating dose (E1 dose) and the open wound is exposed according to surface appearance of healthy red granulation (E1) as opposed to pale grey tissue, slough or eschar (E2–2E4). Dose is further adjusted for wound depth. Treatment is feasible in any healthcare setting, such as in the home, clinic or institution, as equipment is relatively inexpensive as well as portable, and adverse effects have not been reported in the literature.

REFERENCES

Alcantara-Diaz, D., Brena-Valle, M., & Serment-Guerrero, J. (2004). Divergent adaptation of E. coli to cyclic ultraviolet light exposures. *Mutagenesis*, 19, 349–354.

Chandrasekaran, B., Chettri, R., Agrawal, N., & Sathyamoorthy, C. (2012). Short-term multimodal phototherapy approach in a diabetic ulcer patient. *Singapore Medical Journal*, 53(6), e122–124.

Chauvin, D., & LaPier, T. K. (2005). Treatment of a chronic lower extremity ulcer with ultraviolet C light: A case report. *Acute Care Perspectives*, 14(2), 13–19.

Chen, C., Hou, W. H., Chan, E. S. Y., Yeh, M. L., & Lo, H. L. D. (2014). Phototherapy for treating pressure ulcers. *Cochrane Database of Systematic Reviews* (7), CD009224. https://doi.org/10.1002/14651858.CD009224.pub2.

Conner-Kerr, T. A., Sullivan, P. K., Gaillard, J., Franklin, M. E., & Jones, R. M. (1998). The effects of ultraviolet radiation on antibiotic-resistant bacteria. *Ostomy Wound Management*, 44(10), 50–56.

Crous, L. C., & Malherbe, C. P. (1988). Laser and ultraviolet light irradiation in the treatment of chronic ulcers. *Physiotherapy*, 44(3), 73–77.

Dai, T., Vrahas, M. S., Murray, C. K., & Hamblin, M. R. (2012a). Ultraviolet C irradiation: An alternative antimicrobial approach to localized infections? *Expert Review of Anti-infective Therapy*, 10, 185–195.

Dai, T., Garcia, B., Murray, C. K., Vrahas, M. S., & Hamblin, M. R. (2012b). UVC light prophylaxis for cutaneous wound infections in mice. *Antimicrobial Agents and Chemotherapy*, 56(7), 3841–3848.

Dai, T., Tegos, G. P., St Denis, T. G., Anderson, D., Sinofsky, E., & Hamblin, M. R. (2011). Ultraviolet-C irradiation for prevention of central venous catheter-related infections: An in vitro study. *Journal of Photochemistry and Photobiology A*, 87, 250–255.

Devary, Y., et al. (1993). NF-kappa B activation by ultraviolet light not dependent on a nuclear signal. *Science*, 261(5127), 442.

Diffey, B. L., & Farr, P. M. (2017). Ultraviolet erythema: Dose response and mediator diffusion. *Photochemical and Photobiological Sciences*, 17, 1941–1945.

Diffey, B. L., & Oakley, A. M. (1987). The onset of ultraviolet erythema. *British Journal of Dermatology*, 116, 183–187.

Farr, P. M., & Diffey, B. L. (1985). The erythemal response of human skin to ultraviolet radiation. *British Journal of Dermatology*, 113, 65–76.

Freytes, H. A., Fernandez, B., & Fleming, W. C. (1965). Ultraviolet light in the treatment of indolent ulcers. *Southern Medical Journal*, 58(2), 223–226.

High, A. S., & High, J. P. (1983). Treatment of infected skin wounds using ultraviolet radiation – an in-vitro study. *Physiotherapy*, 69, 359–360.

Huang, R.-P., Wu, J.-X., Fan, Y., & Adamson, E. D. (1996). UV activates growth factor receptors via reactive oxygen intermediates. *Journal Cell Biology*, 133, 211–220.

James, L. C., Moore, A. M., Wheeler, L. A., Murphy, G. M., Dowd, P. M., & Greaves, M. W. (1991). Transforming growth factor alpha: In vivo release by normal human skin following UV irradiation and abrasion. *Skin Pharmacology and Physiology*, 4, 61–64.

Kaidbey, K. H., & Klingman, A. H. (1981). Cumulative effects from repeated exposures to ultraviolet radiation. *Inv Dermatology*, 76, 352–355.

Lee, L. D. (2017). Surface and air: What impact does UV-C at the room level have on airborne and surface bacteria? *Canadian Journal of Infection Control*, 32(2), 108–111.

Matz, H. (2010). Phototherapy for psoriasis: What to choose and how to use: Facts and controversies. *Clinics in Dermatology*, 28, 73–80.

Morykwas, M. J., & Mark, M. W. (1998). Effects of ultraviolet light on fibroblast fibronectin production and lattice contraction. *Wounds: A Compendium of Clinical Research and Practice*, 10(4), 111–117.

Nussbaum, E., Biemann, I., & Mustard, B. (1994). Comparison of ultrasound/ultraviolet-C and laser for treatment of pressure ulcers in patients with spinal cord injury. *Physical Therapy*, 74, 812–823.

Nussbaum, E. L., Flett, H., Hitzig, S. L., McGillivray, C. F., Leber, D., Morris, H., et al. (2013). Ultraviolet-C irradiation in the management of pressure ulcers in people with spinal cord injury: A randomized, placebo-controlled trial. *Archives of Physical Medicine and Rehabilitation*, 94, 650–659.

Onigbinde, A. T., Adedoyin, R. A., Ojoawo, O. A., Johnson, O. E., Obembe, A. O., Olafimihan, F. K., et al. (2010). Effects of ultraviolet radiation (type B) on wound exudates, appearance and depth description. *Technology and Health Care*, 18, 297–302.

Parrish, J. A., Jaenicke, K. F., & Anderson, R. R. (1982). Erythema and melanogenesis action spectra of normal human skin. *Photochemistry and Photobiology*, 36, 187–191.

Rao, B. K., Kumar, P., Rao, S., & Gurung, B. (2011). Bactericidal effect of ultraviolet C (UVC), direct and filtered through transparent plastic, on gram-positive cocci: An in vitro study. *Physical Therapy*, 57(7), 46–52.

Rosette, C., & Karin, M. (1996). Ultraviolet light and osmotic stress: Activation of the JNK cascade through multiple growth factor and cytokine receptors. *Science*, 274, 1194–1197.

Sachsenmaier, C., Radler-Pohl, A., Zinck, R., et al. (1994). Involvement of growth factor receptors in the mammalian UVC response. *Cell*, 78, 963–972.

Shelk J, Morgan P. (2000). Narrow-band UVB: A practical approach. *Dermatology Nursing*, 12(6), 407–411.

Shimomura, A., Tahara, D., Tominaga, M., Uchigiri, S., Yamaguchi, Y., Ishioka, H., et al. (1995). The effect of ultraviolet rays on the prevention of exit-site infections. *Advances in Peritoneal Dialysis*, 11, 152–156.

Sullivan, P. K., & Conner-Kerr, T. A. (2000). A comparative study of the effects of UVC irradiation on select procaryotic and eucaryotic wound pathogens. *Ostomy/ Wound Manage*, 46(10), 28–34.

Thai, T. P., Houghton, P. E., Campbell, K. E., & Woodbury, M. G. (2002). Ultraviolet light C in the treatment of chronic wounds with MRSA. *Ostomy Wound Management*, 48, 52–60.

Thai, T. P., Keast, D. H., Campbell, K. E., Woodbury, M. G., & Houghton, P. E. (2005). Effect of ultraviolet light C on bacterial colonization in chronic wounds. *Ostomy Wound Management, 51*, 32–45.

Vangipuram, R., & Feldman, S. R. (2016). Ultraviolet phototherapy for cutaneous diseases: A concise review. *Oral Diseases, 22*(4), 253–259.

Veierød, M. B., Adami, H. O., Lund, E., Armstrong, B. K., & Weiderpass, E. (2010). Sun and solarium exposure and melanoma risk: Effects of age, pigmentary characteristics, and nevi. *Cancer Epidemiology, Biomarkers & Prevention: A Publication of the American Association for Cancer Research, Cosponsored by the American Society of Preventive Oncology, 19*(1), 111–120.

Wills, E. E., Anderson, T. W., Beattie, B. L., & Scott, A. (1983). A randomized placebo-controlled trial of ultraviolet light in the treatment of superficial pressure sores. *Journal of the American Geriatrics Society, 31*, 131–133.

Wysocki, A. B. (2002). Evaluating and managing open skin wounds: Colonization versus infection. *AACN Clinical Issues, 13*(3), 382–397.

Yin, R., Dai, T., Avci, P., Jorge, A. E., de Melo, W. C., Vecchio, D., et al. (2013). Light based anti-infectives: Ultraviolet C irradiation, photodynamic therapy, blue light, and beyond. *Current Opinion in Pharmacology, 13*, 731–762.

12

Magnetic and Pulsed Magnetic (PEMF) Therapies

Oscar Ronzio

CHAPTER OUTLINE

INTRODUCTION – HISTORY

Magnetotherapy includes the use of static magnets and pulsed electromagnetic fields (PEMFs) (Laakso et al 2009). Pulsed EM field applications will be considered in this chapter. Many authors have used the acronym 'PEMF' to describe radio-frequency applications, such as shortwave, which has unfortunately led to some confusion about this term. Whilst there is no universally accepted definition of magnetotherapy, nor indeed PEMFs or PEMFT, in the context of this chapter, it is taken to mean the use of dynamic magnetic fields as a therapeutic application. The use of radio-frequency EM fields (such as shortwave or microwave) are covered elsewhere (Chapter 7). Multiple alternative terms – such as magnetic field therapy (MFT), low field magnetic stimulation (LFMS), electromagnetic pulse therapy (EMPT) and many similar variations – are avoided in this text.

In the early 1900s, with the increased use of electricity, many devices appeared that delivered treatment with PEMF (Rosch & Markov 2004). In the 1950s, Fukada and Yasuda (1957) identified the presence of piezoelectric effects in bone, which are generated in response to physical stress. On the basis that these endogenous currents have an evidenced role in bone healing, clinicians started to employ PEMF generators as a means to stimulate repair after fracture. Early trials (e.g. Bassett 1978; Fukuda & Yasuda 1957) used PEMF to treat delayed union and non-union fractures in preference to the existing direct current applications. The FDA has approved several PEMF devices since that time (Yuan et al 2018).

More recently, high-intensity PEMF (in the range of 2–3 T) have become popular for electrical and transcranial stimulation (Oberman et al 2014; Oberman et al 2016; Pastuszak et al 2016).

PHYSICAL PRINCIPLES

Electromagnetic waves have two components: the electric (E) and the magnetic (M), which are at 90° to each other (Fig. 12.1).

A magnetic field is created when the current flows through a coiled conductor, producing an amplification of the magnetic component (M) (Laakso et al 2009). Its strength used to be expressed in gauss (G), but the actual unit is the tesla (T) and 1 tesla is the equivalent of 10,000 G. Since the intensity in these devices is low, millitesla (mT) is the unit used. The intensity employed in therapy is usually between 1 and 40 mT.

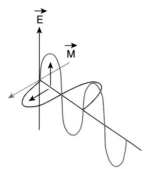

Fig. 12.1 Electric (*E*) and magnetic (*M*) fields.

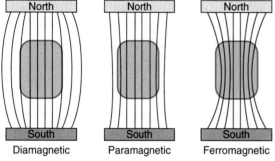

Fig. 12.2 Types of materials.

It is important to differentiate between magnetic field intensity (H) and magnetic field induction (B), which depends on the material magnetic permeability (μ). The formula is expressed:

$$B = \mu \cdot H$$

Materials are classified into diamagnetic (showing no interaction when exposed to a magnetic field), paramagnetic (showing a weak interaction) and ferromagnetic (showing a very strong interaction) (Fig. 12.2). The value for μ depends on the type of material involved.

The most commonly used PEMFs are in the range of 1 to 100 Hz, with a wavelength from 300,000 to 3,000 Km. These types of radiation are included in the 'super extremely low frequency' (1–30 Hz) and 'extremely low frequency' (30–300 Hz) spectrum. Given their frequency, they are a non-thermal agent (Saliev et al 2014; Rosso et al 2015). It is also possible to find other devices with a higher frequency (3000–4000 Hz, in the low frequency spectrum) which have a lower magnetic field (in the range of 1–2 mT).

BIOPHYSICAL EFFECTS, INTERACTIONS AND RESPONSES

The body has both diamagnetic and paramagnetic materials, and therefore some of the tissues show a greater B (induction) than others.

PEMF works by inducing microcurrents in the tissues. In some tissues, mechanical compression and expansion produces electricity due to the piezoelectric phenomenon (Fukuda & Yasuda 1957). In addition, if a magnetic field is applied perpendicular to the transmembrane cation channels, it could affect the ion electrostatic field, thus producing electrical currents as a result of the Hall effect (Balcavage et al 1996; Rodriguez Martin 2014).

Another theory that explains how PEMF works was presented by Liboff. He states that every ion has a specific frequency for its stimulation, according to the 'ion cyclotron resonance' formula. For example, resonance frequency for Ca^{++} is 16 Hz (McLeod & Rubin 1997; Foletti et al 2013).

PEMFs are widely used to promote osteogenesis. It was observed in an in vitro model that an eight-hour exposure to PEMF increases PGE_2 and TGF-β1 (which decreases osteoclastic activity), modulates NO_2- and increases alkaline phosphatase activity (Lohmann et al 2003). Other findings show that PEMFs induce an increase in BMP-2 BMP-4 mRNA levels, which may explain a possible mechanism underlying the osteogenic effects (Bodamyali et al 1998). A systematic review including 42 in vitro studies has shown evidence for an association of PEMFs with internal calcium concentration (Golbach et al 2016). A rat tibial model showed that PEMFs (72 mT, 50 Hz, 30 minutes, 2/day) accelerated bone-healing when compared with the control group (Grana et al 2008). Specific parameters that promote bone differentiation in vitro still have to be translated to clinical trials (Ross et al 2015).

PEMF has been shown to affect cells that might play a role in limiting inflammatory responses. In an in vitro investigation, PEMFs induced apoptotic cell death in T lymphocytes (Nindl et al 2003). This could be beneficial in chronic inflammatory diseases, including osteoarthritis and rheumatoid arthritis (Beaulieu et al 2016). PEMFs also inhibit cAMP accumulation and increase A2A and A3ARs, reducing pro-inflammatory cytokines, and potentially protecting tissues from the catabolic effects of inflammation. This protection may explain why several articles reported chondrocyte proliferation and synthesis of cartilage components, including proteoglycans and collagen type II (Rosso et al 2015; Varani et al 2017). In an in vitro study, nasal and articular chondrocytes were exposed to PEMF (75 Hz, 2.3 mT), inducing an increase in cell proliferation (Pezzetti et al 1999; Ross et al 2015). The effect of PEMFs on inflammation could lead indirectly to pain relief (Beaulieu et al 2016). PEMFs also promote the release of growth factors, such as NGF (Longo et al 1999), IGF-I (Varani et al 2017), IGF-II (Pezzetti et al 1999) and FGF-2 (Tepper et al 2004). Significant changes in blood flow velocity of the smallest superficial observable veins were observed as well.

High-intensity PEMF transcranial magnetic stimulation causes neuron depolarization, thus generating motor, cognitive and emotional effects. Although the mechanisms of action are not yet clear, it is probable that it causes the release of neurotransmitters, modulation of signal transduction pathways, gene transcription and the release of neuroprotective substances (Pastuszak et al 2016).

CLINICAL EVIDENCE

Osteoporosis and Osteogenic Effect

Many reports suggest that PEMFs have a positive impact on osteogenesis. Their use (72 Hz) was observed to significantly increase bone mineral density (Wang et al 2016). Other authors described that PEMFs (8 Hz, 3.82 mT) were as effective in preventing bone loss as alendronate in treating postmenopausal osteoporosis (Wang et al 2016; Zhu et al 2017).

A protocol comparing PEMF application (33 Hz, 50 mT, 30 minutes, 3/week, 12 weeks) with circuit weight training found that both interventions had positive effects on bone mineral density, with a significant difference favouring PEMF in the inter group analysis (Elsisi et al 2015).

Bone Healing

Postoperative exposure to PEMF (4 hours/day, 90 days) following instrumented arthrodesis of the lumbar spine increased consolidation (276% greater chance, OR = 3.76, 16% more consolidation) in the first year after surgery (Risso Neto et al 2017). PEMF stimulus (5–105 Hz, 0.5–2 mT, sinusoidal signals, 1/day, 1 hour, 8 weeks) promotes earlier bone healing compared with placebo in diaphyseal femoral fractures, permitting quicker return to usual daily activities (Martinez-Rondanelli et al 2014).

In scaphoid fractures treated with low-intensity PEMF, fewer work days were lost in the active PEMF group, compared with the placebo group (Hannemann et al 2015). In another clinical trial, this therapy (75 Hz, 1.5 mT, 4 hours daily, 60 days) did not lead to a higher percentage of patients who resumed sports or to earlier resumption of sports after arthroscopic debridement and microfracture of osteochondral talar defects (Reilingh et al 2016). A systematic review and meta-analysis comparing PEMF and LIPUS (Chapter 9) suggests that both interventions could be beneficial for treating acute fractures, shortening time to radiological union (Hannemann et al 2014). Another

review states there is not sufficient evidence to establish the effectiveness of interventions (including PEMF) used in the rehabilitation of adults with fractures of the distal radius (Handoll & Elliott 2015), probably because they only included two articles, each of them with different dose variables (in the first one they used 25 Hz, 6 mT, 30 minutes, concentric coil applicator, 50 cm in diameter and 35 cm high, 5 days a week for 2 weeks; the other one used 50 Hz, 9.9 mT, 30 minutes, u-shaped applicator, with an internal diameter of 12 cm and length of 30 cm, during only 5 consecutive days) (Cheing et al 2005; Lazovic et al 2012).

Knee Arthroplasty

Some clinical trials reported clinical benefit when using PEMF (75 Hz, 1.5–0.3 mT, 4/day, for 60 days) after knee arthroplasty. Pain, knee swelling and functional scores were significantly better in the treated compared with the control group. Pain was still significantly milder at a six-month follow-up. Three years after surgery, severe pain and occasional walking limitations were reported in fewer patients in the treated group. Effects on early control of inflammation may explain the results (Adravanti et al 2014). Another trial showed that this therapy improved functional recovery and restored bone stock. It shows benefits in mobility and pain relief even when applied before surgery (Ibrahim et al 2013).

Osteoarthritis

In knee osteoarthritis, a coil-less device (delivering 8 Hz, 105 mT, twice a day, 5 minutes, for 10 days) showed a highly significant reduction in pain, stiffness and disability in daily activities according to the WOMAC scale (Wuschech et al 2015). Another clinical trial showed that PEMFs (25 Hz, 20 mT, 30 minutes, 3/weeks, during 7 weeks) promote pain reduction and functional capacity (da Silva et al 2016). A meta-analysis, including nine studies with a total of 636 participants, suggests that PEMFs may provide pain relief in osteoarthritis (Li et al 2013).

In hand osteoarthritis, the group that received PEMF (25 Hz, 0.5–8 mT, 20 minutes/day, for 10 days), combined with active range of motion and strengthening, produced pain reduction, improving function and quality of life scores compared with sham group (Kanat et al 2013).

Application of PEMF (15 Hz, 2 mT, 20 minutes) in children with haemophilia was compared with laser therapy. Both were effective in reducing pain and swelling increasing range of movement and improving physical fitness (Eid & Aly 2015).

Tendinopathies

A systematic review found no significant results in pain reduction in elbow tendinopathies (Dingemanse et al 2014).

However, authors included three articles to reach this conclusion. The older two are not available in databases, so the used dose could not be analysed (Chard & Hazleman 1988; Devereaux et al 1985). The third one compares PEMF (6 mT, 25 and 4.6 Hz consecutively, 30 minutes, no waveform informed, 15 sessions, during 3 weeks) versus sham PEMF versus corticosteroid plus anaesthetic injection, showing better long term results for PEMF (Uzunca et al 2007). Another systematic review in subacromial impingement syndrome highlights two clinical trials: one of them showed a positive effect on pain (the original article was not available and the dose was not described) while the other revealed no significant differences (50 Hz, 30 G, 25 minutes per session, 3 weeks, totalling 15 sessions) (Aktas et al 2006; Gebremariam et al 2014). A clinical trial in shoulder impingement showed that the combination of PEMF (30 minutes, 50 Hz, 20 mT) and exercise was effective in improving function, muscle strength and decreasing pain (Galace de Freitas et al 2014). In subacromial pain syndrome, there is strong evidence indicating that PEMF has no effect on pain reduction and moderate evidence showing only a slight effect on functional improvement (Haik et al 2016).

It has to be considered that the biomechanical origin of shoulder impingement could be the reason why the results of PEMF effects are controversial. In this pathology in particular, it is necessary to treat the patient with a biomechanical approach in addition to other appropriate therapies (Seitz et al 2011). Nevertheless, it was suggested that PEMF could have a positive role in tenocyte activation after extracorporeal shockwave therapy (ESWT) (Rosso et al 2015).

Pain

Many studies have evaluated the analgesic effects of PEMF therapy. Positive results have been reported in various pain disorders, such as rheumatoid arthritis, fibromyalgia, polyneuropathy, and persistent neck pain, including inflammatory and postoperative pain conditions (Beaulieu et al 2016).

PEMF application (75 Hz, 1.5 mT) following a rotator cuff repair reduces postoperative pain, the use of analgesics and stiffness in the short term (3 months) (Osti et al 2015). It also reduces postoperative pain, inflammation and the use of narcotics following transverse rectus abdominis flap breast reconstruction (Rohde et al 2015).

Positive effects have been found in clinical trials where PEMF was used to treat patients with fibromyalgia. A very low-intensity PEMF stimulation (8 Hz, 20 minutes, 1/week, 8 weeks, 27 coils, 2 cm each, 43 nT at 1 cm) caused significant improvement regarding somatosensory pain thresholds, the ability to perform daily activities, perceived chronic pain and sleep quality (Maestú et al 2013)

and using higher intensities (1 to 80 Hz, 100 µT, multifrequency, 30 minutes, 3/week, 4 weeks) also showed positive results on pain (Paolucci et al 2016).

PEMF (1 Hz, 0.2 T peak at 5 mm from coil) has been tested in a delayed onset muscle soreness model and was found to be effective in reducing associated physiological deficits and symptoms (Jeon et al 2015).

The direct effect of PEMF (10 minutes, 60 Hz, 0.9 mT, without modulation) was evaluated in a heat pain model (before and after design). The results showed no change in pain intensity or unpleasantness, supporting the idea that PEMFs work in an indirect manner due to their anti-inflammatory effects (Beaulieu et al 2016).

Depression

Some articles suggest that low-strength transcranial PEMF stimulation has an antidepressant effect, even though the mechanism is not yet clear (Van Belkum et al 2016).

Cancer

There are several studies relating to cancer that are not strictly clinical trials The safety of PEMF has been examined using in vitro models and no cytotoxic or genotoxic effects were reported in studies using *Escherichia coli* cultures and plasmid DNA (Froes Meyer et al 2013). Other in vitro studies showed that PEMF increased apoptosis in some tumour types. However, there is no strong evidence to use PEMF in humans; therefore, its use is not currently recommended (Sadeghipour et al 2012; Vadala et al 2016).

THERAPEUTIC EFFECTS AND USES

PEMF effects have been corroborated in daily practice as well as in many types of research models. Unfortunately, clinicians from countries where PEMF use is quite common have not published their results; thus, the number of papers available is not consistent with the number of years this technology has been in use.

The most important effects are inflammation reduction and regeneration. That is why they are so useful in pathologies with inflammatory pain, osteoarthritis, postoperative periods, osteopenia, osteoporosis, bone and soft tissue healing. PEMF-based therapies could also be useful in tendinopathies to modulate the inflammation, but always taking into consideration the tendon pathology models and biomechanical factors for each tendon in particular. Using PEMF as an isolated treatment is not considered an evidenced choice.

Given the diversity of devices available, with different parameters with regard to frequency, pulse length and intensity, it is still difficult to establish the optimum dosage variables. The latest articles indicate, in general, long exposure times and low intensities (1–2 mT) for home-based programmes; in clinic applications, physiotherapists usually apply 30 minutes with higher flux intensities.

High-intensity PEMF (up to 2.5 T) devices, mainly developed to study brain functions, are being used to stimulate spinal cord fibres and peripheral nerves through neuromuscular electrical stimulation by induction. Their effects seems to be similar to those produced by neuromuscular electrical stimulation and transcutaneous electrical stimulation (Kroeling et al 2009). Given the high intensity nature of these treatments, they are unlikely to be employed outside specialist treatment centres in the immediate future.

APPLICATION

Procedures consist of the following steps:
1. **Choose the best coil for your target area**

   This type of device uses coils to generate PEMF. The most commonly used applicators are (a) tunnel-shaped and (b) flat devices. The differences between them are size, shape and the distribution of their magnetic fields. In the tunnel-shaped coil, the field follows the direction of the long axis (Fig. 12.3A). These types of coil have a stronger field towards the borders (represented in the dark-shaded area in Fig. 12.3B). The operator should always place the target area as near as possible to the borders. These kinds of coil are useful for larger treatment areas like the whole lower and upper limbs.

   Flat coils are smaller in size and the field direction is perpendicular to the coil (Fig. 12.4A). These can more easily achieve higher intensities and their field is stronger towards the centre (Fig. 12.4B). Sometimes manufacturers include a ferromagnetic nucleus to further increase the intensity in their centre. If a ferromagnetic nucleus is present, the operator should place the target area as near as possible to the centre of the coil. When there is no nucleus, it should be placed by the side of the centre of the coil. These kinds of coil are useful for smaller treatment areas, such as foot, knee, hip, spine, fingers, hand, elbow and shoulder.

2. **Position the coils**

   Position the stronger-intensity area of the coil on the target tissues and consider Lambert's cosine law.

   It is possible to use just one coil (Fig. 12.5), two in contra planar (Fig. 12.6) or even more in coplanar arrangements. If two or more coils are to be used, the poles should be opposing each other (Fig. 12.6), or else they would repel (Fig. 12.7). Another option is to use a ferromagnetic material to concentrate the field (Fig. 12.8).

3. **Select the waveform**

   When the coil is connected to a direct current it will produce a static field, i.e. not a PEMF. When connected to an alternating or a pulsed current source, it will generate time-varying fields (Fig. 12.9) (Laakso et al 2009).

   Devices can use alternating current (Fig. 12.9A), creating a magnetic field that alternates between north and south poles. Others apply a half-wave rectification (Fig. 12.9C) or a full-wave rectification that transforms 50 Hz into 100 Hz (Fig. 12.9E). When the current is rectified, the coil will have a north and a south side that will not change as it does with alternating current. It is also possible to apply burst-modulations, decreasing the duty cycle (Fig. 12.9B, D and F).

   Other waveforms are employed, such as square and sawtooth-shaped. The therapist should choose the optimal one for the specific treatment objective (Meyer et al 2011).

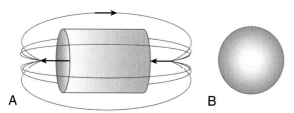

Fig. 12.3 Tunnel-shaped coil: The field follows the long axis direction and the intensity is stronger towards the borders. A: Magnetic field lateral representation. B: Magnetic field representation from an frontal view.

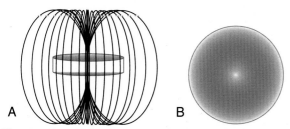

Fig. 12.4 Flat coil: The field is perpendicular to the coil and the intensity is stronger towards the centre. A: Magnetic field lateral representation. B: Magnetic field representation from an upper view.

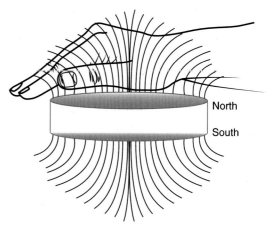

Fig. 12.5 Flat coil application.

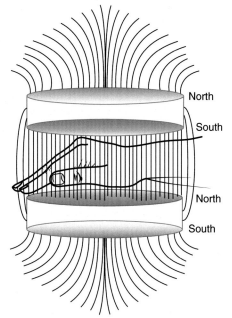

Fig. 12.6 Coils in contra planar with opposite poles. The flux density will be higher than when using just one coil.

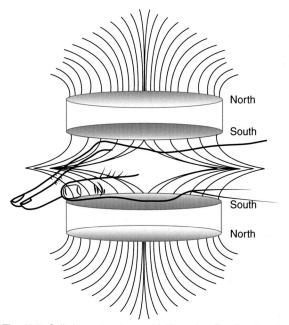

Fig. 12.7 Coils in contra planar with like poles. The flux density will be lower than when using just one coil, therefore, avoid this application.

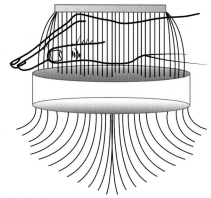

Fig. 12.8 Coil with a ferromagnetic material to increase flux density in the target area.

4. **Select the frequency**

   Select the frequency according to your treatment objective. The most commonly employed frequencies are 50–75 Hz, since these frequencies have been studied the most.

5. **Select the modulation**

   It is possible to modulate or not the emission (see point 3). Burst-modulations reduce coil heating in accordance with Joule's law. When the duty cycle is reduced, this should be compensated by increasing the treatment time. The biophysical effects of modulating or not the emission, could not be the same, but this has not yet been supported by publications.

6. **Set the intensity**

   Intensity should be set according to the cited evidence above and to the type of device available. The normal therapeutic ranges are between 1 mT and 40 mT.

7. **Set the timer**

   Time varies from a 30-minute treatment up to 8 hours/day (in case of a low power, home-based treatment).

8. **Corroborate the emission**

   In Super extremely low frequency and Extremely low frequency PEMF it is possible to test if the device is working by drawing a magnet close to the coils during the emission.

SUMMARY

Magnetotherapy includes the use of static magnets and pulsed electromagnetic fields (PEMFs).

Electromagnetic waves have two components: the electric (E) and the magnetic (M), which are oriented at 90° to each other. A magnetic field is created when the current flows through a coiled conductor, producing an amplification of the magnetic component (M).

The most commonly used PEMFs are in the range of 1 to 100 Hz. These types of radiations are included in the

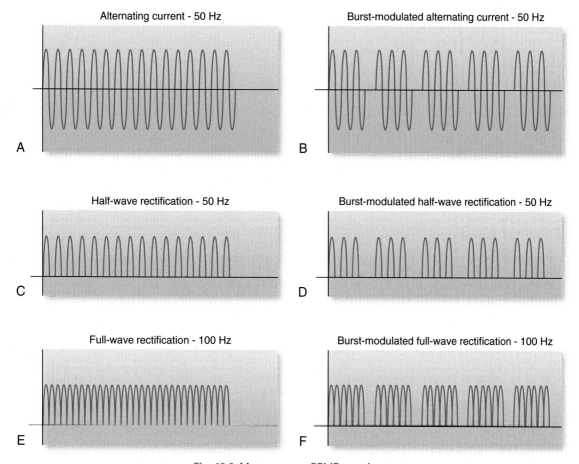

Fig. 12.9 Most common PEMF waveforms.

super extremely low frequency and extremely low frequency spectrum; consequently they are a non-thermal agent. The most studied frequencies are between 50 and 75 Hz. The intensity employed in therapy is usually between 1 and 40 mT.

PEMFs achieve their effects by inducing microcurrents and stimulating the release of growth factors, thereby promoting soft tissue and bone regeneration. They have also been shown to affect inflammatory cells and thus limit inflammation. This effect could lead indirectly to pain relief and tissue protection.

Clinical evidence demonstrates that PEMF-based therapy can be effective in osteoporosis, bone healing, osteoarthritis, knee arthroplasty, inflammatory and pain conditions (such as after a surgical procedure, rheumatoid arthritis, fibromyalgia, polyneuropathy, persistent neck pain). No results have been found in tendinopathies. Their use in depression and cancer is not recommended according the available evidence.

Given the diversity of devices available with different parameters, it is still difficult to establish the optimum dosage variables.

REFERENCES

Adravanti, P., Nicoletti, S., Setti, S., Ampollini, A., & De Girolamo, L. (2014). Effect of pulsed electromagnetic field therapy in patients undergoing total knee arthroplasty: A randomised controlled trial. *International Orthopaedics, 38*(2), 397–403.

Aktas, I., Akgun, K., & Cakmak, B. (2006). Therapeutic effect of pulsed electromagnetic field in conservative treatment of subacromial impingement syndrome. *Clinical Rheumatology, 26*(8), 1234–1239.

Balcavage, W. X., Alvager, T., Swez, J., Goff, C. W., Fox, M. T., Abdullyava, S., et al. (1996). A mechanism for action of extremely low frequency electromagnetic fields on biological systems. *Biochemical and Biophysical Research Communications, 222*(2), 374–378.

Bassett, C. A., S. N. Mitchell, L. Norton and A. Pilla (1978). "Repair of non-unions by pulsing electromagnetic fields." *Acta Orthopaedica Belgica*, 44(5), 706–724.

Beaulieu, K., Beland, P., Pinard, M., Handfield, G., Handfield, N., Goffaux, P., et al. (2016). Effect of pulsed electromagnetic field therapy on experimental pain: A double-blind, randomized study in healthy young adults. *Electromagnetic Biology and Medicine*, 35(3), 237–244.

Bodamyali, T., Bhatt, B., Hughes, F. J., Winrow, V. R., Kanczler, J. M., Simon, B., et al. (1998). Pulsed electromagnetic fields simultaneously induce osteogenesis and upregulate transcription of bone morphogenetic proteins 2 and 4 in rat osteoblasts in vitro. *Biochemical and Biophysical Research Communications*, 250(2), 458–461.

Chard, M., & Hazleman, B. (1988). Pulsed electromagnetic field treatment of chronic lateral humeral epicondylitis. *Clinical & Experimental Rheumatology*, 6(3), 330–332.

Cheing, G. L., Wan, J. W., & Kai Lo, S. (2005). Ice and pulsed electromagnetic field to reduce pain and swelling after distal radius fractures. *Journal of Rehabilitation Medicine: Official Journal of the UEMS European Board of Physical and Rehabilitation Medicine*, 37(6), 372–377.

Devereaux, M., Hazleman, B., & Thomas, P. P. (1985). Chronic lateral humeral epicondylitis--a double-blind controlled assessment of pulsed electromagnetic field therapy. *Clinical & Experimental Rheumatology*, 3(4), 333–336.

Dingemanse, R., Randsdorp, M., Koes, B. W., & Huisstede, B. M. (2014). Evidence for the effectiveness of electrophysical modalities for treatment of medial and lateral epicondylitis: A systematic review. *British Journal of Sports Medicine*, 48(12), 957–965.

Eid, M. A., & Aly, S. M. (2015). LASER versus electromagnetic field in treatment of hemarthrosis in children with hemophilia. *Lasers in Medical Science*, 30(8), 2179–2187.

Elsisi, H. F., Mousa, G. S., & MT, E. L. (2015). Electromagnetic field versus circuit weight training on bone mineral density in elderly women. *Clinical Interventions in Aging*, 10, 539–547.

Foletti, A., Grimaldi, S., Lisi, A., Ledda, M., & Liboff, A. R. (2013). Bioelectromagnetic medicine: The role of resonance signaling. *Electromagnetic Biology and Medicine*, 32(4), 484–499.

Froes Meyer, P., Ronzio, O. A., de Souza da Fonseca, A., Santos-Filho, S. D., & Bernardo-Filho, M. (2013). Cellular and molecular effects of electromagnetic radiation and sonic waves. *South African Journal of Science*, 109(7/8).

Fukuda, E., & Yasuda, I. (1957). On the piezoelectric effect of bone. *Journal of the Physical Society of Japan*, 12, 1158–1162.

Galace de Freitas, D., Marcondes, F. B., Monteiro, R. L., Rosa, S. G., Maria de Moraes Barros Fucs, P., & Fukuda, T. Y. (2014). Pulsed electromagnetic field and exercises in patients with shoulder impingement syndrome: A randomized, double-blind, placebo-controlled clinical trial. *Archives of Physical Medicine and Rehabilitation*, 95(2), 345–352.

Gebremariam, L., Hay, E. M., van der Sande, R., Rinkel, W. D., Koes, B. W., & Huisstede, B. M. (2014). Subacromial impingement syndrome--effectiveness of physiotherapy and manual therapy. *British Journal of Sports Medicine*, 48(16), 1202–1208.

Golbach, L. A., Portelli, L. A., Savelkoul, H. F., Terwel, S. R., Kuster, N., de Vries, R. B., et al. (2016). Calcium homeostasis and low-frequency magnetic and electric field exposure: A systematic review and meta-analysis of in vitro studies. *Environment International*, 92–93, 695–706.

Grana, D. R., Marcos, H., & Kokubu, G. A. (2008). Pulsed electromagnetic fields as adjuvant therapy in bone healing and peri-implant bone formation: An experimental study in rats. *Acta Odontologica Latinoamericana: AOL*, 21(1), 77–83.

Haik, M. N., Alburquerque-Sendin, F., Moreira, R. F., Pires, E. D., & Camargo, P. R. (2016). Effectiveness of physical therapy treatment of clearly defined subacromial pain: A systematic review of randomised controlled trials. *British Journal of Sports Medicine*, 50(18), 1124–1134.

Handoll, H. H., & Elliott, J. (2015). Rehabilitation for distal radial fractures in adults. *Cochrane Database of Systematic Reviews* (9) CD003324.

Hannemann, P. F., Essers, B. A., Schots, J. P., Dullaert, K., Poeze, M., & Brink, P. R. (2015). Functional outcome and cost-effectiveness of pulsed electromagnetic fields in the treatment of acute scaphoid fractures: A cost-utility analysis. *BMC Musculoskeletal Disorders*, 16, 84.

Hannemann, P. F., Mommers, E. H., Schots, J. P., Brink, P. R., & Poeze, M. (2014). The effects of low-intensity pulsed ultrasound and pulsed electromagnetic fields bone growth stimulation in acute fractures: A systematic review and meta-analysis of randomized controlled trials. *Archives of Orthopaedic and Trauma Surgery*, 134(8), 1093–1106.

Ibrahim, M., Twaij, H., Giebaly, D., Nizam, I., & Haddad, F. (2013). Enhanced recovery in total hip replacement: A clinical review. *The Bone & Joint Journal*, 95(12), 1587–1594.

Jeon, H. S., Kang, S. Y., Park, J. H., & Lee, H. S. (2015). Effects of pulsed electromagnetic field therapy on delayed-onset muscle soreness in biceps brachii. *Physical Therapy in Sport*, 16(1), 34–39.

Kanat, E., Alp, A., & Yurtkuran, M. (2013). Magnetotherapy in hand osteoarthritis: A pilot trial. *Complementary Therapies in Medicine*, 21(6), 603–608.

Kroeling, P., Gross, A., Goldsmith, C. H., Burnie, S. J., Haines, T., Graham, N., et al. (2009). Electrotherapy for neck pain. *Cochrane Database of Systematic Reviews* (8), CD004251.

Laakso, L., Lutter, F., & Young, C. (2009). Static magnets: What are they and what do they do? *Brazilian Journal of Physical Therapy*, 13(1), 10–23.

Lazovic, M., Kocic, M., Dimitrijevic, L., Stankovic, I., Spalevic, M., & Ciric, T. (2012). Pulsed electromagnetic field during cast immobilization in postmenopausal women with Colles' fracture. *Srpski Arhiv Za Celokupno Lekarstvo*, 140(9–10), 619–624.

Li, S., Yu, B., Zhou, D., He, C., Zhuo, Q., & Hulme, J. M. (2013). Electromagnetic fields for treating osteoarthritis. *Cochrane Database of Systematic Reviews* (12), CD003523.

Lohmann, C., Schwartz, Z., Liu, Y., Li, Z., Simon, B., Sylvia, V., et al. (2003). Pulsed electromagnetic fields affect phenotype and connexin 43 protein expression in MLO-Y4 osteocyte-like cells and ROS 17/2.8 osteoblast-like cells. *Journal of Orthopaedic Research*, 21(2), 326–334.

Longo, F. M., Yang, T., Hamilton, S., Hyde, J. F., Walker, J., Jennes, L., et al. (1999). Electromagnetic fields influence NGF activity and levels following sciatic nerve transection. *Journal of Neuroscience Research, 55*(2), 230–237.

Maestú, C., Blanco, M., Nevado, A., Romero, J., Rodríguez-Rubio, P., Galindo, J., et al. (2013). Reduction of pain thresholds in fibromyalgia after very low-intensity magnetic stimulation: A double-blinded, randomized placebo-controlled clinical trial. *Pain Research and Management, 18*(6), e101–e106.

Martinez-Rondanelli, A., Martinez, J. P., Moncada, M. E., Manzi, E., Pinedo, C. R., & Cadavid, H. (2014). Electromagnetic stimulation as coadjuvant in the healing of diaphyseal femoral fractures: A randomized controlled trial. *Colombia Médica, 45*(2), 67–71.

McLeod, K. J., & Rubin, C. T. (1997). The effect of low-frequency fields on osteogenesis. *Journal of Bone and Joint Surgery, 74A*, 920–929.

Meyer, P. F., Paiva, A., Cavalcanti, S., da Silva, E. M., da Silva, R. M. V., de Souza Costa, L., et al. (2011). Magnetoterapia: É possível este recurso fazer parte da rotina do fisioterapeuta brasileiro? *Arquivos Brasileiros de Ciências da Saúde, 36*(1).

Nindl, G., Johnson, M. T., & Balcavage, W. X. (2003). *Low frequency electromagnetic field effects on lymphocytes: Potential for treatment of inflammatory diseases. Bioelectromagnetic medicine. R. P and M. M.* USA: Taylor & Francis, 369–391.

Oberman, L. M., Enticott, P. G., Casanova, M. F., Rotenberg, A., Pascual-Leone, A., McCracken, J. T., et al. (2016). Transcranial magnetic stimulation in autism spectrum disorder: Challenges, promise, and roadmap for future research. *Autism Research, 9*(2), 184–203.

Oberman, L. M., Pascual-Leone, A., & Rotenberg, A. (2014). Modulation of corticospinal excitability by transcranial magnetic stimulation in children and adolescents with autism spectrum disorder. *Frontiers in Human Neuroscience, 8*, 627.

Osti, L., Buono, A. D., & Maffulli, N. (2015). Pulsed electromagnetic fields after rotator cuff repair: A randomized, controlled study. *Orthopedics, 38*(3), e223–228.

Paolucci, T., Piccinini, G., Iosa, M., Piermattei, C., de Angelis, S., Grasso, M. R., et al. (2016). Efficacy of extremely low-frequency magnetic field in fibromyalgia pain: A pilot study. *Journal of Rehabilitation Research and Development, 53*(6), 1023–1034.

Pastuszak, Z., Stepien, A., Piusinska-Macoch, R., Brodacki, B., & Tomczykiewicz, K. (2016). Evaluation of repetitive transcranial magnetic stimulation effectiveness in treatment of psychiatric and neurologic diseases. *Polski Merkuriusz Lekarski: Organ Polskiego Towarzystwa Lekarskiego, 40*(240), 388–392.

Pezzetti, F., De Mattei, M., Caruso, A., Cadossi, R., Zucchini, P., Carinci, F., et al. (1999). Effects of pulsed electromagnetic fields on human chondrocytes: An in vitro study. *Calcified Tissue International, 65*(5), 396–401.

Reilingh, M. L., van Bergen, C. J., Gerards, R. M., van Eekeren, I. C., de Haan, R. J., Sierevelt, I. N., et al. (2016). Effects of pulsed electromagnetic fields on return to sports after arthroscopic debridement and microfracture of osteochondral talar defects: A randomized, double-blind, placebo-controlled, multicenter trial. *The American Journal of Sports Medicine, 44*(5), 1292–1300.

Risso Neto, M. I., Zuiani, G. R., Cavali, P. T., Veiga, I. G., Pasqualini, W., Amato Filho, A. C. S., et al. (2017). Effect of pulsed electromagnetic field on the consolidation of postero-lateral arthrodeses in the lumbosacral spine: A prospective, double-blind, randomized study. *Coluna/Columna, 16*(3), 206–212.

Rodriguez Martin, J. M. (2014). *Electroterapia en fisioterapia.* Madrid: Médica Panamericana.

Rohde, C. H., Taylor, E. M., Alonso, A., Ascherman, J. A., Hardy, K. L., & Pilla, A. A. (2015). Pulsed electromagnetic fields reduce postoperative interleukin-1β, pain, and inflammation: A double-blind, placebo-controlled study in TRAM flap breast reconstruction patients. *Ophthalmic Plastic and Reconstructive Surgery, 135*(5), 808e–817e.

Rosch, P. J., & Markov, M. S. (2004). *Bioelectromagnetic medicine.* Informa Healthcare.

Ross, C. L., Siriwardane, M., Almeida-Porada, G., Porada, C. D., Brink, P., Christ, G. J., et al. (2015). The effect of low-frequency electromagnetic field on human bone marrow stem/progenitor cell differentiation. *Stem Cell Research, 15*(1), 96–108.

Rosso, F., Bonasia, D. E., Marmotti, A., Cottino, U., & Rossi, R. (2015). Mechanical stimulation (pulsed electromagnetic fields "PEMF" and extracorporeal shock wave therapy "ESWT") and tendon regeneration: A possible alternative. *Frontiers in Aging Neuroscience, 7*, 211.

Sadeghipour, R., Ahmadian, S., Bolouri, B., Pazhang, Y., & Shafiezadeh, M. (2012). Effects of extremely low-frequency pulsed electromagnetic fields on morphological and biochemical properties of human breast carcinoma cells (T47D). *Electromagnetic Biology and Medicine, 31*(4), 425–435.

Saliev, T., Mustapova, Z., Kulsharova, G., Bulanin, D., & Mikhalovsky, S. (2014). Therapeutic potential of electromagnetic fields for tissue engineering and wound healing. *Cell Proliferation, 47*(6), 485–493.

Seitz, A. L., McClure, P. W., Finucane, S., Boardman, N. D., III, & Michener, L. A. (2011). Mechanisms of rotator cuff tendinopathy: Intrinsic, extrinsic, or both? *Clinical Biomechanics, 26*(1), 1–12.

da Silva, R. M. V., Xavier, W. J. C., Dantas Neto, R. G., de Azevedo, V. M., do Nascimento, B. J. R., d Oliveira, J. F., et al. (2016). Efeitos da magnetoterapia no tratamento da dor na osteoartrose de joelho. *ConScientiae Saúde, 15*(2), 281–287.

Tepper, O. M., Callaghan, M. J., Chang, E. L., Galiano, R. D., Bhatt, K. A., & Baharestani, S. (2004). Electromagnetic fields increase in vitro and in vivo angiogenesis through endothelial release of FGF-2. *The FASEB Journal Express article.* https://doi.org/10.1096/fj.03-0847.

Uzunca, K., Birtane, M., & Tastekin, N. (2007). Effectiveness of pulsed electromagnetic field therapy in lateral epicondylitis. *Clinical Biomechanics, 26*(1), 69–74.

Vadala, M., Morales-Medina, J. C., Vallelunga, A., Palmieri, B., Laurino, C., & Iannitti, T. (2016). Mechanisms and therapeutic effectiveness of pulsed electromagnetic field therapy in oncology. *Cancer Medicine, 5*(11), 3128–3139.

Van Belkum, S., Bosker, F., Kortekaas, R., Beersma, D., & Schoevers, R. (2016). Treatment of depression with low-strength transcranial pulsed electromagnetic fields: A mechanistic point of view. *Progress in Neuro-Psychopharmacology and Biological Psychiatry, 71*, 137–143.

Varani, K., Vincenzi, F., Ravani, A., Pasquini, S., Merighi, S., Gessi, S., et al. (2017). Adenosine receptors as a biological pathway for the anti-inflammatory and beneficial effects of low frequency low energy pulsed electromagnetic fields. *Mediators of Inflammation, 2017*, 2740963.

Wang, R., Wu, H., Yang, Y., & Song, M. (2016). Effects of electromagnetic fields on osteoporosis: A systematic literature review. *Electromagnetic Biology and Medicine, 35*(4), 384–390.

Wuschech, H., von Hehn, U., Mikus, E., & Funk, R. H. (2015). Effects of PEMF on patients with osteoarthritis: Results of a prospective, placebo-controlled, double-blind study. *Bioelectromagnetics, 36*(8), 576–585.

Yuan, J., Xin, F., & Jiang, W. (2018). Underlying signaling pathways and therapeutic applications of pulsed electromagnetic fields in bone repair. *Cellular Physiology and Biochemistry: International Journal of Experimental Cellular Physiology, Biochemistry, and Pharmacology, 46*(4), 1581–1594.

Zhu, S., He, H., Zhang, C., Wang, H., Gao, C., Yu, X., et al. (2017). Effects of pulsed electromagnetic fields on postmenopausal osteoporosis. *Bioelectromagnetics, 38*(6), 406–424.

13

Shockwave

Cliff Eaton, Tim Watson

CHAPTER OUTLINE

INTRODUCTION

A thunder clap is an example of a shockwave in nature. The consensus is that a thunder clap must begin with a shockwave, which is the result of a sudden increase in air pressure and temperature within a lightning bolt (Rakov & Uman 2007). Hot air is expanded outwards where it impacts with cooler air creating a sonic boom, like an explosion or a supersonic aircraft breaking the sound barrier. Ogden et al (2001) describe a shockwave as effectively being a controlled explosion.

In Munich, Germany, during the 1970s, researchers began animal studies to see if focusing this shockwave energy could be used to break down kidney stones (Delius et al 1994). In 1980 they had their first successful transcutaneous treatment in a human patient using one of the world's first lithotripsy machines (Chaussy et al 1980). As an incidental finding during subsequent research it was discovered that there was a dose-related effect: high dosages resulting in a destructive effect and lower dosages leading to a more regenerative effect (Cacchio et al 2009; Huang et al 2013; Wang et al 2005). This finding led to studies using extracorporeal shockwave therapy (ESWT) to treat musculoskeletal conditions. ESWT can nowadays be considered an effective, safe, versatile, repeatable, non-invasive therapy for the treatment of many musculoskeletal diseases (d'Agostino et al 2015).

PHYSICAL PRINCIPLES

There are two different methods that provide extracorporeal 'shockwave' therapy (ESWT): focused shockwave therapy (FSWT) produces true shockwaves and radial pressure waves (RPW) produce pressure waves, which technically are incorrectly referred to as radial shockwaves (Fig. 13.1). RPW is technically more accurate and some authors are adopting this terminology, which will be used in this chapter. Some authors also refer to this technology as extracorporeal pulse activation therapy (EPAT). Authors do not always differentiate between FSWT, RPW or EPAT in the title of their studies, which may cause confusion during literature searches.

The main differences between FSWT and RPW are shown in Table 13.1. FSWT machines create peak pressures in excess of 100 mPa in under 10 ns (Fig. 13.1), which are followed by a negative pressure phase (tensile phase -25 mPa) (Ogden et al 2001; Gerdesmeyer et al 2006). The positive phase produces direct mechanical effects, while during the negative phase, gas bubbles are produced. The cavitation of these bubbles produces secondary pressure waves (Reilly et al 2018). The majority of this cavitation occurs at a focal point within the tissue. Focusing the energy ensures that the treatment can be directed and side effects to unaffected tissue can be minimized. RPW produce much less peak pressure (1mPa), over a longer period

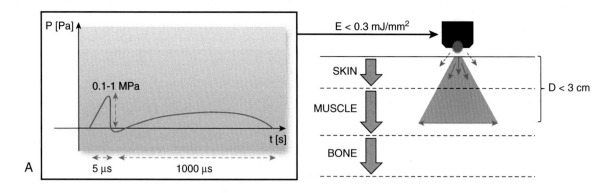

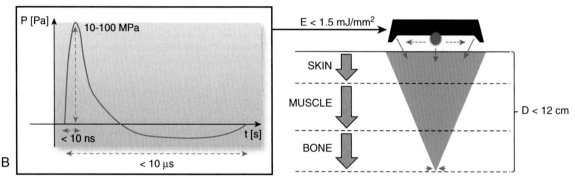

Fig. 13.1 Comparison of wave propagations with physical characteristics of radial pressure wave (RPW) and focused shockwave therapy (FSWT). E; Energy D; Tissue Depth

TABLE 13.1

Focused		Radial
100-1000 bar	PRESSURE	1-10 bar
≈ 0,2 µs	PULSE DURATION	0,2 -0,5 ms
focused	PRESSURE FIELD	radial, divergent
large	PENETRATION DEPTH	small, superficial
cells	EFFECT	tissue

From Novak P 2015.

of time and a smaller tensile phase. The 'focal point' is at the interface between the transmitter and the skin, so any cavitation occurs only superficially. The energy diverges radially, from this point into the tissue.

Focused shockwaves are created using either electrohydraulic, piezoelectric or electromagnetic generators (Fig. 13.2).

The electrohydraulic method produces an electric spark, which is generated between electrode tips in a water filled reflector and a spherical shockwave is released by the rapid vaporization of the water between the tips. The spark discharges are generated at the source and are sent in different directions into the medium. The resulting focal area, which is the largest of all shockwave types (Fig. 13.3), provides the therapeutic energy.

Piezoelectric generators have a few hundred piezoelectric crystals, which are mounted on a spherical surface. When a high voltage pulse is applied to the crystals they immediately expand, generating a low-pressure pulse in the surrounding water. To increase the pulse energy, some piezoelectric shockwave sources consist of a double layer of piezo elements. Piezoelectric shockwaves produce the smallest focal area, so accuracy of placement is important, often requiring the use of in-line ultrasound scanning to determine the position of a lesion.

In the past few years there has been a trend towards electromagnetic generation. Shockwave generation is similar, in principle, to that of a loud speaker with the shockwave transmitted through a paraboloid reflector. The shockwave energy accumulates at a focal point, surrounded by a therapeutic focal area.

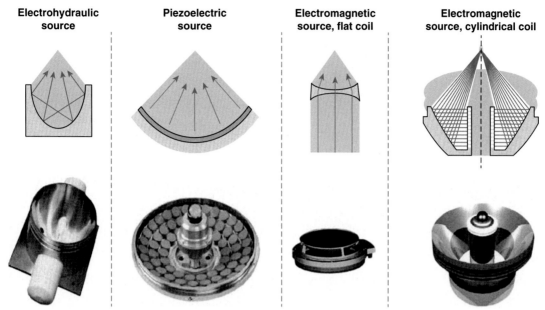

Fig 13.2 Focused shockwaves can be generated by electrohydraulic, piezoelectric or electromagnetic generators.

Focal points cumulate the shockwave energy at a depth of 5–10 cm with a diameter of 5–10 mm (Novak 2015). Therefore, for many years, any larger painful areas were considered as not appropriate for FSWT (Lohrer et al 2016). This treatment principle was upheld until the introduction of RPW therapy. RPW is generated ballistically using compressors, or in a few cases electromagnetics, to accelerate a projectile within a barrel to strike a transmitter. This transmitter converts the kinetic energy into an acoustic pressure wave (Fig 13.4). The shape, size and material of the transmitters affect the amount of energy emitted. The maximum energy is produced at the interface between the transmitter and skin and attenuates as it travels into tissue. Due to the smaller size and lower costs, this technology has been widely embraced (Lohrer et al 2016).

BIOPHYSICAL EFFECTS

ESWT, including both FSWT and RPW, are considered mechanotherapies, which have been defined as "all therapeutic interventions that reduce and reverse injury to damaged tissues or promote the homeostasis of healthy tissues by mechanical means at the molecular, cellular or tissue level" (Huang et al 2013). The importance of mechanical stimuli in both healthy and degenerative tissue has given rise to renewed interest in therapeutic applications, such as exercise prescription (Khan & Scott 2009). Mechanotherapy, whether shockwave or exercise initiated,

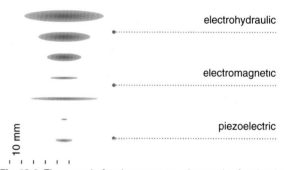

Fig 13.3 Therapeutic focal areas created around a focal point by different focused shockwave generators.

induces mechanotransduction. Mechanotransduction is the mechanism by which cells sense mechanical signals and adapt their biochemical activity, influencing cell migration, proliferation, differentiation and apoptosis. Ingber (2003, 2006, 2008) proposes a series of mechanisms by which these mechanical signals exert influence at a cellular level. Expanded explanations are offered by Dunn and Olmedo (2016), and Wang et al (2010).

During the tensile phase of a shockwave pulse, gas bubbles that are formed in the tissues expand and contract (stable cavitation). With sufficient energy, the gas contained within bubbles can expand so much that the bubbles implode on themselves (unstable cavitation), creating a microjet (Gerdesmeyer et al 2002). The force of this

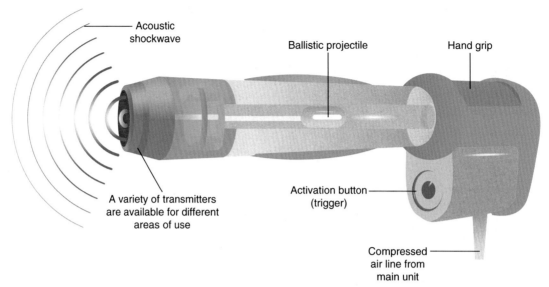

Acoustic shockwave

Ballistic projectile

Hand grip

A variety of transmitters are available for different areas of use

Activation button (trigger)

Compressed air line from main unit

Fig. 13.4 Radial pressure wave emitted from handpiece.

microjet can be destructive, and when occurring near brittle objects, such as kidney stones, they disintegrate. This is the principle used in lithotripsy. Stable cavitation, associated with lower energy values, influences the extracellular matrix (ECM) and cell behaviour by mechanotransduction.

Radial pressure waves also influence cellular activity by mechanotransduction, albeit in a different way. The biological effects of RPW remain less well understood than FSWT. Recent research indicates that the effect is primarily influenced by low frequency (sonic) waves being reflected and refracted at different tissue interfaces. High frequency (ultrasonic) waves appear to have limited penetration depths (Fig. 13.5) so any cavitation will be at a very superficial level (Novak 2013).

Romeo et al (2014) demonstrated the effectiveness of ESWT in stimulating biological events within cells and the ECM. The mechanical stimuli created by ESWT induce some changes in the tridimensional shape of integrins, which are responsible for force transmission between the ECM and the cells (Marshall & Lumpkin 2012). Integrins bind cells to the ECM and, alongside other mediators, act as communicators between cells, and cells to ECM. On sensing changes in force, the integrins instigate biological changes within the cell. Evidence points to mechanotransduction, after ESWT exposure, influencing stem cells, bone marrow and stromal cells, tenocytes, bone cells and their precursors, endothelial cells, fibroblasts and others (Romeo et al 2014; Wang 2012).

Tenocytes, which are known to be sensitive to mechanical stimulation, have received particular attention by

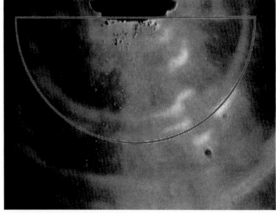

Fig. 13.5 Radial pressure wave showing superficial cavitation. (From Novak P and Verdaasdonk 2013.)

researchers due to the positive results found when using ESWT to treat chronic tendinopathies. In-vitro studies, following ESWT, have shown that there is an expression of proliferating cell nuclear antigen (PCNA), which is essential for DNA replication (Frairia & Berta 2011), an increase in tenocyte proliferation and collagen synthesis (Vetrano et al 2011), and increased expression of transforming growth factor beta-1 (TGF-β1), known to regulate tendon repair (Chen et al 2004). It is therefore hypothesized that ESWT can have an influence on tendon repair. Waugh et al (2015) conducted an in vivo study on both healthy and degenerate human tendons. Their findings suggest that ESWT may initiate tendon regeneration by promoting pro-inflammatory (interleukin-6) and catabolic processes (interleukin-8) to remove damaged matrix constituents. In a chronic pathology, where the normal healing cascade has stalled, the pro-inflammatory effect could be considered as 'rebooting' the healing process.

In recent years there has been interest shown in the role of macrophages in tissue regeneration, especially during the period where an acute condition can continue to resolve or shift to chronicity (e.g. Mantovani et al 2013; Martinez et al 2008). Enhanced macrophage activity in response to a stimulus such as shockwave can result in a pro-inflammatory response and additionally, during later healing phases, macrophages appear to recruit and stimulate stem cells. The combination of the proinflammatory activity combined with stem cell activation may explain in part the beneficial effects observed with shockwave-based therapy.

Animal studies have shown that there is an induced ingrowth of neo-vessels and an increased quantity of capillaries 4 weeks post ESWT at the tendon-bone interfaces (Nishida et al 2004; Wang et al 2002). These findings were related to an increased release of nitric oxide (NO) leading to activation of endothelial nitric oxide synthase (eNOS) and vascular endothelial growth factor (VEGF). The increased blood flow may play a part in pain relief and healing rates of chronic tendinopathies (Frairia & Berta 2011).

Nitric oxide seems to activate latent TGF-β1 and other cytokines, like fibroblast growth factor and insulin-like growth factor to promote collagen synthesis. Fibroblasts are the most common cells found in connective tissue types: tendon, ligaments, skin and even visceral tissue. Frairia et al (2011) propose that shockwave stimulates fibroblast proliferation, collagen synthesis and growth factor cytokine expression.

Studies in bone metabolism have also demonstrated the involvement of ESWT induced NO in bone healing (Evans & Ralston 1996). Yin et al (2011) reported that post ESWT there was enhanced angiogenesis and osteogenesis gene expression in hip osteonecrosis through the NO-mediated pathway. Fibroblast growth factor-2 and TGF-β1, which are important elements in bone growth, have also been shown to be increased after ESWT (Hausdorf et al 2011). Other influences of ESWT on bone and periosteum have been shown, including direct stimulation of osteoblasts and periosteal cells (Martini et al 2003; Tam et al 2008), osteogenic differentiation of mesenchymal cells (Wang et al 2002), accelerated migration of osteoblasts (Xu et al 2012), and reduction of osteoclast activity (Tamma et al 2009). Frairia and Berta (2011) report on a growing number of studies that show the positive effects of ESWT on non-union fractures and callus formation due to the increased production of NO.

Wound healing has also been shown to be enhanced by ESWT intervention, improving blood flow through an ingrowth of new capillary beds accompanied by fibroblast proliferation, which will assist in the formation of granulation tissue. During the remodelling phase fibroblasts can also assist to maintain collagen production (Doan et al 1999). ESWT studies have shown the influence of NO-mediators on wound tissue VEGF, the most potent angiogenic initiator. There is also evidence to show that the effects of ESWT extend beyond the ischaemic area, which also influences the surrounding tissue (Mittermayr et al 2012). Zhang et al (2016) recently compiled a systematic review and meta-analysis for the use of shockwave in wound healing studies. They conclude that the addition of shockwave to standard care improves the healing response in chronic wounds.

ESWT is reported to have a local analgesic effect, notably in myofascial pain (Lohrer et al 2016). Local myofascial trigger points (MTP) demonstrate local tissue contracture and ischaemia (Lohrer et al 2016; Ramon et al 2015). The use of RPW at 15 Hz and above appears to have a clinically beneficial effect on myofascial pain, potentially achieved through a mechanical separation of inappropriately fixed actin-myosin links (Gleitz & Hornig 2012) combined with a local hyperaemia and angiogenic response (Kuo 2009).

In addition to mechanotransduction mediated analgesia, Gleitz and Hornig (2012) report on other mechanisms for pain relief. There is a transient analgesic effect modulated by the 'pain gate theory'. A longer lasting analgesic effect is achieved when ESWT is used as a noxious stimulus. A noxious stimulus is responsible for the release of the neuropeptides substance P and calcitonin gene related peptides (CGRP). In response there is local vasodilation, which creates a 'wash out' or flushing effect, diminishing the sensitivity of vasoneuroactive substances like prostaglandin and histamine. The selective degeneration of C-afferent nerve fibres has also been described by Hausdorf et al (2008). The authors point out that the effects on pain relief have been reported on both muscular and non-muscular tissue using both FSWT and RPW. The analgesic effects are similar to those associated with dry needling, as described by Shah et al (2008) but are non-invasive and non-traumatic.

As ESWT is considered as a noxious stimulus, in the early 1990s it was suggested that full, regional or local anaesthesia was administered before ESWT. As a consequence, several randomized controlled trials (RCTs) reported no significantly positive outcomes when comparing ESWT to sham treatments (Lohrer et al 2016). It was not until 2005 that two studies on plantar fasciitis demonstrated the reduced effectiveness of ESWT after the administration of anaesthesia, explained because anaesthesia suppresses substance P and thereby negates some of the positive effects of ESWT.

Since that time, analgesia is not recommended for soft tissue ESWT treatments (Schmitz et al 2015) although some level of anaesthesia is still regarded as beneficial for FSWT applied to bone lesions (Schaden et al 2015).

Although some biophysical responses are still under investigation, it is clear ESWT can provide pain relief, positively regulate inflammation, promote angioneogenesis, induce stem cell activities and thereby improve tissue healing and regeneration (d'Agostino et al 2015).

CLINICAL EVIDENCE

Whilst the shockwave literature includes a high volume of publications (given the relative youth of this clinical intervention) (Dreisilker 2015) there is currently little consensus with regard to treatment parameters: energy flux density (EFD), number of shocks, ESWT generation and treatment frequency. There is also a wide range of clinical outcomes employed in trials, and this combination makes it problematic for clinicians to identify clear clinical guidelines (Lohrer et al 2016).

Literature Reviews for Musculoskeletal Conditions

The literature includes numerous systematic and narrative reviews looking at the overall effectiveness of ESWT in musculoskeletal conditions. The overall findings are positive for ESWT in "treating a subset of chronic tendon and plantar fasciitis diseases for a subset of patients" (Reilly et al 2018). The findings of individual reviews are very much dependent on the parameters used for outcomes and inclusion/exclusion criteria.

Speed (2014), updating an earlier review (2004), conducted a systematic review of ESWT for musculoskeletal conditions. A thorough search of the usual databases, medical journals and shockwave literature was performed between the years 1980 and 2012. In the study, 130 articles were retrieved with 26 satisfying the author's inclusion criteria. The studies involved plantar fasciitis (10), insertional Achilles tendinopathy (1), mid portion Achilles tendinopathy (3), calcific (4) and non-calcific (3) rotator cuff tendinopathies and lateral epicondylitis (5). Articles were excluded if they were: "Uncontrolled or had lack of sham control (67); small sample size (3); statistical errors (6); high dropout (5); lack of blinding (4); randomisation errors (2); lack of similarity of groups at baseline (4) and miscellaneous (not in English)" (Speed 2014). The principle outcome measure was patient's pain at 12 weeks.

The author concluded that there is good evidence for:
- High-dose FSWT and RPW in plantar fasciitis, although there was only one level 1 RCT for RPW.
- Lack of benefit for low-dose FSWT in plantar fasciitis.

- FSWT in calcific tendinopathy of the rotator cuff, especially in high doses.

While accepting that there is no consensus in the literature to define 'high and low' energy ESWT, the author provided a guideline of <0.12 mJ/mm^2 as low and >0.12 mJ/mm^2 as high.

There is some evidence for:
- High-dose FSWT in mid portion and insertional Achilles tendinopathies, but no benefit for low dose FSWT in this condition.
- Benefit of RPW in calcific tendinopathy.
- Lack of benefit of FSWT in non-calcific tendinopathy of the rotator cuff.
- There is no evidence to support or refute the effects of FSWT or RPW in other conditions.
- There is mixed evidence for the effects of low-dose FSWT in common extensor tendinopathy.

With respect to FSWT and RPW, Speed (2014) stated that "Both treatments offer an alternative to surgery in the management of recalcitrant conditions" and suggested the establishment of an industry standard in sham therapy to facilitate comparison among ESWT studies. The assumption that FSWT and RPW should be considered equivalent in this regard has been criticized (Gleitz 2011).

It has been suggested that RPW is the better choice for myalgia and myofascial trigger points and FSWT for tendinopathies (Gleitz 2011). Although one study contradicts this viewpoint, showing no significant difference in outcomes between FSWT and RPW for patella tendinopathies (van der Worp et al 2014). Simons et al (1998) theorized that active myofascial trigger points are the cause of insertional tendinopathies. Dreisilker (2010) suggests that treating both the tendon and the associated myofascial area provides the best outcomes. This has not been demonstrated in clinical trials and should be something to consider when developing the 'optimal protocol'.

Mani-Babu et al (2015), using different protocol criteria than Speed (2014), reviewed the effectiveness of ESWT concentrating on the lower limb. A literature search identified 255 articles of which 20 were included in the study. The aim was to look at the effectiveness at <12 months and >12 months post intervention for greater trochanteric pain syndrome (GTPS) (two studies), patella tendinopathy (PT) (seven studies) and Achilles tendinopathy (11 studies). The selected studies comprised nine RCTs, six single-cohort prospective studies and five retrospective studies. No animal studies were included, and those not available in English were also excluded. There was no limit on the publication year.

Mani-Babu et al (2015) concluded that there was moderate-level evidence to support the use of ESWT for the three reviewed lower limb tendinopathies. In agreement with other authors, they conceded that there are too few high-quality studies for lower limb tendinopathies, noting the need for larger sample sizes and better controls; furthermore, stating the need for comparison of the parameters used in ESWT to identify "the optimal protocols" for clinicians to use. From those high-quality studies that were analysed, it was clear that combining ESWT with progressive loading strategies and flexibility training provided superior results to either modality used in isolation. They suggested that ESWT could be used for the first 3 weeks in patient management in combination with a progressive loading regime. This viewpoint is supported by Cook (2011) who stated that "monotherapies are rarely used in clinical practice".

Reilly et al (2018), like Speed (2015), reviewed articles that studied musculoskeletal conditions for both the upper and lower limbs, including tendinopathies and plantar fasciitis. However, this review included both retrospective and prospective studies, noting whether they used a control group, were blinded, or used a placebo and also included the primary and secondary findings. In 2017 a PubMed search was performed using these keywords: shock wave therapy, ESWT, extracorporeal shockwave therapy, tendinopathy, and fasciopathy. Although reference is made to low-energy radial shockwave outcomes it is not apparent whether omitting from the search the terms radial pressure wave or extracorporeal pulsed activation therapy (EPAT) introduced any bias. Both these terms have been used in studies as they better describe the properties of 'radial shockwave'. For lateral epicondylitis, six studies using FSWT were reviewed but none for RPW, despite there being RPW studies that would appear to fulfil the inclusion criterion (Beyazal & Devrimsel 2015; Ilieva et al 2012; Spacca et al 2005). Similar selective inclusion criteria appear for rotator cuff studies (three FSWT versus one RPW) and plantar fasciitis (seven FSWT versus one RPW).

Reilly et al (2018) set out to review the treatment of musculoskeletal conditions with ESWT and included a quality score (PEDro scale) in their consideration. All of the papers considered in the narrative review scored a high-quality score, bar one, which fell just below this level.

Reilly et al (2018) concluded that the current evidence does suggest ESWT may be a reasonable treatment to consider for management of chronic musculoskeletal conditions that fail to respond to conservative care, with a low risk of side effects. The use of RPW was supported for most applications that were reviewed while rotator cuff lesions with calcification responded best to high-energy FSWT. It was also noted that there were mixed outcomes for the conditions reviewed and even studies demonstrating favourable outcomes did not report consistent improvement for

all patients. As with previous reviews the authors point to the lack of "optimal protocols", which may have a bearing on this finding: the various EFDs used, number of shocks, types of shockwave machines, generation of shockwaves, number of treatment sessions and interval between sessions. The latter was the only variable showing some consistency between studies, with all studies separating treatment sessions by 1 week.

The difficulty in adopting a 'best practice' approach owing to the inconsistencies in research protocols does consistently appear in ESWT literature reviews. Having established that 80% of the studies in PEDro demonstrated that ESWT provided better outcomes than placebo, Schmitz et al (2015) felt a clinical review would be more appropriate than a meta-analysis to reduce the confusion. The authors pointed out that previous systematic reviews had added to the confusion by not defining terminology, and by not distinguishing between different types of ESWT. Using a PEDro search in 2015 they found 106 suitable studies involving non-operative tendinopathy and musculoskeletal pathologies to compare ESWT with other treatments, FSWT versus RPW and RPW and high energy versus low energy ESWT. The PEDro search did not include the terms radial pressure wave or extracorporeal pulse activation therapy (EPAT). The selected studies were divided into those with positive outcomes (FSWT = 66, RPW = 23) and those with negative outcomes (FSWT = 15, RPW = 3). One study compared FSWT to RPW so was included in both groups.

The study considered the following variables:
- Number of treatment sessions
- Interval time between sessions
- Number of shocks per treatment
- The EFD for each treatment
- The total energy administered during the course of treatment
- PEDro score from 0–10.

The review proposes that the optimal treatment protocol for treating musculoskeletal conditions is: three treatment sessions, administering 2000 shocks per treatment at the highest tolerable EFD. The proposal was made on the basis of analysing the data from one plantar fasciitis study using RPW (Chow & Cheing 2007) and one FSWT study on calcific rotator cuff (Loew et al 1999), which found "more is better". The authors then pointed out that there is not one RCT in the PEDro database that contradicts this statement.

The findings of the review showed that for plantar fasciitis, non-calcific supraspinatus and calcific rotator cuffs, the PEDro criteria for type of RCT and highest PEDro scores were fulfilled. For all other conditions treated with ESWT there were not enough RCTs for FSWT or RPW to draw meaningful conclusions.

Contrary to the reported belief that higher quality RCTs demonstrate that ESWT is ineffective, it was found that the RCTs with both positive or negative outcomes averaged the same PEDro score (Schmitz et al 2015). When consideration was given to the different types of FSWT generation, no significant difference was observed in either positive or negative outcome studies, thus no generation mechanism superiority was demonstrated.

The review by Schmitz et al (2015) shows ESWT as an effective and safe, non-invasive treatment option for chronic recalcitrant tendinopathies and other musculoskeletal conditions. Twenty-three out of 26 (88%) RPW studies and 66 out of 81 (72%) for FSWT provide positive outcomes compared to placebo or alternative interventions. Not one study on the PEDro database showed any serious adverse events during or after ESWT intervention.

In agreement with other ESWT reviewers the authors suggest trying to establish "optimal protocols" to assist clinicians and, additionally, to have more direct comparisons using the same EFDs between FSWT and RPW, as it is suggested that there is no scientific evidence in favour of either FSWT or RPW with respect to treatment outcomes.

Proximal Hamstring Tendinopathy

Forty professional athletes with chronic proximal hamstring tendinopathy were included in a randomized controlled clinical study generating level 1 evidence (Cacchio et al 2011). The aim of the study was to consider the effectiveness of ESWT in the treatment of proximal insertional hamstring tendinopathy. Two groups of 20 were randomly assigned for either shockwave therapy or conservative treatment consisting of NSAIDs, physiotherapy and exercise. Evaluations for pain were taken before treatment, at weeks 1 and 3 and months 6 and 12 after treatment. RPW was administered for 4 sessions at weekly intervals, applying 2500 shocks at an equivalent of 0.18m J/mm². At 3 months post treatment, 17 of 20 (85%) in the RPW group and two of the 20 in the control group had achieved at least 50% reduction in pain, using visual analogue scale (VAS) and the Nirschl phase rating scale (NPRS). The authors reasonably concluded that shockwave therapy is a safe and effective treatment for patients with chronic proximal hamstring tendinopathy.

Notable Evidence for Other Musculoskeletal Treatments Using ESWT

Osgood Schlatter's Disease

Lohrer et al (2012) conducted a pilot study to analyse the safety and effectiveness of RPW in the treatment of Osgood Schlatter's disease (translated from German). Fourteen adolescent subjects were treated with RPW once a week over 5–7 weeks using 2000 shocks with a range of EFD of 0.06 to 0.09 mJ/mm². A 5.6 year follow up showed that 12 of the 16 knees (75%) attained a score of 100% in a Visa P-G validated questionnaire. In the case of four knees, the patients reported persistent tibial tuberosity pain when playing sport. In the case of four knees that caused distal patella tendon pain, the patients changed their sporting activity. Apart from demonstrating the effectiveness of RPW in this pilot study, it also showed the safety of RPW in treating this condition. Therapists are generally advised to err on the side of caution when treating over epiphyseal growth plates. Not one of the cohort reported any side effects or long-term complications of having had RPW treatment. Subsequent studies by the same authors confirmed these findings for both Osgood Schlatter's disease and Sever's disease (Lohrer et al 2012; Lohrer & Nauck 2015).

Osteochondrosis of the Hip

A systematic review of 17 articles including two case reports, nine open label trials, two cohorts, and six randomized controlled trials has been completed considering the effect of ESWT for osteochondrosis of the hip (Zhang et al 2016). Fourteen articles provided the energy intensity of ESWT, all of which exceeded 0.18 mJ/mm² and nine were 0.62 mJ/mm². Unfortunately, the authors only used the term 'ESWT', neglecting to state whether the studies used FSWT or RPW, and if FSWT, then what type of generation. Analysis of the reviewed studies showed that studies using high energy intensities (0.62 mJ/mm²) used electrohydraulic generated FSWT found in hospitals, with the patient anaesthetised in supine position (Wang et al 2005). At least one study did use RPW, which was a case study, looking at the long-term use of RPW for this condition (Ma et al 2016). The affected hip was treated with 6000 shocks of RPW at 10 Hz with an intensity ranging from 2.5 to 4.0 bar at 7-day intervals for 24 months. No equivalent EFD was quoted. MRI scans demonstrated that joint effusion was reduced, there was no longer bone oedema and the gluteal muscles were more developed. While potentially offering a non-invasive, safe treatment, the long-term course of treatment may prove not to be a practical option.

Zhang et al (2016) additionally consider that ESWT is a safe and effective treatment to improve motor function and provide pain relief for patients with avascular necrosis of the hip, especially in the early stages. This conclusion was tempered by recognizing the low-quality of the reviewed studies.

Chronic Facet Joint Pain

A retrospective study of 62 patients with unilateral facet joint pain was conducted to consider whether RPW would have a positive outcome on reducing pain. RPW group was compared to a corticosteroid group and a radiofrequency neurotomy group, the latter being considered as the gold standard treatment for this condition but with potential risks of complications. Pain scales were used before treatments and compared to follow-up at 2, 6 and 12 months. Twenty-one patients were selected for the RPW group and received 3000 shocks, once a week for 5 weeks with an equivalent EFD of 0.12 mJ/mm^2. The treatment was assisted with initial ultrasound guidance to ensure the correct angle of delivery.

The study demonstrated that RPW showed better long-term nociceptive pain relief compared to steroid injections and only slightly less pain relief compared to the invasive procedure of radiofrequency. It was also observed that for the RPW and radiofrequency groups their activities of daily living were less restricted due to back pain. Neuropathic pain was unchanged with RPW at 6 and 12 months but radiofrequency provided long-term relief. The authors concluded that shockwave therapy had shown reasonable efficacy in treatment of chronic lumbar facet joint pain.

Carpal Tunnel Syndrome (CTS)

In 2017 there was a published systematic review of RCTs considering the effectiveness of physical therapy and electrophysical therapy for CTS (Huisstede et al 2017). One high-quality RCT compared RPW plus a night splint (n=20) with placebo RPW and night splint (n=20). 2000 shocks at a pressure of 4 bar (no equivalent EFD provided) and a frequency of 5Hz were administered once a week for 3 weeks (Wu et al 2016). A significant difference in pain relief was found at 11 weeks and 15 weeks follow-up compared to the control group. There was no change in pinch grip strength.

The systematic review also considered two RCTs (one high-quality and one low-quality) comparing ESWT to injection therapy. No significant difference between groups was found in either study for pain, function or recovery at 1, 2, 4 or 6 months.

In contrast, a more recent paper showed significant benefit using one session of RPW compared to injection therapy over a 24-week period (Atthakomol et al 2018). The prospective RCT enlisted 25 subjects (13 = RPW, 12 = injection) complaining of mild to moderate CTS symptoms. Each RPW patient received a single treatment of 5000 shocks at 4 bar (no equivalent EFD) 15 Hz followed by an ice pack. There was a significant difference between the groups for pain severity and function at both 12 and 24 weeks follow up and compared to baseline. The study concluded that a single dose RPW treatment is an appropriate treatment for mild to moderate CTS with the benefits lasting longer than an injection intervention.

Myalgia and MTPs

Gleitz (2008) conducted a study with the aim of identifying whether RPW could improve calf extensibility in patients with chronic Achilles pain. A total of 102 patients (63 males, 39 females) with less than 20 degrees of active dorsiflexion associated with Achilles pain were recruited for the study. All subjects received between 4000 and 6000 shocks at 15 Hz at maximum tolerable intensity over a course of treatment lasting on average 4.4 sessions. Immediately after the end of the course of treatment patients had gained on average an additional 9 degrees of active dorsiflexion, which lasted several months. When compared to a conventional stretching programme the RPW approach proved far superior in terms of range of movement and duration of effectiveness.

Gleitz and other authors have also found that ESWT can be very effective in the treatment of myofascial trigger points (Damian & Zalpour 2011; Gleitz & Hornig 2012). Ramon et al (2015) reviewed the use of ESWT for both myofascial pain syndrome (for which it appears to be of clinical benefit) and for fibromyalgia (in which the results remain equivocal).

ESWT for Spasticity

There appears to be strong evidence to support the use of ESWT in reducing muscle hypertonia. Studies have demonstrated increased ranges of movement following ESWT intervention in spastic plantar flexors in childhood cerebral palsy (Gonkova et al 2013; Wang et al 2016) and adult stroke patients (Sawan et al 2017; Wu et al 2017). Stroke patients with upper limb spasticity have also benefitted from ESWT to increase range of movement and reduce pain (Kim et al 2013; Li et al 2016). Most studies prefer the use of RPW to FSWT to reduce hypertonia. This choice of RPW appears to provide greater passive range of movement gains in the plantar flexors than FSWT (Wu et al 2018). The number and frequency of treatments, the treatment frequency (Hz) and the treatment area (musculotendinous junction or muscle belly) have yet to be determined to establish the optimal protocol (Xiang 2018).

THERAPEUTIC USES

In 1985, researchers with concerns over the effects on the hip whilst treating lower ureteral stones made a new discovery. There was no adverse effect to the bone after lithotripsy; indeed clinicians found that there was an increase in bone density (Graff et al 1988). A few years later, Valchanou and Michailov (1991) reported on FSWT using high energy providing successful outcomes for delayed and non-union fractures.

ESWT is currently applied to a wide range of pathologies, both in orthopaedics and rehabilitative medicine (Cacchio et al 2009; d'Agostino et al 2014; Romeo et al 2014; Wang 2012), dermatology/wound healing (Mittermayr et al 2012; Saggini et al 2008), neurology (spastic hypertonia and related syndromes) (Amelio & Manganotti 2010; Lee et al 2014), dentistry (Sathishkumar 2008; Novak 2008) and urology (Chung & Cartmill 2015; Paulis & Brancato 2012). Regenerative and trophic effects have also been demonstrated in ischaemic heart diseases, although, at present, ESWT application in this field is still to be considered experimental (Ito et al 2011). The evidence reviewed in this chapter concentrates on applications in orthopaedic and rehabilitative medicine. The indications for ESWT, based on the quality and quantity of the available evidence, are provided by the International Society for Medical Shockwave Therapy (ISMST) (Table 13.2).

In line with the evidence for other electrophysical modalities, there appears to be a dose-dependent response when ESWT is employed clinically. Energy values used in orthopaedics and rehabilitative medicine are of low- or medium-energy intensity. This brings into question

---

TABLE 13.2   Indications for ESWT Recommended by the International Society for Medical Shockwave Therapy (2016)

1. Approved Standard Indications	2. Empirically Tested Clinical Uses
1.1.0. Chronic Tendinopathies	2.1.0. Tendinopathies
1.1.1. Calcifying tendinopathy of the shoulder	2.1.1. Non calcifying shoulder tendinopathy
1.1.2. Lateral epicondylopathy of the elbow	2.1.2. Medial epicondylopathy of the elbow
1.1.3. Greater trochanter pain syndrome	2.1.3. Adductor tendinopathy syndrome
1.1.4. Patellar tendinopathy	2.1.4. Pes-Anserinus tendinopathy syndrome
1.1.5. Achilles tendinopathy	2.1.5. Peroneal tendinopathy
1.1.6. Plantar fasciitis, with or without heel spur	2.1.6. Foot and ankle tendinopathies
1.2.0. Bone pathologies	2.2.0. Bone pathologies
1.2.1. Delayed bone healing	2.2.1. Bone marrow oedema
1.2.2. Bone non-union (pseudarthroses)	2.2.2. Osgood Schlatter disease
1.2.3. Stress fracture	2.2.3. Tibial stress syndrome (shin splint)
1.2.4. Avascular bone necrosis without articular derangement	2.3.0. Muscle pathologies
1.2.5. Osteochondritis Dissecans (OCD) without articular derangement	2.3.1. Myofascial Syndrome
1.3.0. Skin Pathologies	2.3.2. Muscle sprain without discontinuity
1.3.1. Delayed or non-healing wounds	2.4.0. Skin pathologies
1.3.2. Skin ulcers	2.4.1. Cellulite
1.3.3. Non-circumferential burn wounds	
3. Exceptional Indications	**4. Experimental Indications**
3.1.0. Musculoskeletal Pathologies	4.1.0. Heart Muscle Ischemia
3.1.1. Osteoarthritis	4.2.0. Peripheral nerve lesions
3.1.2. Dupuytren disease	4.3.0. Pathologies of the spinal cord and brain
3.1.3. Plantar fibromatosis (Ledderhose disease)	4.4.0. Skin calcinosis
3.1.4. De Quervain disease	4.5.0. Periodontal disease
3.1.5. Trigger finger	4.6.0. Jawbone pathologies
3.2.0. Neurological pathologies	4.7.0. Complex Regional Pain Syndrome (CRPS)
3.2.1. Spasticity	4.8.0. Osteoporosis
3.2.2. Polyneuropathy	
3.2.3. Carpal Tunnel Syndrome	
3.3.0. Urologic pathologies	
3.3.1. Pelvic chronic pain syndrome (abacterial prostatitis)	
3.3.2. Erectile dysfunction	
3.3.3. Peyronie disease	
3.4.1. Lymphoedema	

what constitutes low, medium and high energy values. Unfortunately, there is no consensus in the literature, or indeed among the scientific advisory groups, on what these are. There are a number of parameters attributed to the production of a shockwave:

- Peak positive and negative acoustic pressure
- Derived pulse intensity integral (energy density = ED)
- Total energy (−6dB)
- Focal extension in x-, y- and z-direction
- Number of pulses
- Pulse repetition rate (Hz).

The convention is to use energy flux density (EFD), measured in mJ/mm^2, as the comparable parameter (Lohrer et al 2016), as this indicates that the shockwave energy 'flows' through an area perpendicular to the direction of propagation (Rompe et al 1998).

In Rompe et al's (1998) study they compared three EFDs (0.08, 0.28 and 0.60 mJ/mm^2) of FSWT on rabbits' Achilles tendons. They found that the lowest EFD had no effect, the middle EFD produced a slight inflammatory effect, while the higher EFD produced significant inflammation and evidence of cell necrosis. The authors recommended that EFDs of over 0.28 mJ/mm^2 should not be used when treating tendon disorders. Based on the findings of this study it could be considered that the following ranges are reasonable (Rompe et al 1998):

- Low (up to 0.08 mJ/mm^2)
- Medium (up to 0.28 mJ/mm^2)
- High (over 0.6 mJ/mm^2)

Scientific advisory groups in some countries have published their own recommendations. The Chinese Shockwave Association (CSA) in 2018 recommended these intensities to its members:

- Low (0.06–0.11 mJ/mm^2)
- Medium (0.12–0.25 mJ/mm^2)
- High (0.26–0.39 mJ/mm^2)

Contraindications for FSWT and RPW are discussed in Chapter 22. As most contraindications for therapeutic use are listed for high energy intensities the consensus on high intensity is particularly relevant.

It should be stated that the contraindications suggested by scientific advisory bodies will differ from those provided by most machine manufacturers. The reason for this is that manufacturers must demonstrate that their machine will not cause harm before being awarded a licence to sell in different countries. To avoid the expense of meaningful clinical trials it is often easier for a manufacturer to advocate blanket contraindications, for example pregnancy.

Furthermore, when an ESWT clinician is looking for supportive evidence for their clinical practice, they must take into consideration the dosages that are provided by the authors. The dosages are often quoted in mJ/mm^2, yet

for RPW users, the machines they use only provide bar pressure (the pressure within the handpiece). The energy transmitted from the RPW transmitter will vary depending on the bar pressure, but also on the size, material and shape of the transmitter.

APPLICATION

Shockwaves transmit well through water and less so through air. To ensure coupling to the patient's body, ultrasound gel is used. Care should be taken to use plenty of gel, while ensuring minimal air bubbles within it. Some authors (e.g. Maier et al. 1999) have suggested the use of oil as a coupling medium, though this is not widely used in clinical practice.

The technique for application of FSWT and RPW differs. As FSWT cumulates to a focal point at a given depth, the handpiece is kept still in direct line with the lesion. As piezoelectric generators produce a small focal area, it is generally accepted that the combined use of in-line ultrasound imaging is recommended. Less accuracy is required with electrohydraulic and electromagnetic generators as they have larger focal areas. A scanning technique to localize the treatment area can be used, and a more precise location can then be achieved by tilting the head at the site (Fig. 13.6). This technique for identifying painful areas has been shown to be more effective than simply using anatomical landmarks or ultrasound imaging alone (Buchbinder et al 2002; Sems et al 2006).

Good contact with the patient's skin is ensured by applying light pressure. The transmitter is then moved along the muscle when treating myalgia or reduced muscle extensibility. Localized areas of treatment, such as myofascial trigger points (MTPs) or tendons, require the shockwaves to be applied with small oscillatory movements.

The desired EFD to be delivered with FSWT is set, along with the number of shocks and their frequency. What is the most effective EFD is open to debate as various cell types react differently to ESWT. It is accepted that high energy levels can damage cell structure, while low energy values enhance biochemical processes within cells (Mariotto et al 2005; Speed 2004). The debate revolves around what constitutes low and high energy values, which has been discussed earlier in this chapter. Anecdotally, a range of 1000 to 2000 shocks appears to provide the best results for MTP and tendinopathies. Frequency, the number of shocks delivered per second (Hz), is not a variable that has been considered in the literature and does not appear to be a critical clinical parameter. Clinicians do, however, report that patients find higher frequencies more tolerable, so the alteration of pulse frequency to match patient-reported comfort appears to be a viable pragmatic approach. These parameters still require further research to determine the most effective approach for pathologies at different stages of healing (Mani-Babu et al 2015).

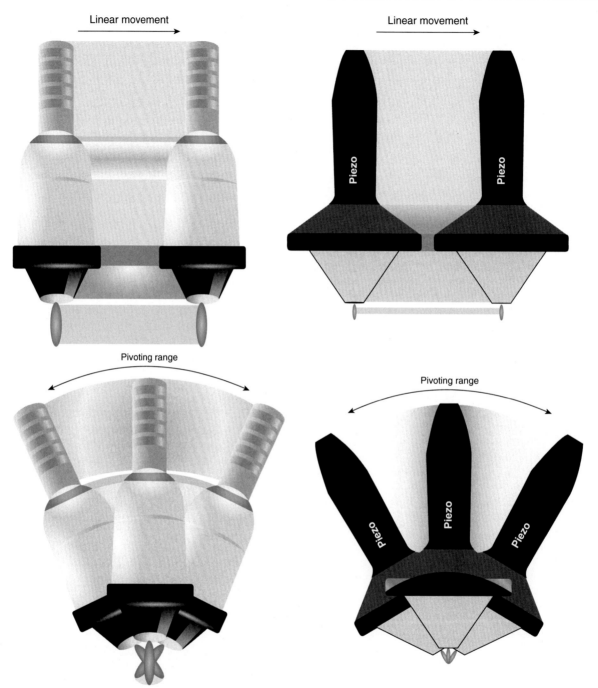

Fig.13.6 Comparison of electromagnetic and piezoelectric applications using scanning or pivoting technique for localizing treatment area.

Providing a desired EFD at a given depth when using RPW is more problematic. Manufacturers can only provide information on the amount of bar pressure within the handpiece. The EFD at the surface is determined by the size, material and shape of the transmitter. There is a difference between the EFD emitted from manufacturer's transmitters at the same bar pressure. Therefore, bar pressure cannot be used as a determinant for energy intensity in comparative studies.

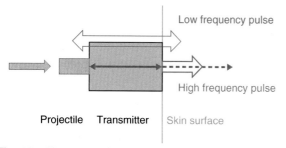

Fig. 13.7 Illustration of high frequency (ultrasonic) and low frequency (sonic) waves emitted from RPW transmitter. (From Novak P 2015.)

A radial pressure wave consists of high frequency oscillations (ultrasonic) and low frequency oscillations (sonic), which comprises longitudinal and elastic (or shear) waves (Fig. 13.7). Until recently, only one component, the ultrasonic pulse, has been considered for the evaluation of the radial pressure waves. The impact of the projectile striking the transmitter generates a longitudinal acoustic wave, which passes into the tissue as a high frequency ultrasonic wave (100 Hz depending on the transmitter). This ultrasonic pulse can be measured in a water bath, at least approximately, by hydrophone (Cleveland et al 2007). It has been shown that the penetration of the ultrasonic pulse can be quite small. Penetration depth (the depth at which the maximal intensity at skin surface becomes 50% reduced) differs from transmitter to transmitter. A standard 15 mm transmitter (Storz R15) was shown to penetrate only 6 mm (see Fig. 13.8) and a larger transmitter (Storz D20) to a depth of 16 mm (Novak & Verdaasdonk 2013).

Whilst the use of a hydrophone describes the effect of focused shockwaves, it has limitations for radial pressure waves, as the results do not sufficiently reflect the in-vivo conditions owing to the difference between the behaviour of water and tissue at low frequencies (Novak & Verdaasdonk 2013). The elastic waves can be seen in a closed water bath, appearing almost simultaneously with the ultrasonic wave (Fig. 13.9).

Further investigations on the penetration depths of elastic waves were conducted using a tissue gel block owing to its more appropriate elastic properties. Consideration was given to penetration depth allowing for attenuation of the pressure wave. Using Biological Oxygen Demand imaging, the attenuation of the elastic wave has been quantified by measuring the grey level of the propagating wave; the elastic wave appears as the dark segment (Fig. 13.10). The effect of increasing the pressure on intensity and penetration was illustrated with the darkness and width of this segment tracked over timed-lapsed shots of 0.5 ms (Fig. 13.11). Using the same two transmitters used to measure ultrasonic wave penetration, the penetration depth for sonic waves was measured at 26 mm and 76 mm respectively, a lot more than

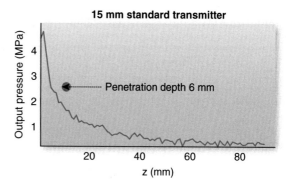

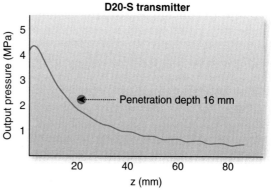

Fig. 13.8 Examples of pressure profiles along Z axis for two transmitters (Storz Technology) quantified at best by penetration depth (at −6db pressure level) using 1 bar (4Mpa). (From Novak P and Verdaasdonk 2013.)

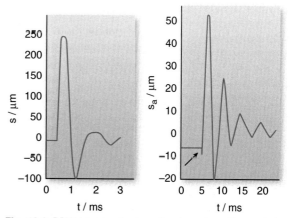

Fig. 13.9 RPW impulse in air and water where the sonic low frequency wave can be seen (*arrow*).

ultrasonic waves (Table 13.3). Due to its greater penetration depth, the shear component of the pressure wave might be the most important component of the radial pressure wave (Novak & Verdaasdonk 2013).

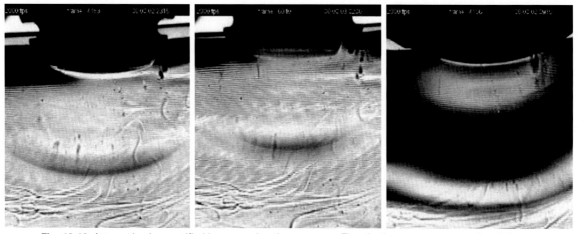

Fig. 13.10 Attenuation is quantified by measuring the grey area. The elastic wave appears as the dark segment. The intensity increases with the width of this segment and differs between transmitters. (From Novak P and Verdaasdonk 2013.)

Elastic wave

1 bar

2 bar

3 bar

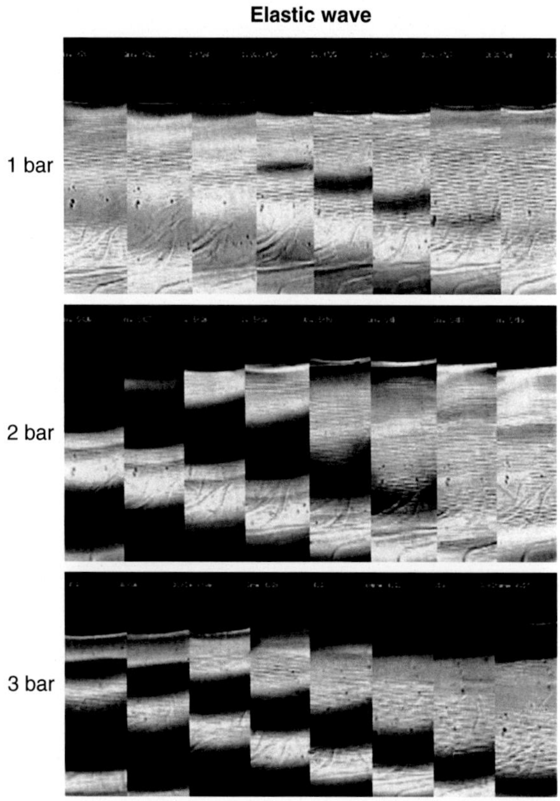

Fig. 13.11 Illustration of attenuation (*grey area*), greater intensity and penetration depth with increased pressure (*black area*). Each column represents a time lapse of 0.5 ms. (From Novak P and Verdaasdonk 2013.)

TABLE 13.3 Penetration Depth of the Components of a Radial Pressure Wave in Two Transmitters (Storz Technology) Illustrating the Significance of Elastic Waves			
RPW component		**Penetration depth (mm)**	
	Transmitter	Ø15 mm standard	D20-S
Ultrasonic wave		5.9	16
Sonic wave			
	Force (small reference area, Ø 9 mm)	10	12
	Force (large reference area, Ø 50 mm)	23	25
Elastic wave		26	76

From Novak P and Verdaasdonk 2013.

The findings of this study may also provide support to Schmitz et al's (2015) systematic review on the desired treatment parameters for ESWT, recommending three treatment sessions at 1-week intervals, with 2000 impulses per session and the highest energy flux density the patient can tolerate. Whilst this statement conflicts with earlier reports, recent research appears to support Schmitz et al's proposal. There is evidence to show that the number of treatment sessions can be reduced by increasing the EFD (Lee et al 2014;

Malliaropoulos et al 2016). Using a target VAS score of 7/10 is becoming popular with clinicians using ESWT to ensure a noxious stimulus to promote an analgesic effect, while staying within the patient's tolerance levels.

Whilst specific dose parameters continue to be researched and debated, it is important to recognize that when employing shockwave-based treatments for tendinopathy, the ESWT should be an adjunct to a graduated loading strategy, which also influences mechanotransduction and has a demonstrable benefit in tendinopathy management. Exercise prescription will require several weeks for its effects to be manifest; Alfredson et al (1998) suggest 12 weeks of eccentric exercise for Achilles tendinopathy. ESWT typically requires 3 weeks, at weekly intervals to 'reboot' the normal healing cascade. A combined, individualized exercise programme should be considered, depending on the pathology (Cook & Purdam 2009), using ESWT initially, alongside the graduated loading programme (Mani-Babu et al 2015). There is evidence that demonstrates this combination confers benefit (Rompe et al 2008). This element in patient management is not generally considered in randomized controlled studies.

SUMMARY

ESWT can be delivered in two modes: Focused Shockwave Therapy (FSWT) involves the delivery of mechanical energy such that at some point in the tissue, the energy concentration is greater than that which is delivered at the skin surface. In radial mode, often called radial shockwave, but more properly termed radial pressure wave therapy (RPW), the energy production mode is different from FSWT with a key difference that the energy travelling into the tissue never reaches a concentration greater than that delivered at the surface. The energy levels used in FSWT can be of high value, used for bone healing, wound healing and lithotripsy, or like RPW, low/medium for musculoskeletal practice.

For musculoskeletal practice, a range of applications dominates the literature. The use of shockwave in tendinopathy related lesions (including plantar fasciitis and Achilles tendinopathy) dominates. Used in conjunction with existing best evidenced therapy (e.g. exercise, managed loading), there is an advantage to the patient in terms of their recovery. Other applications for which sufficiently strong evidence is published includes greater trochanteric pain syndrome, compromised wound and bone healing (high energy), myalgia and trigger point therapy, and calcific rotator cuff pathology. There is a growing body of evidence to support the use of ESWT in Central Nervous System related muscle spasticity.

Whilst further research would be welcomed in all clinical application areas, refinement of clinical optimal doses will emerge with increased publication. Given the relative youth of this modality, the research to date supports its judicious application, primarily in urology as well as musculoskeletal practice.

REFERENCES

Alfredson, O. H., Pietilä, T., Jonsson, P., & Lorentzon, R. (1998). Heavy-load eccentric calf muscle training for the treatment of chronic Achilles tendinosis. *The American Journal of Sports Medicine, 26*, 360.

Amelio, E., & Manganotti, P. (2010). Effect of shock wave stimulation on hypertonic plantar flexor muscles in patients with cerebral palsy: A placebo-controlled study. *Journal of Rehabilitation Medicine, 42*(4), 339–343.

Atthakomol, P., Manosroi, W., Phanphaisarn, A., Phrompaet, S., Iammatavee, S., & Tongprasert, S. (2018). Comparison of single-dose radial extracorporeal shock wave and local corticosteroid injection for treatment of carpal tunnel syndrome including mid-term efficacy: A prospective randomized controlled trial. *BMC Musculoskeletal Disorders, 19*, 32.

Beyazal, M. S., & Devrimsel, G. (2015). Comparison of the effectiveness of local corticosteroid injection and extracorporeal shock wave therapy in patients with lateral epicondylitis. *Journal of Physical Therapy Science, 27*(12), 3755–3758.

Buchbinder, R., Ptasznik, R., Gordon, J., Buchanan, J., Prabaharan, V., & Forbes, A. (2002). Ultrasound-guided extracorporeal shockwave therapy for plantar fasciitis: A randomized controlled trial. *The Journal of Medical Association, 288*(11), 1364–1372.

Cacchio, A., Giordano, L., & Oet al, C. (2009). Extracorporeal shock-wave therapy compared with surgery for hypertrophic long-bone nonunions. *Journal of Bone and Joint Surgery. American Volume, 91*(11), 2589–2597.

Cacchio, A., Rompe, J. D., Furia, J. P., Susi, P., & Santilli V De Paulis, F. (2011). Shockwave therapy for the treatment of chronic proximal hamstring tendinopathy in professional athletes. *American Journal of Sports Medicine, 39*(1), 146–153.

Chaussy, C., Brendel, W., & Schmiedt, E. (1980). Extracorporeally induced destruction of kidney stones by shockwaves. *The Lancet, 316*(8207), 1265–1268.

Chen, Y. J., Wang, C. J., & Yang, KD. al (2004). Extracorporeal shock waves promote healing of collagenase-induced Achilles tendinitis and increase TGF-beta1 and IGF-I expression. *Journal of Orthopaedic Research, 22*, 854–861.

Chow, I. H. W., & Cheing, G. L. Y. (2007). Comparison of different energy densities of extracorporeal shock wave therapy (ESWT) for the management of chronic heel pain. *Clinical Rehabilitation, 21*, 131–141.

Chung, E., & Cartmill, R. (2015). Evaluation of clinical efficacy, safety and patient satisfaction rate after low-intensity extracorporeal shockwave therapy for the treatment of male erectile dysfunction: An Australian first open-label single-arm prospective clinical trial. *BJU International, 115*(Suppl. 5), 46–49.

Cleveland, R. O., Chitnis, P. V., & McClure, S. R. (2007). Acoustic field of ballistic shock wave therapy device. *Ultrasound in Medicine and Biology, 33*(8), 1327–1335.

Cook, J. (2011). Tendinopathy: No longer a 'one size fits all' diagnosis. *British Journal of Sports Medicine, 45*(5), 385.

Cook, J. L., & Purdam, C. R. (2009). Is tendon pathology a continuum? A pathology model to explain the clinical presentation of load-induced tendinopathy. *British Journal of Sports Medicine, 43*(6), 409–416.

d'Agostino, C., Romeo, P., Lavanga, V., Pisani, S., & Sansone, V. (2014). Effectiveness of extracorporeal shock wave therapy in bone marrow edema syndrome of the hip. *Rheumatology International, 34*(11).

d'Agostino, M. C., Craig, K., Tibalta, E., and Respizz, S. (2015). Shockwave as biological therapeutic tool: From, mechanical stimulation to recovery and healing, through mechanotransduction, *International Journal of Surgery*, 1–7.

Damian, M., & Zalpour, C. (2011). *Trigger point treatment with radial shock waves in musicians with nonspecific shoulder-neck pain.* Medical Problems of Performing Artists, 211–217.

Delius, M., Ueberle, F., & Gambihler, S. (1994). Destruction of gallstones and model stones by extracorporeal shock waves. *Ultrasound in Medicine and Biology, 20*(3), 251–258.

Doan, N., Reher, P., Meghji, S., & Harris, M. (1999). In vitro effects of therapeutic ultrasound on cell proliferation, protein synthesis, and cytokine production by human fibroblasts, osteoblasts, and monocytes. *Journal of Oral and Maxillofacial Surgery, 57*, 409–419.

Dreisilker, U. (2010). *Shockwave therapy in practice: Enthesiopathies.* Hielbronn, Germany: Level 10 Buchverlag, Daniela Bamburg.

Dreisilker, U. (2015). *Shockwave therapy in practice: Enthesiopathies II, radial shockwave treatment of tendinopathies.* Heilbronn, Germany: Level 10 Buchverlag, Daniela Bamburg.

Dunn, S., L & Olmedo, M., L. (2016). Mechanotransduction: Relevance to physical therapist practice-understanding our ability to affect genetic expression through mechanical forces. *Physical Therapy, 96*(5): 712–21.

Evans, D. M., & Ralston, S. H. (1996). Nitric oxide and bone. *Journal of Bone and Mineral Research, 11*, 300–305.

Friara, R., & Berta, L. (2011). Biological effects of extracorporeal shock waves on fibroblasts. A review. *Muscles, Ligaments and Tendons Journal, 1*(4) 138-114.

Gerdesmeyer, L., Henne, M., Gobel, M., & Diehl, P. (2006). Physical principles and generation of shock waves. In *Extracorporeal shock wave therapy clinical results, technologies, basics* (pp. 11–20). Towson USA: Data Trace Publishing Company.

Gerdesmeyer, L., Maier, M., Haake, M., et al. (2002). Physical technical principles of extracorporeal shockwave therapy (ESWT). *Orthopäde, Der, 31*, 610–617.

Gleitz, M. (2008). Translated from: "Verbesserung der aktiven Wadenmuskeldehnfähigkeit mittels radialer Stosswellen bei chronischen Achillodynien"; In: Orthopädie-Report Sonderheft; pp. 176–178.

Gleitz. (2011). *Shockwave therapy in practice: Myofascial syndromes and trigger points.* Germany: Leveho Buchverlag Daniela Bamberg.

Gleitz, M., & Hornig, K. (2012). Trigger points – diagnosis and treatment concepts with special reference to extracorporeal shock waves. *Orthopäde, Der, 41*, 113–125 2012.

Gonkova, M. I., Elena, M., Ilieva, E. M., Giorgio Ferriero, G., & Chavdarov, I. (2013). Effect of radial shock wave therapy on muscle spasticity in children with cerebral palsy. *International Journal of Rehabilitation Research.*

Graff, J., Richter, K. D., & Pastor, J. (1988). Effect of high energy shock waves on bony tissue. *Urological Research, 16*, 252–258.

Hausdorf, J., Lemmens, M. A., Heck, K. D., et al. (2008). Selective loss of unmyelinated nerve fibers after extracorporeal shockwave application to the musculoskeletal system. *Neuroscience, 155*(1), 138–144.

Hausdorf, J., Sievers, B., Schmitt-Sody, M., Jansson, V., Maier, M., & Mayer-Wagner, S. (2011). Stimulation of bone growth factor synthesis in human osteoblasts and fibroblasts after extracorporeal shock wave application. *Archives of Orthopaedic and Trauma Surgery, 131*, 303–309.

Huang, C., Holfeld, J., Schaden, W., Orgill, D., & Ogawa, R. (2013). Mechanotherapy: Revisiting physical therapy and recruiting mechanobiology for a new era in medicine. *Trends in Molecular Medicine, 19*(9), 555–564.

Huissstede, B. M., Hoogvliet, P., Franke, T. P., Randsdorp, M. S., & Koes, B. W. (2017). Carpal tunnel syndrome: Effectiveness of physical therapy and electrophysical modalities. An updated systematic review of randomized controlled trials. *Archives of Physical Medicine and Rehabilitation, 99*(8), 1623–1634.

Ilieva, E. M., Minchev, R. M., & Petrova, N. S. (2012). Radial shock wave therapy in patients with lateral epicondylitis. *Folia Medica, 54*(3), 35–41.

Ingber, D. E. (2003). Tensegrity II. How structural networks influence cellular information processing networks, *Journal of Cell Science*, 15;116(Pt 8)1397-408.

Ingber, D. E. (2006). Cellular mechanotransduction: Putting all the pieces together again. *FASEP Journal, 20*(7).

Ingber, D. E. (2008). Tensegrity and mechanotransduction. *J Bodyw Mov Ther*, 12(3):198–200.

ISMST website. Available: https://www.shockwavetherapy.org/home/ 30 Sept 2018.

Ito, K., Fukumoto, Y., & Shimokawa, H. (2011). Extracorporeal shock wave therapy for ischemic cardiovascular disorders. *American Journal of Cardiovascular Drugs, 11*(5), 295–302.

Khan, K. M., & Scott, A. (2009). Mechanotherapy: How physical therapists' prescription of exercise promotes tissue repair. *British Journal of Sports Medicine, 43*(4), 247–252.

Kim, Y. W., Shin, J. C., Yoon, J. G., Kim, Y. K., & Lee, S. C. (2013). Usefulness of radial extracorporeal shock wave therapy for the spasticity of the subscapularis in patients with stroke: A pilot study. *Chinese Medical Journal, 126*(24), 4638-4643.

Kuo, Y. R., Wang, C. T., Wang, F. S., et al. (2009). Extracorporeal shockwave therapy enhanced wound healing via increasing topical blood perfusion and tissue regeneration in a rat model of STZ-induced diabetes. *Wound Repair and Regeneration, 17*(4), 522–530.

Lee, J. Y., Kim, S. N., Lee, I. S., Jung, H., Lee, K. S., & Koh, S. E. (2014). Effects of extracorporeal shock wave therapy on spasticity in patients after brain injury: A meta-analysis. *Journal of Physical Therapy Science, 26*(10), 1641–1647.

Li, T. Y., Chang, C. Y., Chou, Y. C., et al. (2016). Effect of radial shock wave therapy on spasticity of the upper limb in patients with chronic stroke: A prospective, randomized, single blind, controlled trial. *Medicine, 95*(18), e3544.

Loew, M., Daecke, W., Kusnierczak, D., et al. (1999). Shockwave therapy is effective for chronic calcifying tendinitis of the shoulder. *The Journal of Bone and Joint Surgery. British Volume, 81*, 863–867.

Lohrer, H., & Nauck T, T. (2015). Radial shock wave therapy for patients with apophysitis calcanei. *Deutsche Zeitschrift für Sportmedizin, 66*(3), 60–63.

Lohrer, H., Nauck, T., Korakakis, V., & Malliaropoulos, N. (2016). Historical ESWT paradigms are overcome: A narrative review. *BioMed Research International.* https://doi.org/10.1155/2016/3850461.

Lohrer, H., Nauck, T., Schöll, J., Zwerver, J., & Malliaropoulos, N. (2012). Extracorporeal shock wave therapy for patients suffering from recalcitrant Osgood-Schlatter disease. *Sportverletzung Sportschaden, 26*(4), 218–222.

Ma, Y. W., Jiang, D. L., Zhang, D., Wang, X. B., & Yu, X. T. (2016). Radial extracorporeal shock wave therapy in a person with advanced osteonecrosis of the femoral head. *American Journal of Physical Medicine & Rehabilitation, 95*(9), 133–139.

Maier, M., Staupendahl, D., Duerr, H. R., Refior, H. J., (2016). Castor oil decreases pain during extracorporeal shock wave application. *Archives of Orthopaedic and Trauma Surgery, 119*(7-8), 423–7.

Malliaropoulos, N., Crate, G., Meke, M., et al. (2016). Success and recurrence rate after radial extracorporeal shock wave therapy for plantar fasciopathy: A retrospective study. *BioMed Research International, 3*(1), 1–18.

Mani-Babu, S., Morrissey, D., Waugh, D., Screen, H., & Barton, C. (2015). The effectiveness of extracorporeal shock wave therapy in lower limb tendinopathy. *The American Journal of Sports Medicine, 43*(3), 752–761.

Mantovani, A., Biswas, S. K., Galdiero, M. R., Sica, A., & Locati, M. (2013). Macrophage plasticity and polarization in tissue repair and remodelling. *The Journal of Pathology, 229*(2), 176–185.

Mariotto, S., Cavalieri, E., Amelio, E., et al. (2005). Extracorporeal shock waves: From lithotripsy to anti-inflammatory action by NO production. *Nitric Oxide, 12*, 89–96.

Marshall, K. L., & Lumpkin, E. A. (2012). The molecular basis of mechanosensory transduction. In C. López-Larrea (Ed.), *Sensing in nature* (pp. 142–155). New York: Springer.

Martinez, F. O., Sica, A., Mantovani, A., & Locati, M. (2008). Macrophage activation and polarization. *Frontiers in Bioscience, 13*(1), 453–461.

Martini, L., Giavaresi, G., & al, F. M. (2003). Effect of extracorporeal shock wave therapy on osteoblastlike cells. *Clinical Orthopaedics and Related Research, 413*, 269–280.

Mittermayr, R., Antonic, V., Hartinger, J., et al. (2012). Extracorporeal shock wave therapy (ESWT) for wound healing: Technology, mechanisms, and clinical efficacy. *Wound Repair and Regeneration, 20*(4), 456–465.

Nishida, T., Shimokawa, H., Keiji Oi, K., et al. (2004). Extracorporeal cardiac shock wave therapy markedly ameliorates ischemia-induced myocardial dysfunction in pigs in vivo. *Circulation, 110*, 3055–3061.

Novak, K. F., Govindaswami, M., Ebersole, J. L., Schaden, W., House, N., & Novak, M. J. (2008). Effects of low-energy shock waves on oral bacteria. *Journal of Dental Research, 87*(10):928–931.

Novak, P. (2015). Physics: F-SW and R-SW. Basic information on focused and radial shock wave physics. In H. Lohrer & L. Gerdesmeyer (Eds.), *Multidisciplinary medical applications* (pp. 28–49). Heilbronn, Germany: level 10 Buchverlag Daniela Bamberg.

Novak, P., & Verdaasdonk (2013). Radial ESWT update: New observations to explain positive treatment outcomes in sports medicine. In H. Lohrer & T. Nuack (Eds.), *Shockwave in sports medicine* (pp. 129–157). Heilbronn, Germany: Level10 Buchverlag.

Ogden, J. A., Toth-Kischkat, A., & Schulteiss, R. (2001). Principles of shock wave therapy. *Clinical Orthopaedics and Related Research, 387*, 8–17.

Paulis, G., & Brancato, T. (2012). Inflammatory mechanisms and oxidative stress in Peyronie's disease: Therapeutic "rationale" and related emerging treatment strategies. *Inflammation and Allergy - Drug Targets, 11*(1), 48–57.

PEDro Scale. (2017). Available: www.pedro.org.au/ english/ downloads/pedro-scale/.

Rakov, V. A., & Uman, M. A. (2007). *Lightning: Physics and effects.* Cambridge, England: Cambridge University Press, 378.

Ramon, S., Gleitz, M., Hernandez, L., & Romero, L. D. (2015). Update on the efficacy of extracorporeal shockwave treatment for myofascial pain syndrome and fibromyalgia. *International Journal of Surgery, 24*(Pt B), 201–206.

Reilly, J. M., Bluman, E., & Tenforde, A. S. (2018). Narrative review on the effect of shockwave treatment for management of upper and lower extremity musculoskeletal conditions. *American Academy of Physical Medicine and Rehabilitation, 18* 1934-1482.

Romeo, P., Lavanga, V., Pagani, D., & Sansone, V. (2014). Extracorporeal shock wave therapy in musculoskeletal disorders: A review. *Medical Principles and Practice, 23*(1), 7–13.

Rompe, J. D., Cacchio, A., Furia, J. P., & Maffulli, N. (2008). Controlled trial chronic insertional Achilles tendinopathy. A randomized, eccentric loading compared with shock wave treatment. *Journal of Bone and Joint Surgery, 90*, 52–61.

Rompe, J. D., Kirkpatrick, C. J., Kullmer, K., Schwitalle, M., & Krischek, O. (1998). Dose-related effects of shock waves on rabbit tendo Achillis: A sonographic and histological study. *The Journal of Bone and Joint Surgery. British Volume, 80-B*, 546–552.

Saggini, R., Figus, A., Troccola, A., Cocco, V., Saggini, A., & Scuderi, N. (2008). Extracorporeal shock wave therapy for management of chronic ulcers in the lower extremities. *Ultrasound in Medicine and Biology, 34*(8), 1261–1271.

Sathishkumar, S., Meka, A., Dawson, D., House, N., Schaden, W., Novak, M, J., Ebersole, J. L., Kesavalu, L. (2008). Extracorporeal shock wave therapy induces alveolar bone regeneration, Journal of Dental Research, 87(7): 687–91.

Sawan, S., Abd-Allah, F., Hegazy, M. M., Farrag, M. A., & Sharf El-Den, N. H. (2017). Effect of shock wave therapy on ankle planter flexors spasticity in stroke patients. *NeuroRehabilitation, 40*(1), 115–118.

Schaden, W., Mittermayr, R., Haffner, N., Smolen, D., Gerdesmeyer, L., & Wang, C. J. (2015). Extracorporeal shock-wave therapy (ESWT)—first choice treatment of fracture non-unions? *International Journal of Surgery, 24*, 179–183.

Schmitz, C., Császár, N. B. M., Milz, S., et al. (2015). Efficacy and safety of extracorporeal shock wave therapy for orthopedic conditions: A systematic review on studies listed in the PEDro database. *British Medical Bulletin, 116*(1), 115–138.

Sems, A., Dimeff, R., & Iannotti, J. P. (2006). Extracorporeal shockwave therapy in the treatment of chronic tendinopathies. *Journal of the American Academy of Orthopaedic Surgeons, 14*(4), 195–204.

Shah, J. P., Danoff, J. V., Desai, M. J., et al. (2008). Biochemicals associated with pain and inflammation are elevated in sites near to and remote from active myofascial trigger points. *Archives of Physical Medicine and Rehabilitation, 89*(1), 16–23.

Simons, D. G., Travell, J. G., & Simons, L. S. (1998). *Myofascial pain and dysfunction: The trigger point. Manual V1* (2nd ed.).

Spacca, G., Necozione, S., & Cacchio, A. (2005). Radial shock wave therapy for lateral epicondylitis: A prospective randomised controlled single-blind study. *European Journal of Physical and Rehabilitation Medicine, 41*(1), 17–25 2005.

Speed, C. A. (2004). Extracorporeal shock wave therapy in management of chronic soft-tissue conditions. *The Journal of Bone and Joint Surgery. British Volume, 86*, 165–171.

Speed, C. (2014). A systematic review of shockwave therapies in soft tissue conditions: Focusing on the evidence. *British Journal of Sports Medicine, 48*, 1538–1542.

Tam, K. F., Cheung, W. H., Lee, K. M., Qin, L., & Leung, K. S. (2008). Osteogenic effects of low intensity pulsed ultrasound, extracorporeal shockwaves and their combination – an in vitro comparative study on human periosteal cells. *Ultrasound in Medicine and Biology, 34*(12), 1957–1965.

Tamma, R., dell'Endice, S., Notarnicola, A., Moretti, L., Patella, S., Patella, V., et al. (2009). Extracorporeal shock waves stimulate osteoblast activities. *Ultrasound in Medicine and Biology, 35*(12), 2093–2100.

Valchanou, V. D., & Michailov, P. (1991). High energy shock waves in the treatment of delayed and nonunion of fractures. *International Orthopaedics, 15*(3), 181–184.

Vetrano, M., d'Alessandro, F., Torrisi, M. R., Ferretti, A., Vulpiani, M. C., & Visco, V. (2011). Extracorporeal shock wave therapy promotes cell proliferation and collagen synthesis of primary cultured human tenocytes. *Knee Surgery, Sports Traumatology, Arthroscopy, 19*, 2159–2168.

Wang, C. J. (2012). Extracorporeal shockwave therapy in musculoskeletal disorders. *Journal of Orthopaedic Surgery and Research, 7*, 11.

Wang, T., Du, L., Shan, L., Dong, H., Feng, J., Kiessling, M. C., et al. (2016). A prospective case-control study of radial extracorporeal shock wave therapy for spastic plantar flexor muscles in very young children with cerebral palsy. *Medicine, 95*(19), e3649.

Wang, C. J., Huang, H. Y., & Pai, C. H. (2002). Shock wave–enhanced neovascularization at the tendon-bone junction: An experiment in dogs. *The Journal of Foot and Ankle Surgery, 41*, 16–22.

Wang, C. J., Wang, F. S., Huang, C. C., Yang, K. D., Weng, L. H., & Huang, H. Y. (2005). Treatment for osteonecrosis of the femoral head: Comparison of extracorporeal shockwaves with core decompression and bone-grafting. *The Journal of Bone and Joint Surgery. American Volume, 87*(11), 2380–2387.

Wang, F. S., Yang, K. D., Chen, R. F., et al. (2002). Extracorporeal shock wave promotes growth and differentiation of bone marrow stromal cells towards osteoprogenitors associated with induction of TGF- β 1. *The Journal of Bone and Joint Surgery. British Volume, 84*, 457–461.

Waugh, C. M., Morrissey, D., Jones, E., Riley, G. P., Langberg, H., & Screen, H. R. C. (2015). In vivo biological to extracorporeal shockwave therapy in human tendinopathy. *European Cells and Materials, 29*, 268–280.

van der Worp, H., Zwerver, J., Hamstra, M., et al. (2014). No difference in effectiveness between focused and radial shockwave therapy for treating patellar tendinopathy: A randomized controlled trial. *Knee Surgery, Sports Traumatology, Arthroscopy, 22*, 2026–2032.

Wu, Y. T., Chang, C. N., Chen, Y. M., & Hu, G. C. (2018). Comparison of the effect of focused and radial extracorporeal shock waves on spastic equinus in patients with stroke – A randomized controlled trial. *European Journal of Physical and Rehabilitation Medicine, 54*(4), 518–525.

Wu, Y. T., Ke, M. J., Chou, Y. C., Chang, C. Y., Lin, C. Y., Li, T. Y., et al. (2016). Effect of radial shock wave therapy for carpal tunnel syndrome: A prospective randomized, double-blind, placebo-controlled trial. *Journal of Orthopaedic Research, 34*(6) 977–84.

Xu, J. K., Chen, H. J., Li, X. D., Huang, Z. L., Xu, H., Yang, H. L., et al. (2012). Optimal intensity shock wave promotes the adhesion and migration of rat osteoblasts via integrin b1-mediated expression of phosphorylated focal adhesion kinase. *Journal of Biological Chemistry, 287*(31), 26200–26212.

Yin, T. C., Wang, C. J., Yang, K. D., Wang, F. S., & Sun, Y. C. (2011). Shockwaves enhance the osteogenetic gene expression in marrow stromal cells from hips with osteonecrosis. *Chang Gung Medical Journal, 34*, 367–374.

Zhang, Q., Liu, L., Sun, W., Gao, F., Cheng, L., & Li, Z. (2016). Extracorporeal shockwave therapy in osteonecrosis of femoral head: A systematic review of now available clinical evidences. *Medicine, 96*(4), 1–8.

Vibration

Marco Y. C. Pang, Freddy M. H. Lam

INTRODUCTION

The use of vibration as a treatment modality has a long history. Focal muscle vibration has been used in physical therapy since the 1950s (Bishop 1975; Eklund & Hagbarth 1966), when several treatment approaches specifically designed to address neurological disability came into being, including the Bobath (Bobath 1955), Brunnstrom (Perry 1967), and Rood (Stockmeyer 1967) approaches. In the 1970s, the application of vibration as an exercise intervention to enhance muscle strength and power in well-trained individuals was studied by Russian scientists (Issurin et al 1994; Issurin & Tennenbaum 1999). In earlier research and clinical applications, muscle vibrations were applied locally by means of manual vibrators, vibrating cables and vibrating dumbbells (Bobath 1955; Bishop 1975; Issurin et al 1994; Issurin & Tennenbaum 1999; Cardinale and Bosco 2003) (Fig. 14.1A).

Animal research in the 1990s and 2000s found that high-frequency dynamic mechanical loading was a potent stimulus for bone formation (Flieger et al 1998; Hsieh & Turner 2001; Ozcivici et al 2007; Robling et al 2001; Rubin et al 2001; Turner & Robling 2003; Umemura et al 1997). These discoveries sparked the development of platforms that could deliver whole-body vibrations (WBV) (Fig. 14.1B), although the concept of applying vibrations to the whole body can be dated back to the 19th century, when vibratory chairs were used to treat Parkinson's disease by Jean-Martin Charcot (Goetz 2009). Different from focal muscle vibrations, exercising on the vibration platform would allow the delivery of mechanical vibrations throughout the body, thereby potentially inducing more systemic effects not only on the muscles, but also on other soft tissues (e.g. bones, cartilages), as well as the neural, cardiovascular and hormonal systems (Cardinale and Bosco 2003; Musumeci 2017; Pang 2010). Nowadays, whole-body vibration (WBV), defined as a mechanical stimulus characterized by oscillatory motion delivered to the entire body, is commonly used in physical therapy as a treatment tool in a variety of patient populations (Rauch et al 2010).

PHYSICAL PRINCIPLES

Mechanical vibrations are characterized by two important parameters, namely frequency and amplitude (Rauch et al 2010). Focal muscle vibrations used in various

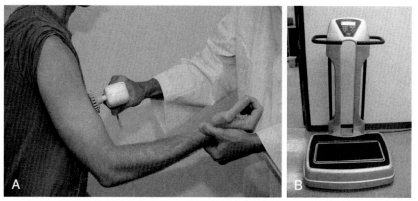

Fig. 14.1 (A) Manual vibrator. (B) Whole-body vibration platform.

neurofacilitation treatment approaches are delivered by manual vibrators. High-frequency vibrations typically involve a frequency range of 100–200 Hz and amplitude of 0.2–0.3 mm, whereas low-frequency stimulations involve a frequency range of 5–50 Hz (Murillo et al 2014). There are two common types of platform available commercially for whole-body vibrations: (1) sinusoidal (i.e. generation of a constant vibration frequency) (Rauch et al 2010; Torvinen et al 2003; Verschueren et al 2004; von Stengel et al 2011) and (2) stochastic resonance (i.e. with random vibration frequencies and harmonics) (Rogan et al 2011, 2012; Rogan & Hilfiker 2015). Sinusoidal vibration platforms have two subtypes. In rotational/side-alternating vibration devices, there is reciprocating displacement of the plate on the left and right side of a fulcrum (axis of rotation) and thus a mediolateral component of the force is also produced (Cardinale & Wakeling 2005) (Fig. 14.2A). Thus, the amplitude of the vibration would depend on the position of the feet. In vertical/synchronous vibration devices, the whole plate oscillates uniformly up and down (Fig. 14.2B). The frequencies and amplitudes commonly used in previous research were 20–60 Hz and 2–5 mm respectively for sinusoidal platforms, compared with 1–12 Hz and 3–6 mm for stochastic resonance vibration devices (Lam et al 2012; Lau et al 2011a; Liao et al 2014a; Rogan et al 2015). The theoretical peak acceleration, which is often used as a measure of vibration intensity/magnitude, can be calculated as: $A(2\pi f)^2$ where A and f represent the amplitude and frequency of the vibration signals respectively (Kiiski et al 2008). The key parameters of WBV are illustrated in Table 14.1 and Fig. 14.3. As the vibrations are transmitted from the feet upwards to the rest of the body, there should be attenuation of signals (Huang et al 2018; Kiiski et al 2008; Lam et al 2018a). However, at certain frequencies, particularly when the applied frequency is near the

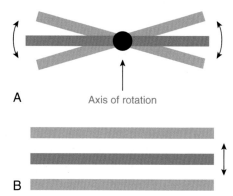

Fig. 14.2 (A) Side-alternating/rotational vibrations. (B) Vertical vibrations.

natural frequency of the tissue, there may be amplifications of the signals (Huang et al 2018; Kiiski et al 2008; Lam et al 2018a). Distortion of the sinusoidal waveforms is also more pronounced with signals of higher amplitude (Kiiski et al 2008).

BIOPHYSICAL EFFECTS, INTERACTIONS AND RESPONSES

Sensory Responses

Vibration is a form of sensory stimulation because cutaneous mechanoreceptors, such as Merkel disks, Meissner corpuscles and Pacinian corpuscles, are sensitive to low (5–15 Hz), medium (20–50 Hz) and high (60–400 Hz) vibratory frequencies, respectively (Darian-Smith 1984; Poenaru et al 2016). Vibration also stimulates the muscle spindles, which relay proprioceptive information. It has thus been used to create a movement illusion to assess balance control strategies (Claeys et al 2011).

TABLE 14.1 Parameters of Whole-Body Vibration

Vibration Parameters	Description
Amplitude	Amount of vertical displacement (mm)
Frequency	Number of impulses per second (Hz)
Magnitude	Acceleration of movement, in g (1 g = acceleration due to Earth's gravitational field, 9.8 m/s^2)
Duration	Total amount of time that a person is exposed to WBV treatment

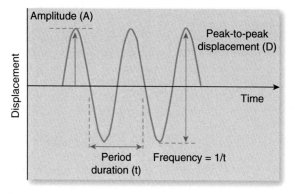

Fig. 14.3 Parameters of whole-body vibration. Frequency = 1/t.

The neural signals generated from vibratory stimulation are transmitted by the large-diameter mechanosensitive afferents. Hence, vibrations can potentially inhibit transmission of nociceptive information at the dorsal horn of the spinal cord involving the pain gating mechanism similar to that observed with transcutaneous electrical nerve simulation (TENS) (Braz et al 2014). Indeed, vibration stimulation has been shown to increase pain threshold, especially in women (Dahlin 2006).

The vibratory information ultimately reaches the cortex, through cortical projections from the thalamus to the primary somatosensory S1 area in the postcentral gyrus (Peonaru et al 2016). It was suggested that there are inhibitory interactions between the brain region responsible for pain (area 3a) and for non-nociresponsive stimulation (areas 3b and 1), including vibration (Vierck et al 2013).

Neuromuscular Responses

Tonic vibration reflex can be elicited by applying focal vibration on musculotendinous junctions (Eklund 1966). The primary Ia afferents of the muscle spindles are very sensitive to vibrations, and reflex muscle contractions are induced through their connections with the motor neurons in the spinal cord. Generally, vibration frequencies between 100–150 Hz elicit the classic tonic vibratory reflex, with augmentation of electromyographic (EMG) activity and synchronization of motor units (Martin 1997; Homma 1972).

Whole-body vibration has also been consistently shown to increase the EMG activity of the stimulated muscles (Cardinale and Lim 2003; Hazell et al 2007, 2010; Lam et al 2016; Liao 2014b, 2015a; Pollock et al 2010; Ritzmann et al 2010, 2013). It should not be confused with the tonic vibration reflex, because the typical frequency range used in WBV (20–60 Hz) is well below that which is effective in inducing the tonic vibration reflex (100–150 Hz). The neural mechanisms underlying WBV-induced increase in muscle activity must be more complex than that involved in the tonic vibration reflex, as multiple muscles are simultaneously stimulated by WBV.

As the nerve fibres relaying the vibratory information have extensive connections with motor neurons and interneurons at different levels, vibration stimulation can also modulate the excitability of the spinal motoneuronal pool (Kipp et al 2011; Rittweger et al 2003; Sayenko et al 2010) and corticomotor neurons (Christova et al 2010; Mileva et al 2009), thereby influencing the motor output. Presynaptic inhibition (Burke et al 1996; Kipp et al 2011; Sayenko et al 2010), intracortical facilitation (Marconi et al 2008; Mileva et al 2009) and intracortical inhibition (Marconi et al 2008; Mileva et al 2009) have been suggested as some of the potential mechanisms involved.

Osteogenic Responses

Being a form of dynamic mechanical stimulation, vibration is a potent stimulus for bone tissue (Burr et al 2002; Robling et al 2000, 2001; Rubin et al 2002a, 2002b; Turner & Robling 2003). Ample animal work has shown that low-magnitude, dynamic mechanical stimulation can induce osteogenesis (Turner & Robling 2003). Through the process of mechanotransduction, the biophysical force applied to the bone tissue is converted into a cellular response by the osteoblasts, which are responsible for osteogenesis (Qin et al 2003; Turner & Pavalko 1998). Whole-body vibration has also been shown to promote fracture healing in various animal models (Chow et al 2011, 2016; Chung et al 2014; Leung et al 2009; Shi et al 2010; Wei et al 2016), through enhancing expression of the genes related to callus formation (Chow et al 2016; Chung et al 2014) and mesenchymal stem cell recruitment (Wei et al 2016), and increasing angiogenesis (Cheung et al 2012).

Cardiovascular Responses

The cardiovascular system also responds to vibrations (Cochrane et al 2008; Fuller et al 2013; Hazell et al 2008, 2012; Kang et al 2016; Liao et al 2015b; Rittweger et al 2000, 2001, 2002a, 2010; Robbins et al 2014; Vissers et al 2009; Yarar-Fisher et al 2014). Whole-body vibration has been shown to increase blood flow, blood flow velocity and diameter of the blood vessels in the stimulated area (Fuller et al 2013; Kerschan-Schindl et al 2001; Lythgo et al 2009). Oxygenation of the stimulated muscle is also enhanced in the initial phase (30 seconds) of exposure to WBV (Rittweger et al 2010). Increase in oxygen consumption rate (VO_2) and heart rate (Hazell et al 2012; Kang et al 2016; Liao et al 2015b; Rittweger et al 2001) can be induced by WBV, but the magnitude of the responses seems to highly depend on the type (static versus dynamic) and intensity of exercise performed on the platform, as well as the intensity of WBV (Cochrane et al 2008; Hazell et al 2008; Liao et al 2015b; Rittweger et al 2002a). Generally, the change in heart rate, VO_2 and blood pressure associated with WBV is modest (Avelar et al 2011a; Cochrane et al 2008; Hazell et al 2008; Liao et al 2015b).

Hormonal Responses

Whole-body vibration exercise may also induce acute changes in blood hormone concentrations, such as increases in growth hormone, noradrenaline and testosterone levels, and reduction in cortisol level (Bosco et al 2000). This phenomenon is similar to the rapid hormonal responses observed in short-term intensive exercises (e.g. weight lifting) (Bosco et al 1996; Kraemer et al 1990; Schwab et al 1993). The effect of WBV on inducing hormonal response remains largely controversial as other studies could not replicate the findings (Di Loreto et al 2004; Erskine et al 2007).

Summary

In summary, because of the influence of vibrations on the sensori-motor, cardiovascular and musculoskeletal systems, it may have potential applications in modifying muscle flexibility/strength/power, spasticity, pain, circulation and bone health.

CLINICAL EVIDENCE

Focal Vibration

Pain Relief

Focal vibration has been used to treat different types of pain. Research studies showed that 70% of patients suffering from acute/chronic pain due to a variety of causes reported a decrease in pain level during vibratory stimulation (Lundeberg 1983). The pain reduction was more than 50% for patients with light to moderate pain and 50% or less for those reporting moderate to severe pain before stimulation. The effect of pain relief could last for 3 hours and up to more than 12 hours (Lundeberg 1983). Vibration stimulation attenuates the pain induced by heat stimulation on the forearm in healthy people, and people with chronic pain or fibromyalgia (Staud et al 2011). Evidence on reduction of sharp pain (e.g. induced by injection, staple or suture removal) was largely similar (Eichhorn et al 2016; Nanitsos et al 2009). Vibration reduced sharp pain by up to 44% (Eichhorn et al 2016).

Neuromuscular Function

Brief sessions of focal vibration applied to contracted quadriceps were found to improve lower limb power and balance in older women, whereas vibration applied to non-contracted quadriceps had no significant effect (Filippi et al 2009). Adding vibration to a submaximal quadriceps contraction significantly improved balance and mobility in patients with osteoarthritis compared with submaximal contraction alone without vibration (Rabini et al 2015). A similar finding was observed in postmenopausal women (Brunetti et al 2015; Celletti 2015). Improvement in upper limb function was also reported in healthy individuals (Aprile et al 2006). Focal vibration has been used extensively in various neurological conditions, including stroke, spinal cord injury, Parkinson's disease, and multiple sclerosis (Murillo et al 2014). Significant reduction in spasticity, and improvement in movement and gait quality, was observed after brief sessions of vibratory stimulation (Camerota et al 2016). Some studies suggested that the effect of vibration on physical functions can last for months (Brunetti et al 2015; Rabini et al 2015).

Bone Health

There is preliminary evidence that focal vibration can improve bone quality of the upper limbs in disabled children and prevent the decline in hip bone density in osteoporotic women (Brunetti et al 2015; Reyes et al 2011) but the effect of focal vibration on bone health requires further investigation.

Whole-Body Vibration (WBV)

Sensory Function and Pain Relief

The effects of WBV on proprioception is inconclusive (Dickin et al 2012; Games & Sefton 2013; Hannah et al 2013; Pollock et al 2011). Fontana et al (2005) found a significant improvement in lumbosacral proprioception, as indicated by the lumbosacral repositioning error, following 5 minutes of rotational WBV (18 Hz) among healthy individuals. However, using a similar protocol, Lee and

Chow (2013) found no significant change in lumbar repositioning error. Whole-body vibration was reported to be superior to conventional exercise training in improving knee proprioception in athletes who had undergone ACL reconstruction surgery (Moezy et al 2008). However, other studies reported no such benefits in young adults and people with knee osteoarthritis (Hannah et al 2013; Pollock et al 2011; Trans et al 2009). Cutaneous sensation in the foot and ankle was found to be reduced immediately post-WBV. The effect was more prolonged and widespread if a higher amplitude protocol (8 mm) was used (Pollock et al 2011).

The use of WBV in pain modulation has been investigated in patients with prolonged bed rest (Miokovic et al 2014), osteoporosis (Iwamoto et al 2005), low back pain (del Pozo-Cruz et al 2011; Rittweger et al 2002b), knee osteoarthritis (Avelar et al 2011b; Park et al 2013; Simão et al 2012; Trans et al 2009), fibromyalgia (Alentorn-Geli et al 2008), chronic Achilles tendinopathy (Horstmann et al 2013) and general musculoskeletal pain (Elfering et al 2013). Adding WBV to resistive exercise had no additional effect on pain level for people undergoing bed rest (Miokovic et al 2014). Adding WBV (20 Hz, 0.7–4.2 mm, side-alternating) to alendronate treatment resulted in greater reduction in pain in postmenopausal women with osteoporosis than alendronate treatment alone (Iwamoto et al 2005). In terms of its effect on low back pain and fibromyalgia, WBV treatment (18–20 Hz) was not different from active exercises (Alentorn-Geli et al 2008; Rittweger et al 2002b), but was superior to usual activity or no-intervention (Alentorn-Geli et al 2008; del Pozo-Cruz et al 2011). The use of WBV to reduce pain in people with knee osteoarthritis has been explored in a few studies (Avelar et al 2011b; Park et al 2013; Simão et al 2012; Trans et al 2009; Wang et al 2015), and the results were conflicting, regardless of the nature of the comparison group. Whole-body vibration (16–21 Hz, 0.5–0.8 mm, side-alternating) was found to result in a similar degree of pain reduction in the midsection of the Achilles tendon as eccentric exercise training in patients with chronic Achilles tendinopathy, but eccentric training was more effective in reducing pain at the musculotendinous junction and also lessened the impact of pain on running training (Horstmann et al 2013). Stochastic resonance WBV was shown to be effective when treating general musculoskeletal pain in young adults (Elfering et al 2011, 2013), with a mean frequency of 5 Hz being more effective than 1.5 Hz (Elfering et al 2011). In summary, there are some preliminary findings to suggest that WBV may have some benefits on reducing pain in people with osteoporosis or musculoskeletal pain. Otherwise, there was no strong evidence demonstrating the effectiveness of WBV in pain management.

Muscle Strength and Power

Quite consistent evidence shows that WBV exposure has acute effect on muscle strength/power performance, in a phenomenon often described as post-activation potentiation (Avelar et al 2014). Whole-body vibration has been used in preconditioning exercise to improve subsequent muscle performance in athletes and non-athletes (Annino 2017 et al; Avelar et al 2014; Dallas et al 2014; Duc et al 2017; Kelly et al 2010; Rønnestad et al 2016). However, the type of preconditioning exercise seems to have an impact. Bush et al (2015) showed that post-activation potentiation occurred only when WBV was combined with dynamic exercise, but not static exercise.

The effects of long-term WBV training on neuromuscular function in able-bodied individuals (Bautmans et al 2005; Delecluse et al 2003; Kvorning et al 2006; Lau et al 2011a; Mahieu et al 2006; Marin & Rhea 2010a, 2010b; Mikhael et al 2010; Osawa et al 2011, 2013b; Perchthaler et al 2015; Petit et al 2010; Rees et al 2007; Rehn et al 2007; Russo et al 2003; Sitjà-Rabert et al 2012a, 2012b; von Stengel et al 2012; Wyon et al 2010) have been well studied. The majority of these studies reported beneficial effects on leg muscle strength. Based on the results from several meta-analyses (Calendo et al 2014; Lau et al 2011a; Manimmanakorn et al 2014; Osawa et al 2013b), it can be concluded that WBV induced additional beneficial effects on leg muscle power (often measured as jump height) compared with no exercise, or identical conditions without WBV, or with cardiovascular exercise. Greater benefits were associated with a higher WBV frequency (>30 Hz), higher amplitude (>3 mm), longer duration of WBV exposure (>10 minutes per session), and longer treatment period (>12 weeks). In addition, non-athletes had greater benefit for jump height improvement than athletes (Manimmanakorn et al 2014). Vertical WBV (frequencies: 30.0 to 40.0 Hz; 3 sessions per week; 15 minutes per session) was found to increase the isometric maximal voluntary contraction (by 15–17%) and dynamic maximal strength (8–17%) (Calendo et al 2014). The gain in isometric strength seemed to be greater with a lower frequency at 12.5 Hz (26.6%) (Calendo et al 2014). The acute effect of WBV exercise on lower limb muscle activity was also stronger in the older population than in their younger counterparts (Lienhard et al 2017).

Increasing research has explored the use of WBV to improve muscle strength in patients with clinical conditions, including stroke (Liao et al 2014a), Parkinson's disease (Lau et al 2011b), knee osteoarthritis (Park et al 2013), low back pain (del Pozo-Cruz et al 2011), COPD (Broekmans et al 2010; Gloeckl et al 2015; Pleguezuelos et al 2013), and multiple sclerosis (Claerbout et al 2012; Jackson et al 2008; Sitjà-Rabert et al 2012a). No consistent evidence was demonstrated.

Muscle Flexibility, Spasticity and Rigidity

The effect of WBV on muscle flexibility is quite well studied. A meta-analysis conducted by Osawa & Oguma (2013a) revealed that WBV had significant additive effects on flexibility compared with the same condition without WBV.

The effect of WBV on spasticity has been studied in patients with cerebral palsy (Ahlborg et al 2006; Cheng et al 2015; Ibrahim et al 2014), multiple sclerosis (Schyns et al 2009), spinocerebellar ataxia (Kaut et al 2014) and stroke (Brogårdh et al 2012; Chan et al 2012; Pang et al 2013; Tankisheva et al 2014). A systematic review (Huang et al 2017) demonstrated that WBV may be useful in reducing leg muscle spasticity in patients with cerebral palsy. As the available studies have serious methodological flaws, the benefit of WBV in spasticity management following cerebral palsy will need further investigations. Evidence is inadequate to support or refute the notion that WBV can modify spasticity in other neurological conditions.

Due to the conflicting findings (Gaßner et al 2014; Haas et al 2006; Kaut et al 2011), there is no overall evidence to support the use of WBV in reducing rigidity in Parkinson's disease.

Balance and Mobility

WBV training could improve relatively basic dynamic balance ability and mobility in older adults, with the frailer individuals showing more improvement (Lam et al 2012). Side-alternating vibration might be better than vertical vibration in improving balance ability in the elderly, probably due to the added mediolateral instability (Lam et al 2012). However, WBV was often used in conjunction with exercise training (Furness et al 2010; Machado et al 2010), and it was difficult to delineate the effect of WBV stimulation. More recent trials that were able to delineate the effect of WBV tended to report insignificant effect (Lam et al 2018b; Sievänen et al 2014; Sitjà-Rabert et al 2015). Similar findings have also been reported in other populations, including stroke, osteoarthritis, Parkinson's disease, fibromyalgia, and post anterior cruciate ligament reconstruction surgery (Berschin et al 2014; Lau et al 2011b; Liao et al 2014a; Sañudo et al 2013; Simão et al 2012). Whether WBV stimulation, when added to regular exercise training, could augment the training effects on balance and mobility function remains uncertain.

Bone Health

Based on the results from several meta-analyses, WBV can improve bone density of the lumbar spine and hip compared with a control group among postmenopausal women (Calendo et al 2014; Lau et al 2011a; Oliveira et al 2016; Slatkovska et al 2011). The optimal frequency/magnitude was not clear, although side-alternating vibration seemed to be more effective (Oliveira et al 2016). The increase in bone density of the lumbar spine was generally less than 1% after more than 6 months of WBV intervention (Calendo et al 2014).

Few randomized controlled studies have examined the effects of WBV on bone health in patients with disability. The results in children with disabling conditions were conflicting (Ruck et al 2010; Ward et al 2004). Only one study has examined the effect of WBV on bone health in chronic stroke, and found no changes in bone resorption and formation markers after 8 weeks of WBV intervention (Pang et al 2013).

Although ample animal work has shown the benefits of WBV on bone fracture healing (Wang et al 2017), no randomized controlled trials to date have examined the effects of WBV on bone healing after fracture in humans.

Cardiovascular Health

Research on the long-term effects of WBV on the cardiovascular system is scarce (Beijer et al 2015; Bogaerts et al 2009; van Duijnhoven et al 2010; Weber et al 2013). Six weeks of resistive exercise training with WBV (20–40 Hz, 6 mm, 9 minutes/session) increased the resting diameter of the superficial femoral artery in young healthy men to a similar degree as resistive exercise without WBV (Weber et al 2013). However, adding vibration was found to be more effective in attenuating the reduction in dilatory capacity and diameter of the superficial femoral artery induced by bed rest, relative to resistive exercise alone (van Duijnhoven et al 2010). Adding WBV to resistive exercise can enhance the blood volume by 27% and the vasodilator response by 14% in the gastrocnemius muscle after 6 weeks of training (Beijer et al 2015).

Only one study (Bogaerts et al 2009) has assessed the effect of long-term WBV therapy on VO_{2peak}, which is considered a gold standard measure of cardiorespiratory fitness. It was found that WBV intervention (40 minutes/session, 3 sessions/week for 1 year) induced similar gains in VO_{2peak} as a fitness programme consisting of cardiovascular, resistance, balance and flexibility exercises in older adults. The improvement in VO_{2peak} in these two groups was significantly better than in a non-intervention control group. However, it is not known whether the improvement is related to the WBV itself or the exercises performed while receiving WBV. The six-minute walk test (6MWT) is often used as an indicator of cardiovascular fitness. In patients with chronic obstructive pulmonary disease (COPD) (Braz Júnior et al 2015; Furness et al 2014; Gloeckl et al 2015; Greulich et al 2014; Pleguezuelos et al 2013), there is some evidence that WBV can improve 6MWT performance after 3–6 weeks of training (Gloeckl et al 2015; Pleguezuelos et al 2013).

Overall, whether long-term WBV training has any additional benefit on improving VO$_{2peak}$ is unclear, although some benefits on muscle blood flow are reported.

THERAPEUTIC EFFECTS AND USES

Focal Vibration

There is evidence to support the use of focal vibration on both slow conducting (e.g. heat) and fast conducting (e.g. sharp) pain. It could be applied in chronic pain conditions in the extremities, trunk, and orofacial regions (Lundeberg 1983). It can also reduce sharp pain during injection or surgery (Eichhorn et al 2016).

Focal vibration could improve muscle power, motor control and balance with evidence mostly in the elderly population (Brunetti et al 2015; Celletti et al 2015). In the neurological population, vibration treatment could reduce spasticity (Murillo et al 2014). Its effect might have implications for improving movement control and gait quality. The evidence on bone health is relatively scarce and requires more research (Reyes et al 2011).

Whole-Body Vibration

Exercising on the WBV platform augments muscle activation levels during exercise. Regarding the therapeutic effects of WBV, improvement in leg muscle strength and power has the most supportive evidence (Lau et al 2011a; Liao et al 2014a; Osawa et al 2013b). Whole-body vibration appears to have a similar effect on improving muscle strength and power to conventional muscle strength training. Incorporating WBV into warm-up or preconditioning exercise has beneficial effects on flexibility and subsequent muscle performance (Osawa & Oguma 2013a)

Performing simple exercise on the WBV platform may also improve balance and mobility, particularly for those who are frail (Lam et al 2012). For bone health, evidence suggests that WBV might induce a modest increase in bone mineral density (BMD) of the lumbar spine and hip in postmenopausal women (Oliveira et al 2016).

WBV may reduce pain in people with general musculoskeletal pain. However, whether WBV is superior to active exercise treatment on pain relief remains unclear (Alentorn-Geli et al 2008; del Pozo-Cruz et al 2011). There is preliminary evidence that WBV intervention could improve spasticity in cerebral palsy (Huang et al 2017). However, further high-quality research is required to confirm this finding.

Overall, WBV might be useful in improving muscle strength/power/flexibility, balance, mobility and bone health in frailer people who cannot undergo conventional exercise training or those who have low activity levels.

APPLICATION

Focal Vibration

For focal vibration intervention that targets muscle stimulation, focal vibration is often imposed on the muscle belly or musculotendinous junction (Cochrane 2011). The frequency is commonly set at 60–200 Hz, with an amplitude ranging from 0.1 mm to 0.25 mm (Aprile et al 2006; Filippi et al 2009). The training programme usually lasted for 30 mins a day consecutively for 3 days (Brunetti et al 2015; Filippi et al 2009). A submaximal voluntary contraction should be performed when receiving the vibratory stimulation. The precise contraction intensity was suggested to be not important (Brunetti et al 2015). For treating spasticity and reducing muscle tone, studies often used an amplitude of 0.1–1 mm. The training duration was usually around 5 to 10 minutes (Murillo et al 2014) (Table 14.2).

For the purpose of pain relief, focal vibration is often administered by pressing the vibrator on the skin adjacent to the painful site (e.g. site of injection) (Eichhorn et al 2016; Nanitsos et al 2009). The frequency used typically ranges from 20–200 Hz (Hollins et al 2014; Lundeberg 1984; Staud et al 2011). Higher vibration frequencies (100–200 Hz) are more effective than low frequency (20 Hz) (Lundeberg 1984). Hollins et al (2014) have used an amplitude of 0.3 mm. The vibration intensity can be adjusted according to the sensation threshold of the patient (Staud et al 2011). Most studies that used focal vibration for acute/chronic musculoskeletal pain management had delivered vibration close to the painful region (Hollins et al 2014; Lundeberg 1983, 1984; Staud et al 2011). Other application sites that were found effective included antagonistic muscle, or a trigger point near the area of pain, or even remote region from the painful region (e.g. opposite arm) (Lundeberg 1984; Staud et al 2011). To maximize the duration of pain relief, the vibration stimulation has to be applied for 30–45 minutes (Lundeberg 1983). For treating sharp pain during injection, vibration was often applied shortly before and during the injection (Table 14.2).

Whole-Body Vibration

For relieving musculoskeletal pain, the frequency and amplitude used was typically around 20 Hz and <1 mm respectively. The side-alternating vibration platform was more commonly used (Alentorn-Geli et al 2008; del Pozo-Cruz et al 2011; Horstmann et al 2013; Rittweger et al 2002b). Stochastic resonance WBV with a mean frequency of 5 Hz has also been used (Elfering et al 2013) (Table 14.2).

For muscle stimulation, higher vibration amplitude (1–4 mm) is often used to induce a greater level of neuromuscular activation. For side-alternating platforms, the feet position is particularly important as it determines the vibration amplitude delivered. The further the feet are away from the pivot, the larger the vibration amplitude. The frequency range is typically 20 Hz–40 Hz for vertical vibration and slightly lower at 10 Hz–30 Hz for side-alternating platform (Lam et al 2012; Lau et al 2011a). To avoid strong signal transmission to the upper body, especially the head, the knees should be slightly bent, particularly when high-intensity WBV is used. This is to allow muscle activation and joint motions to damp the signals transmitted to the upper body (Lam et al 2018a). Vibration training could also be coupled with other exercises on the platform. Commonly used postures/exercises include static/dynamic squats, single leg standing, and lunges (Lam et al 2016; Liao et al 2014a) (Table 14.2).

For the purpose of enhancing bone health, there are two major types of training protocol. Low-magnitude, high-frequency vibration is often used. The vibration frequency used is around 35 Hz with a much lower amplitude of <0.1 mm (Leung et al 2014). For low-magnitude vibration training, the individual could stand upright on the platform without bending the knees to facilitate the transmission of the signals to the common treatment target areas (lumbar spine, hip), as the signal intensity measured at the level of the head should be minimal with a low-intensity protocol (Kiiski et al 2008; Lam et al 2018a; Rubin et al 2003). Another type of WBV training protocol is largely similar to the one used for muscle stimulation (Table 14.2).

TABLE 14.2   Summary of Vibration Protocols Used for Different Purposes

	Vibration frequency (Hz)	Vibration amplitude (mm)	Vibration bout per session	Duration per bouts	Treatment period	Remarks
Focal muscle vibration						
Muscle stimulation	60–200	0.1–0.25	3	10 mins	Consecutively for 3 days	• Submaximal voluntary contraction during vibratory stimulation
Pain relief	100–200	0.3 or adjust to the sensation threshold of the patient	1	• 30–45 mins for chronic pain • shortly before and during the induction of pain (e.g., injection)	-	• Effect of pain relief for chronic pain may last for several hours
Whole-body vibration						
Musculoskeletal pain	Side-alternating: 20–35 Vertical: 35 Stochastic: 5 (mean)	0.7–5	3–36	30–60s	2–3 days per week, for weeks to months	• Knees should be slightly bent to damp the vibration signals transmitted to the head, especially for higher intensity protocols
Muscle stimulation	Vertical: 20–40 Side-alternating: 10–30	1–4	2–10	30–60s	2–3 times per week, lasted from weeks to months	• Knee should be slightly bent to damp the vibration signal transmitted to the upper body • Performing other exercises on the platform (e.g., static / dynamic squats, single leg standing, and lunges)

TABLE 14.2 Summary of Vibration Protocols Used for Different Purposes—Cont'd

	Vibration frequency (Hz)	Vibration amplitude (mm)	Vibration bout per session	Duration per bouts	Treatment period	Remarks
Bone health	Vertical: 30–40	0.05–0.1	1–2	10–20mins	2–7 times per week, lasted from 6–18 months	• Standing up-right without bending knees
	Vertical: 30–40 Side-alternating: 12–30	1–4	3–10	30–60s		• Performing other exercise on the platform with knee bent

SUMMARY

Vibration has been used in physiotherapy since the 1950s. There are two major modes of vibration application – focal vibration and whole-body vibration (WBV). Both modes of application involve delivering vibratory signals directly to the human body.

Several types of body tissues respond to vibratory stimulation. Vibration is a form of sensory stimulation. Research work, particularly in focal vibration, suggests that vibration has an analgesic effect. Vibration stimulation also triggers reflex muscle activity through stimulating the muscle spindles, which may lead to improvement in muscle strength and power, and thus modification of other motor functions, such as balance and mobility. In neurological conditions, brief sessions of vibratory stimulation have been shown to reduce spasticity. Being a form of dynamic mechanical stimulation, vibration is also a potent stimulus for bone tissue. There is preliminary evidence that WBV can improve bone quality. Whole-body vibration may provide a systemic stimulation that might also induce cardiovascular and hormonal changes.

The protocol of vibration stimulation is mainly governed by five parameters – type of vibration, vibration amplitude, vibration frequency, duration, and location of the application. These parameters may vary largely according to the specific treatment goals.

REFERENCES

Ahlborg, L., Andersson, C., & Julin, P. (2006). Whole-body vibration training compared with resistance training: Effect on spasticity, muscle strength and motor performance in adults with cerebral palsy. *Journal of Rehabilitation Medicine, 38*, 302–308.

Alentorn-Geli, E., Padilla, J., Moras, G., Lázaro Haro, C., & Fernández-Solà (2008). J Six weeks of whole-body vibration exercise improves pain and fatigue in women with fibromyalgia. *Journal of Alternative and Complementary Medicine, 14*, 975–981.

Annino, G., Iellamo, F., Palazzo, F., et al. (2017). Acute changes in neuromuscular activity in vertical jump and flexibility after exposure to whole body vibration. *Medicine (Baltimore), 96*(33), e7629.

Aprile I, Di Sipio E, Germanotta M, Simbolotti C Padua L (2006). Muscle focal vibration in healthy subjects: evaluation of the effects on upper limb motor performance measured using a robotic device. *European Journal of Applied Physiology, 116*, 729–737.

Avelar, N. C., Salvador, F. S., Ribeiro, V. G., et al. (2014). Whole body vibration and post-activation potentiation: A study with repeated measures. *International Journal of Sports Medicine, 35*, 651–657.

Avelar, N. C., Simão, A. P., Tossige-Gomes, R., et al. (2011a). Oxygen consumption and heart rate during repeated squatting exercises with or without whole-body vibration in the elderly. *The Journal of Strength & Conditioning Research, 25*, 3495–3500.

Avelar, N. C., Simão, A. P., Tossige-Gomes, R., et al. (2011b). The effect of adding whole-body vibration to squat training on the functional performance and self-report of disease status in elderly patients with knee osteoarthritis: A randomized, controlled clinical study. *Journal of Alternative & Complementary Medicine, 17*, 1149–1155.

Bautmans, I., Van Hees, E., Lemper, J. C., et al. (2005). The feasibility of whole body vibration in institutionalised elderly persons and its influence on muscle performance, balance and mobility: A randomised controlled trial. *BMC Geriatrics, 5*, 7.

Beijer, Å., Degens, H., Weber, T., et al. (2015). Microcirculation of skeletal muscle adapts differently to a resistive exercise intervention with and without superimposed whole-body vibrations. *Clinical Physiology and Functional Imaging, 35*(6), 425–435.

Berschin, G., Sommer, B., Behrens, A., & Sommer, H. M. (2014). Whole body vibration exercise protocol versus a standard exercise protocol after ACL reconstruction: A clinical randomized controlled trial with short term follow-up. *Journal of Sports Science and Medicine, 13*(3), 580–589.

Bishop, B. (1975). Vibratory stimulation. Part III. Possible applications of vibration in treatment of motor dysfunctions. *Physical Therapy, 55*, 139–143.

Bobath, B. (1955). The treatment of motor disorders of pyramidal and extra-pyramidal origin by reflex inhibition and by facilitation of movements. *Physiotherapy, 41*, 146–153.

Bogaerts, A. C., Delecluse, C., Claessens, A. L., et al. (2009). Effects of whole body vibration training on cardiorespiratory fitness and muscle strength in older individuals (a 1-year randomised controlled trial). *Age and Ageing, 38*, 448–454.

Bosco, C., Iacovelli, M., Tsarpela, O., et al. (2000). Hormonal responses to whole-body vibration in men. *European Journal of Applied Physiology, 81*, 449–454.

Bosco, C., Tihanyi, J., Rivalta, L., et al. (1996). Hormonal responses to strenuous jumping effort. *The Japanese Journal of Physiology, 46*, 93–98.

Braz Júnior, D. S., Dornelas de Andrade, A., Teixeira, A. S., et al. (2015). Whole-body vibration improves functional capacity and quality of life in patients with severe chronic obstructive pulmonary disease (COPD): A pilot study. *International Journal of Chronic Obstructive Pulmonary Disease, 10*, 125–132.

Braz, J., Solorzano, C., Wang, X., & Basbaum, A. (2014). Transmitting pain and itch messages: A contemporary view of the spinal cord circuits that generate gate control. *Neuron, 82*(3), 522–536.

Broekmans, T., Roelants, M., Alders, G., et al. (2010). Exploring the effects of a 20-week whole-body vibration training programme on leg muscle performance and function in persons with multiple sclerosis. *Journal of Rehabilitation Medicine, 42*, 866–872.

Brogårdh, C., Flansbjer, U. B., & Lexell, J. (2012). No specific effect of whole-body vibration training in chronic stroke: A double-blind randomized controlled study. *Archives of Physical Medicine and Rehabilitation, 93*, 253–258.

Brunetti, O., Botti, F. M., Brunetti, A., et al. (2015). Effects of focal vibration on bone mineral density and motor performance of postmenopausal osteoporotic women. *The Journal of Sports Medicine and Physical Fitness, 55*(1–2), 118–127.

Burke, J. R., Schutten, M. C., Koceja, D. M., et al. (1996). Age-dependent effects of muscle vibration and the Jendrassik maneuver on the patellar tendon reflex response. *Archives of Physical Medicine and Rehabilitation, 77*, 600–604.

Burr, D. B., Robling, A. G., & Turner, C. H. (2002). Effects of biomechanical stress on bones in animals. *Bone, 30*, 781–786.

Bush, J. A., Blog, G. L., Kang, J., Faigenbaum, A. D., & Ratamess, N. A. (2015). Effects of quadriceps strength after static and dynamic whole-body vibration exercise. *The Journal of Strength & Conditioning Research, 29*, 1367–1377.

Calendo, L. R., Taeymans, J., & Rogan, S. (2014). Does muscle activation during whole-body vibration induce bone density improvement in postmenopausal women? A systematic review. *Sportverletzung - Sportschaden, 28*, 125–131.

Camerota, F., Celletti, C., Suppa, A., et al. (2016). Focal muscle vibration improves gait in Parkinson's disease: A pilot randomized, controlled trial. *Movement Disorders Clinical Practice, 3*(6), 559–566.

Cardinale, M., & Bosco, C. (2003). The use of vibration as an exercise intervention. *Exercise and Sport Sciences Reviews, 31*, 3–7.

Cardinale, M., & Lim, J. (2003). Electromyographic activity of vastus lateralis muscle during whole-body vibrations of different frequencies. *The Journal of Strength & Conditioning Research, 17*, 621–624.

Cardinale, M., & Wakeling, J. (2005). Whole body vibration exercise: Are vibrations good for you? *British Journal of Sports Medicine, 39*, 585–589.

Celletti, C., Fattorini, L., Camerota, F., et al. (2015). Focal muscle vibration as a possible intervention to prevent falls in elderly women: A pragmatic randomized controlled trial. *Aging Clinical and Experimental Research, 27*(6), 857–863.

Chan, K. S., Liu, C. W., Chen, T. W., Weng, M. C., Huang, M. H., & Chen, C. H. (2012). Effects of a single session of whole body vibration on ankle plantarflexion spasticity and gait performance in patients with chronic stroke: A randomized controlled trial. *Clinical Rehabilitation, 26*, 1087–1095.

Cheng, H. Y., Ju, Y. Y., Chen, C. L., Chuang, L. L., & Cheng, C. H. (2015). Effects of whole body vibration on spasticity and lower extremity function in children with cerebral palsy. *Human Movement Science, 39*, 65–72.

Cheung, W. H., Sun, M. H., Zheng, Y. P., et al. (2012). Stimulated angiogenesis for fracture healing augmented by low-magnitude, high-frequency vibration in a rat model-evaluation of pulsed wave Doppler, 3-D power Doppler ultrasonography and micro-CT microangiography. *Ultrasound in Medicine and Biology, 38*, 2120–2129.

Chow, S. K., Leung, K. S., Qin, J., et al. (2016). Mechanical stimulation enhanced estrogen receptor expression and callus formation in diaphyseal long bone fracture healing in ovariectomy-induced osteoporotic rats. *Osteoporosis International, 27*, 2989–3000.

Chow, D. H., Leung, K. S., Qin, L., Leung, A. H., & Cheung, W. H. (2011). Low-magnitude high-frequency vibration (LMHFV) enhances bone remodeling in osteoporotic rat femoral fracture healing. *Journal of Orthopaedic Research, 29*, 746–752.

Christova, M., Rafolt, D., Mayr, W., et al. (2010). Vibration stimulation during non-fatiguing tonic contraction induces outlasting neuroplastic effects. *Journal of Electromyography and Kinesiology, 20*, 627–635.

Chung, S. L., Leung, K. S., & Cheung, W. H. (2014). Low-magnitude high-frequency vibration enhances gene expression related to callus formation, mineralization and remodeling during osteoporotic fracture healing in rats. *Journal of Orthopaedic Research, 32*, 1572–1579.

Claerbout, M., Gebrara, B., Ilsbroukx, S., et al. (2012). Effects of 3 weeks' whole body vibration training on muscle strength and functional mobility in hospitalized persons with multiple sclerosis. *Multiple Sclerosis, 18*, 498–505.

Claeys, K., Brumagne, S., Dankaerts, W., Kiers, H., & Janssens, L. (2011). Decreased variability in postural control strategies in young people with non-specific low back pain is associated with altered proprioceptive reweighting. *European Journal of Applied Physiology, 111*(1), 115–123.

Cochrane, D. J. (2011). The potential neural mechanisms of acute indirect vibration. *Journal of Sports Science and Medicine, 10*(1), 19–30.

Cochrane, D. J., Stannard, S. R., Sargeant, A. J., & Rittweger, J. (2008). The rate of muscle temperature increase during acute whole-body vibration exercise. *European Journal of Applied Physiology*, 103, 441–448.

Dahlin, L., Lund, I., Lundeberg, T., & Molander, C. (2006). Vibratory stimulation increase the electro-cutaneous sensory detection and pain thresholds in women but not in men. *BMC Complementary and Alternative Medicine*, 6, 20.

Dallas, G., Kirialanis, P., & Mellos, V. (2014). The acute effect of whole body vibration training on flexibility and explosive strength of young gymnasts. *Biology of Sport*, 31(3), 233–237.

Darian-Smith, I. (1984). The sense of touch: Performance and peripheral neural processes. In J. M. Brookhart & V. B. Mountcastle (Eds.), *Handbook of Physiology Section I: The nervous system. Vol. III. Sensory Processes, part 2* (pp. 739–788). Bethesda, MD: American Physiological Society.

Delecluse, C., Roelants, M., & Verschueren, S. (2003). Strength increase after whole-body vibration compared with resistance training. *Medicine and Science in Sports and Exercise*, 35, 1033–1041.

Di Loreto, C., Ranchelli, A., Lucidi, P., et al. (2004). Effects of whole-body vibration exercise on the endocrine system of healthy men. *Journal of Endocrinological Investigation*, 27, 323–327.

Dickin, D. C., McClain, M. A., Hubble, R. P., et al. (2012). Changes in postural sway frequency and complexity in altered sensory environments following whole body vibrations. *Human Movement Science*, 31(5), 1238–1246.

Duc, S., Rønnestad, B. R., & Bertucci, W. (2017). Adding whole body vibration to preconditioning squat exercise increases cycling sprint performance. *The Journal of Strength & Conditioning Research*.

van Duijnhoven, N. T., Thijssen, D. H., Green, D. J., et al. (2010). Resistive exercise versus resistive vibration exercise to counteract vascular adaptations to bed rest. *Journal of Applied Physiology*, 108, 28–33.

Eichhorn, M. G., Karadsheh, M. J., Krebiehl, J. R., & Ford, D. M. (2016). Ford RD Vibration for pain reduction in a plastic surgery clinic. *Plastic Surgical Nursing*, 36(2), 63–68.

Eklund, G., & Hagbarth, K. E. (1966). Normal variability of tonic vibration reflexes in man. *Experimental Neurology*, 16, 80–92.

Elfering, A., Arnold, S., Schade, V., Burger, C., & Radlinger, L. (2013). Stochastic resonance whole-body vibration, musculoskeletal symptoms, and body balance: A worksite training study. *Safety and Health at Work*, 4(3), 149–155.

Elfering, A., Thomann, J., Schade, V., & Radlinger, L. (2011). Stochastic resonance whole body vibration reduces musculoskeletal pain: A randomized controlled trial. *World Journal of Orthopedics*, 2(12), 116–120.

Erskine, J., Smillie, I., Leiper, J., Ball, D., & Cardinale, M. (2007). Neuromuscular and hormonal responses to a single session of whole body vibration exercise in healthy young men. *Clinical Physiology and Functional Imaging*, 27(4), 242–248.

Filippi, G. M., Brunetti, O., Botti, F. M., et al. (2009). Improvement of stance control and muscle performance induced by focal muscle vibration in young-elderly women: A randomized controlled trial. *Archives of Physical Medicine and Rehabilitation*, 90(12), 2019–2025.

Flieger, J., Karachalios, T., Khaldi, L., Raptou, P., & Lyritis, G. (1998). Mechanical stimulation in the form of vibration prevents postmenopausal bone loss in ovariectomized rats. *Calcified Tissue International*, 63, 510–514.

Fontana, T. L., Richardson, C. A., & Stanton, W. R. (2005). The effect of weight-bearing exercise with low frequency, whole body vibration on lumbosacral proprioception: A pilot study on normal subjects. *Australian Journal of Physiotherapy*, 51(4), 259–263.

Fuller, J. T., Thomson, R. L., Howe, P. R., & Buckley, J. D. (2013). Effect of vibration on muscle perfusion: A systematic review. *Clinical Physiology and Functional Imaging*, 33, 1–10.

Furness, T., Joseph, C., Naughton, G., et al. (2014). Benefits of whole-body vibration to people with COPD: A community-based efficacy trial. *BMC Pulmonary Medicine*, 14, 38.

Furness, T. P., Maschette, W. E., Lorenzen, C., Naughton, G. A., & Williams, M. D. (2010). Efficacy of a whole-body vibration intervention on functional performance of community-dwelling older adults. *Journal of Alternative & Complementary Medicine*, 16(7), 795–797.

Games, K. E., & Sefton, J. M. (2013). Whole-body vibration influences lower extremity circulatory and neurological function. *Scandinavian Journal of Medicine and Science in Sports*, 23(4), 516–523.

Gaßner, H., Janzen, A., Schwirtz, A., & Jansen, P. (2014). Random whole body vibration over 5 weeks leads to effects similar to placebo: A controlled study in Parkinson's disease. *Parkinson's Disease*, 386495 2014.

Gloeckl, R., Heinzelmann, I., & Kenn, K. (2015). Whole body vibration training in patients with COPD: A systematic review. *Chronic Respiratory Disease*, 12(3), 212–221.

Goetz, C. G. (2009). Jean-Martin Charcot and his vibratory chair for Parkinson disease. *Neurology*, 73, 475–478.

Greulich, T., Nell, C., Koepke, J., et al. (2014). Benefits of whole body vibration training in patients hospitalised for COPD exacerbations – a randomized clinical trial. *BMC Pulmonary Medicine*, 14, 60.

Haas, C. T., Turbanski, S., Kessler, K., & Schmidtbleicher, D. (2006). The effects of random whole-body-vibration on motor symptoms in Parkinson's disease. *NeuroRehabilitation*, 21, 29–36.

Hannah, R., Minshull, C., & Folland, J. P. (2013). Whole-body vibration does not influence knee joint neuromuscular function or proprioception. *Scandinavian Journal of Medicine and Science in Sports*, 23(1), 96–104.

Hazell, T. J., Jakobi, J. M., & Kenno, K. A. (2007). The effects of whole-body vibration on upper- and lower-body EMG during static and dynamic contractions. *Applied Physiology, Nutrition, and Metabolism*, 32, 1156–1163.

Hazell, T. J., Kenno, K. A., & Jakobi, J. M. (2010). Evaluation of muscle activity for loaded and unloaded dynamic squats during vertical whole-body vibration. *The Journal of Strength & Conditioning Research*, 24, 1860–1865.

Hazell, T. J., & Lemon, P. W. (2012). Synchronous whole-body vibration increases VO2 during and following acute exercise. *European Journal of Applied Physiology*, 112, 413–420.

Hazell, T. J., Thomas, G. W., Deguire, J. R., et al. (2008). Vertical whole-body vibration does not increase cardiovascular stress to static semi-squat exercise. *European Journal of Applied Physiology, 104,* 903–908.

Hollins, M., McDermott, K., & Harper, D. (2014). How does vibration reduce pain? *Perception, 43*(1), 70–84.

Homma, S., Kanda, K., & Watanabe, S. (1972). Integral pattern of coding during tonic vibration reflex. In G. G. Somjen (Ed.), *Neurophysiology studied in man* (pp. 345–349). Amsterdam: Experta Medica.

Horstmann, T., Jud, H. M., Fröhlich, V., Mündermann, A., & Grau, S. (2013). Whole-body vibration versus eccentric training or a wait-and-see approach for chronic Achilles tendinopathy: A randomized clinical trial. *Journal of Orthopaedic and Sports Physical Therapy, 43,* 794–803.

Hsieh, Y. F., & Turner, C. H. (2001). Effects of loading frequency on mechanically induced bone formation. *Journal of Bone and Mineral Research, 16,* 918–924.

Huang, M., Liao, L. R., & Pang, M. Y. (2017). Effects of whole body vibration on muscle spasticity for people with central nervous system disorders: A systematic review. *Clinical Rehabilitation, 31,* 23–33.

Huang, M., Tang, C. Y., & Pang, M. Y. C. (2018). Use of whole body vibration in individuals with chronic stroke: Transmissibility and signal purity. *Journal of Biomechanics, 73,* 80–91.

Ibrahim, M. M., Eid, M. A., & Moawd, S. A. (2014). Effect of whole-body vibration on muscle strength, spasticity, and motor performance in spastic diplegic cerebral palsy children – effect of whole-body vibration. *Egyptian Journal of Medical Human Genetics, 15,* 173–179.

Issurin, V. B., Liebermann, D. G., & Tenenbaum, G. (1994). Effect of vibratory stimulation training on maximal force and fleibility. *Journal of Sports Sciences, 12,* 561–566.

Issurin, V. B., & Tenenbaum, G. (1999). Acute and residual effects of vibratory stimulation on explosive strength in elite and amateur athletes. *Journal of Sports Sciences, 17,* 177–182.

Iwamoto, J., Takeda, T., Sato, Y., & Uzawa, M. (2005). Effect of whole-body vibration exercise on lumbar bone mineral density, bone turnover, and chronic back pain in post-menopausal osteoporotic women treated with alendronate. *Aging Clinical and Experimental Research, 17,* 157–163.

Jackson, K. J., Merriman, H. L., Vanderburgh, P. M., et al. (2008). Acute effects of whole-body vibration on lower extremity muscle performance in persons with multiple sclerosis. *Journal of Neurologic Physical Therapy, 32*(4), 171–176.

Kang, J., Porfido, T., Ismaili, C., et al. (2016). Metabolic responses to whole-body vibration: Effect of frequency and amplitude. *European Journal of Applied Physiology, 116*(9), 1829–1839.

Kaut, O., Allert, N., Coch, C., et al. (2011). Stochastic resonance therapy in Parkinson's disease. *NeuroRehabilitation, 28,* 353–358.

Kaut, O., Jacobi, H., & Coch, C. (2014). A randomized pilot study of stochastic vibration therapy in spinocerebellar ataxia. *The Cerebellum, 13,* 237–242.

Kelly, S. B., Alvar, B. A., Black, L. E., Dodd, D. J., Carothers, K. F., & Brown, L. E. (2010). The effect of warm-up with whole-body vibration vs. cycle ergometry on isokinetic dynamometry. *The Journal of Strength & Conditioning Research, 24,* 3140–3143.

Kerschan-Schindl, K., Grampp, S., Henk, C., et al. (2001). Whole body vibration exercise leads to alterations in muscle blood volume. *Clinical Physiology, 21,* 377–382.

Kiiski, J., Heinonen, A., Jarvinen, T. L., et al. (2008). Transmission of vertical whole body vibration to the human body. *Journal of Bone and Mineral Research, 23,* 1318–1325.

Kipp, K., Johnson, S. T., Doeringer, J. R., et al. (2011). Spinal reflex excitability and homosynaptic depression after a bout of whole-body vibration. *Muscle & Nerve, 43,* 259–262.

Kraemer, W. J., Marchitelli, L., Gordon, S. E., et al. (1990). Hormonal and growth factor responses to heavy resistance exercise protocols. *Journal of Applied Physiology, 69,* 1442–1450.

Kvorning, T., Bagger, M., Caserotti, P., et al. (2006). Effects of vibration and resistance training on neuromuscular and hormonal measures. *European Journal of Applied Physiology, 96,* 615–625.

Lam, F. M. H., Lau, R. W. K., Chung, R. C. K., & Pang, M. Y. C. (2012). The effect of whole body vibration on balance, mobility and falls in older adults: A systematic review and meta-analysis. *Maturitas, 72,* 206–213.

Lam, F. M., Liao, L. R., Kwok, T. C., & Pang, M. Y. C. (2016). The effect of vertical whole-body vibration on lower limb muscle activation in elderly adults: Influence of vibration frequency, amplitude and exercise. *Maturitas, 88,* 59–64.

Lam, F. M. H., Tang, C. Y., Kwok, T. C. Y., & Pang, M. Y. C. (2018a). Transmissibility and waveform purity of whole-body vibrations in older adults. *Clinical Biomechanics, 51,* 82–90.

Lam, F. M., Chan, P. F., Liao, L., et al. (2018b). Effects of whole-body vibration on balance and mobility in institutionalized older adults: A randomized controlled trial. *Clinical Rehabilitation, 32*(4), 462–472.

Lau, R. W. K., Liao, L. R., Yu, F., Teo, T., Chung, R. C. K., & Pang, M. Y. C. (2011a). The effects of whole body vibration therapy on bone mineral density and leg muscle strength in older adults: A systematic review and meta-analysis. *Clinical Rehabilitation, 25,* 975–988.

Lau, R. W. K., Teo, T., Yu, F., Chung, R. C. K., & Pang, M. Y. C. (2011b). Effects of whole-body vibration on sensorimotor performance in people with Parkinson disease: A systematic review. *Physical Therapy, 91*(2), 198–209.

Lee, T. Y., & Chow, D. H. (2013). Effects of whole body vibration on spinal proprioception in normal individuals (2013). *Conference Proceedings: Annual International Conference of the IEEE Engineering in Medicine and Biology Society,* 4989–4992.

Leung, K. S., Li, C. Y., Tse, Y. K., et al. (2014). Effects of 18-month low-magnitude high-frequency vibration on fall rate and fracture risks in 710 community elderly – a cluster-randomized controlled trial. *Osteoporosis International, 25*(6), 1785–1795.

Leung, K. S., Shi, H. F., Cheung, W. H., Qin, L., Ng, W. K., Tam, K. F., et al. (2009). Low-magnitude high-frequency vibration accelerates callus formation, mineralization, and fracture healing in rats. *Journal of Orthopaedic Research, 27,* 458–465.

Liao, L. R., Huang, M., Lam, F. M., & Pang, M. Y. (2014a). Effects of whole-body vibration therapy on body functions and structures, activity, and participation poststroke: A systematic review. *Physical Therapy, 94*, 1232–1251.

Liao, L. R., Lam, F. M. H., Pang, M. Y. C., Jones, A. Y. M., & Ng, G. Y. F. (2014b). Leg muscle activity during whole-body vibration in individuals with chronic stroke. *Medicine and Science in Sports and Exercise, 46*, 537–545.

Liao, L. R., Ng, G. Y. F., Jones, A. Y. M., Chung, R. C. K., & Pang, M. Y. C. (2015a). Effect of vibration intensity, exercise and motor impairment on leg muscle activity induced by whole-body vibration in people with stroke. *Physical Therapy, 95*, 1617–1627.

Liao, L. R., Ng, G. Y. F., Jones, A. Y. M., & Pang, M. Y. C. (2015b). Cardiovascular stress induced by whole-body vibration exercise in individuals with chronic stroke. *Physical Therapy, 95*, 966–977.

Lienhard, K., Vienneau, J., Nigg, S., Friesenbichler, B., & Nigg, B. M. (2017). Older adults show higher increases in lower-limb muscle activity during whole-body vibration exercise. *Journal of Biomechanics, 52*, 55–60.

Lundeberg, T. C. (1983). Vibratory stimulation for the alleviation of chronic pain. *Acta Physiologica Scandinavica - Supplementum, 523*, 1–51.

Lundeberg, T. C. (1984). The pain suppressive effect of vibratory stimulation and transcutaneous electrical nerve stimulation (TENS) as compared to aspirin. *Brain Research, 294*(2), 201–209.

Lythgo, N., Eser, P., de Groot, P., et al. (2009). Whole-body vibration dosage alters leg blood flow. *Clinical Physiology and Functional Imaging, 29*, 53–59.

Machado, A., García-López, D., González-Gallego, J., & Garatachea, N. (2010). Whole-body vibration training increases muscle strength and mass in older women: A randomized-controlled trial. *Scandinavian Journal of Medicine and Science in Sports, 20*(2), 200–207.

Mahieu, N. N., Witvrouw, E., Van de Voorde, D., et al. (2006). Improving strength and postural control in young skiers: Whole-body vibration versus equivalent resistance training. *Journal of Athletic Training, 41*, 286–293.

Manimmanakorn, N., Hamlin, M. J., Ross, J. J., & Manimmanakorn, A. (2014). Long-term effect of whole body vibration training on jump height: Meta-analysis. *The Journal of Strength & Conditioning Research, 28*(6), 1739–1750.

Marconi, B., Filippi, G. M., Koch, G., et al. (2008). Long-term effects on motor cortical excitability induced by repeated muscle vibration during contraction in healthy subjects. *Journal of the Neurological Sciences, 275*(1–2), 51–59.

Marin, P. J., & Rhea, M. R. (2010a). Effects of vibration training on muscle power: A meta-analysis. *The Journal of Strength & Conditioning Research, 24*, 871–878.

Marín, P. J., & Rhea, M. R. (2010b). Effects of vibration training on muscle strength: A meta-analysis. *The Journal of Strength & Conditioning Research, 24*(2), 548–556.

Martin, B. J., & Park, H. S. (1997). Analysis. Hee-sok P analysis of the tonic vibration: Influence of vibration variables on motor unit synchronization and fatigue. *European Journal of Applied Physiology, 75*(6), 504–511.

Mikhael, M., Orr, R., & Fiatarone Singh, M. A. (2010). The effect of whole body vibration exposure on muscle or bone morphology and function in older adults: A systematic review of the literature. *Maturitas, 66*(2), 150–157.

Mileva, K. N., Bowtell, J. L., & Kossev, A. R. (2009). Effects of low-frequency whole-body vibration on motor-evoked potentials in healthy men. *Experimental Physiology, 94*, 103–116.

Miokovic, T., Armbrecht, G., Gast, U., et al. (2014). Muscle atrophy, pain, and damage in bed rest reduced by resistive (vibration) exercise. *Medicine and Science in Sports and Exercise, 46*, 1506–1516.

Moezy, A., Olyaei, G., Hadian, M., et al. (2008). A comparative study of whole body vibration training and conventional training on knee proprioception and postural stability after anterior cruciate ligament reconstruction. *British Journal of Sports Medicine, 42*, 373–378.

Murillo, N., Valls-Sole, J., Vidal, J., Opisso, E., Medina, J., & Kumru, H. (2014). Focal vibration in neurorehabilitation. *European Journal of Physical and Rehabilitation Medicine, 50*, 231–242.

Musumeci, G. (2017). The use of vibration as physical exercise and therapy. *Journal of Functional Morphology and Kinesiology, 2*, 17.

Nanitsos, E., Vartuli, R., Forte, A., Dennison, P. J., & Peck, C. C. (2009). The effect of vibration on pain during local anaesthesia injections. *Australian Dental Journal, 54*(2), 94–100.

Oliveira, L. C., Oliveira, R. G., & Pires-Oliveira, D. A. A. (2016). Effects of whole body vibration on bone mineral density in postmenopausal women: A systematic review and meta-analysis. *Osteoporosis International, 27*(10), 2913–2933.

Osawa, Y., & Oguma, Y. (2013a). Effects of vibration on flexibility: A meta-analysis. *Journal of Musculoskeletal and Neuronal Interactions, 13*, 442–453.

Osawa, Y., Oguma, Y., & Ishii, N. (2013b). The effects of whole-body vibration on muscle strength and power: A meta-analysis. *Journal of Musculoskeletal and Neuronal Interactions, 13*, 380–390.

Osawa, Y., Oguma, Y., & Onishi, S. (2011). Effects of whole-body vibration training on bone-free lean body mass and muscle strength in young adults. *Journal of Sports Science and Medicine, 10*, 97–104.

Ozcivici, E., Garman, R., & Judex, S. (2007). High-frequency oscillatory motions enhance the simulated mechanical properties of non-weight bearing trabecular bone. *Journal of Biomechanics, 40*, 3404–3411.

Pang, M. Y. C. (2010). Whole body vibration therapy in fracture prevention among adults with chronic disease. *World Journal of Orthopedics, 1*, 20–25.

Pang, M. Y., Lau, R. W., & Yip, S. P. (2013). The effects of whole-body vibration therapy on bone turnover, muscle strength, motor function, and spasticity in chronic stroke: A randomized controlled trial. *European Journal of Physical and Rehabilitation Medicine, 49*, 439–450.

Park, Y. G., Kwon, B. S., Park, J. W., et al. (2013). Therapeutic effect of whole body vibration on chronic knee osteoarthritis. *Annals of Rehabilitation Medicine, 37*, 505–515.

Perchthaler, D., Grau, S., & Hein, T. (2015). Evaluation of a six-week whole-body vibration intervention on neuromuscular performance in older adults. *The Journal of Strength & Conditioning Research, 29*(1), 86–95.

Perry, C. E. (1967). Principles and techniques of the Brunnstrom approach to the treatment of hemiplegia. *American Journal of Physical Medicine, 46,* 789–815.

Petit, P. D., Pensini, M., Tessaro, J., et al. (2010). Optimal whole-body vibration settings for muscle strength and power enhancement in human knee extensors. *Journal of Electromyography and Kinesiology, 20,* 1186–1195.

Pleguezuelos, E., Pérez, M. E., Guirao, L., et al. (2013). Effects of whole body vibration training in patients with severe chronic obstructive pulmonary disease. *Respirology, 18*(6), 1028–1034.

Poenaru, D., Cinteza, D., Petrusca, I., Cioc, L., & Dumitrascu, D. (2016). Local application of vibration in motor rehabilitation – scientific and practical consideration. *Médica, 11,* 227–231.

Pollock, R. D., Provan, S., Martin, F. C., et al. (2011). The effects of whole body vibration on balance, joint position sense and cutaneous sensation. *European Journal of Applied Physiology, 111*(12), 3069–3077.

Pollock, R. D., Woledge, R. C., Mills, K. R., et al. (2010). Muscle activity and acceleration during whole body vibration: Effect of frequency and amplitude. *Clinical Biomechanics, 25,* 840–846.

del Pozo-Cruz, B., Hernández Mocholí, M. A., Adsuar, J. C., Parraca, J. A., Muro, I., & Gusi, N. (2011). Effects of whole body vibration therapy on main outcome measures for chronic non-specific low back pain: A single-blind randomized controlled trial. *Journal of Rehabilitation Medicine, 43*(8), 689–694.

Qin, Y. X., Kaplan, T., Saldanha, A., & Rubin, C. (2003). Fluid pressure gradients, arising from oscillations in intramedullary pressure, is correlated with the formation of bone and inhibition of intracortical porosity. *Journal of Biomechanics, 36,* 1427–1437.

Rabini, A., de Sire, A., Marzetti, E., et al. (2015). Effects of focal muscle vibration on physical functioning in patients with knee osteoarthritis: A randomized controlled trial. *European Journal of Physical and Rehabilitation Medicine, 51*(5), 513–520.

Rauch, F., Sievänen, H., Boonen, S., et al. (2010). Reporting whole-body vibration intervention studies: Recommendations of the International Society of Musculoskeletal and Neuronal Interactions. *Journal of Musculoskeletal and Neuronal Interactions, 10,* 193–198.

Rees, S., Murphy, A., & Watsford, M. (2007). Effects of vibration exercise on muscle performance and mobility in an older population. *Journal of Aging and Physical Activity, 15*(4), 367–381.

Rehn, B., Lidström, J., Skoglund, J., et al. (2007). Effects on leg muscular performance from whole-body vibration exercise: A systematic review. *Scandinavian Journal of Medicine and Science in Sports, 17,* 2–11.

Reyes, M. L., Hernández, M., Holmgren, L. J., Sanhueza, E., & Escobar, R. G. (2011). High-frequency, low-intensity vibrations increase bone mass and muscle strength in upper limbs, improving autonomy in disabled children. *Journal of Bone and Mineral Research, 26*(8), 1759–1766.

Rittweger, J., Beller, G., & Felsenberg, D. (2000). Acute physiological effects of exhaustive whole-body vibration exercise in man. *Clinical Physiology, 20,* 134–142.

Rittweger, J., Ehrig, J., Just, K., et al. (2002a). Oxygen uptake in whole-body vibration exercise: Influence of vibration frequency, amplitude, and external load. *International Journal of Sports Medicine. 23,* 428–432.

Rittweger J, Just K, Kautzsch K, Reeg P, Felsenberg D. (2002b). Treatment of chronic lower back pain with lumbar extension and whole-body vibration exercise: a randomized controlled trial. *Spine, 27*(17), 1829–1834.

Rittweger, J., Moss, A. D., Colier, W., et al. (2010). Muscle tissue oxygenation and VEGF in VO-matched vibration and squatting exercise. *Clinical Physiology and Functional Imaging, 30,* 269–278.

Rittweger, J., Mutschelknauss, M., & Felsenberg, D. (2003). Acute changes in neuromuscular excitability after exhaustive whole body vibration exercise as compared to exhaustion by squatting exercise. *Clinical Physiology and Functional Imaging, 2,* 81–86.

Rittweger, J., Schiessl, H., & Felsenberg, D. (2001). Oxygen uptake during whole-body vibration exercise: Comparison with squatting as a slow voluntary movement. *European Journal of Applied Physiology, 86,* 169–173.

Ritzmann, R., Gollhofer, A., & Kramer, A. (2013). The influence of vibration type, frequency, body position and additional load on the neuromuscular activity during whole body vibration. *European Journal of Applied Physiology, 113,* 1–11.

Ritzmann, R., Kramer, A., Gruber, M., et al. (2010). EMG activity during whole body vibration: Motion artifacts or stretch reflexes? *European Journal of Applied Physiology, 110,* 143–151.

Robbins, D., Yoganathan, P., & Goss-Sampson, M. (2014). The influence of whole body vibration on the central and peripheral cardiovascular system. *Clinical Physiology and Functional Imaging, 34,* 364–369.

Robling, A. G., Burr, D. B., & Turner, C. H. (2000). Partitioning a daily mechanical stimulus into discrete loading bouts improves the osteogenic response to loading. *Journal of Bone and Mineral Research, 15,* 1596–1602.

Robling, A. G., Duijvelaar, K. M., Geevers, J. V., Ohashi, N., & Turner, C. H. (2001). Modulation of appositional and longitudinal bone growth in the rat ulna by applied static and dynamic force. *Bone, 29,* 105–113.

Rogan, S., & Hilfiker, R. (2012). Training methods – increase muscle strength due to whole-body vibration – force with Hz. *Sportverletzung - Sportschaden, 26,* 185–187.

Rogan, S., Hilfiker, R., Herren, K., Radlinger, L., & de Bruin, E. D. (2011). Effects of whole-body vibration on postural control in elderly: A systematic review and meta-analysis. *BMC Geriatrics, 11,* 72.

Rogan, S., Radlinger, L., Hilfiker, R., Schmidtbleicher, D., de Bie, R. A., & de Bruin, E. D. (2015). Feasibility and effects of applying stochastic resonance whole-body vibration on untrained elderly: A randomized crossover pilot study. *BMC Geriatrics, 15,* 25.

Rønnestad, B. R., Slettaløkken, G., & Ellefsen, S. (2016). Adding whole body vibration to preconditioning exercise increases subsequent on-ice sprint performance in ice-hockey players. *The Journal of Strength & Conditioning Research*, 30, 1021–1026.

Rubin, C., Pope, M., Fritton, J. C., Magnusson, M., Hansson, T., & McLeod, K. (2003). Transmissibility of 15-hertz to 35-hertz vibrations to the human hip and lumbar spine: Determining the physiologic feasibility of delivering low-level anabolic mechanical stimuli to skeletal regions at greatest risk of fracture because of osteoporosis. *Spine*, 28, 2621–2627.

Rubin, C., Turner, A. S., Bain, S., Mallinckrodt, C., & McLeod, K. (2001). Anabolism. Low mechanical signals strengthen long bones. *Nature*, 412, 603–604.

Rubin, C., Turner, A. S., Mallinckrodt, C., et al. (2002a). Mechanical strain, induced noninvasively in the high-frequency domain, is anabolic to cancellous bone, but not cortical bone. *Bone*, 30, 445–452.

Rubin, C., Turner, S., Muller, R., et al. (2002b). Quantity and quality of trabecular bone in the femur are enhanced by a strongly anabolic, noninvasive mechanical intervention. *Journal of Bone and Mineral Research*, 17, 349–357.

Ruck, J., Chabot, G., & Rauch, F. (2010). Vibration treatment in cerebral palsy: A randomized controlled pilot study. *Journal of Musculoskeletal and Neuronal Interactions*, 10, 77–83.

Russo, C. R., Lauretani, F., Bandinelli, S., et al. (2003). High-frequency vibration training increases muscle power in postmenopausal women. *Archives of Physical Medicine and Rehabilitation*, 84, 1854–1857.

Sañudo, B., Carrasco, L., De Hoyo, M., Oliva-Pascual-Vaca Á, & Rodríguez-Blanco, C. (2013). Changes in body balance and functional performance following whole-body vibration training in patients with fibromyalgia syndrome: A randomized controlled trial. *Journal of Rehabilitation Medicine*, 45(7), 678–684.

Sayenko, D. G., Masani, K., Alizadeh-Meghrazi, M., et al. (2010). Acute effects of whole body vibration during passive standing on soleus H-reflex in subjects with and without spinal cord injury. *Neuroscience Letters*, 482, 66–70.

Schwab, R., Johnson, G. O., Housh, T. J., et al. (1993). Acute effects of different intensities of weight-lifting on serum testosterone. *Medicine and Science in Sports and Exercise*, 25, 1381–1386.

Schyns, F., Paul, L., Finlay, K., Ferguson, C., & Noble, E. (2009). Vibration therapy in multiple sclerosis: A pilot study exploring its effects on tone, muscle force, sensation and functional performance. *Clinical Rehabilitation*, 23, 771–781.

Shi, H. F., Cheung, W. H., Qin, L., Leung, A. H., & Leung, K. S. (2010). Low-magnitude high-frequency vibration treatment augments fracture healing in ovariectomy-induced osteoporotic bone. *Bone*, 46, 1299–1305.

Sievänen, H., Karinkanta, S., Moisio-Vilenius, P., & Ripsaluoma, J. (2014 Oct). Feasibility of whole-body vibration training in nursing home residents with low physical function: A pilot study. *Aging Clinical and Experimental Research*, 26(5), 511–517.

Simão, A. P., Avelar, N. C., Tossige-Gomes, R., et al. (2012). Functional performance and inflammatory cytokines after squat exercises and whole-body vibration in elderly individuals with knee osteoarthritis. *Archives of Physical Medicine and Rehabilitation*, 93(10), 1692–1700.

Sitjà-Rabert, M., Martínez-Zapata, M. J., Fort Vanmeerhaeghe, A., Rey Abella, F., Romero-Rodríguez, D., & Bonfill, X. (2015). Effects of a whole body vibration (WBV) exercise intervention for institutionalized older people: A randomized, multicentre, parallel, clinical trial. *Journal of the American Medical Directors Association*, 16(2), 125–131.

Sitjà-Rabert, M., Rigau, D., Fort Vanmeerghaeghe, A., et al. (2012a). Efficacy of whole body vibration exercise in older people: A systematic review. *Disability & Rehabilitation*, 34(11), 883–893.

Sitjà-Rabert, M., Rigau-Comas, D., Fort-Vanmeerhaeghe, A., et al. (2012b). Whole-body vibration training for patients with neurodegenerative disease. *Cochrane Database of Systematic Reviews* (2), CD009097.

Slatkovska, L., Alibhai, S. M., Beyene, J., et al. (2011). Effect of 12 months of whole-body vibration therapy on bone density and structure in postmenopausal women: A randomized trial. *Annals of Internal Medicine*, 155(10), 668–679, W205.

Staud, R., Robinson, M. E., Goldman, C. T., & Price, D. D. (2011). Attenuation of experimental pain by vibro-tactile stimulation in patients with chronic local or widespread musculoskeletal pain. *European Journal of Pain*, 15(8), 836–842.

von Stengel, S., Kemmler, W., Bebenek, M., Engelke, K., & Kalender, W. A. (2011). Effects of whole-body vibration training on different devices on bone mineral density. *Medicine and Science in Sports and Exercise*, 43, 1071–1079.

von Stengel, S., Kemmler, W., Engelke, K., et al. (2012). Effect of whole-body vibration on neuromuscular performance and body composition for females 65 years and older: A randomized-controlled trial. *Scandinavian Journal of Medicine and Science in Sports*, 22(1), 119–127.

Stockmeyer, S. A. (1967). An interpretation of the approach of Rood to the treatment of neuromuscular dysfunction. *American Journal of Physical Medicine*, 46, 900–961.

Tankisheva, E., Bogaerts, A., Boonen, S., Feys, H., & Verschueren, S. (2014). Effects of intensive whole-body vibration training on muscle strength and balance in adults with chronic stroke: A randomized controlled pilot study. *Archives of Physical Medicine and Rehabilitation*, 95, 439–446.

Torvinen, S., Kannus, P., Sievanen, H., et al. (2003). Effect of 8-month vertical whole body vibration on bone, muscle performance, and body balance: A randomized controlled study. *Journal of Bone and Mineral Research*, 8, 876–884.

Trans, T., Aaboe, J., Henriksen, M., et al. (2009). Effect of whole body vibration exercise on muscle strength and proprioception in females with knee osteoarthritis. *The Knee*, 16, 256–261.

Turner, C. H., & Pavalko, F. M. (1998). Mechanotransduction and functional response of the skeleton to physical stress: The mechanisms and mechanics of bone adaptation. *Journal of Orthopaedic Science*, 3, 346–355.

Turner, C. H., & Robling, A. G. (2003). Designing exercise regimens to increase bone strength. *Exercise and Sport Sciences Reviews*, 31, 45–50.

Umemura, Y., Ishiko, T., Yamauchi, T., Kurono, M., & Mashiko, S. (1997). Five jumps per day increase bone mass and breaking force in rats. *Journal of Bone and Mineral Research, 12,* 1480–1485.

Verschueren, S. M., Roelants, M., Delecluse, C., et al. (2004). Effect of 6-month whole body vibration training on hip density, muscle strength, and postural control in postmenopausal women: A randomized controlled pilot study. *Journal of Bone and Mineral Research, 19,* 352–359.

Vierck, C. J., Whitsel, B. L., Favorov, O. V., Brown, A. W., & Tommerdahl, M. (2013). Role of primary somatosensory cortex in the coding of pain. *Pain, 154*(3), 334–344.

Vissers, D., Baeyens, J. P., Truijen, S., et al. (2009). The effect of whole body vibration short-term exercises on respiratory gas exchange in overweight and obese women. *The Physician and Sportsmedicine, 37,* 88–94.

Wang, J., Leung, K. S., Chow, S. K. H., & Cheung, W. H. (2017). The effect of whole body vibration on fracture healing – a systematic review. *European Cells and Materials, 34,* 108–127.

Wang, P., Yang, X., Yang, Y., et al. (2015). Effects of whole body vibration on pain, stiffness and physical functions in patients with knee osteoarthritis: A systematic review and meta-analysis. *Clinical Rehabilitation, 29*(10), 939–951.

Ward, K., Alsop, C., Caulton, J., et al. (2004). Low magnitude mechanical loading is osteogenic in children with disabling conditions. *Journal of Bone and Mineral Research, 19,* 360–369.

Weber, T., Beijer, Å., Rosenberger, A., et al. (2013). Vascular adaptations induced by 6 weeks WBV resistance exercise training. *Clinical Physiology and Functional Imaging, 33*(2), 92–100.

Wei, F. Y., Chow, S. K., Leung, K. S., et al. (2016). Low-magnitude high-frequency vibration enhanced mesenchymal stem cell recruitment in osteoporotic fracture healing through the SDF-1/CXCR4 pathway. *European Cells and Materials, 31,* 341–354.

Wyon, M., Guinan, D., & Hawkey, A. (2010). Whole-body vibration training increases vertical jump height in a dance population. *The Journal of Strength & Conditioning Research, 24,* 866–870.

Yarar-Fisher, C., Pascoe, D. D., Gladden, L. B., et al. (2014). Acute physiological effects of whole body vibration (WBV) on central hemodynamics, muscle oxygenation and oxygen consumption in individuals with chronic spinal cord injury. *Disability & Rehabilitation, 36,* 136–145.

Electrical Stimulation

Transcutaneous Electrical Nerve Stimulation (TENS)

Mark I. Johnson

CHAPTER OUTLINE

INTRODUCTION

Transcutaneous electrical nerve stimulation (TENS) is a simple, non-invasive analgesic technique that is used for the symptomatic management of acute and non-malignant chronic pain (Box 15.1) (Johnson 2014f; Sluka 2016). TENS is also used in palliative care to manage pain caused by metastatic bone disease and neoplasms (Johnson 2012; Loh & Gulati 2015). It is claimed that TENS also has antiemetic and tissue-healing effects, and that it can improve some of the neurophysiological and behavioural effects of dementia (see Johnson 2014g). It is used less often for these non-analgesic actions.

During TENS, pulsed electrical currents are generated by a portable pulse generator and delivered across the intact surface of the skin via conducting electrodes (Fig. 15.1). The conventional way of administering TENS is to generate strong but comfortable electrical paraesthesia within, or close to, the site of pain, akin to electrically 'rubbing pain away'. Surveys show that TENS is one of the most frequently used electrotherapies for pain relief because it is inexpensive, non-invasive, easy to administer, has few side effects and has no drug interactions (Chipchase et al 2009). TENS effects are rapid in onset for most patients, so benefit can be achieved almost immediately. There is no potential for toxicity or overdose. TENS may be prescribed by healthcare professionals and can also be purchased without the need for a medical prescription. It is preferable for patients to administer TENS for themselves following assessment by a practitioner to ensure that TENS is an appropriate treatment.

History

The use of electricity to relieve pain is an age-old technique dating back to the ancient Egyptians who treated ailments using electrogenic fish (Gildenberg 2006). In modern times, interest in the use of electricity to relieve pain was re-awakened in 1965 by the publication of *Pain mechanisms: a new theory* by Melzack and Wall (1965). They suggested that electrically stimulating large-diameter peripheral afferents

BOX 15.1 Common Medical Conditions for Which TENS Has Been Used

Analgesic Effects of TENS
Relief of Acute Pain
- Postoperative pain
- Labour pain
- Dysmenorrhoea
- Angina pectoris
- Orofacial pain, including dental procedures
- Physical trauma, including fractured ribs and minor medical procedures

Relief of Chronic Pain
- Low back pain
- Arthritic pain, including osteoarthritis, rheumatoid arthritis
- Muscle pain, including myofascial pain, muscle tension, post-exercise soreness
- Neuropathic pain, including post amputation pain, postherpetic, trigeminal neuralgia
- Cancer pain, including metastatic bone pain
- Complex regional pain syndrome

Non-Analgesic Effects of TENS
Neuropsychological and Behavioural Effects
- Reducing symptoms of Alzheimer's dementia

Neuromuscular Stimulating Effects
- Faecal and urinary incontinence

Antiemetic Effects
- Nausea from pregnancy, travelling, chemotherapy, postoperative opioid medication
- Improving blood flow
- Raynaud's disease
- Wound healing
- Ischaemia due to reconstructive surgery

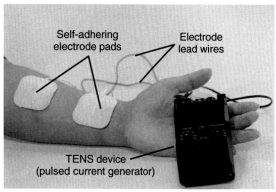

Fig. 15.1 A standard device delivering TENS to the arm.

term 'TENS' to describe electrical currents administered using a 'standard TENS device' (Fig. 15.1). The standard device is portable and battery-powered, and produces monophasic or biphasic waveforms of pulsed current in a repetitive manner (Johnson 2014e). The main components of a standard TENS device are:

- A power source to generate current, usually a 9V PP3 or 2 × AA 1.5 V batteries.
- DC oscillators to transform direct current (DC) from batteries to a pulsed output, and to determine the rate (pulses per second (pps), Hz) and pattern (mode) of pulses.
- An amplifier to amplify battery power to maximum peak-to-peak amplitude of approximately 60 milliamperes (mA) into a 1 kilohm load.

Standard TENS devices are characterized by their technical output characteristics (Table 15.1, Fig. 15.3). Design may vary between manufacturers but these variations are minor and appear to have limited impact on the physiological effects produced. Developments in electronic technology have flooded the market with a variety of TENS-like devices whose technical output specifications and generic name differ from those of TENS (Table 15.2) (Johnson 2014d). The remainder of this chapter will focus on TENS admi nistered using a standard TENS device.

PHYSICAL PRINCIPLES

TENS is a technique-based intervention with outcome influenced by the number, type and site of electrodes, the electrical characteristics of currents (i.e. pulse amplitude, frequency, pattern and duration) and the dosing regimen (i.e. how often and for how long). The physiological intention of TENS when used for pain relief is to selectively activate different populations of nerve fibres to initiate antinociceptive mechanisms. The electrical characteristics of TENS influence which population of nerve fibres are activated.

could inhibit transmission of noxious information and thus alleviate pain (Fig. 15.2). In 1967 percutaneous electrical stimulation was shown to alleviate chronic neuropathic pain (Wall & Sweet 1967) and electrical stimulation of the dorsal columns was shown to alleviate pain associated with cancer (Shealy et al 1967). Initially, TENS was used to predict the success of dorsal column stimulation implants until it was realized that TENS could alleviate pain in its own right (Long 1974).

The Standard TENS Device

By strict definition, TENS is anything that delivers electricity across the intact surface of the skin to stimulate underlying nerves. However, healthcare professionals use the

B

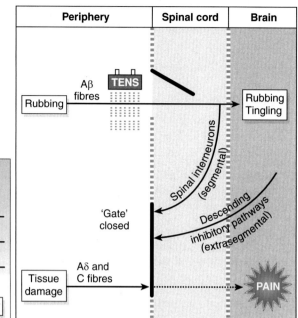

A

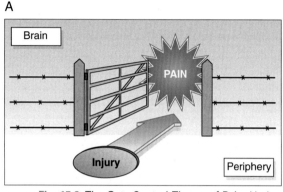

Fig. 15.2 The Gate Control Theory of Pain. Under normal physiological circumstances, incoming noxious information arising from stimuli such as tissue damage may contribute to the generation of pain by the brain. If noxious information is to reach the brain it must pass through a metaphorical 'gate', which is located in lower levels of the central nervous system. In physiological terms, the gate is excitatory and inhibitory synapses regulating the flow of neural information through the central nervous system. This 'gate' has a tendency to be opened by noxious events in the periphery and a tendency to be closed by activation of mechanoreceptors by 'rubbing the skin' or by activation of large-diameter Aβ peripheral afferents by TENS. This closing of the 'gate' reduces noxious information reaching the brain. The neuronal circuitry involved is segmental in its organization. The aim of conventional TENS is to activate Aβ fibres using electrical currents. The 'gate' can also be closed by the activation of inhibitory pathways, which originate in the brain and descend to the spinal cord through the brain stem (extrasegmental circuitry). These pathways become active during psychological activities, such as motivation, and when small-diameter peripheral fibres are excited physiologically. The aim of AL-TENS is to excite small-diameter peripheral fibres to activate the descending inhibitory pathways.

Principles of Nerve Fibre Activation

When the pulse amplitude (intensity) of TENS is increased, low threshold, large-diameter, non-nociceptive nerve fibres (mechanoreceptive Aβ fibres) are activated and the user experiences a non-painful 'tingling' under the electrodes (see Chapter 4). If the pulse amplitude (intensity) of TENS is increased further, higher threshold, small-diameter nociceptive nerve fibres (Aδ and C fibres) are activated and the user experiences a painful 'tingling' under the electrodes. In principle, pulsed currents with small amplitudes (i.e. low intensity) and durations between 50 and 500 microseconds would be best to activate large-diameter fibres (Aβ) without activating small-diameter nociceptive fibres (Aδ and C)

(Fig. 15.4). Increasing the pulse frequency of TENS should increase the rate of nerve impulses generated, although this is limited by the absolute and relative refractory periods for the axon (Johnson 2014e). The waveform of pulsed current used in TENS devices varies between manufacturers (Fig. 15.5). If the device delivers a monophasic pulsed wave, the cathode (traditionally the black lead) is placed proximal to the anode because the cathode activates the axonal membrane, leading to an action potential (Fig. 15.6). Many TENS devices use biphasic waveforms, which results in zero net current flow, reducing the risk of adverse skin reactions due to a build-up of ion concentrations beneath electrodes (Kantor et al 1994b). Electrode positioning with

TABLE 15.1	Typical Features on TENS Devices
Feature	**Examples**
Weight	50–250 g
Dimensions	6×5×2 cm (small device)
	12×9×4 cm (large device)
Cost	£30–150
Pulse waveform (fixed)	Monophasic
	Symmetrical biphasic
	Asymmetrical biphasic
Pulse amplitude (adjustable)	1–50 mA into a 1 kΩ load
Pulse duration (often fixed)	50–500 μs
Pulse frequency (adjustable)	1–200 pps
Pulse pattern	Continuous, burst, modulation (modulated amplitude, modulated frequency, modulated pulse duration)
Channels	1 or 2
Batteries	PP3 (9 V), rechargeable
Additional features	Timer
	Most devices deliver constant current output

these biphasic waveforms is less critical given the zero net DC element. Some TENS devices have modulated pulse patterns which have been used to reduce nervous system habituation (Fig. 15.7).

The exact nature and distribution of currents through the skin is difficult to predict due to the complex and non-homogeneous impedance of the tissue underlying electrodes (Demmink 1995). The skin offers high impedance to pulse frequencies used during TENS, so it is likely that currents will remain superficial, stimulating cutaneous nerve fibres rather than the more deep-seated visceral and muscle nerve fibres. Interestingly, however, evidence from animal studies suggests that activity in deeper afferents may be partly responsible for the antinociceptive effects of TENS (Radhakrishnan & Sluka 2005). Evidence suggests that skin impedance may not be a critical factor in hypoalgesia during TENS (Vance et al 2015).

Principles Underpinning Types of TENS Technique

The most common types of TENS technique described in the literature are conventional TENS (Fig. 15.8), acupuncture-like TENS (AL-TENS) (Fig. 15.9) and intense TENS (Fig. 15.10) (Johnson 2014e). The characteristics

of different TENS techniques are provided in Table 15.3. In clinical practice, patients most commonly use conventional TENS, whereas AL-TENS and intense TENS tend to be used only in specific situations. There is a paucity of research to determine the relative effectiveness and analgesic profiles of different TENS techniques.

Conventional TENS

The intention of conventional TENS is to selectively activate large-diameter Aβ fibres (touch-related) without concurrently activating small-diameter Aδ and C fibres (pain-related), or muscle efferents, as this has been shown to inhibit onward transmission of nociceptive information in the spinal cord and to reduce central sensitization (Garrison & Foreman 1994; Ma & Sluka 2001; Matsuo & Sluka 2014) (Fig. 15.8). Studies on healthy human participants exposed to experimentally induced pain in laboratory settings demonstrate that TENS applied at a strong but comfortable level produces hypoalgesic effects over and above those seen with sham (placebo) TENS (Moran et al 2011; Pantaleao et al 2011).

Acupuncture-Like TENS (AL-TENS)

The intention of AL-TENS, as described by the opinion leaders who developed it, is to generate activity in muscle afferents that arise from ergoreceptors in response to muscle 'twitching' (Eriksson & Sjölund 1976; also see Francis & Johnson 2011) (Fig. 15.9). This includes large-diameter myelinated type Ia and type II afferents arising from muscle spindles that monitor changes in muscle length and velocity of contraction, and type Ib afferents arising from Golgi tendon organs that monitor changes in muscle tension. Small-diameter thinly myelinated (type III) and unmyelinated (type IV) muscle afferents may also become active (Mense 1993). The impulses generated in small-diameter muscle afferents initiate extrasegmental antinociceptive mechanisms and the release of endogenous opioid peptides in a manner similar to that suggested for acupuncture (Meyerson 1983). Burst patterns of pulse delivery were originally incorporated into TENS devices as they were found to be more comfortable than low-frequency single pulses in producing muscle twitches (Eriksson & Sjölund 1976). Some commentators describe AL-TENS as the delivery of TENS over acupuncture points irrespective of muscle activity, although this technique has also been described as Acu-TENS and transcutaneous acupoint stimulation (TEAS) (Yu & Jones 2014). It is possible that there are differences in physiological action when TENS is applied over acupuncture points in this way (see reviews by Francis and Johnson 2011; Johnson 1998; Johnson 2014e; Walsh 1996).

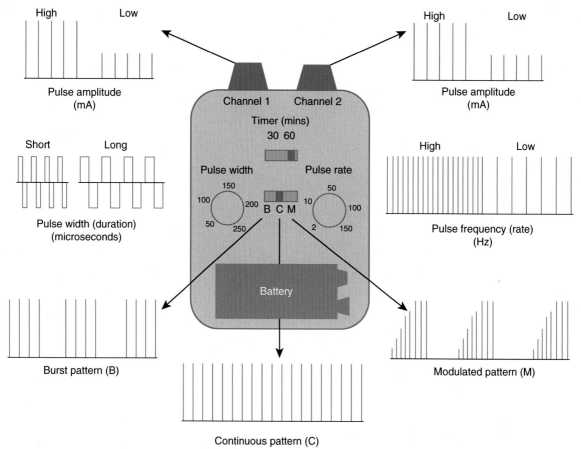

Fig. 15.3 The output characteristics of a standard TENS device (each vertical line represents one pulse of current). The current amplitude dials are used to control the intensity of individual pulses; the pulse frequency control dial regulates the rate of pulse delivery (Hz or pulses per second; pps) and the pulse width control dial regulates the time duration of each pulse (microseconds). Most TENS devices offer patterns of pulse delivery such as burst, continuous and modulated (e.g. amplitude modulated).

Intense TENS

The intention of intense TENS is to activate small-diameter Aδ afferents to block transmission of nociceptive information in peripheral nerves and to initiate extrasegmental antinociceptive mechanisms via counter irritation (Chung et al 1984a; Ignelzi & Nyquist 1979) (Fig. 15.10). Intense TENS can only be delivered for short periods of time (Levin & Hui Chan 1993) but has been used for minor surgical procedures, such as wound dressing and suture removal.

BIOLOGICAL EFFECTS

TENS effects can be subdivided into analgesic and non-analgesic (see Box 15.1). Research from basic sciences suggests that TENS alters cardiovascular physiology with tentative evidence that pulsate (low-frequency) TENS increases microperfusion and reduces heart rate and systolic and diastolic blood pressure (Campos et al 2016). TENS has been used to restore blood flow to ischaemic tissue and to improve oxygenation of tissue in arterial insufficiency and claudication due to arterial and neuropathic diseases. Parasympathetic nerves have been a target for invasive and non-invasive electrical stimulation techniques because they exert local reflex control over many visceral functions counteracting detrimental effects associated with constipation, urinary retention and the consequences of elevated sympathetic tone. Research findings are inconclusive.

TABLE 15.2 Characteristics of Some of the Commercially Available TENS-Like Devices

Device	Experimental Work	Manufacturers Claim	Typical Stimulating Characteristics
Action potential simulation (APS)	Odendaal & Joubert (1999)	Pain relief Improve mobility Improve circulation Reduce inflammation	Monophasic square pulse with exponential decay Delivered by two electrodes Pulse amplitude low (<25 mA), duration long (800 μs–6.6 ms), frequency fixed at 150 pps
Codetron	Pomeranz & Niznick (1987) Fargas-Babjak et al (1989, 1992)	Pain relief Reduce habituation	Square wave Delivered randomly to one of 6 electrodes Pulse amplitude low, duration long (1 ms), frequency low (2 pps)
H-wave stimulation	McDowell et al (1995; 1999)	Pain relief Improve mobility Improve circulation Reduce inflammation Promote wound healing	'Unique' biphasic wave with exponential decay Delivered by 2 electrodes Pulse amplitude low (<10 mA), Duration long (fixed at 16 ms), frequency low and high (2–60 pps)
Interferential therapy (interference currents)	See Chapter 18	Pain relief Improve mobility Improve circulation Reduce inflammation Promote wound healing Muscle re-education	Two out of phase sinusoidal currents which interfere with each other to produce an amplitude modulated wave Traditionally, delivered by 4 electrodes; Some devices have amplitude modulated waves that are premodulated within the device (two electrodes) Pulse amplitude low, amplitude modulated frequency 1–200 Hz (carrier wave frequencies approximately 2–4 KHz)
Microcurrent, including transcranial stimulation and 'acupens'	Johannsen et al (1993) Johnson et al (1997)	Promote wound healing Pain relief Other indications often claimed	modified square direct current with monophasic or biphasic pulses Changing polarity at regular intervals (0.4 s) Delivered by 2 electrodes Pulse amplitude low (1–600 μA with no paraesthesia), frequency depends on manufacturer (1–5000 pps) Many variants exist (e.g. transcranial stimulation for migraine and insomnia; acupens for pain)
Transcutaneous Spinal Electroanalgesia (TSE)	Macdonald & Coates (1995)	Pain relief, especially allodynia and hyperalgesia due to central sensitization	Differentiated wave Delivered by two electrodes positioned on spinal cord at T1 and T12 or straddling C3–C5. Pulse amplitude high (although no paraesthesia), duration very short (1.5–4 μs), frequency high (600–10000 pps)
Pain®Gone	Asbjorn (2000) Ivanova-Stoilova & Howells (2002)	Pain relief Could be non-invasive acupuncture	Hand-held pen device using piezoelectric elements Low-ampere high-voltage (e.g. 6 μA/15000 V) single monophasic spiked pulse Delivered by giving 30–40 individual shocks at the site of pain or on acupuncture points to generate non-noxious to mild noxious pin-prick sensation; repeated whenever pain returns

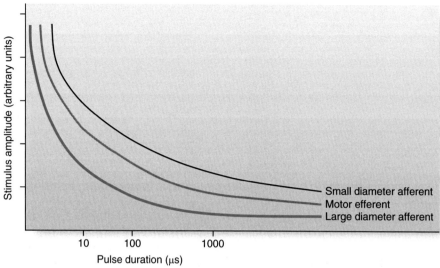

Fig. 15.4 Strength–duration curve for fibre activation. As pulse duration increases, less current amplitude is needed to excite an axon to generate an action potential. Small pulse durations are unable to excite nerve axons even at high current amplitudes. Large-diameter axons require lower current amplitudes than small-diameter fibres. Thus, passing pulsed currents across the surface of the skin excites large-diameter non-noxious sensory nerves first (paraesthesia), followed by motor efferents (muscle contraction) and small-diameter noxious afferents (pain). Alteration of pulse duration is one means to help in the selective recruitment of different types of nerve fibre. For example, intense TENS should use long pulse durations (>500 microseconds) as they activate small-diameter afferents more readily. During conventional TENS pulse durations ~100–200 microseconds are used as there is a large separation (difference) in the amplitude needed to recruit different types of fibre. This enables greater precision when using the intensity (amplitude) dial so that a strong but comfortable paraesthesia can be achieved without muscle contraction or pain.

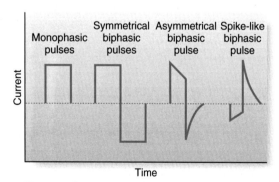

Fig. 15.5 Common pulse waveforms used in TENS.

Mechanism of Action for Analgesic Effects

TENS is predominantly used for symptomatic relief of pain via neuromodulation of nociceptive input via peripheral, segmental and extrasegmental mechanisms. The main action of conventional TENS is segmental in nature and mediated by neural activity in large-diameter

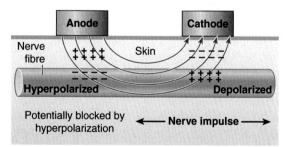

Fig. 15.6 Fibre activation by TENS. When devices use waveforms that produce net DC outputs that are not zero, the cathode excites (depolarization) the axon and the nerve impulse will travel in both directions along the axon. The anode tends to inhibit the axon (hyperpolarization), which could extinguish the nerve impulse. Thus, during conventional TENS the cathode should be positioned proximal to the anode so that the nerve impulse is transmitted to the central nervous system unimpeded. However, during AL-TENS the cathode should be placed distally or over the motor point, as the purpose of AL-TENS currents is to activate a motor efferent.

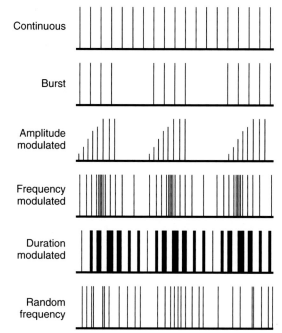

Fig. 15.7 Novel pulse patterns available on TENS devices. Modulated patterns fluctuate between upper and lower limits over a fixed period of time; this is usually preset in the design of the TENS device.

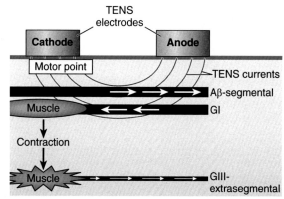

Fig. 15.9 The aim of AL-TENS is to selectively activate group I (GI/A-α) efferents, producing a muscle contraction that results in activity in ergoreceptors and group III (GIII) afferents. Activity in GIII afferents has been shown to activate descending inhibitory pathways that contribute to analgesia. Cutaneous afferents (Aβ and Aδ) will also be activated during AL-TENS. Note the position of the cathode.

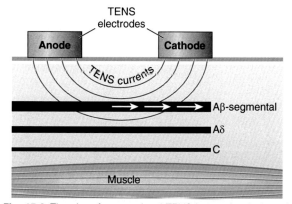

Fig. 15.8 The aim of conventional TENS is to selectively activate Aβ afferents producing segmental analgesia.

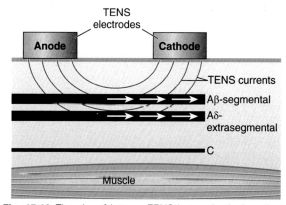

Fig. 15.10 The aim of intense TENS is to selectively activate Aδ afferents leading to extrasegmental analgesia. Aβ afferents will also be activated, producing segmental analgesia.

non-noxious afferents (Sjölund 1985; Woolf et al 1980, 1988) (Fig. 15.13). Garrison and Foreman (1994, 1996) found that TENS inhibited dorsal horn nociceptive transmission cells when applied to somatic receptive fields even after transection of the spinal cord. TENS has been found to reduce inflammation-induced sensitization of dorsal horn neurons in anaesthetized rats (Ma & Sluka 2001). The main action of AL-TENS is extrasegmental in nature and mediated by neural activity in small-diameter cutaneous and deeper-seated muscle afferents associated with ergoreceptors. TENS-induced activity in small-diameter peripheral afferents (Aδ) has been shown to inhibit central nociceptive transmission cells, and this inhibitory effect is reduced by spinal transection, suggesting a role for extrasegmental structures (Chung et al 1984a, 1984b; Woolf et al 1980) (Fig. 15.14). The main action of intense TENS is extrasegmental in nature and mediated by neural activity in small-diameter cutaneous afferents. TENS-induced activity in small-diameter cutaneous afferents produces long-term inhibition of central nociceptive transmission cells that persists up to 2 hours poststimulation (Macefield & Burke 1991;

TABLE 15.3   The Characteristics of Different Types of TENS

	Purpose of TENS	Physiological intention of TENS (fibre type responsible for hypoalgesic effects)	Desired outcome/patient experience	Optimal electrical characteristics	Electrode position	Analgesic profile	Duration of treatment	Main mechanism of analgesic action
Conventional TENS	Selective activation of large-diameter non-noxious afferents	Generate nerve impulses in large-diameter non-noxious cutaneous afferents (Aβ) arising from mechanoreceptors	Strong comfortable electrical paraesthesia with minimal muscle activity	High frequency/low intensity Amplitude='low' Duration=usually 100-200 μs Frequency= 10-200 pps Pattern=continuous	Over site of pain Dermatomal	Rapid onset <30 minutes after switch-on Rapid offset <30 minutes after switch-off	Continuously when in pain	Segmental
AL-TENS	Selective activation of motor efferents to produce phasic muscle twitch (cause GIII afferent activity)	Generate nerve impulses in small-diameter non-noxious muscle afferents GIII arising from ergoreceptors. Cutaneous afferents (Aβ and Aδ) will also be active.	Strong comfortable phasic muscle contraction	Low frequency/high intensity Amplitude='high' Duration= usually 100-200 μs Frequency=~100 pps within burst Pattern=burst (2-5bps)	Over motor point/muscle at site of pain Myotomal	Delayed onset >30 minutes after switch-on Delayed offset >1 hour after switch-off	~30 minutes/session	Extrasegmental Segmental
Intense TENS	Activation of small-diameter noxious afferents	Generate nerve impulses in small-diameter cutaneous afferents (Aδ), some arising from nociceptors	Very strong electrical paraesthesia that is tolerable and with minimal muscle contraction	High frequency/high intensity Amplitude='high' Duration = usually >500 μs Frequency= ~50-200 pps Pattern=continuous	Over site of pain or proximal over main nerve bundle	Rapid onset <30 minutes after switch-on Delayed offset > 1 hour after switch-off experience	~15 minutes/session	Blockade of peripheral nociceptive input Extrasegmental Segmental

AL-TENS, Acupuncture-like TENS; GIII, Group III afferents. pps, pulses per second: bps, bursts per second.

Sandkühler 2000; Sandkühler et al 1997). Thus, a brief period of intense TENS immediately after conventional TENS (e.g. 'sequential TENS') may prolong poststimulation analgesia.

TENS may produce peripheral blockade in large-diameter non-noxious fibres (Nardone & Schieppati 1989; Walsh et al 1998) and small-diameter nociceptive fibres (Ignelzi & Nyquist 1976). This is because delivery of electrical currents over a nerve fibre provokes nerve impulses that travel in both directions along the nerve axon. Nerve impulses travelling away from the central nervous system will collide and extinguish afferent impulses arising from tissue damage (Fig 15.12).

Neuropharmacology of TENS

TENS suppresses the expression and production of biomarkers pivotal in the central transmission of nociceptive information. A systematic review of five studies (240 participants) found that TENS reduced blood levels of the pro-inflammatory

cytokine interleukin-6 in individuals with pain (do Carmo Almeida et al 2018). Chen et al (2014, 2015) found that high-frequency TENS reduced mechanical hypersensitivity associated with skin/muscle incision and retraction models of post-operative nociception in rats by inhibiting up-regulation of substance P, N-methyl-D-aspartate receptor 1, and cytokines (interleukins 1β and 6, tumour necrosis factor 1α) in dorsal root ganglion and spinal cord. Fang et al (2013) found that TENS suppressed expression of p-extracellular signal–regulated kinase 1/2 and cyclooxygenase-2 in the dorsal horn, suggesting that the mechanism of action involved inhibition of activity in the spinal extracellular signal–regulated kinase 1/2-cyclooxygenase-2 pathway. Some effects are frequency dependent as high-frequency, but not low-frequency, TENS has been shown to reduce aspartate and glutamate release in the spinal cord dorsal horn (Sluka et al 2005).

A complex interplay between excitatory and inhibitory neurotransmitters and neuromodulators mediates inhibition of central nociceptive transmission by TENS. Much

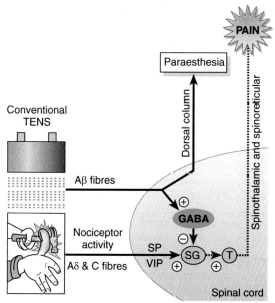

Fig. 15.11 Neurophysiology of conventional TENS analgesia. Activity in Aδ and C fibres from nociceptors leads to excitation (+) of interneurons in the substantia gelatinosa (SG) of the spinal cord via neurotransmitter-like substance P (SP, cutaneous nociceptors) or vasoactive intestinal peptide (VIP, visceral nociceptors). Central nociceptive transmission neurons (T) project to the brain via spinoreticular and spinothalamic tracts contributing to the experience of pain. TENS-induced activity in A-β afferents leads to the inhibition (–) of SG and T cells (dotted line) via the release of gamma amino butyric acid (GABA, black interneuron). Paraesthesia associated with TENS is generated by information travelling to the brain via the dorsal columns.

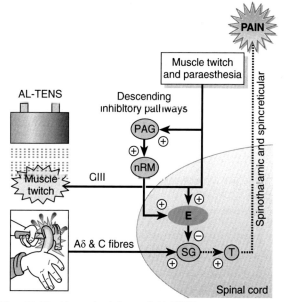

Fig. 15.12 Neurophysiology of AL-TENS analgesia. Activity in Aδ and C fibres from nociceptors leads to excitation (+) of central nociceptive transmission neurons (T), which project to the brain contributing to the experience of pain. TENS-induced activity in small-diameter muscle afferents (GIII) leads to the activation of brainstem nuclei such as the periaqueductal grey (PAG) and nucleus raphe magnus (nRM). These nuclei form the descending inhibitory pathways, which excite interneurons that inhibit (–) SG and T cells (*dotted line*) via the release of met-enkephalin (E interneuron). It is likely that paraesthesia and sensations related to the muscle twitch are relayed to the brain via the dorsal columns.

attention has focused on the role of opioids released at spinal and brainstem sites (Ainsworth et al 2006; Kalra et al 2001). Originally, it was suggested AL-TENS – but not conventional TENS – was mediated by endorphins (Sjölund et al 1977; Sjölund & Eriksson 1979; Thompson 1989) but more recently, the findings of animal studies suggest that antinociceptive effects associated with low-frequency TENS involve μ opioid receptors, and high-frequency TENS involves δ opioid receptors (Kalra et al 2001; Sluka et al 1998, 1999). Tolerance in μ and δ opioid receptors may develop with repeated TENS administration (Chandran & Sluka 2003; Lima et al 2015) and the antihyperalgesic effects

of low- but not high-frequency TENS have been shown to diminish in morphine-tolerant rats (Sluka et al 2000).

Maeda et al (2007) have found that high-but not low-frequency TENS increased levels of extracellular spinal cord GABA and that spinal blockade of $GABA_A$ receptors reversed reductions in hyperalgesia by both high- and low-frequency TENS. High- and low-frequency TENS also involves spinal muscarinic receptors M1 and M3 (Radhakrishnan & Sluka 2003) and peripheral $alpha_{2A}$ adrenergic receptors (King et al 2005). Combining clonidine, a centrally acting $alpha_2$ adrenoceptor agonist, augmented TENS-induced antihyperalgesia (Sluka & Chandran 2002). $5\text{-}HT_2$ and $5\text{-}HT_3$ receptors may be involved in antihyperalgesia produced by low- but not high-frequency TENS (Radhakrishnan & Sluka 2003).

Relationships Between Electrical Characteristics and Biological Effects

The effectiveness of TENS is dependent on the use of appropriate technique. Many of the claims about using specific electrical characteristics of TENS for different painful conditions are unfounded because remarkably few studies have systematically investigated the analgesic profiles of TENS pulse frequencies, pulse durations and pulse patterns when all other stimulating characteristics are fixed. Existing research is conflicting, confusing and generally of very poor quality, and systematic reviews have been unable to confirm with any degree of certainty dose-related effects of specific electrical characteristics of TENS on chronic pain patients or healthy individuals exposed to experimentally induced pain (Claydon & Chesterton 2008; Claydon et al 2011). This has opened the way for clinical practice based on ritual and mystique. In clinical practice it is likely that pulse amplitude will be the key electrical characteristic because of its relationship to fibre recruitment. Simple

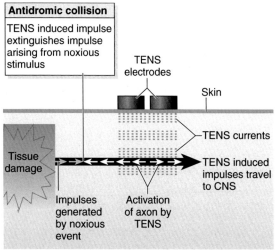

Fig. 15.13 TENS-induced blockade of peripheral transmission. Impulses generated by TENS will travel in both directions along an axon. Impulses generated by TENS travelling towards the periphery extinguish impulses arising from somatosensory receptors travelling towards the central nervous system (CNS).

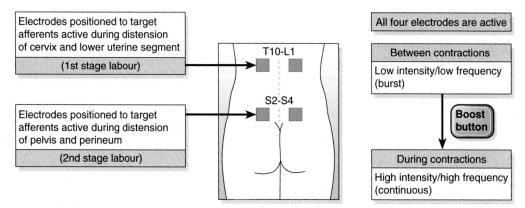

Fig. 15.14 The position of electrodes and the electrical characteristics of TENS when used to manage pain during labour.

titration of pulse amplitude coupled with the patient's report of TENS intensity enables selective activation of nerve fibres in line with the principles discussed earlier.

Pulse Amplitude (Intensity)

Pulse amplitude refers to the magnitude of current (mA) or voltage (V) and is the key determinant of outcome because sufficient current is necessary to activate the targeted nerve. There is a positive correlation between pulse amplitude (intensity), hypoalgesia (Aarskog et al 2007; Hughes et al 2013; Lazarou et al 2009; Moran et al 2011), and clinical outcome (Bennett et al 2011; Bjordal et al 2003). The intensity of TENS sensation subsides over time due to habituation, so it may be necessary to increase pulse amplitude to maintain the intensity of TENS at a strong but comfortable level which is needed to achieve pain relief (Pantaleao et al 2011).

Pulse Frequency

The frequency of electrical pulses is measured in pulses per second (pps) and this unit of measure will be used throughout the chapter rather than Hz, which describes the frequency of a Hertzian wave. Increasing pulse frequency, labelled 'rate' on some TENS devices, causes the pulsate sensation during TENS to shift from slow to fast. At frequencies above ~60 pps it is not possible to distinguish individual electrical pulses and a sensation of electrical paraesthesia develops with kinaesthetic sensations of body movement (Geng et al 2011). Increasing pulse frequency also produces stronger TENS sensations and lowers perception thresholds (Jelinek & McIntyre 2010).

A great many studies have compared the analgesic effects of two pulse frequencies (usually high ~100pps and low ~2 pps) in animals, healthy individuals and patients in pain. Research from animal studies suggests that the pulse frequency of TENS influences neuropharmacology and physiological effects (for a review, see DeSantana et al 2008b). The findings of studies using healthy participants exposed to experimental pain are too variable to make definitive conclusions about the efficacy of pulse frequency. For example, a systematic review of head-to-head comparisons of pulse frequency when the intensity of TENS was standardized found no difference in hypoalgesia between TENS frequencies during conventional TENS in ten studies (Chen et al 2008). Likewise, there is a paucity of systematic research into the relationship between pulse frequency and pain relief in clinical populations when intensity is standardized; the available evidence from randomized controlled trials (RCTs) is inconclusive. Johnson et al (1991b) found that there was no relationship between patient, electrical characteristics of TENS, and outcome variables in a sample of 179 chronic pain patients using

TENS successfully on a long-term basis. As evidence is inconclusive, individuals using conventional TENS are advised to select pulse frequencies that are comfortable for them at that moment in time. If using AL-TENS, individuals select low-frequency single pulsed currents or burst patterns to generate pulsate sensation with accompanying muscle contractions/twitching.

Pulse Pattern

Pulses may be delivered using a variety of patterns (Fig. 15.7). Burst patterns deliver trains of pulses interrupted by periods of no current output. The frequency of the burst is usually preset in TENS devices at 2–4 bursts per second (bps), although the frequency of pulses contained within each burst (the internal pulse frequency) can be adjusted according to the upper and lower limits of the device. Modulated patterns produce pre-programmed fluctuations of electrical parameters by, say, ± 25 per cent of the dial setting and include amplitude modulation (e.g. 0.0–25 mA over 3 seconds followed by a 2-second period of no current), frequency modulation (e.g. 20–100 pps and back over 12 seconds), and duration modulation (e.g. 50–250 μs and back over 12 seconds). Some devices also provide alternating patterns that switch a variable, usually frequency, duration, or pattern at fixed time points (e.g. 2 pps for 3 seconds followed by 110 pps for 3 seconds).

There is a paucity of experimental and clinical studies that have systematically investigated the effect of pulse patterns with other electrical characteristics held constant and those that exist are inconsistent in findings (Chen & Johnson 2009; Hamza et al 1999; Johnson 1991a, 1991b; Law & Cheing 2004; Tong et al 2007; Tulgar et al 1991a, 1991b). Hence, it seems reasonable to advise patients to use conventional TENS with a continuous pattern of pulses and then to experiment with other patterns to find which pattern produces a pleasant TENS sensation and/or pain relief for that moment in time.

Pulse Duration

Pulse duration, sometimes improperly referred to as pulse width, is the time interval between the leading and trailing edge of a pulsed current. In clinical practice, pulse durations between 50<500 microseconds are commonly used and patients are encouraged to experiment with pulse durations to find which produces a pleasant TENS sensation and/or pain relief at that moment in time because of a paucity of research on the influence of pulse duration when other electrical characteristics remain constant. Generally, longer pulse durations are recommended to generate hyperstimulation associated with AL-TENS or intense

TENS. Shorter pulse durations are recommended to facilitate delivery of currents to deeper tissue.

Pulse Waveform

The majority of standard TENS devices do not allow adjustment of pulse waveform. There is a paucity of experimental studies that have systematically investigated the effect of TENS waveforms on pain. Symmetrical biphasic waveforms require less pulse charge to excite peripheral nerves compared with amplitude-modulated sinusoidal waveforms or bursts of symmetrical pulses (Kantor et al 1994a) and produce fewer adverse skin reactions than monophasic waveforms (Fary & Briffa 2011). Monophasic square waves have been found to produce more discomfort than sine wave, Russian, and interferential waveforms (Petrofsky et al 2009).

EVIDENCE

Evidence-Based Practice

From a scientific perspective the electrical currents are the active ingredient for TENS so clinical efficacy is derived by comparing effects achieved during the delivery of active TENS with those achieved while receiving placebo TENS using a sham device. In other words, 'Do you need batteries in the TENS device to alleviate pain?'

There is extensive literature on the clinical effectiveness of TENS, although the majority of reports are anecdotal or of clinical trials lacking control groups or valid sample sizes. These reports are of limited use because they cannot account for normal fluctuations in patients' symptoms, the treatment effects of concurrent interventions or patients' expectation of treatment success. Randomized, placebo-controlled clinical trials are needed to determine effects due to the active ingredient of TENS (i.e. the electrical currents). A cursory search of literature in PubMed using the medical subject heading (MeSH) term 'transcutaneous electric nerve stimulation' conducted in May 2018 resulted in over 7000 hits, with ~1800 of these hits categorized as clinical trials, ~1400 as RCTs and ~85 as meta-analyses. This is an overwhelming amount of information facing the practitioner. A summary of systematic reviews is presented in Table 15.6 for acute pain and Table 15.7 for chronic pain. Although efficacy has been evaluated on a wide range of conditions, there is a paucity of good quality research to make a confident judgement on outcome. For some conditions, evidence appears to have changed over time due to the publication of new studies with larger sample sizes and more robust methodologies. When reasonable quality evidence is available, the judgements of reviewers tend towards superiority for TENS compared with placebo, providing appropriate TENS technique has been used.

TENS and Acute Pain

TENS is used extensively for acute nociceptive or inflammatory pain, although opinion is divided about whether it is effective. The first systematic review on TENS for acute pain associated with a variety of conditions was published by Reeve et al (1996) and the reviewers judged evidence to be inconclusive. The most recent Cochrane Review on TENS as a sole treatment for acute pain was published in 2015 and included 19 studies with over one thousand participants experiencing pain associated with cervical laser surgery, venepuncture, sigmoidoscopy, post-partum uterine contractions and rib fractures (Johnson et al 2015b). Many RCTs were excluded from the review because it was impossible to isolate the effect of TENS in those studies in which participants combined other treatments with TENS. Data pooled from six studies (seven comparisons) found an overall reduction of pain intensity favouring TENS compared with placebo of approximately 25 mm on a 100 mm visual analogue scale, although there was a major risk of bias due to the small sample size. The reviewers concluded that the analysis provided tentative evidence that TENS reduced pain intensity compared with placebo TENS when administered as a stand-alone treatment for acute pain in adults. Guidelines from the Australian and New Zealand College of Anaesthetists and Faculty of Pain Medicine recommend TENS for acute pain, including pain after thoracic surgery (Schug et al 2016).

TENS and Postoperative Pain

Early reports suggested that TENS reduced postoperative pain and opioid consumption (Hymes et al 1974), but systematic reviews performed in the mid-1990s were less favourable (Johnson 2017). Carroll et al (1996) reported that TENS did not produce significant postoperative pain relief in 15/17 RCTs. However, the use of pain relief as the primary outcome measure may have been compromised because patients in some of the included trials had access to additional analgesic drugs, enabling patients in sham and active TENS groups to titrate analgesic consumption to achieve similar levels of pain relief. Furthermore, some RCTs used suboptimal TENS technique and doses. A subsequent meta-analysis of 21 RCTs that accounted for these issues found that the mean reduction in analgesic consumption after TENS was 26.5% (range 26 to 15.1%) better than placebo (Bjordal et al 2003). Importantly, a subgroup analysis of 11 trials (964 patients) that met criteria for optimal TENS dosage (i.e. a strong, subnoxious electrical stimulation at the site of pain) reported a mean weighted reduction in analgesic consumption of 35.5%

TABLE 15.4 Suggested Characteristics to Use for a Patient Trying TENS for the First Time

	Conventional TENS	AL-TENS	Intense TENS
Electrode placement	Straddling site of pain or over main nerve bundle proximal to pain	Over muscle or motor point myotomally related to the site of pain	Straddling site of pain or over main nerve bundle proximal to pain
Pulse pattern	Continuous	Burst	Continuous
Pulse frequency	80–100 pps	80–100 pps	200 pps
Pulse duration	200μs	200μs	1000μs
Pulse amplitude (intensity)	Increase intensity to produce a strong but comfortable tingling	Increase intensity to produce a strong but comfortable muscle twitch	Increase intensity to produce an uncomfortable tingling that is bearable
Duration of stimulation in first instance	At least 30 minutes	No more than 20 minutes	No more than 5 minutes

TABLE 15.5 Suggested Advice Following the Initial Trial

	Conventional TENS	AL-TENS	Intense TENS
Electrode positions	Straddle site of pain but if not successful try main nerve bundle, across spinal cord or contralateral positions; dermatomal	Over muscle belly at site of pain but if not successful try motor point at site of pain, contralateral positions; myotomal	Straddle site of pain but if not successful try over main nerve bundle
Pulse pattern	Patient preference	Burst but if not successful or uncomfortable try amplitude modulated	Continuous but if not successful or uncomfortable try frequency or duration modulated
Pulse frequency	Patient preference usually 10–200 pps	Above fusion frequency of muscle 80–100 pps within the burst	High, e.g. 200 pps
Pulse duration	Patient preference usually 50–200μs	Patient preference 200μs	Highest possible but if uncomfortable gradually reduce duration
Pulse amplitude (intensity)	Strong but comfortable sensation without visible muscle contraction	Strong but comfortable sensation with visible muscle contraction	Highest tolerable sensation with limited muscle contraction
Dosage	As much and as often as is required; have a break every hour or so	About 30 minutes at a time as fatigue may develop with ongoing muscle contractions	15 minutes at a time as the stimulation may be uncomfortable
Analgesic effects	Occur when stimulator on	Occur when stimulator on and for a while after stimulator has been switched off May exacerbate pain	Occur when stimulator on and for a while once the stimulator has been switched off May exacerbate pain
General advice	Experiment with settings to maintain strong comfortable sensation	Experiment with settings (except burst) to maintain a phasic twitch	Experiment with settings to maintain highest tolerable sensation

(range 14–51%) better than placebo. In the trials without explicit confirmation of optimal TENS dosage, the mean weighted analgesic consumption was 4.1% (range 210 to 129%) in favour of active TENS. This was the first review to demonstrate the importance of using appropriate outcome measures and the need to consider the appropriateness of TENS technique when pooling results for the purposes of meta-analyses. In 2010, Freynet and Falcoz (2010)

TABLE 15.6 Outcomes of Systematic Reviews on Acute Pain

Reference	Scope of Review	TENS Data Set Method of Analysis	Conclusion for Pain Outcome
Johnson et al (2015b)	Various acute pains Cochrane Review	19 RCTs Meta-analysis	Evidence towards efficacy – sufficient data to judge
Simpson et al (2014)	Various acute pains in prehospital emergency medical services	4 RCTs Meta-analysis	Evidence towards efficacy – insufficient data to judge
Reeve et al (1996)	Various acute pains	39 studies (34 RCTs) Descriptive analysis	Evidence inconclusive – sufficient data to judge
Kerai et al (2014)	Various postoperative pains	8 RCTs Descriptive analysis	Evidence towards efficacy – insufficient data to judge
Bjordal et al (2003)	Various postoperative pains	21 RCTs Meta-analysis	Evidence towards efficacy – sufficient data to judge
Carroll et al (1996)	Various postoperative pains	17 RCTs Descriptive analysis	Evidence towards no efficacy – sufficient data to judge
Sbruzzi et al (2012)	Post-thoracotomy or sternotomy pain	11 RCTs Meta-analysis	Evidence towards efficacy – insufficient data to judge
Freynet and Falcoz (2010)	Post thoracic surgery pain	9 RCTs Descriptive analysis	Evidence towards efficacy – insufficient data to judge
Yue et al (2018)	Total knee arthroplasty Comparative effectiveness of neuromuscular electrical stimulation (8 RCTs), electroacupuncture (2 RCTs) and TENS (7 RCTs)	7 RCTs Descriptive analysis	Evidence towards efficacy – insufficient data to judge
Li and Song (2017)	Total knee arthroplasty	5 RCTs Meta-analysis	Evidence towards efficacy – insufficient data to judge
Zhu et al (2017)	Total knee arthroplasty	6 RCTs Meta-analysis	Evidence towards efficacy – insufficient data to judge
Beckwee et al (2014)	Total knee arthroplasty	5 RCTs Descriptive analysis	Evidence inconclusive – insufficient data to judge
Bedwell et al (2011)	Labour pain Update of (Dowswell et al 2009)	14 RCTs Descriptive analysis	Evidence inconclusive – sufficient data
Mello et al (2011)	Labour pain	9 RCTs Meta-analysis	Evidence towards no efficacy – sufficient data to judge
Dowswell et al (2009)	Labour pain Cochrane Review	17 RCTs Meta-analysis	Evidence inconclusive – sufficient data
Carroll et al (1997)	Labour pain	10 RCTs Meta-analysis	Evidence towards no efficacy – sufficient data to judge
Igwea et al (2016)	Primary dysmenorrhoea TENS or heat therapy	6 RCTs Descriptive analysis	Evidence towards efficacy – insufficient data to judge
Proctor et al (2003)	Primary dysmenorrhoea Cochrane Review	7 RCTs Descriptive analysis	Evidence towards efficacy (HF TENS) – insufficient data to judge
Abou-Setta et al (2011)	Pain after hip fracture 83 studies (64 RCTs) of various pharmacologic and non-pharmacologic interventions including TENS (2 RCTs)	2 RCTs Meta-analysis	Evidence inconclusive – insufficient data to judge
Gajjar et al (2016)	Pain during and after colposcopy treatment for cervical intraepithelial neoplasia Variety of interventions (19 RCTs) Cochrane Review	1 RCT Descriptive analysis	Evidence towards no efficacy – insufficient data to judge

TABLE 15.7   Outcomes of Systematic Reviews on Chronic Pain

Reference	Scope of Review	TENS Data Set Method of Analysis	Conclusion for Pain Outcome
Almeida et al (2018)	Various acute and chronic pain Cochrane Review	8 RCTs Meta-analysis	Evidence towards efficacy – insufficient data to judge
Nnoaham and Kumbang (2008)	Various chronic pains	25 RCTs Descriptive analysis	Evidence inconclusive – sufficient data to judge
Claydon and Chesterton (2008)	Various chronic pains Overview of systematic reviews	6 systematic reviews Descriptive analysis	Evidence inconclusive – insufficient data to judge
Canadian Agency for Drugs and Technologies in Health (2016)	Various chronic musculoskeletal pains TENS used at home	2 RCTs, 2 cohort studies Descriptive analysis	Evidence inconclusive – insufficient data to judge
Johnson and Martinson (2007)	Various chronic musculoskeletal pains TENS (32 RCTs) or percutaneous electrical nerve stimulation (6 RCTs)	32 RCTs Meta-analysis	Evidence towards efficacy – sufficient data to judge
Resende et al (2018)	Chronic low back (8 RCTs) and/ or neck pain (1 RCT)	9 RCTs Meta-analysis	Evidence inconclusive – insufficient data to judge
Wu et al (2018)	Chronic low back pain	12 RCTs Meta-analysis	Evidence towards no effect – insufficient data to judge
Jauregui et al (2016)	Chronic low back pain	9 RCTs, 4 cohort studies Meta-analysis	Evidence towards efficacy – insufficient data to judge
Chou et al (2010)	Chronic low back pain	1 Cochrane Review and 1 additional RCT	Evidence inconclusive – insufficient data to judge
Dubinsky and Miyasaki (2010)	Chronic low back pain	2 RCTs Descriptive analysis	Evidence towards no effect – insufficient data to judge
Machado et al (2009)	Chronic and acute low back pain Various treatments (76 RCTs)	4 RCTs Meta-analysis	Evidence towards efficacy – insufficient data to judge
Khadilkar et al (2008)	Chronic low back pain Cochrane Review	3 RCTs Descriptive analysis	Evidence inconclusive – Insufficient data to judge
Poitras and Brosseau (2008)	Chronic low back pain	6 RCTs Descriptive analysis	Evidence towards efficacy – insufficient data to judge
Kroeling et al (2013)	Mechanical and whiplash associated disorders Various electrotherapies (20 RCTs) Cochrane Review	7 RCTs Descriptive analysis	Evidence inconclusive – insufficient data to judge
Desmeules et al (2016)	Rotator cuff tendinopathy	6 RCTS Descriptive analysis	Evidence inconclusive - insufficient data to judge
Page et al (2016)	Rotator cuff disease Various electrotherapies (47 RCTs/quasi-RCTs) Cochrane Review	8 studies Descriptive analysis	Evidence inconclusive – insufficient data to judge
Page et al (2014)	Adhesive capsulitis Various modalities 19 RCTs (1249 participants)	4 RCTs Descriptive analysis	Evidence inconclusive – insufficient data to judge

Continued

TABLE 15.7   Outcomes of Systematic Reviews on Chronic Pain—cont'd

Reference	Scope of Review	TENS Data Set Method of Analysis	Conclusion for Pain Outcome
Johnson et al (2017)	Fibromyalgia Cochrane Review	7 RCTs, one quasi-RCT Descriptive analysis	Evidence inconclusive – insufficient data to judge
Salazar et al (2017)	Fibromyalgia Various electrotherapies (9 RCTs)	6 RCTs Meta-analysis	Evidence inconclusive – insufficient data to judge
Zeng et al (2015)	Knee osteoarthritis Various electrotherapies (27 RCTs)	13 RCTs Meta(network)-analysis	Evidence towards efficacy – insufficient data to judge
Rutjes et al (2009)	Knee osteoarthritis Cochrane Review	18 RCTs Descriptive analysis	Evidence inconclusive – insufficient data to judge
Bjordal et al (2007)	Knee osteoarthritis	7 RCTs Meta-analysis	Evidence towards efficacy – insufficient data to judge
Brosseau et al (2003)	Rheumatoid arthritis Cochrane Review	3 RCTs Meta-analysis	Evidence towards efficacy – insufficient data to judge
Wu et al (2015)	Palliative care of cancer Acupuncture and related therapies (23 systematic reviews)	1 Cochrane Review Descriptive analysis	Evidence inconclusive – insufficient data to judge
Hurlow et al (2012)	Cancer pain Cochrane Review	3 studies Descriptive analysis	Evidence inconclusive – insufficient data to judge
Dingemanse et al (2014)	Epicondylitis Various electrophysical treatments (2 reviews, 20 RCTs)	1 RCT Descriptive analysis	Evidence inconclusive – insufficient data to judge
Gibson et al (2017)	Various neuropathic pains Cochrane Review	5 RCTs Meta-analysis	Evidence inconclusive – insufficient data to judge
Cruccu et al (2007)	Various neuropathies	9 studies Descriptive analysis	Evidence towards efficacy – insufficient data to judge
Dubinsky and Miyasaki (2010)	Painful diabetic neuropathy	3 RCTs Descriptive analysis	Evidence towards efficacy – insufficient data to judge
Jin et al (2010)	Painful diabetic neuropathy	3 RCTs Meta-analysis	Evidence towards efficacy – insufficient data to judge
Pieber et al (2010)	Painful diabetic neuropathy Various electrotherapies (15 RCTs/retrospective analysis)	4 RCTs + 1 retrospective analysis	Evidence towards efficacy – insufficient data to judge
Sawant et al (2015)	Central pain associated with multiple sclerosis	4 studies (case-control/RCT) Meta-analysis	Evidence towards efficacy – insufficient data to judge
Jawahar et al (2014)	Central neuropathic pain associated with multiple sclerosis Various non-pharmacological interventions (13 RCTs)	2 RCTs Descriptive analysis	Evidence towards efficacy – insufficient data to judge
Harvey et al (2016)	Spinal cord injury Physiotherapy interventions (38 RCTs)	2 RCTs Meta-analysis	Evidence towards efficacy – insufficient data to judge
Boldt et al (2014)	Spinal cord injury Various treatments (16 RCTs) Cochrane Review	1 RCT Descriptive analysis	Evidence inconclusive – insufficient data to judge

TABLE 15.7   Outcomes of Systematic Reviews on Chronic Pain—cont'd

Reference	Scope of Review	TENS Data Set Method of Analysis	Conclusion for Pain Outcome
Fattal et al (2009)	Spinal cord injury Various electrotherapies (17 controlled trials)	4 RCTs Descriptive analysis	Evidence towards efficacy – insufficient data to judge
Price and Pandyan (2000)	Post-stroke shoulder pain Surface electrical stimulation (4 RCTs) Cochrane Review	4 RCTs Descriptive analysis	Evidence inconclusive – insufficient data to judge
Johnson et al (2015a)	Post amputation pain Cochrane Review	0 RCTs	Insufficient data to judge
Huisstede et al (2017)	Carpal tunnel syndrome Various electrotherapies and physical therapy (2 reviews, 22 RCTs)	1 RCT Descriptive analysis	Insufficient data to judge
Bronfort et al (2004)	Chronic headache Non-invasive physical treatments (22 RCTs/quasi-RCTs) Cochrane Review	2 RCTs Descriptive analysis	Evidence inconclusive – insufficient data to judge
Tao et al (2018)	Migraine	4 RCTs Meta-analysis	Evidence towards efficacy – insufficient data to judge

published a systematic review that found that TENS was effective on its own for video-assisted thoracoscopy incision (mild post-thoracotomy pain), and as an adjunct to opioid analgesics for muscle-sparing thoracotomy incision (moderate post-thoracotomy pain). In 2012, Sbruzzi et al (2012) published a meta-analysis that found that TENS combined with analgesics reduced thoracotomy or sternotomy pain compared with placebo TENS combined with analgesics. However, TENS was not found to be beneficial for pulmonary function. In 2017, two systematic reviews were published that suggested that TENS reduced postsurgical pain and analgesic consumption following total knee arthroplasty (Li & Song 2017; Zhu et al 2017).

TENS and Labour Pain

Augustinsson et al (1977) pioneered the use of TENS in obstetrics by applying TENS to dermatomes that correspond to the input of nociceptive afferents associated with the first and second stages of labour (T10–L1 and S2–S4, respectively; Fig. 15.15). Specially designed obstetric TENS devices followed with dual channels and a 'boost' control button for contraction pain. Nowadays, there is widespread use of TENS for pain during childbirth.

Early systematic reviews concluded that evidence for TENS analgesia during labour was weak (Table 15.6), although women receiving TENS were more 'satisfied' with treatment than those receiving placebo. The most recent Cochrane Review, published in 2009, included 19 studies (1671 women) and found no differences between TENS and controls (mostly placebo TENS) for pain ratings or other outcomes in labour (Dowswell et al 2009). The use of TENS at home in early labour was not evaluated. In 2011, an update of the Cochrane Review (14 studies, 1256 women) did not alter the conclusion (Bedwell et al 2011) and a non-Cochrane Review that included a meta-analysis (nine studies, 1076 women) found no differences in pain relief during labour or the need of additional analgesia between TENS and no TENS treatment or placebo TENS (Mello et al 2011). There are many confounders that undermine confidence in study findings, including difficulty of taking self-reports of pain when women are experiencing fluctuating physical and emotional conditions during childbirth, not evaluating TENS in the early stages of labour where it is more likely to be effective, the use of concurrent analgesic medication, and the inclusion of non-standard TENS devices. At present, NICE recommend that TENS should not be offered to women in established labour, although it may be beneficial in the early stages of labour (National Institute for Health and Clinical Excellence 2007).

TENS and Dysmenorrhoea, Angina and Other Painful Acute Conditions

There is weak evidence from a Cochrane Review of seven RCTs (213 patients) published in 2003 that high-frequency, but not low-frequency, TENS is superior to sham

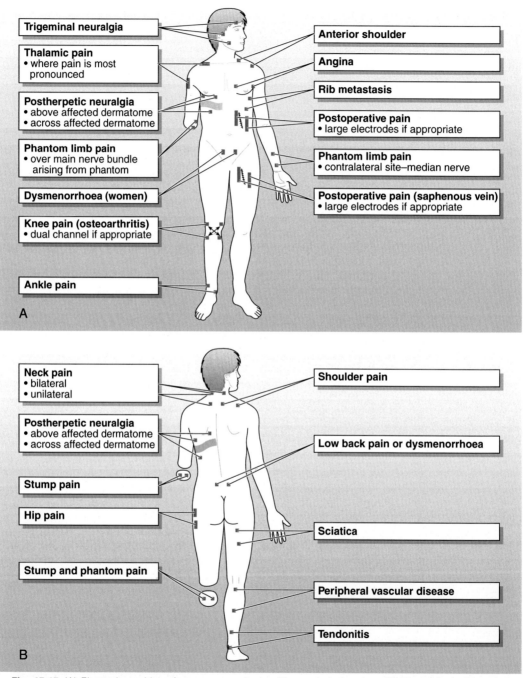

Trigeminal neuralgia

Thalamic pain
• where pain is most pronounced

Postherpetic neuralgia
• above affected dermatome
• across affected dermatome

Phantom limb pain
• over main nerve bundle arising from phantom

Dysmenorrhoea (women)

Knee pain (osteoarthritis)
• dual channel if appropriate

Ankle pain

A

Anterior shoulder

Angina

Rib metastasis

Postoperative pain
• large electrodes if appropriate

Phantom limb pain
• contralateral site–median nerve

Postoperative pain (saphenous vein)
• large electrodes if appropriate

Neck pain
• bilateral
• unilateral

Postherpetic neuralgia
• above affected dermatome
• across affected dermatome

Stump pain

Hip pain

Stump and phantom pain

B

Shoulder pain

Low back pain or dysmenorrhoea

Sciatica

Peripheral vascular disease

Tendonitis

Fig. 15.15 (A) Electrode positions for common pain conditions – anterior view. (B) Electrode positions for common pain conditions – posterior view.

at reducing pain associated with primary dysmenorrhoea when electrodes are applied over the lower thoracic spine and sometimes on acupuncture points (Proctor et al 2002). In 2016, a systematic review that included a descriptive analysis of six low quality RCTs on TENS provided weak evidence of efficacy (Igwea et al 2016). There is insufficient good quality evidence to determine whether TENS is beneficial for angina when administered directly over the painful area of the chest, although clinical studies with small sample sizes have found TENS to reduce the frequency of angina attacks and nitroglycerin consumption compared to control groups (Borjesson et al 1997). NICE recommend that TENS should not be offered to patients for the management of stable angina due to insufficient cost-effectiveness data (National Institute for Health and Clinical Excellence 2011). There are published reports of clinical studies on the use of TENS for pain associated with lacerations, fractures, hematomas, contusions, orofacial pain and dental procedures. Most findings are in favour of TENS but studies have inadequate samples sizes to make definitive conclusions.

TENS and Chronic Pain

There are a large number of clinical trials and systematic reviews with meta-analyses on the efficacy of TENS for chronic pain of nociceptive, neuropathic and musculoskeletal origin (Table 15.7). An overview of six systematic reviews on mixed populations of chronic pain patients published in 2008 found evidence in three systematic reviews that TENS was superior to placebo and that higher intensities of TENS generated greater pain relief (Claydon & Chesterton 2008). The most recent Cochrane Review of TENS for chronic pain associated with a variety of conditions was also published in 2008 (Nnoaham & Kumbang 2008). TENS was superior to inactive TENS controls in 13 out of 22 studies using single dose and eight out of 15 studies using multiple doses. There were no differences in pain outcome in comparisons of high-frequency and low-frequency TENS. The review was subsequently withdrawn in 2014 and replaced by an overview of Cochrane Reviews that found that although the methodological quality of reviews was good the quality of RCTs was too low to judge whether TENS was efficacious for people with chronic pain (Gibson et al 2019).

TENS and Musculoskeletal Pain

The largest meta-analysis to date found that TENS alleviated chronic musculoskeletal pain from a variety of conditions (29 RCTs, 32 comparisons), although the review was criticized for combining multiple diseases at the expense of homogeneity (Johnson & Martinson 2007). There are many systematic reviews on specific conditions contributing to chronic musculoskeletal pain.

TENS and back, neck and shoulder pain. There is a paucity of RCTs on which to judge efficacy of TENS for chronic low back pain, although this has not prevented the publication of countless systematic reviews. The most recent Cochrane Review was published in 2008: the authors concluded that there was conflicting evidence for reducing pain intensity (four studies, 585 patients) and consistent evidence (two studies, 410 patients) that TENS did not improve back-specific functional status (Khadilkar et al 2008). Recent systematic reviews found that TENS did not improve lower back pain but may offer short-term improvement of functional disability (12 studies, 700 patients) (Wu et al 2018) and that TENS improved chronic low back pain during but not immediately after stimulation compared with placebo TENS (meta-analysis of seven studies, 655 participants) (Resende et al 2018). In 2009, Machado et al published a comparison of the efficacy of 34 treatments for non-specific, chronic low back pain (Machado et al 2009). They gathered data from four trials (178 participants) on TENS and estimated that mean pain reduction was between 10 and 20% and comparable to other treatments, including muscle relaxants and NSAIDs.

In the UK, the NICE recommends that TENS is not offered for early management of persistent non-specific low back pain due to an absence of evidence to make a judgement (National Institute for Health and Care Excellence 2016). However, the American Society of Anesthesiologists Task Force on Chronic Pain Management and American Society of Regional Anesthesia and Pain Medicine recommended that: *"TENS should be used as part of a multimodal approach to pain management for patients with chronic back pain and may be used for other pain conditions, including neck and phantom limb pain"* (American Society of Anesthesiologists 2010, p. 816). The impact of basing clinical recommendations on too few studies of low quality has been discussed by Johnson and Walsh (2010) and Sluka et al (2013).

The most recent Cochrane Review on various types of electrotherapy for neck pain with and without radiculopathy or cervicogenic headache in adults (20 RCTs, 1239 people) found very low quality evidence that TENS was more effective than placebo (Kroeling et al 2013). A recent Cochrane Review on electrotherapy modalities for rotator cuff disease found insufficient evidence to judge the clinical efficacy of TENS (Page 2016).

Non-inflammatory rheumatic diseases. The most recent Cochrane Review of TENS for knee osteoarthritis was published in 2009 and was inconclusive (Rutjes et al 2009). The meta-analysis found surface electrical nerve stimulation (TENS, interferential current therapy or pulsed electrostimulation) to be superior to placebo/control at alleviating pain, but this effect disappeared when meta-regression techniques were used to minimize biases associated with inadequate study sample sizes. A systematic review that included a meta-analysis of seven RCTs using adequate TENS technique found reductions in pain of 22.2 mm (95% CI: 18.1– 26.3) on a 100 mm visual analogue scale compared with placebo (Bjordal et al 2007). A systematic review with network meta-analysis of any surface electrical stimulation was unable to judge the efficacy of TENS and suggested that interferential currents was the most promising intervention for the management of pain associated with knee osteoarthritis (Zeng et al 2015). In the UK, the NICE recommended that TENS should be offered as an adjunct to core treatment for short-term relief of osteoarthritic knee pain (National Institute for Health and Care Excellence 2014). An analysis of the cost-effectiveness of non-pharmacological interventions to alleviate pain associated with osteoarthritis of the knee found TENS to have an incremental cost-effectiveness ratio of £2,690 per Quality-Adjusted Life Year when compared with usual care, and this rates favourably with the NICE threshold of £20,000 per Quality-Adjusted Life Year (Woods et al 2017).

Inflammatory rheumatic diseases. The most recent Cochrane Review of TENS for rheumatoid arthritis of the hand was published in 2003, included three RCTs (78 patients) and was inconclusive (Brosseau et al 2003). In the UK, the NICE recommends that TENS should be used as an adjunct to core treatment for short-term relief of rheumatoid arthritis of the hand (National Institute for Health and Clinical Excellence 2009). There is a paucity of evidence for soft-tissue periarticular disorders. A systematic review of the effect of various electrophysical techniques on epicondylitis included one RCT on TENS that found TENS on acupuncture points was superior to placebo TENS (Dingemanse et al 2014). A pragmatic randomized controlled trial found no additional benefit when TENS was used as an adjunct to primary-care management of tennis elbow (Chesterton et al 2013).

Fibromyalgia and myofascial pain syndromes. A Cochrane Review on TENS for fibromyalgia in adults found insufficient high-quality evidence to make a judgement about efficacy (Johnson 2017). RCTs on myofascial pain syndrome are generally positive (Dissanayaka et al 2016).

TENS and Neuropathic Pain

Clinical experience suggests that TENS may be useful for neuropathic pain whether or not there is a sympathetic component. TENS is likely to be more effective for neuropathic pains of peripheral rather than central origin because of the more localized nature of peripheral neuropathic pain. TENS has been reported to be beneficial for peripheral neuropathic pain due to post-herpetic neuralgia, trigeminal neuralgia, phantom limb and stump pain, painful diabetic neuropathy, entrapment neuropathies (carpal tunnel syndrome), radiculopathies (cervical, thoracic and lumbar), and complex regional pain syndromes type I and type II (for review, see Johnson and Bjordal 2011).

A Cochrane Review of pain associated with various neuropathic conditions included 15 studies (724 participants), but there was insufficient good quality evidence on which to make a judgement about efficacy (Gibson et al 2017). A meta-analysis of five of these studies found a mean difference in pain reduction in favour of TENS compared with placebo TENS although this effect estimate had a high risk of bias due to methodological shortcomings in RCTs. The European Federation of Neurological Societies Task Force for neurostimulation therapy for neuropathic pain recommended that TENS may be useful as a preliminary or add-on therapy, but available evidence for efficacy was weak (Cruccu et al 2007). A recent update of these guidelines did not include TENS (Cruccu et al 2016).

Peripheral neuropathic pain conditions. A number of systematic reviews suggest that TENS is superior to placebo TENS for painful diabetic neuropathy but findings are based on inadequate sample sizes (Dubinsky & Miyasaki 2010; Jin et al 2010; Pieber et al 2010). A Cochrane Review found that there were no RCTs to judge the efficacy of TENS for pain following amputation (Johnson et al 2015a) and there are no systematic reviews on TENS for complex regional pain syndrome, or post-herpetic and trigeminal neuralgias. The findings of the few RCTs that have been published to date are contradictory (Johnson & Bjordal 2011).

Central neuropathic pain conditions. A Cochrane Review on various forms of surface electrical stimulation for post-stroke shoulder pain included four trials on TENS (170 patients) and found no significant change in pain incidence or intensity (Price & Pandyan 2000). Systematic reviews evaluating TENS for neuropathic pain associated with spinal cord injuries have failed to find sufficient RCTs on which to make a judgement (Boldt et al 2014; Fattal et al 2009; Harvey et al 2016). A systematic review of four studies published in 2015 suggested that TENS may be beneficial for the management of central pain associated with multiple sclerosis (Sawant et al 2015). In 2003, NICE recommended that TENS should be considered for patients with musculoskeletal pain associated with multiple sclerosis (National Institute for Health and Clinical Excellence and Conditions 2003), although a recent update of the guidelines made no reference to TENS. A systematic review has provided weak evidence for beneficial effects of TENS for the management of limb spasticity associated with damage to the central nervous system (Mills & Dossa 2016).

TENS and Cancer Pain

Success with TENS has been reported in the palliative care setting in both adults and children. TENS can be used for metastatic bone disease, for pains caused by secondary deposits and for pains due to nerve compression by a neoplasm (for review, see Johnson et al 2012). In these circumstances, electrodes are placed on healthy skin near to the painful area or metastatic deposit provided sensory function is preserved, or alternatively on the affected dermatome. TENS has been used for neuropathic cancer pain caused by nerve compression by a neoplasm or infiltration by a tumour, and for iatrogenic neuralgias, such as postmastectomy and post-thoracotomy pains. The most recent Cochrane Review on TENS for cancer-related pain found that there was insufficient data to make a meaningful judgement on clinical efficacy (Hurlow et al 2012).

Miscellaneous

Cochrane reviews have found insufficient evidence on which to judge the efficacy of chronic headache (Bronfort et al 2004) or carpal tunnel syndrome (Huisstede et al 2017). A non-Cochrane Review with a meta-analysis of four studies suggested that TENS may be efficacious for individuals with migraine but there were insufficient participants on which to base a definitive conclusion (Tao et al 2018).

Shortcomings of Systematic Reviews and Clinical Trials

The methodological quality of RCTs on TENS is weak with inadequate sample sizes in individual trials and pooled-analyses remaining a problem. Bennett et al (2011) quantified sources of bias from 38 RCTs from Cochrane Reviews on TENS for acute, chronic, and cancer pain and identified factors that introduce bias towards underestimating the size of treatment effects. These include inadequate TENS technique, under dosing TENS, failing to account for the effects of concurrent medication and failure to measure TENS outcome during stimulation when TENS effects are maximal. There needs to be at least 200 participants per treatment arm in single studies and 500 participants per treatment arm in meta-analyses to assure any level of confidence in estimates of treatment effect (Moore et al 1998). The impact of inappropriate randomization in TENS trials was demonstrated by Carroll et al (1996) who found that 17 of 19 non-randomized controlled trials reported that TENS relieved postoperative pain, whereas 15 of 17 RCTs reported that TENS did not.

Risk of bias associated with inadequate blinding of interventions is common in TENS trials because it is not possible to blind participants to whether or not they receive a strong, non-painful TENS sensation. This makes the design and operationalization of an authentic placebo TENS challenging. Commonly, sham TENS devices with no current output are used to deliver placebo TENS. Active TENS devices that deliver currents below sensory-detection threshold or deliver currents for a short period of time before fading away to zero current output have also been used (Rakel et al 2010). These approaches can be viable if study participants are uncertain about whether a strong, non-painful TENS sensation is a pre-requisite for treatment effects. Such uncertainty can be introduced through carefully worded study briefings and the selection of naive participants (Bennett et al 2011; Johnson 2014b). Gladwell et al (2013) have suggested that outcome measures used in previously published RCTs have limited capacity to capture the breadth of benefits reported by patients and that future RCTs should utilize a context-mechanism-outcome model to assess TENS outcomes. Bennett et al (2011) have published requirements for a robust clinical trial of TENS for pain, including operational explanations.

THERAPEUTIC EFFECTS AND USES

The main therapeutic use of TENS is to alleviate pain. However, electrical nerve stimulation techniques, including TENS, are also used to alleviate symptoms and improve functional outcomes associated with faecal and urinary incontinence, constipation, nausea and vomiting, xerostomia, peripheral ischaemia and Reynaud's syndrome, dementia, stroke (neuromuscular condition and neglect), oedema, wound healing, tissue regeneration (nerve, soft tissue, skin, and bone), reduction of tissue necrosis, sleep, fatigue, depression, and coma. The use of TENS in these conditions is underpinned by physiological rationale and research from the basic sciences with only tentative evidence provided from clinical research. A discussion of the use of TENS in these conditions lies outside of the scope of this chapter (for review, see Johnson 2014g).

The main use of TENS is to alleviate pain irrespective of origin (i.e. nociceptive, neuropathic and nociplastic). Physiological evidence suggests that TENS modulates nociceptive system activity rather than healing tissue so it provides symptom relief and is not curative. There are no robust indicators to predict response in individual patients so any type of pain may respond to TENS. The desirable characteristics of national pain strategies published by the International Association for the Study of Pain recommends that pain be managed using a biopsychosocial model of care and combinations of pharmacological and non-pharmacological methods. Neuromodulation techniques, such as TENS, are recommended for medicine, physiotherapy and nursing. Self-administered treatments, such as TENS, empower patients to take control of their pain management and remove the need for patients to be supervised or to have to travel to clinic for treatment. This means that patients can administer treatment immediately without the need of a practitioner. TENS meets the requirements of an ideal self-administered treatment because there is minimal potential for harm, toxicity, overdose, abuse, or interactions with other treatments or lifestyle.

APPLICATION

It is important to assess patients using TENS for the first time and to instruct them on the safe use of TENS including safety procedures (see Chapter 22). TENS may worsen pain in some individuals and because this could be due to a wide variety of reasons, careful assessment is necessary.

TENS is not appropriate for patients who do not cooperate with or understand instructions (e.g. patients with learning difficulties, mental illness or phobias about electricity). TENS can be used on children as young as four years of age, providing they understand what to expect and can tolerate sensations during TENS (Merkel et al 1999). Patients are advised not to use TENS in the shower or bath and not to use TENS when operating vehicles or potentially hazardous equipment. Drivers of motor vehicles are advised not to use TENS while driving because a surge of current could cause distraction. TENS can be used at bedtime provided the device has a timer so that it switches off automatically.

Contraindications, Precautions and Adverse Effects

Decisions on whether to prescribe TENS to a patient are taken according to the professional judgement of the healthcare professional. Contraindications to TENS are few and mostly hypothetical (see Chapter 22). A detailed review of contraindications, precautions and adverse events is available in Johnson (2014c) and safety guidelines published by professional bodies available in Robertson et al (2001), Chartered Society of Physiotherapy (2006) and Houghton et al (2010).

Electrode Positions
Normal Skin Sensation

TENS electrodes are positioned on healthy innervated skin where sensation is intact, so it is important to check skin sensation prior to application. For most types of pain, TENS electrodes are placed around the site of pain so that paraesthesia can be directed into the painful area (Fig. 15.11). This is because conventional TENS is operating via

a segmental mechanism so electrodes are placed to stimulate Aβ fibres, which enter the same spinal segment as the nociceptive fibres associated with the origin of the pain.

Heightened Skin Sensation (Allodynia)

TENS may aggravate the pain when skin sensation has been heightened and allodynia and/or hyperalgesia exist, as may be the case when there is mechanical (tactile) allodynia. In these situations, electrodes are positioned along the main nerves well proximal to the site of pain. Interestingly, TENS does not always exacerbate pain in the presence of mechanical allodynia.

Diminished Skin Sensation (Hypoaesthesia)

TENS is likely to be ineffective when applied over skin that has diminished sensation and is numb and insensitive to touch, as may be the case in chronic neuropathic wounds. In these situations, TENS electrodes are positioned along the main nerves well proximal to the site of pain.

Other Situations

Electrodes are positioned along the main nerves proximal to the site of pain when it is not possible to deliver currents within the site of pain, due to absence of a body part following amputation or the presence of a skin lesion. Alternatively, electrodes are applied paravertebrally at spinal segments related to origin of pain or at contralateral dermatomes. This may be appropriate in conditions such as trigeminal neuralgia where the affected side of the face may be sensitive to touch.

Dual Channel Devices

Dual channel devices using four electrodes or large electrodes can be used for pain covering large areas. However, if the pain is generalized and widespread over a number of body parts it may be more appropriate to use AL-TENS at the relevant myotome, as this may produce a more generalized analgesic effect. Dual channel stimulators are useful for patients with multiple pains, such as low back pain and sciatica, or for pains which change in their location and quality over a short time period, e.g. during childbirth.

Accurate Placement of Pads

Accurate placement of pads can be time-consuming. Berlant (1984) described a useful method of determining optimal electrode sites for TENS. The therapist applies one TENS electrode to the patient at a potential placement site, holds the second electrode and uses his or her index finger to probe the patient's skin to locate the best site to place it. When the TENS device is switched on and the amplitude slowly increased, the patient and/or therapist will feel TENS paraesthesia when the circuit is made by touching the patient's skin. As the therapist probes the patient's skin, the intensity of TENS paraesthesia will increase whenever nerves on the patient's skin run superficially. This will help to target an effective electrode site.

Electrical Characteristics of TENS

The potential number of combinations of electrical characteristics of TENS is vast. No relationships have been found between pulse frequency and pattern used by patients and the magnitude of analgesia or their medical diagnosis. The relationship between electrical characteristics of TENS and selective activation of nerve fibres was discussed previously and the patient's report of the sensation produced by TENS is the easiest means of assessing the type of fibre activity (Table 15.3). For conventional TENS, patients are instructed to titrate the intensity of currents to achieve a strong but comfortable electrical paraesthesia without muscle contraction. In practice, patients have individual preferences for their selection of electrical characteristics of TENS and these seem to be based on the comfort of the electrical paraesthesia. Encouraging patients to experiment with TENS settings will produce the most effective outcome.

Timing and Dosage

Laboratory and clinical evidence suggest that TENS analgesia is maximal when the stimulator is switched on, irrespective of the type of TENS used (for review, see Johnson 2014a). Dosing regimens of 20 minutes at daily, weekly or monthly intervals are likely to be ineffective for conventional TENS and patients may need to keep the device switched on whenever the pain is present to achieve pain relief. For ongoing chronic pain this may mean that patients use TENS over the entire day. In a study of long-term users of TENS, Johnson et al (1991b) reported that 75% used TENS on a daily basis and 30% reported using TENS for more than 49 hours a week. Patients can leave electrodes in situ and administer TENS intermittently throughout the day providing they attend to skin care underneath the electrodes, as minor skin irritation may occur. Patients are advised to take regular (although short) breaks from stimulation, to wash their skin after TENS and to apply electrodes to adjacent fresh skin on a regular basis.

Some patients report poststimulation analgesia, although reports of the duration of these poststimulation effects vary widely, from 18 hours (Augustinsson et al 1976) to 2 hours (Johnson et al 1991b). It is claimed that post-TENS analgesia is longer for AL-TENS than conventional TENS, and is due to segmental mechanisms generating long-term depression inhibition (depression) of central nociceptive transmission cells and activation of descending pain inhibitory pathways. However, reports that AL-TENS produces prolonged poststimulation analgesia may also reflect natural fluctuations in symptoms and the patients' expectation

of treatment duration rather than specific TENS-induced effects.

Declining Response to TENS

Woolf and Thompson (1994) claimed that the magnitude of pain relief from TENS declined by up to 40% over a period of 1 year, although there has been no systematic investigation to support this claim. Reasons for a decline in response include dead batteries, perished leads, a worsening pain problem or waning of the initial enthusiasm for a new treatment. Revisiting patient expectation of TENS is often a good first step to resolve the situation.

Some patients report that TENS sensations fade within treatment sessions and analgesic response declines over successive treatments (i.e. tolerance). This may be a result of the nervous system habituating to the repetitive non-noxious electrical pulses of TENS (Pomeranz & Niznick 1987). Repeated daily application of high-frequency TENS produced opioid tolerance by day 4 and repeated daily application of low-frequency TENS by day 5 (Chandran & Sluka 2003; Liebano et al 2011) with cholecystokinin (DeSantana et al 2010) and N-methyl-D-aspartate receptors (Hingne & Sluka 2008) implicated. If a patient reports that they are responding less well to TENS over time it may be worth experimenting with electrode placements or the electrical characteristics of TENS. Gradually increasing the intensity or using frequencies that alternate over short periods of time (e.g. from 4 pps to 100 pps every 10 minutes) or longer periods of time (4 pps on one day, 100 pps on the next day) (DeSantana et al 2008a; Lima et al 2015; Sato et al 2012) are potential solutions. Combining TENS with therapies such as cold, heat, massage or acupuncture that generate input from other types of afferents, may also be worth considering. However, it is important not to place an icepack over the electrodes and cool to the point of numbness because that would defeat the purpose of TENS. Temporarily withdrawing TENS treatment so that an objective assessment of the contribution of TENS to pain relief is also an option. When this is done patients may report that their pain worsens in the absence of TENS, demonstrating that TENS was in fact beneficial.

Other Practicalities

It is recommended that new patients are given a supervised trial of TENS to ensure that TENS does not aggravate pain and to give careful instruction on equipment use and expected therapeutic outcome. It is advisable to use conventional TENS on a new patient and to encourage patients to experiment with all stimulator settings (i.e. pulse frequency, pattern and duration) so that they achieve optimal pain relief and a pleasant TENS sensation (Table 15.4). A set of audio speakers (or headphones) can be plugged into the output sockets of some TENS devices to demonstrate the sound of pulses and improve patient understanding of TENS output characteristics. Patients are advised to self-administer TENS in 30-minute sessions until they have familiarized themselves with equipment, after which they are encouraged to use TENS as much as they like (Table 15.5).

An early review of progress, ideally within a few weeks, can serve to ensure correct application, provide further instruction and to recall TENS devices that are no longer required. Assessing TENS effectiveness at regular intervals is vital for tracking the location and continued use of devices. Some clinics and manufacturers allow patients to borrow TENS devices for a limited period with a view to purchasing the device. A point of contact should always be made available for patients who encounter problems. It is important to explore possible reasons for patients who claim they are not responding to TENS. It may be necessary to revisit treatment goals if the patient has unrealistic expectations of outcome and to re-assess lifestyle factors that mask potential improvements from TENS. The patient may be using inappropriate technique, electrode positions or dosage or may have lost motivation to use TENS because of the effort involved to apply treatment.

Gladwell et al (2013, 2015, 2016) have investigated the experiences of TENS users with chronic musculoskeletal pain and found that they were very strategic in their use of TENS. Users reported a broad spectrum of benefits including pain relief, reducing sensations of muscle tension and spasm, reducing medication, achieving specific functional goals and enhancing rest periods. Electrode positioning and TENS settings needed to be personalized and readjusted over time, suggesting the need for a learning phase to allow patients to optimize this complex pattern of TENS usage. Positioning TENS electrodes can be awkward and inconvenient and targeting currents to the area of pain can take time. Recent developments include electrodes woven into clothing, smart TENS electrodes with algorithms and electrode arrays for precise targeting of currents, and interfacing the TENS device with mobile technology. Data capture systems time-linked to TENS use could be a useful way to facilitate adherence and implementation monitoring of self-administered TENS (Pallett et al 2014).

SUMMARY

TENS is used extensively in healthcare for pain relief because it is inexpensive, safe, and can be administered by the patients themselves. Success with TENS depends on appropriate application, and therefore patients and therapists need an understanding of the principles of application. When used in its conventional form TENS is delivered to selectively activate Aβ afferents leading to inhibition of nociceptive transmission in the central nervous system. It is claimed that the mechanism of action and analgesic profile of AL-TENS and intense TENS differs from conventional TENS and may prove useful when conventional TENS is providing limited benefit. Systematic reviews of RCTs are compromised by insufficient high-quality RCTs and this has led to review conclusions that are inconsistent and which contrast with clinical experience. It would be inappropriate to dismiss the use of TENS until the reasons for the discrepancy in experience and published evidence are fully explored. Better-quality trials are required to determine differences in the effectiveness of different types of TENS and to compare the cost-effectiveness of TENS with other analgesic interventions, including other electrotherapies.

REFERENCES

Aarskog, R., Johnson, M. I., Demmink, J. H., et al. (2007). Is mechanical pain threshold after transcutaneous electrical nerve stimulation (TENS) increased locally and unilaterally? A randomized placebo-controlled trial in healthy subjects. *Physiotherapy Research International, 12*(4), 251–263.

Abou-Setta, A. M., Beaupre, L. A., Rashiq, S., et al. (2011). Comparative effectiveness of pain management interventions for hip fracture: A systematic review. *Annals of Internal Medicine, 155*(4), 234–2345.

Ainsworth, L., Budelier, K., Clinesmith, M., et al. (2006). Transcutaneous electrical nerve stimulation (TENS) reduces chronic hyperalgesia induced by muscle inflammation. *Pain, 120*(1–2), 182–187.

Almeida, C. C., Silva, V., Junior, G. C., Liebano, R. E., & Durigan, J. L. Q. (2018). Transcutaneous electrical nerve stimulation and interferential current demonstrate similar effects in relieving acute and chronic pain: A systematic review with meta-analysis. *Brazilian Journal of Physical Therapy, 22*(5), 347–354.

American Society of Anesthesiologists. (2010). Practice guidelines for chronic pain management: An updated report by the American Society of Anesthesiologists Task Force on Chronic Pain Management and the American Society of Regional Anesthesia and Pain Medicine. *Anesthesiology, 112*(4), 810–833.

Asbjorn, O. (2000) Treatment of tennis elbow with transcutaneous nerve stimulation (TNS). http://www.paingone.com/.

Augustinsson, L., Bohlin, P., Bundsen, P., et al. (1977). Pain relief during delivery by transcutaneous electrical nerve stimulation. *Pain, 4*(1), 59–65.

Augustinsson, L., Carlsson, C., & Pellettieri, L. (1976). Transcutaneous electrical stimulation for pain and itch control. *Acta Neurochirurgica, 33*, 342.

Beckwée, D., Bautmans, I., Swinnen, E., et al. (2014). A systematic review investigating the relationship between efficacy and stimulation parameters when using transcutaneous electrical nerve stimulation after knee arthroplasty. *SAGE Open Med, 2*, 2050312114539318.

Bedwell, C., Dowswell, T., Neilson, J. P., & Lavender, T. (2011). The use of transcutaneous electrical nerve stimulation (TENS) for pain relief in labour: A review of the evidence. *Midwifery, 27*(5), e141–148.

Bennett, M. I., Hughes, N., & Johnson, M. I. (2011). Methodological quality in randomised controlled trials of transcutaneous electric nerve stimulation for pain: Low fidelity may explain negative findings. *Pain, 152*(6), 1226–1232.

Berlant, S. R. (1984). Method of determining optimal stimulation sites for transcutaneous electrical nerve stimulation. *Physical Therapy, 64*(6), 924–928.

Bjordal, J. M., Johnson, M. I., & Ljunggreen, A. E. (2003). Transcutaneous electrical nerve stimulation (TENS) can reduce postoperative analgesic consumption. A meta-analysis with assessment of optimal treatment parameters for postoperative pain. *European Journal of Pain, 7*(2), 181–188.

Bjordal, J. M., Johnson, M. I., Lopes-Martins, R. A., Bogen, B., Chow, R., & Ljunggren, A. E. (2007). Short-term efficacy of physical interventions in osteoarthritic knee pain. A systematic review and meta-analysis of randomised placebo-controlled trials. *BMC Musculoskeletal Disorders, 8*, 51.

Boldt, I., Eriks-Hoogland, I., Brinkhof, M. W., de Bie, R., Joggi, D., & Elm, E. (2014). Non-pharmacological interventions for chronic pain in people with spinal cord injury. *Cochrane Database of Systematic Reviews* (11), CD009177.

Borjesson, M., Eriksson, P., Dellborg, M., Eliasson, T., & Mannheimer, C. (1997). Transcutaneous electrical nerve stimulation in unstable angina pectoris. *Coronary Artery Disease, 8*(8–9), 543–550.

Bronfort, G., Nilsson, N., Haas, M., et al. (2004). Non-invasive physical treatments for chronic/recurrent headache. *Cochrane Database of Systematic Reviews* (3), CD001878.

Brosseau, L., Judd, M. G., Marchand, S., Robinson, V. A., Tugwell, P., Wells, G., et al. (2003). Transcutaneous electrical nerve stimulation (TENS) for the treatment of rheumatoid arthritis in the hand. *Cochrane Database of Systematic Reviews* (3), CD004377.

Canadian Agency for Drugs and Technologies in Health. (2016). *Home transcutaneous electrical nerve stimulation for chronic pain: A review of the clinical effectiveness.* Ottawa (ON): CADTH Rapid Response Reports.

Campos, F. V., Neves, L. M., Da Silva, V. Z., et al. (2016). Hemodynamic effects induced by transcutaneous electrical nerve stimulation in apparently healthy individuals: A systematic review with meta-analysis. *Archives of Physical Medicine and Rehabilitation, 97*(5), 826–835.

do Carmo Almeida, T. C., Dos Santos Figueiredo, F. W., Barbosa Filho, V. C., de Abreu, L. C., Fonseca, F. L. A., & Adami, F. (2018). Effects of transcutaneous electrical nerve stimulation on proinflammatory cytokines: Systematic review and meta-analysis. *Mediators of Inflammation,* 1094352.

Carroll, D., Moore, A., Tramer, M., & McQuay, H. (1997). Transcutaneous electrical nerve stimulation does not relieve in labour pain: Updated systematic review. *Contemporary Reviews in Obstetrics and Gynecology, September,* 195–205.

Carroll, D., Tramer, M., McQuay, H., Nye, B., & Moore, A. (1996). Randomization is important in studies with pain outcomes: Systematic review of transcutaneous electrical nerve stimulation in acute postoperative pain. *British Journal of Anaesthesia, 77*(6), 798–803.

Chandran, P., & Sluka, K. A. (2003). Development of opioid tolerance with repeated transcutaneous electrical nerve stimulation administration. *Pain, 102*(1–2), 195–201.

Chartered Society of Physiotherapy (2006). *Guidance for the clinical use of electrophysical agents.* London: Chartered Society of Physiotherapy.

Chen, C. C., & Johnson, M. I. (2009). An investigation into the effects of frequency-modulated transcutaneous electrical nerve stimulation (TENS) on experimentally-induced pressure pain in healthy human participants. *The Journal of Pain, 10*(10), 1029–1037.

Chen, C. C., Tabasam, G., & Johnson, M. I. (2008). Does the pulse frequency of transcutaneous electrical nerve stimulation (TENS) influence hypoalgesia? A systematic review of studies using experimental pain and healthy human participants. *Physiotherapy, 94*(1), 11–20.

Chen, Y. W., Tzeng, J. I., Lin, M. F., Hung, C. H., Hsieh, P. L., & Wang, J. J. (2014). High-frequency transcutaneous electrical nerve stimulation attenuates postsurgical pain and inhibits excess substance P in rat dorsal root ganglion. *Regional Anesthesia and Pain Medicine, 39*(4), 322–328.

Chen, Y. W., Tzeng, J. I., Lin, M. F., Hung, C. H., & Wang, J. J. (2015). Transcutaneous electrical nerve stimulation attenuates postsurgical allodynia and suppresses spinal substance P and proinflammatory cytokine release in rats. *Physical Therapy, 95*(1), 76–85.

Chesterton, L. S., Lewis, A. M., Sim, J., et al. (2013). Transcutaneous electrical nerve stimulation as adjunct to primary care management for tennis elbow: Pragmatic randomised controlled trial (TATE trial). *BMJ (Clinical Research Ed.), 347,* f5160.

Chipchase, L. S., Williams, M. T., & Robertson, V. J. (2009). A national study of the availability and use of electrophysical agents by Australian physiotherapists. *Physiotherapy Theory and Practice, 25*(4), 279–296.

Chou, R. (2010) Low back pain (chronic). *Clinical Evidence (Online)* 2010.

Chung, J. M., Fang, Z. R., Hori, Y., Lee, K. H., & Willis, W. D. (1984a). Prolonged inhibition of primate spinothalamic tract cells by peripheral nerve stimulation. *Pain, 19*(3), 259–275.

Chung, J. M., Lee, K. H., Hori, Y., Endo, K., & Willis, W. D. (1984b). Factors influencing peripheral nerve stimulation produced inhibition of primate spinothalamic tract cells. *Pain, 19*(3), 277–293.

Claydon, L. S., & Chesterton, L. S. (2008). Does transcutaneous electrical nerve stimulation (TENS) produce 'dose-responses'? A review of systematic reviews on chronic pain. *Physical Therapy Reviews, 13*(6), 450–463.

Claydon, L. S., Chesterton, L. S., Barlas, P., & Sim, J. (2008). Effects of simultaneous dual-site TENS stimulation on experimental pain. *European Journal of Pain, 12*(6), 696–704.

Claydon, L. S., Chesterton, L. S., Barlas, P., & Sim, J. (2011). Dose-specific effects of transcutaneous electrical nerve stimulation (TENS) on experimental pain: A systematic review. *The Clinical Journal of Pain, 27*(7), 635–647.

Cruccu, G., Aziz, T. Z., Garcia-Larrea, L., et al. (2007). EFNS guidelines on neurostimulation therapy for neuropathic pain. *European Journal of Neurology, 14*(9), 952–970.

Cruccu, G., Garcia-Larrea, L., Hansson, P., et al. (2016). EAN guidelines on central neurostimulation therapy in chronic pain conditions. *European Journal of Neurology, 23*(10), 1489–1499.

Demmink, J.H. (1995) The effect of a biological conducting medium on the pattern of modulation and distribution in a two-circuit static interferential field. In: Proceedings of the 12th International Conference of the World Confederation for Physical Therapy (pp. 583); Jun 25-30; Washington DC. Alexandria (VA): American Physical Therapy Association.

DeSantana, J. M., da Silva, L. F., & Sluka, K. A. (2010). Cholecystokinin receptors mediate tolerance to the analgesic effect of TENS in arthritic rats. *Pain, 148*(1), 84–93.

DeSantana, J. M., Santana-Filho, V. J., & Sluka, K. A. (2008a). Modulation between high- and low-frequency transcutaneous electric nerve stimulation delays the development of analgesic tolerance in arthritic rats. *Archives of Physical Medicine and Rehabilitation, 89*(4), 754–760.

DeSantana, J. M., Walsh, D. M., Vance, C., Rakel, B. A., & Sluka, K. A. (2008b). Effectiveness of transcutaneous electrical nerve stimulation for treatment of hyperalgesia and pain. *Current Rheumatology Reports, 10*(6), 492–499.

Dingemanse, R., Randsdorp, M., Koes, B. W., & Huisstede, B. M. (2014). Evidence for the effectiveness of electrophysical modalities for treatment of medial and lateral epicondylitis: A systematic review. *British Journal of Sports Medicine, 48*(12), 957–965.

Dissanayaka, T. D., Pallegama, R. W., Suraweera, H. J., Johnson, M. I., & Kariyawasam, A. P. (2016). Comparison of the effectiveness of transcutaneous electrical nerve stimulation and interferential therapy on the upper trapezius in myofascial pain syndrome: A randomized controlled study. *American Journal of Physical Medicine & Rehabilitation, 95*(9), 663–672.

Dowswell, T., Bedwell, C., Lavender, T., & Neilson, J. P. (2009). Transcutaneous electrical nerve stimulation (TENS) for pain relief in labour. *Cochrane Database of Systematic Reviews* (2), CD007214.

Dubinsky, R. M., & Miyasaki, J. (2010). Assessment: Efficacy of transcutaneous electric nerve stimulation in the treatment of pain in neurologic disorders (an evidence-based review): Report of the Therapeutics and Technology Assessment Subcommittee of the American Academy of Neurology. *Neurology, 74*(2), 173–176.

Eriksson, M., & Sjölund, B. (1976). Acupuncture-like electroanalgesia in TNS resistant chronic pain. In Y. Zotterman (Ed.), *Sensory functions of the skin* (pp. 575–581). Oxford/New York: Pergamon Press.

Fang, J. F., Liang, Y., Du, J. Y., & Fang, J. Q. (2013). Transcutaneous electrical nerve stimulation attenuates CFA-induced hyperalgesia and inhibits spinal ERK1/2-COX-2 pathway activation in rats. *BMC Complementary and Alternative Medicine, 13*, 134.

Fary, R. E., & Briffa, N. K. (2011). Monophasic electrical stimulation produces high rates of adverse skin reactions in healthy subjects. *Physiotherapy Theory and Practice, 27*(3), 246–251.

Fattal, C., Kong, A. S. D., Gilbert, C., Ventura, M., & Albert, T. (2009). What is the efficacy of physical therapeutics for treating neuropathic pain in spinal cord injury patients? *Annals of Physical and Rehabilitation Medicine, 52*(2), 149–166.

Francis, R. P. & Johnson, M. I. (2011). The characteristics of acupuncture-like transcutaneous electrical nerve stimulation (acupuncture-like TENS): A literature review. *Acupuncture and Electro-Therapeutics Research, 36*(3–4), 231–258.

Freynet, A., & Falcoz, P. E. (2010). Is transcutaneous electrical nerve stimulation effective in relieving postoperative pain after thoracotomy? *Interactive Cardiovascular and Thoracic Surgery, 10*(2), 283–288.

Gajjar, K., Martin-Hirsch, P. P., Bryant, A., & Owens, G. L. (2016). Pain relief for women with cervical intraepithelial neoplasia undergoing colposcopy treatment. *Cochrane Database of Systematic Reviews, 7* CD006120.

Garrison, D. W., & Foreman, R. D. (1994). Decreased activity of spontaneous and noxiously evoked dorsal horn cells during transcutaneous electrical nerve stimulation (TENS). *Pain, 58*(3), 309–315.

Gibson, W., Wand, BM, Meads, C., Catley, MJ, & O'Connell, NE. (2019). Transcutaneous electrical nerve stimulation (TENS) for chronic pain - an overview of Cochrane Reviews. *Cochrane Database of Systematic Reviews*, (2), Art. No.: CD011890. https://doi.org/10.1002/14651858.CD011890.pub2.

Garrison, D. W., & Foreman, R. D. (1996). Effects of transcutaneous electrical nerve stimulation (TENS) on spontaneous and noxiously evoked dorsal horn cell activity in cats with transected spinal cords. *Neuroscience Letters, 216*(2), 125–128.

Geng, B., Yoshida, K., & Jensen, W. (2011). Impacts of selected stimulation patterns on the perception threshold in electrocutaneous stimulation. *Journal of NeuroEngineering and Rehabilitation, 8*, 9.

Gibson, W., Wand, B. M., & O'Connell, N. E. (2017). Transcutaneous electrical nerve stimulation (TENS) for neuropathic pain in adults. *Cochrane Database of Systematic Reviews, (9)* CD011976.

Gildenberg, P. L. (2006). History of electrical neuromodulation for chronic pain. *Pain Medicine, 7*(Suppl. 1), S7–S13.

Gladwell, P. W. (2013). *Focusing outcome measurement for transcutaneous electrical nerve stimulation evaluation: Incorporating the experiences of TENS users with chronic musculoskeletal pain* PhD Thesis, University of the West of England.

Gladwell, P. W., Badlan, K., Cramp, F., & Palmer, S. (2015). Direct and indirect benefits reported by users of transcutaneous electrical nerve stimulation for chronic musculoskeletal pain: Qualitative exploration using patient interviews. *Physical Therapy, 95*(11), 1518–1528.

Gladwell, P. W., Badlan, K., Cramp, F., & Palmer, S. (2016). Problems, solutions, and strategies reported by users of transcutaneous electrical nerve stimulation for chronic musculoskeletal pain: Qualitative exploration using patient interviews. *Physical Therapy, 96*(7), 1039–1048.

Hamza, M. A., White, P. F., Ahmed, H. E., & Ghoname, E. A. (1999). Effect of the frequency of transcutaneous electrical nerve stimulation on the postoperative opioid analgesic requirement and recovery profile. *Anesthesiology, 91*(5), 1232–1238.

Harvey, L. A., Glinsky, J. V., & Bowden, J. L. (2016). The effectiveness of 22 commonly administered physiotherapy interventions for people with spinal cord injury: A systematic review. *Spinal Cord, 54*(11), 914–923.

Hingne, P. M., & Sluka, K. A. (2008). Blockade of NMDA receptors prevents analgesic tolerance to repeated transcutaneous electrical nerve stimulation (TENS) in rats. *The Journal of Pain, 9*(3), 217–225.

Houghton, P., Nussbaum, E., & Hoens, A. (2010). Electrophysical agents. contraindications and precautions: An evidence-based approach to clinical decision making in physical therapy. *Physiotherapy Canada, 62*(5), 1–80.

Hughes, N., Bennett, M. I., & Johnson, M. I. (2013). An investigation into the magnitude of the current window and perception of transcutaneous electrical nerve stimulation (TENS) sensation at various frequencies and body sites in healthy human participants. *The Clinical Journal of Pain, 29*(2), 146–153.

Huisstede, B. M., Hoogvliet, P., Franke, T. P., Randsdorp, M. S., & Koes, B. W. (2017). Carpal tunnel syndrome: Effectiveness of physical therapy and electrophysical modalities. an updated systematic review of randomized controlled trials. *Archives of Physical Medicine and Rehabilitation, 99*(8), 1623–1634 e23.

Hurlow, A., Bennett, M. I., Robb, K. A., Johnson, M. I., Simpson, K. H., & Oxberry, S. G. (2012). Transcutaneous electric nerve stimulation (TENS) for cancer pain in adults. *Cochrane Database of Systematic Reviews* (3), CD006276.

Ivanova-Stoilova, T. & Howells, D. (2002). The usefulness of PainGone pain killing pen for self-treatment of chronic musculoskeletal pain - a pilot study. The Pain Society. Annual Scientific Meeting. Bournemouth UK.

Ignelzi, R. J., & Nyquist, J. K. (1976). Direct effect of electrical stimulation on peripheral nerve evoked activity: Implications in pain relief. *Journal of Neurosurgery, 45*(2), 159–165.

Ignelzi, R. J., & Nyquist, J. K. (1979). Excitability changes in peripheral nerve fibers after repetitive electrical stimulation. Implications in pain modulation. *Journal of Neurosurgery, 51*(6), 824–833.

Igwea, S. E., Tabansi-Ochuogu, C. S., & Abaraogu, U. O. (2016). TENS and heat therapy for pain relief and quality of life improvement in individuals with primary dysmenorrhea: A systematic review. *Complementary Therapies in Clinical Practice, 24*, 86–91.

Jauregui, J. J., Cherian, J. J., Gwam, C. U., et al. (2016). A meta-analysis of transcutaneous electrical nerve stimulation for chronic low back pain. *Surgical Technology International, 28*, 296–302.

Jelinek, H. F., & McIntyre, R. (2010). Electric pulse frequency and magnitude of perceived sensation during electrocutaneous forearm stimulation. *Archives of Physical Medicine and Rehabilitation, 91*(9), 1378–1382.

Jin, D. M., Xu, Y., Geng, D. F., & Yan, T. B. (2010). Effect of transcutaneous electrical nerve stimulation on symptomatic diabetic peripheral neuropathy: A meta-analysis of randomized controlled trials. *Diabetes Research and Clinical Practice, 89*(1), 10–15.

Johnson, M. I. (1998). Acupuncture-like transcutaneous electrical nerve stimulation (AL-TENS) in the management of pain. *Physical Therapy Reviews, 3*, 73–93.

Johnson, M. I. (2014a). Appropriate electrode sites and electrical characteristics for TENS. In M. I. Johnson (Ed.), *Transcutaneous electrical nerve stimulation (TENS). Research to support clinical practice* (pp. 64–92). Oxford, UK: Oxford University Press.

Johnson, M. I. (2014b). Clinical research on the efficacy of TENS. In M. I. Johnson (Ed.), *Transcutaneous electrical nerve stimulation (TENS). Research to support clinical practice* (pp. 147–171). Oxford, UK: Oxford University Press.

Johnson, M. I. (2014c). Contraindications, precautions, and adverse events. In M. I. Johnson (Ed.), *Transcutaneous electrical nerve stimulation (TENS). Research to support clinical practice* (pp. 93–115). Oxford, UK: Oxford University Press.

Johnson, M. I. (2014d). TENS-like devices. In M. I. Johnson (Ed.), *Transcutaneous electrical nerve stimulation (TENS). Research to support clinical practice* (pp. 203–212). Oxford, UK: Oxford University Press.

Johnson, M. I. (2014e). TENS equipment, techniques, and biophysical principles. In M. I. Johnson (Ed.), *Transcutaneous electrical nerve stimulation (TENS). Research to support clinical practice* (pp. 34–63). Oxford, UK: Oxford University Press.

Johnson, M. I. (2014f). *Transcutaneous electrical nerve stimulation (TENS). Research to support clinical practice.* Oxford, UK: Oxford University Press.

Johnson, M. I. (2014g). The use of TENS for non-painful conditions. In M. I. Johnson (Ed.), *Transcutaneous electrical nerve stimulation (TENS). Research to support clinical practice* (pp. 193–202). Oxford, UK: Oxford University Press.

Johnson, M. I. (2017). Transcutaneous electrical nerve stimulation (TENS) as an adjunct for pain management in perioperative settings: A critical review. *Expert Review of Neurotherapeutics, 17*(10), 1013–1027.

Johnson, M. I., Ashton, C. H., Bousfield, D. R., & Thompson, J. W. (1991a). Analgesic effects of different pulse patterns of transcutaneous electrical nerve stimulation on cold-induced pain in normal subjects. *Journal of Psychosomatic Research, 35*(2–3), 313–321.

Johnson, M. I., Ashton, C. H., & Thompson, J. W. (1991b). An in-depth study of long-term users of transcutaneous electrical nerve stimulation (TENS). Implications for clinical use of TENS. *Pain, 44*(3), 221–229.

Johannsen, F., Gam, A., Hauschild, B., Mathiesen, B. & Jensen, L. (1993) Rebox: an adjunct in physical medicine? Arch Phys Med Rehabil *74*(4), 438–40.

Johnson, M. I., Penny, P. & Sajawal, M. A. (1997). An examination of the analgesic effects of microcurrent stimulation (MES) on cold-induced pain in healthy subjects. *Physiotherapy Theory and Practice, 13*, 293–301.

Johnson, M. I., & Bjordal, J. M. (2011). Transcutaneous electrical nerve stimulation for the management of painful conditions: Focus on neuropathic pain. *Expert Review of Neurotherapeutics, 11*(5), 735–753.

Johnson, M. I., Claydon, L. S., Herbison, G. P., Jones, G., & Paley, C. A. (2017). Transcutaneous electrical nerve stimulation (TENS) for fibromyalgia in adults. *Cochrane Database of Systematic Reviews (10)*, CD012172.

Johnson, M. I., Filshie, J., & Thompson, J. W. (2012). Transcutaneous electrical nerve stimulation and acupuncture. In J. Hester Sykes, N., & Peat, S. (Eds.), *Interventional pain control in cancer pain management* (pp. 235–258). Oxford, UK: Oxford University Press.

Johnson, M., & Martinson, M. (2007). Efficacy of electrical nerve stimulation for chronic musculoskeletal pain: A meta-analysis of randomized controlled trials. *Pain, 130*(1–2), 157–165.

Johnson, M. I., Mulvey, M. R., & Bagnall, A. M. (2015a). Transcutaneous electrical nerve stimulation (TENS) for phantom pain and stump pain following amputation in adults. *Cochrane Database of Systematic Reviews (8)*, CD007264.

Johnson, M. I., Paley, C. A., Howe, T. E., & Sluka, K. A. (2015b). Transcutaneous electrical nerve stimulation for acute pain. *Cochrane Database of Systematic Reviews (6)*, CD006142.

Johnson, M. I., & Walsh, D. M. (2010). Pain: Continued uncertainty of TENS' effectiveness for pain relief. *Nature Reviews Rheumatology, 6*(6), 314–316.

Jawahar, R., Oh, U., Yang, S. & Lapane, K. L. (2014). Alternative approach: a systematic review of non-pharmacological non-spastic and non-trigeminal pain management in multiple sclerosis. European Journal of Physical and Rehabilitation Medicine 2014 Oct, 50(5), 567–557.

Kalra, A., Urban, M. O., & Sluka, K. A. (2001). Blockade of opioid receptors in rostral ventral medulla prevents antihyperalgesia produced by transcutaneous electrical nerve stimulation (TENS). *Journal of Pharmacology and Experimental Therapeutics, 298*(1), 257–263.

Kantor, G., Alon, G., & Ho, H. (1994a). The effects of selected stimulus waveforms on pulse and phase characteristics at sensory and motor thresholds. *Physical Therapy, 74*(10), 951–962.

Kantor, G., Alon, G., & Ho, H. S. (1994b). The effects of selected stimulus waveforms on pulse and phase characteristics at sensory and motor thresholds. *Physical Therapy, 74*(10), 951–962.

Kerai, S., Saxena, K. N., Taneja, B., & Sehrawat, L. (2014). Role of transcutaneous electrical nerve stimulation in post-operative analgesia. *Indian Journal of Anaesthesia, 58*(4), 388–393.

Khadilkar, A., Odebiyi, D. O., Brosseau, L., & Wells, G. A. (2008). Transcutaneous electrical nerve stimulation (TENS) versus placebo for chronic low-back pain. *Cochrane Database of Systematic Reviews* (4), CD003008.

King, E. W., Audette, K., Athman, G. A., Nguyen, H. O., Sluka, K. A., & Fairbanks, C. A. (2005). Transcutaneous electrical nerve stimulation activates peripherally located alpha-2A adrenergic receptors. *Pain, 115*(3), 364–373.

Kroeling, P., Gross, A., Graham, N., et al. (2013). Electrotherapy for neck pain. *Cochrane Database of Systematic Reviews* (8), CD004251.

Law, P. P., & Cheing, G. L. (2004). Optimal stimulation frequency of transcutaneous electrical nerve stimulation on people with knee osteoarthritis. *Journal of Rehabilitation Medicine, 36*(5), 220–225.

Lazarou, L., Kitsios, A., Lazarou, I., Sikaras, E., & Trampas, A. (2009). Effects of intensity of transcutaneous electrical nerve stimulation (TENS) on pressure pain threshold and blood pressure in healthy humans: A randomized, double-blind, placebo-controlled trial. *The Clinical Journal of Pain, 25*(9), 773–780.

Levin, M., & Hui-Chan, C. (1993). Conventional and acupuncture-like transcutaneous electrical nerve stimulation excite similar afferent fibers. *Archives of Physical Medicine and Rehabilitation, 74*(1), 54–60.

Liebano, R. E., Rakel, B., Vance, C. G., Walsh, D. M., & Sluka, K. A. (2011). An investigation of the development of analgesic tolerance to TENS in humans. *Pain, 211*, 335–342.

Lima, L. V., Cruz, K. M., Abner, T. S., Mota, C. M., Agripino, M. E., Santana-Filho, V. J., et al. (2015). Associating high intensity and modulated frequency of TENS delays analgesic tolerance in rats. *European Journal of Pain, 19*(3), 369–376.

Li, J., & Song, Y. (2017). Transcutaneous electrical nerve stimulation for postoperative pain control after total knee arthroplasty: A meta-analysis of randomized controlled trials. *Medicine (Baltimore), 96*(37), e8036.

Loh, J., & Gulati, A. (2015). The use of transcutaneous electrical nerve stimulation (TENS) in a major cancer center for the treatment of severe cancer-related pain and associated disability. *Pain Medicine, 16*(6), 1204–1210.

Long, D. M. (1974). Cutaneous afferent stimulation for relief of chronic pain. *Clinical Neurosurgery, 21*, 257–268.

Macefield, G., & Burke, D. (1991). Long-lasting depression of central synaptic transmission following prolonged high-frequency stimulation of cutaneous afferents: A mechanism for post-vibratory hypaesthesia. *Electroencephalography and Clinical Neurophysiology, 78*(2), 150–158.

Machado, L. A., Kamper, S. J., Herbert, R. D., Maher, C. G., & McAuley, J. H. (2009). Analgesic effects of treatments for non-specific low back pain: A meta-analysis of placebo-controlled randomized trials. *Rheumatology, 48*(5), 520–527.

Macdonald, A. R. J. & Coates, T. W. (1995). The discovery of transcutaneous spinal electroanalgesia and its relief of chronic pain. *Physiotherapy, 81*, 653–660.

Maeda, Y., Lisi, T. L., Vance, C. G., & Sluka, K. A. (2007). Release of GABA and activation of GABA(A) in the spinal cord mediates the effects of TENS in rats. *Brain Research, 1136*(1), 43–50.

Ma, Y. T., & Sluka, K. A. (2001). Reduction in inflammation-induced sensitization of dorsal horn neurons by transcutaneous electrical nerve stimulation in anesthetized rats. *Experimental Brain Research, 137*(1), 94–102.

Matsuo, H., Uchida, K., Nakajima, H., Guerrero, A. R., Watanabe, S., Takeura, N., et al. (2014). Early transcutaneous electrical nerve stimulation reduces hyperalgesia and decreases activation of spinal glial cells in mice with neuropathic pain. *Pain, 155*(9), 1888–1901.

Mello, L. F., Nobrega, L. F., & Lemos, A. (2011). Transcutaneous electrical stimulation for pain relief during labor: A systematic review and meta-analysis. *Revista Brasileira de Fisioterapia.* 15(3), 175–184.

Melzack, R., & Wall, P. D. (1965). Pain mechanisms: A new theory. *Science,* 150(3699), 971–979.

Mense, S. (1993). Nociception from skeletal muscle in relation to clinical muscle pain. *Pain,* 54(3), 241–289.

Merkel, S. I., Gutstein, H. B., & Malviya, S. (1999). Use of transcutaneous electrical nerve stimulation in a young child with pain from open perineal lesions. *Journal of Pain and Symptom Management,* 18(5), 376–381.

Meyerson, B. (1983). Electrostimulation procedures: Effects presumed rationale, and possible mechanisms. In J. Bonica, U. Lindblom, & A. Iggo (Eds.), *Advances in pain research and therapy* (Vol. 5) (pp. 495–534). New York: Raven.

Mills, P. B., & Dossa, F. (2016). Transcutaneous electrical nerve stimulation for management of limb spasticity: A systematic review. *American Journal of Physical Medicine & Rehabilitation,* 95(4), 309–318.

Moore, R. A., Gavaghan, D., Tramer, M. R., Collins, S. L., & McQuay, H. J. (1998). Size is everything – large amounts of information are needed to overcome random effects in estimating direction and magnitude of treatment effects. *Pain,* 78(3), 209–216.

Moran, F., Leonard, T., Hawthorne, S., Hughes, C. M., McCrum-Gardner, E., Johnson, M. I., et al. (2011). Hypoalgesia in response to transcutaneous electrical nerve stimulation (TENS) depends on stimulation intensity. *The Journal of Pain,* 12(8), 929–935.

Nardone, A., & Schieppati, M. (1989). Influences of transcutaneous electrical stimulation of cutaneous and mixed nerves on subcortical and cortical somatosensory evoked potentials. *Electroencephalography and Clinical Neurophysiology,* 74(1), 24–35.

National Institute for Health and Care Excellence. (2014). *Osteoarthritis: Care and management.* London: NICE guidelines [CG177].

National Institute for Health and Care Excellence. (2016). *Low back pain and sciatica in over 16s: Assessment and management. Clinical guideline [NG59].* National Institute for Health and Care Excellence (NICE).

National Institute for Health and Clinical Excellence. (2007). *NICE clinical guideline 55 Intrapartum care: Care of healthy women and their babies during childbirth* (London).

National Institute for Health and Clinical Excellence. (2009). *NICE clinical guideline 79 Rheumatoid arthritis: The management of rheumatoid arthritis in adults* (London).

National Institute for Health and Clinical Excellence. (2011). *NICE clinical guideline 126. Management of stable angina* (London).

National Institute for Health and Clinical Excellence and Conditions. (2003). *NICE clinical guideline 8. Multiple Sclerosis. National clinical guideline for diagnosis and management in primary and secondary care.*

Nnoaham, K. E., & Kumbang, J. (2008). Transcutaneous electrical nerve stimulation (TENS) for chronic pain. *Cochrane Database of Systematic Reviews* (3), CD003222.

Page, M. J., Green, S., Kramer, S., Johnston, R. V., McBain, B., & Buchbinder, R. (2014). Electrotherapy modalities for adhesive capsulitis (frozen shoulder). *Cochrane Database of Systematic Reviews* (10), CD011324.

Odendaal, C. & Joubert, G. (1999) APS Therapy - A new way of treating chronic headache - a pilot study. South African Journal of Anaesthesiology and Analgesia 5(1), 1-3.

Page, M. J., Green, S., Mrocki, M. A., Surace, S. J., Deitch, J., McBain, B., et al. (2016). Electrotherapy modalities for rotator cuff disease. *Cochrane Database of Systematic Reviews* (6), CD012225.

Pallett, E. J., Rentowl, P., Johnson, M. I., & Watson, P. J. (2014). Implementation fidelity of self-administered transcutaneous electrical nerve stimulation (TENS) in patients with chronic back pain: An observational study. *The Clinical Journal of Pain,* 30(3), 224–231.

Pantaleao, M. A., Laurino, M. F., Gallego, N. L., Cabral, C. M., Rakel, B., Vance, C., et al. (2011). Adjusting pulse amplitude during transcutaneous electrical nerve stimulation (TENS) application produces greater hypoalgesia. *The Journal of Pain,* 12(5), 581–590.

Petrofsky, J., Laymon, M., Prowse, M., Gunda, S., & Batt, J. (2009). The transfer of current through skin and muscle during electrical stimulation with sine, square, Russian and interferential waveforms. *Journal of Medical Engineering & Technology,* 33(2), 170–181.

Pieber, K., Herceg, M., & Paternostro-Sluga, T. (2010). Electrotherapy for the treatment of painful diabetic peripheral neuropathy: A review. *Journal of Rehabilitation Medicine,* 42(4), 289–295.

Poitras, S., & Brosseau, L. (2008). Evidence-informed management of chronic low back pain with transcutaneous electrical nerve stimulation, interferential current, electrical muscle stimulation, ultrasound, and thermotherapy. *The Spine Journal,* 8(1), 226–233.

Pomeranz, B., & Niznick, G. (1987). Codetron, a new electrotherapy device overcomes the habituation problems of conventional TENS devices. *American Journal of Electromedicine First Quarter,* 22–26.

Price, C. I., & Pandyan, A. D. (2000). Electrical stimulation for preventing and treating post-stroke shoulder pain. *Cochrane Database of Systematic Reviews* (4), CD001698.

Proctor, M. L., Smith, C. A., Farquhar, C. M., & Stones, R. W. (2002). Transcutaneous electrical nerve stimulation and acupuncture for primary dysmenorrhoea. *Cochrane Database of Systematic Reviews* (1), CD002123.

Proctor, M. L., Smith, C. A., Farquhar, C. M., & Stones, R. W. (2003). Transcutaneous electrical nerve stimulation and acupuncture for primary dysmenorrhoea (Cochrane Review). *Cochrane Database of Systematic Reviews* (1), CD002123.

Radhakrishnan, R., & Sluka, K. A. (2003). Spinal muscarinic receptors are activated during low or high-frequency TENS-induced antihyperalgesia in rats. *Neuropharmacology,* 45(8), 1111–1119.

Radhakrishnan, R., & Sluka, K. A. (2005). Deep tissue afferents, but not cutaneous afferents, mediate transcutaneous electrical nerve stimulation-Induced antihyperalgesia. *The Journal of Pain,* 6(10), 673–680.

Rakel, B., Cooper, N., Adams, H. J., Messer, B. R., Frey Law, L. A., Dannen, D. R., et al. (2010). A new transient sham TENS device allows for investigator blinding while delivering a true placebo treatment. *The Journal of Pain*, 11(3), 230–238.

Reeve, J., Menon, D., & Corabian, P. (1996). Transcutaneous electrical nerve stimulation (TENS): A technology assessment. *International Journal of Technology Assessment in Health Care*, 12(2), 299–324.

Resende, L., Merriwether, E., Rampazo, E. P., Dailey, D., Embree, J., Deberg, J., et al. (2018). Meta-analysis of transcutaneous electrical nerve stimulation for relief of spinal pain. *European Journal of Pain*, 22(4), 663–678.

Robertson, V., Chipchase, L., & Laakso, E. (2001). *Guidelines for the clinical use of electrophysical agents*. Melbourne: Australian Physiotherapy Association.

Rutjes, A. W., Nuesch, E., Sterchi, R., Kalichman, L., Hendriks, E., Osiri, M., et al. (2009). Transcutaneous electrostimulation for osteoarthritis of the knee. *Cochrane Database of Systematic Reviews* (4), CD002823.

Salazar, A. P., Stein, C., Marchese, R. R., Plentz, R. D., & Pagnussat, A. S. (2017). Electric stimulation for pain relief in patients with fibromyalgia: A systematic review and meta-analysis of randomized controlled trials. *Pain Physician*, 20(2), 15–25.

Sandkühler, J. (2000). Long-lasting analgesia following TENS and acupuncture: Spinal mechanisms beyond gate control. *9th World Congress on Pain: Progress in pain research and management* (Vol. 16). Austria: IASP Press.

Sandkühler, J., Chen, J. G., & Cheng, G. (1997). Low-frequency stimulation of afferent Adelta -fibers induces long-term depression at primary afferent synapses with substantia gelatinosa neurons in the rat. *Journal of Neuroscience*, 17(16), 6483–6491.

Sato, K. L., Sanada, L. S., Rakel, B. A., & Sluka, K. A. (2012). Increasing intensity of TENS prevents analgesic tolerance in rats. *The Journal of Pain*, 13(9), 884–890.

Sawant, A., Dadurka, K., Overend, T., & Kremenchutzky, M. (2015). Systematic review of efficacy of TENS for management of central pain in people with multiple sclerosis. *Multiple Sclerosis and Related Disorders*, 4(3), 219–227.

Sbruzzi, G., Silveira, S. A., Silva, D. V., Coronel, C. C., & Plentz, R. D. (2012). Transcutaneous electrical nerve stimulation after thoracic surgery: Systematic review and meta-analysis of 11 randomized trials. *Revista Brasileira de Cirurgia Cardiovascular*, 27(1), 75–87.

Schug, S. A., Palmer, G. M., Scott, D. A., Halliwell, R., & Trinca, J. (2016). Acute pain management: Scientific evidence, fourth edition, 2015. *Medical Journal of Australia*, 204(8), 315–317.

Shealy, C. N., Mortimer, J. T., & Reswick, J. B. (1967). Electrical inhibition of pain by stimulation of the dorsal columns: Preliminary clinical report. *Anesthesia & Analgesia*, 46(4), 489–491.

Simpson, P. M., Fouche, P. F., Thomas, R. E., & Bendall, J. C. (2014). Transcutaneous electrical nerve stimulation for relieving acute pain in the prehospital setting: A systematic review and meta-analysis of randomized-controlled trials. *European Journal of Emergency Medicine*, 21(1), 10–17.

Sjölund, B. H. (1985). Peripheral nerve stimulation suppression of C-fiber-evoked flexion reflex in rats. Part 1: Parameters of continuous stimulation. *Journal of Neurosurgery*, 63(4), 612–616.

Sjölund, B. H., & Eriksson, M. B. (1979). The influence of naloxone on analgesia produced by peripheral conditioning stimulation. *Brain Research*, 173(2), 295–301.

Sjölund, B., Terenius, L., & Eriksson, M. (1977). Increased cerebrospinal fluid levels of endorphins after electro-acupuncture. *Acta Physiologica Scandinavica*, 100(3), 382–384.

Sluka, K. A., Bailey, K., Bogush, J., Olson, R., & Ricketts, A. (1998). Treatment with either high or low frequency TENS reduces the secondary hyperalgesia observed after injection of kaolin and carrageenan into the knee joint. *Pain*, 77(1), 97–102.

Sluka, K. A., Bjordal, J. M., Marchand, S., & Rakel, B. A. (2013). What makes transcutaneous electrical nerve stimulation work? Making sense of the mixed results in the clinical literature. *Physical Therapy*, 93(10), 1397–1402.

Sluka, K. A., & Chandran, P. (2002). Enhanced reduction in hyperalgesia by combined administration of clonidine and TENS. *Pain*, 100(1–2), 183–190.

Sluka, K. A., Deacon, M., Stibal, A., Strissel, S., & Terpstra, A. (1999). Spinal blockade of opioid receptors prevents the analgesia produced by TENS in arthritic rats. *Journal of Pharmacology and Experimental Therapeutics*, 289(2), 840–846.

Sluka, K. A., Judge, M. A., McColley, M. M., Reveiz, P. M., & Taylor, B. M. (2000). Low frequency TENS is less effective than high-frequency TENS at reducing inflammation-induced hyperalgesia in morphine-tolerant rats. *European Journal of Pain*, 4(2), 185–193.

Sluka, K. A., Vance, C. G., & Lisi, T. L. (2005). High-frequency, but not low-frequency, transcutaneous electrical nerve stimulation reduces aspartate and glutamate release in the spinal cord dorsal horn. *Journal of Neurochemistry*, 95(6), 1794–1801.

Sluka, K., & Walsh, D. (2016). Chapter 8: Transcutaneous electrical nerve stimulation and interferential therapy. In S. Ka (Ed.), *Mechanisms and management of pain for the physical therapist* (2nd ed.) (pp. 203–224). Philadelphia: IASP Press.

Tao, H., Wang, T., Dong, X., Guo, Q., Xu, H., & Wan, Q. (2018). Effectiveness of transcutaneous electrical nerve stimulation for the treatment of migraine: A meta-analysis of randomized controlled trials. *The Journal of Headache and Pain*, 19(1), 42.

Thompson, J. (1989). The pharmacology of transcutaneous electrical nerve stimulation (TENS). *Intractable Pain Society Forum*, 7, 33–39.

Tong, K. C., Lo, S. K., & Cheing, G. L. (2007). Alternating frequencies of transcutaneous electric nerve stimulation: Does it produce greater analgesic effects on mechanical and thermal pain thresholds? *Archives of Physical Medicine and Rehabilitation*, 88(10), 1344–1349.

Tulgar, M., McGlone, F., Bowsher, D., & Miles, J. B. (1991a). Comparative effectiveness of different stimulation modes in relieving pain. Part I. A pilot study. *Pain*, 47(2), 151–155.

Tulgar, M., McGlone, F., Bowsher, D., & Miles, J. B. (1991b). Comparative effectiveness of different stimulation modes in relieving pain. Part II. A double-blind controlled long-term clinical trial. *Pain*, 47(2), 157–162.

Vance, C. G., Rakel, B. A., Dailey, D. L., & Sluka, K. A. (2015). Skin impedance is not a factor in transcutaneous electrical nerve stimulation effectiveness. *Journal of Pain Research, 8*, 571–580.

Wall, P. D., & Sweet, W. H. (1967). Temporary abolition of pain in man. *Science, 155*(758), 108–109.

Walsh, D. M. (1996). Transcutaneous electrical nerve stimulation and acupuncture points. *Complementary Therapies in Medicine, 4*(2), 133–137.

Walsh, D. M., Lowe, A. S., McCormack, K., Willer, J. C., Baxter, G. D., & Allen, J. M. (1998). Transcutaneous electrical nerve stimulation: Effect on peripheral nerve conduction, mechanical pain threshold, and tactile threshold in humans. *Archives of Physical Medicine and Rehabilitation, 79*(9), 1051–1058.

Woods, B., Manca, A., Weatherly, H., Saramago, P., Sideris, E., Giannopoulou, C., et al. (2017). Cost-effectiveness of adjunct non-pharmacological interventions for osteoarthritis of the knee. *PLoS One, 12*(3), e0172749.

Woolf, C. J., Mitchell, D., & Barrett, G. D. (1980). Antinociceptive effect of peripheral segmental electrical stimulation in the rat. *Pain, 8*(2), 237–252.

Woolf, C., & Thompson, J. (1994). Segmental afferent fibre-induced analgesia: Transcutaneous electrical nerve stimulation (TENS) and vibration. In P. Wall & R. Melzack (Eds.), *Textbook of pain* (pp. 1191–1208). Edinburgh: Churchill Livingstone.

Woolf, C. J., Thompson, S. W., & King, A. E. (1988). Prolonged primary afferent induced alterations in dorsal horn neurones, an intracellular analysis in vivo and in vitro. *Journal de Physiologie, 83*(3), 255–266.

Wu, X., Chung, V. C., Hui, E. P., Ziea, E. T., Ng, B. F., Ho, R. S., et al. (2015). Effectiveness of acupuncture and related therapies for palliative care of cancer: Overview of systematic reviews. *Scientific Reports, 5*, 16776.

Wu, L. C., Weng, P. W., Chen, C. H., Huang, Y. Y., Tsuang, Y. H., & Chiang, C. J. (2018). Literature review and meta-analysis of transcutaneous electrical nerve stimulation in treating chronic back pain. *Regional Anesthesia and Pain Medicine, 43*(4), 425–433.

Yue, C., Zhang, X., Zhu, Y., Jia, Y., Wang, H., & Liu, Y. (2018). Systematic review of three electrical stimulation techniques for rehabilitation after total knee arthroplasty. *Journal of Arthroplasty, 33*(7)2330–2337.

Yu, D. T., & Jones, A. Y. (2014). Are physiological changes experienced by healthy subjects during Acu-TENS associated with acupuncture point sensations? *Acupuncture in Medicine, 32*(1), 28–36.

Zeng, C., Li, H., Yang, T., Deng, Z. H., Yang, Y., Zhang, Y., et al. (2015). Electrical stimulation for pain relief in knee osteoarthritis: Systematic review and network meta-analysis. *Osteoarthritis and Cartilage, 23*(2), 189–202.

Zhu, Y., Feng, Y., & Peng, L. (2017). Effect of transcutaneous electrical nerve stimulation for pain control after total knee arthroplasty: A systematic review and meta-analysis. *Journal of Rehabilitation Medicine, 49*(9), 700–704.

16

Neuromuscular Electrical Stimulation (NMES)

Joseph Anthony

CHAPTER OUTLINE

BRIEF HISTORY

Artificial contraction of the muscles of frogs' legs had been achieved using a metallic couple to provide an external electric charge for well over a century before Luigi Galvani (1737–1798), the Italian physician, physicist, biologist and philosopher, correctly explained the mechanism by which skeletal muscle could be made to contract by the application of external electricity (Cambridge 1977).

Almost fifty years previously, Johann Gottlob Krüger (1715–1759) had speculated that electricity might be useful in medicine, writing, "The best effect would be found in paralyzed limbs to restore sensation and re-establish the power of motion" (Petrofsky 2004).

John Wesley (1704–1791), having become enthused by the demonstrations of Benjamin Franklin, saw potential for electricity to have a therapeutic effect. Wesley procured an apparatus in 1756 and started treating patients (Tyerman 1890).

The founder of modern electrotherapy is considered to be the French neurologist Guillaume-Benjamin-Armand Duchenne de Boulogne (1806–1875) (Cambridge 1977). Beginning in about 1833, and building on the work of Franklin, Wesley and Krüger, Duchenne devoted himself to the study of the "curative value of electricity", as well as to the use of electricity for investigation and classification of motor deficiencies, taking induced current, or faradism (the term was coined by Duchenne), as a new means of investigation (Poore 1883). Duchenne developed the application of "cutaneous local faradization", as distinct from "general", using a symmetric biphasic waveform and moist pads on the skin to cause contraction of specific muscles (Duchenne 1871; Licht 1967).

Electricity was used to improve muscle function by Jackson and Seddon (1945), who successfully reduced muscle wasting associated with peripheral nerve injuries during the Second World War (Jackson & Seddon 1945).

In 1961, Liberson and colleagues reported an experiment using electrical stimulation (ES) of the peroneal nerve in patients suffering from foot-drop related to hemiplegia (Liberson 1961).

The term neuromuscular electrical stimulation (NMES), used to describe electrical stimulation of muscle contraction that can be used for 'functional' purposes, may be found in the literature as early as 1964 (Valenti 1964).

PHYSICAL PRINCIPLES

In general, the goal of NMES is tetanic contraction of muscle fibres in response to depolarization of motor nerves, using surface electrodes.

The nature of a muscle contraction caused by electrical stimulation (ES) will depend on the frequency of the stimulating pulses, the intensity of ES, pulse duration and, to some degree, the location and size of the electrodes; all of which determine the number and location of nerve fibres to be depolarized, and the strength and frequency of the subsequent muscle contraction.

The pulse waveform for NMES is usually rectangular, symmetric or asymmetric biphasic (for description of waveforms see Chapter 4). Some devices will allow the operator to choose between symmetric and asymmetric biphasic waveforms. The shape of the waveform may have an impact on the amount of torque developed, and the comfort of the application (see later in this chapter).

Muscle stimulation may also be achieved using currents such as low frequency, burst mode, alternating current (AC) or Russian current (RC). These waveforms are described in Chapter 4.

While it is possible in the case of denervated muscle to depolarize skeletal muscle sarcolemma directly using surface electrodes, this requires a pulse duration longer than that possible with most NMES stimulators. This chapter is primarily concerned with the use of ES to achieve a nerve mediated effect on muscle.

When using a monophasic or asymmetric biphasic current, the negatively charged cathode is said to be slightly more effective at causing nerve depolarization (i.e. this electrode is more 'active') (Guyton 1976). However, in practice, clinicians find that there is not a lot of observable difference, especially when using a symmetric biphasic current.

Stimulus intensity, or current amplitude, determines (a) the presence or absence of a motor response to ES, and (b) the intensity of any motor response. Current intensity that is too low will fail to cause depolarization of nerves – either sensory or motor. In order to cause nerve depolarization, current must reach an intensity sufficient to cause ionic displacement great enough to reduce the potential difference across the nerve cell membrane to about -55 mV, allowing nerve depolarization to occur.

According to Coulomb's law, the strength of the electric field and, therefore, the current density under the electrode, decreases by a factor of 4 as the distance from the electrode is doubled. Conversely, current density increases by a factor of 4 if the distance to the electrode is halved. This explains why those nerves closest to the electrodes will be more readily stimulated, and why it is important to place electrodes as close as possible to the target nerves.

BIOPHYSICAL EFFECTS

In order to depolarize nerves, electric current must traverse the skin, which forms a barrier to exogenous energy. Skin resistance to electric current is non-linear. Resistance varies with current intensity, pulse duration, duration of application, and the nature of the skin itself.

Skin is comprised of epidermis and dermis, and has variable properties in different locations throughout the body (Keller & Kuhn 2008). Outermost is the layered epidermis, the stratum corneum, which consists of a lipid-corneocyte matrix traversed by appendages such as sweat ducts and hair follicles (Chizmadzhev et al 1998). The stratum corneum has high resistance to the passage of electric current due to dry keratin layers, however current of sufficient intensity will overcome this resistance. It is believed that therapeutic electric current crosses the skin primarily via two parallel pathways – the lipid-corneocyte matrix of the stratum corneum, and the skin appendages (sweat ducts and hair follicles). This being said, in most clinical applications, NMES current will pass across the skin predominantly via skin appendages, leading to inhomogeneity in the distribution of current density, with the potential to affect stimulation efficiency and patient comfort. Readers are referred to Chizmadzhev et al (1998) for a more detailed discussion of this topic.

The frequency of the electrical pulses determines whether the muscle contraction will be a twitch (i.e. individual contractions at the frequency of the depolarizing current), or tetany (Watanabe et al 2017). Fusion of individual impulses usually occurs somewhere between 5 and 25 Hz. The exact fusion frequency is dependent on the muscle fibre composition, but below the fusion frequency, each electrical pulse will usually cause a separate muscle contraction of every motor unit supplied by the depolarized motor nerve, followed by a relaxation, with the muscle force returning to resting tone. However, at a frequency somewhere between 5 and 25 Hz, depending on the muscle, the muscle fibres will not be able to relax sufficiently between stimulating electrical pulses, and muscle force will not return to resting between electrical pulses. This effect is due to the physical characteristics of actin and myosin filaments sliding over one another. Fast, glycolytic muscle fibre contractions generally last about 40 ms after ES, and slow, oxidative motor units contract for about 100 ms after stimulation. At some point the fibres cannot respond quickly enough and the muscle cannot relax between stimulation. Increasing the frequency further results in a tetanic contraction, or tetany. See Chapter 4 for further details.

When stimulating peripheral nerves via the skin, the amount of current flowing through two different sized neurons will not be equal, but rather will be determined by the diameter of the neuron, with a greater change in voltage occurring for a larger neuron than a smaller one (Blair & Erlanger 1933; Solomonow 1984). This leads to a positive relationship between axonal diameter and conduction velocity (Solomonow 1984) and between axonal diameter and axial resistance, making large diameter axons more easily excited by external electric fields (Enoka 2002; Feiereisen et al 1997; Gersh 1992; Garnett & Stephens 1981; Knaflitz et al 1990). Further details are given in Chapter 4.

Differences Between Physiological Muscle Contractions and Stimulated Muscle Contractions

During a voluntary (physiological) contraction, motor unit recruitment proceeds according to the size principle, from smallest motor units, to largest motor units. This was first described by Henneman (Henneman et al 1965, Henneman, 1957), and has been confirmed by others.

Electrically stimulated (evoked) muscle contractions differ from physiological muscle contractions in four ways: temporal recruitment, spatial recruitment, fibre order recruitment, and metabolic demand. Current best evidence suggests that recruitment of motor units during stimulated contraction, rather than being a true reversal of physiological recruitment order, as was once believed, is non-selective, random, disorderly, spatially fixed and temporally synchronous (Bickel et al 2011; Jubeau et al 2007). The implication is that NMES can activate both fast and slow motor units, even at low stimulation levels, and this may be more related to the location of the nerve with respect to the stimulating electrode than nerve size (Maffiuletti 2010). Stimulated contractions are different from physiological contractions, and surface stimulation engages a different motor unit recruitment pattern than stimulation via a nerve trunk directly, which may explain some of the differences reported in the literature. Further details may be found in Chapter 4.

In order to strengthen muscle most effectively with NMES the force developed by NMES stimulation needs to be maximized. There is a positive correlation between strength gains during voluntary contraction following treatment with NMES and the ES-induced contraction intensity and duration used during the strength training (Maffiuletti 2010; Scott et al 2009; Selkowitz 1985; Stevens-Lapsley et al 2012b).

Torque developed during muscle contraction is dependent on motor unit activity. Torque is proportional to the number of motor units active and the rate of motor unit discharge (Vanderthommen & Duchateau 2007). However, there does seems to be a natural variability in anatomy and physiology, which account for a large proportion of the variability in response to ES of muscle contraction – this is to say that not all factors affecting strength of stimulated muscle contraction will be within the clinician's control (Lieber & Kelly 1991).

Of those factors that are within the clinician's control, the most important related to torque production are: intensity, frequency and pulse duration. It is thought that current amplitude (intensity) increases the force of contraction by stimulating a greater number of motor units, leading to contraction of more muscle fibres. Increasing the frequency of stimulating pulses results in more force by causing summation of the contractions of the same stimulated muscle fibres. An increase in muscle force development has also been observed with an increase in pulse duration, perhaps due to increased stimulation of fast-twitch fibres with longer pulse durations (Gorgey et al 2006).

Torque production will also be dependent to a lesser extent on waveform, electrode size, electrode position, and the superposition of voluntary contraction. These factors are considered in the following paragraphs.

Voluntary Contraction

NMES is less effective than voluntary control for generating a maximum muscle contraction. This is probably due to the limited portion of target muscle fibres that can be activated by NMES within tolerable levels of stimulation (Adams et al 1993; Kramer et al 1984; Vanderthommen & Duchateau 2007). With the caveat that most studies have been carried out using subjects without pathology or muscle weakness, when comparing maximum torque produced by voluntary contraction (MVT) with torque developed by ES, using current at the maximum tolerable intensity, the evoked muscle contraction generally produces torque in the range from 25% to 90% of MVT. While there are scattered reports in the literature of subjects eliciting torque from an evoked contraction that exceeds MVT, these reports are thought to involve isolated individuals, or specific applications that are not clinically applicable (Bellew et al 2014; Vanderthommen & Duchateau 2007).

Waveform

Several studies have examined the contribution of waveform to the generation of force produced by electrically stimulated muscle contraction (Kramer et al 1984; Walmsley et al 1984; Snyder-Mackler et al 1989). When compared with other waveforms, an asymmetric biphasic waveform has been shown to develop more torque, especially in larger muscle groups (Kramer et al 1984). However, it does seem that motor unit activation (consequently torque) is more closely related to the total pulse charge of the waveform than the waveform shape *per se*, with stimulation of larger muscles requiring a greater total pulse charge (Bickel et al 2011).

Duchenne chose a symmetric biphasic waveform, generated by fairly primitive equipment, as he had determined that this was more comfortable, allowing higher intensity current to flow before stimulating nociceptors (Licht 1967). Of course, Duchenne was comparing this waveform not with an asymmetrical biphasic waveform, but with galvanic (i.e. direct) current (Licht 1967). Studies have since examined the effect of waveform on patient comfort during stimulation (Baker et al 1988; Bowman & Baker 1985; Delitto & Rose 1986; Kantor et al 1994; McNeal & Baker 1988). This effect seems to vary according to the muscle groups being stimulated, which may imply that there is a relationship between comfort and total phase charge – larger muscle groups (e.g. the quadriceps) requiring a greater phase charge to develop a strong stimulated contraction, and this being more comfortable when delivered via a symmetric biphasic square wave. For smaller muscles, such as the wrist flexor and extensor muscles, which require less phase charge to cause a strong contraction, an asymmetric, balanced,

biphasic, square wave is both comfortable and clinically effective (Baker et al 1988). In summary, for large muscle groups, requiring higher intensity stimulation, a symmetric biphasic waveform is usually found to be more comfortable, although more torque may be developed by the use of an asymmetric waveform. For smaller muscle groups, waveform seems to be less important with regard to comfort.

Intensity

As expected, a higher intensity of NMES stimulation leads to greater muscle cross-sectional area activation, and greater torque production (Gorgey et al 2006). In fact, Adams and co-authors (1993) were able to propose a formula to predict the activated cross-sectional area of a muscle in relation to the stimulus intensity. Based on the linear relationship between electrically-stimulated torque as a percent of maximum voluntary torque and the activated cross-sectional area of the muscle, the authors calculate that NMES could elicit torque commensurate with maximum voluntary torque when 71.1% of the muscle cross-sectional area is stimulated. Given that most NMES training intensities fall within the range of 40–60% of MVC, the amount of cross-sectional area activated by NMES would only be in the range 29–43% (Maffiuletti 2010).

Pulse Duration

Pulse duration is related to maximum torque developed during the stimulation (Scott et al 2009). Gorgey et al (2006) were able to increase torque by 55%, and increase the amount of muscle activated by 40%, by increasing the pulse duration from 150 μs to 450 μs. Further, shortening the pulse duration from 450 μs to 150 μs not only decreased torque, but decreased the area of activated muscle, and the specific tension developed by the muscle. These authors were able to demonstrate that the highest levels of stimulated torque could be generated only when a long pulse duration was combined with an increased frequency of pulses.

Hultman and co-workers (1983) investigated the effect on muscle tension of pulse durations up to 10 ms. These authors found that stimulated muscle tension increased markedly throughout the range from 200 μs to 1 ms, but that tension then plateaued for pulse durations longer than 1 ms. Pulses in this range (above 200 μsec) allowed for a lower stimulating voltage to be used, and longer pulse durations (greater than 1 ms) were associated with increased discomfort (Hultman et al 1983). Bowman and colleagues (1985) have demonstrated that shorter pulse durations (50 μs) are also uncomfortable. Consequently, it might be expected to see pulse durations in the range of about 200 μs to about 450 μs most commonly used in the clinic.

Frequency of Stimulation

Within limits, the amount of torque developed is correlated with the frequency of stimulation (Dreibati et al 2010; Gorgey et al 2006; Lieber et al 1993; Zhou et al 1987). However, higher frequencies are associated with greater fatigue. Studies reporting effective use of NMES show a range of stimulation frequencies generally between 20 Hz and 100 Hz, with most studies falling in the range 35–50 Hz.

Size of Electrodes

The size of electrodes used for stimulation will determine current density, nociception and, in some cases, effectiveness of the stimulation. Recall that lower current density is more comfortable, however a low current density can also limit the effectiveness of the stimulation. Larger electrodes have been shown to have lower impedance and more evenly distribute the current density across the electrode, generally being more comfortable (Lindemans & Zimmerman 1979).

Alon and co-workers (1994) were able to show, using four different sizes of surface electrodes, that when stimulus intensity was normalized to produce the same amount of muscle force, the comfort of stimulation for the same amount of muscle force improved significantly as electrode size became larger. Further, as electrode size was increased, the ability to discriminate between nerve fibre types improved and it became easier to discriminate between motor threshold and pain threshold. As expected, larger electrodes (20.25 cm² and 40.3 cm² in the study) were not only more comfortable, but were also associated with the development of greater muscle force. However, the effects were not linear. For example, between 2.25 cm² and 9 cm² there was no significant increase in contraction force or pain threshold. However, for 20.25 cm² and 40.3 cm² both pain threshold and generated muscle force were significantly improved. In this study, which focused on stimulation of the gastrocnemius, there was no significant difference between the 20.25-cm² and the 40.3-cm² electrodes. Since the largest electrode required more electrical energy to achieve the clinical results, the 20.25-cm² electrode was recommended as optimum size. However, the authors noted that large electrodes can cause contraction of unwanted muscles near the target muscle, and (especially with battery-operated portable devices) may not deliver sufficient current density to maximize muscle contraction. This is an important point. Small battery-powered NMES devices may not be able to produce sufficient current to effectively depolarize large muscle groups. In this case, it is suggested that a mains-operated NMES device be used.

While electrode size and current density are important, electrode shape seems to be immaterial. Square, round or oval shapes seem to have no effect on the strength of contraction or the stimulation of nociceptors (Forrester & Petrofsky 2004). Lastly, there is evidence to suggest that resistance at the electrode-tissue interface decreases as electrode size increases (Alon et al 1994).

In general, the recommendation is to use large (e.g. 5 × 10 cm) or very large electrodes (e.g. 10 × 10 cm) for large muscle groups, such as the quadriceps femoris, and smaller electrodes (e.g. 5 × 5 cm) for smaller muscles, such as the wrist flexors or extensors. Again, it is a question of finding the balance between an electrode that is so large that it picks up unwanted muscles and an electrode that is so small that the current density required to cause a muscle contraction is high enough to cause discomfort.

Electrical stimulation of muscles, when combined with voluntary contraction, may generate more torque, and hence provide a stronger stimulus for muscle growth (Kramer 1987; Kramer et al 1984). Many authors consider NMES to be more effective when combined in this way (Hainaut & Duchateau 1992; Paillard 2008; Williams et al 1976). While maximum torque during treatment may be increased by superimposing a voluntary contraction onto a stimulated contraction, the evidence that this approach creates additional muscle strengthening beyond what might be achieved by stimulated contraction alone is weak.

Minimizing Fatigue with NMES

NMES stimulation is fatiguing. There are at least three reasons for increased fatigue found with external stimulation of motor contraction: (i) altered motor recruitment – probably not a pure reversal of the Henneman size principle, but rather a non-selective, disorderly recruitment (Gregory & Bickel 2005); (ii) all motor units stimulated by the applied external field depolarize at the same time. This is in contrast to the asynchronous recruitment in a physiological contraction, during which fibres alternately depolarize and rest. Lastly, (iii) ES using surface electrodes recruits only superficial fibres, closest to the electrodes, leaving activation of deeper muscles, or deeper portions of muscles, difficult or impossible. Hence greater fatigue is the result of the inability to alter recruitment patterns of motor units and the inability to modulate firing frequency. NMES recruitment of muscle is superficial, fixed and incomplete (Doucet et al 2012; Maffiuletti 2010, Vanderthommen 2000). Muscle fatigue in response to ES is dependent on both frequency and intensity of stimulation (Binder-Macleod & Snyder-Mackler 1993). Higher frequencies (>50 Hz) are associated with greater fatigue (Bigland-Ritchie et al 1979; Dreibati et al 2010; Jones et al 1979), as are lower frequencies (<30 Hz) (Edwards et al

1977; Garland et al 1988). Edwards et al (1977) showed that frequencies below 25 Hz may induce a prolonged fatigue called 'low-frequency fatigue' that may last several hours.

Fatigue is minimized when the stimulating frequency approximates the physiological rate of motor unit discharge – in the range of 30–40 Hz for many muscles (Fuglevand et al 1992). A study by Zhou and colleagues (1987), involving the gastrocnemius muscle of the cat, showed that a frequency of 40 Hz was associated with the lowest levels of fatigue. Binder-Macleod and Snyder-Mackler (1993) suggest that to minimize fatigue, the parameters be set to use the lowest frequency and the highest intensity that will produce the amount of force required to achieve the therapeutic goals. However, higher frequencies, while more fatiguing, are more comfortable.

CLINICAL EVIDENCE

The therapeutic purpose of NMES will generally be to activate, strengthen or retrain innervated skeletal muscles for the purpose of improving clinical outcomes or to achieve treatment goals more quickly.

A significant body of literature supports the application of NMES in this regard for specific orthopaedic and neurological conditions, as well as in critical illness, some paediatric conditions, some genitourinary muscular disorders, and others.

An overview of this literature is presented below.

Application in Orthopaedic Conditions
Post-Operative Management of ACL Reconstruction

Indications, rationale and literature support. Muscle inhibition is commonly encountered post trauma or surgery. Inhibition of muscle contraction in response to pain, joint effusion and joint trauma, such as ACL injury, leads via presynaptic muscle inhibition to muscle atrophy (Durigan et al 2014), particularly of fast-twitch fibres (Konishi et al 2002). Following ACL injury and surgery, ongoing quadriceps inhibition has been reported to be associated with changes in neuromuscular activation that affect lower body joint mobility and tissue extensibility, leading to compromised joint protection and function (Nyland et al 2016). NMES for muscle strengthening is indicated following ACL reconstruction to augment voluntary contraction and strengthen the quadriceps (Fitzgerald et al 2003; Hasegawa et al 2011; Lepley et al 2015; Rebai et al 2002; Taradaj et al 2013).

A recent review of the literature suggests that the addition of NMES to a rehabilitation programme can improve both strength and function at 6–8 weeks post-operatively but is inconclusive for functional performance at 6 weeks

and self-reported function at 12–16 weeks post-operatively (Nussbaum et al 2017). There is evidence that using NMES in conjunction with an active exercise programme (not simultaneously) has better results than using NMES alone (Kim et al 2010).

Benefits. Benefits that have been shown from the use of NMES post-ACL surgery include: reduced pain, improved muscle strength (both isometric and isokinetic), reduction in loss of muscle volume or thickness, self-reported function, gait parameters, achieving clinical milestones, limb circumference and functional performance (Ediz et al 2012; Fitzgerald et al 2003; Hasegawa et al 2011; Lepley et al 2015; Rebai et al 2002; Taradaj et al 2013).

Parameter recommendations. Goals of treatment have changed since the 1980s, when a prolonged period of immobilization followed ACL repair, and NMES was used primarily to reduce muscle atrophy. Modern rehabilitation protocols usually involve accelerated rehabilitation with shorter periods of immobilization, and NMES is used to re-establish voluntary quadriceps control (Wilk et al 2012). NMES protocols have evolved as well – earlier studies tend to report the use of slightly lower frequencies and somewhat shorter pulse durations than more recent studies, although this is by no means a rule.

Many reported studies have used Burst Mode AC or RC (Russian Current), and so there are not a lot of published NMES studies on which to base recommendations. The only two systematic reviews identified are now almost a decade old. Individual studies do show limitations, and not all parameters are recorded. As well, it is not possible to conduct a blinded study involving electrical muscle stimulation. There are reports of mixed results, but generally NMES is found to be a useful modality to improve strength, improve torque, increase muscle thickness or circumference, and reduce pain. Where reported, there does seem to be more variability in benefit for functional outcomes.

While not standardized in the literature, placement of electrodes is frequently recorded as one of: (1) over the femoral nerve or muscle belly of rectus femoris or vastus intermedius and on motor point or muscle belly of vastus medialis or (2) electrodes as in (1) and also on hamstrings (over muscle bellies of biceps femoris and semitendinosis or semimembranosis). Some studies placed electrodes on vastus lateralis (VL). Note that VL should not be stimulated alone (i.e. without other quadriceps muscles) as this may cause patella subluxation. Generally, the starting position is with the knee flexed to about 65 degrees to facilitate maximum force production.

Where recorded, the NMES waveform is most frequently symmetric or asymmetric biphasic, with a frequency in the range of 30–50 Hz (there are two studies using 20 Hz, and one reporting 200 Hz, with all recording positive effects).

The pulse duration is usually in the range of 250–400 μs. Current amplitude should be to the individual maximum tolerated intensity; at the least, causing a strong but comfortable muscle contraction. On:Off ratios are recorded in the ranges 6–10:12–50 s. It is recommended to use a lower duty cycle (e.g. work–rest 1:3–1:5) if the muscle is weaker, to limit fatigue associated with an electrically induced muscle contraction. Treatment should be initiated early. Many studies report starting treatment on post-operative day one (POD1) certainly within one week post-operatively. Sessions should involve 10–15 contractions, delivered three times per week over a period of 4–6 weeks.

Pre- and Post-Surgical Care After Joint (Hip and Knee) Arthroplasty

Indications, rationale and literature support. End-stage osteoarthritis of either the knee or hip is usually associated with significant muscle weakness, especially of the *quadriceps femoris* (Bade et al 2010). Post-operatively a pronounced failure of activation of the quadriceps muscle, with knee extension force deficits of 30–40%, persists for months to years (Mizner et al 2003). Patients with total joint arthroplasty will usually obtain additional benefit from a rehabilitation programme that includes more than just volitional quadriceps exercise. Including NMES in the post-operative rehabilitation of lower limb joint arthroplasties has been shown to confer additional benefits (Bistolfi et al 2018; Hauger et al 2018; Yue et al 2018).

One study showed that the use of ES for pre-operative quadriceps strengthening prior to total joint arthroplasty resulted in a significant increase (28%) in *quadriceps femoris* muscle strength (pre-habilitation) and significantly greater strength and functional recovery from 6–12 weeks post-total knee arthroplasty (Walls et al 2010).

Studies that applied NMES using low contraction–repetition rates on 3 days/week showed improved strength, muscle activation, and function during follow-up at 6 months (Stevens et al 2004) or 12 months (Petterson et al 2009; Stevens-Lapsley et al 2012a), with some loss to follow-up at the 12 month review.

Benefits. Benefits that have been shown from the use of NMES post-total joint arthroplasty surgery include: improved muscle strength and activation, reduction in loss of muscle volume or thickness, improved self-reported function or disability, improved function, improved walking speed, and perceived health status (Avramidis et al 2011; Levine et al 2013; Petterson 2009; Stevens et al 2004; Stevens-Lapsley 2012a; Walls et al 2010).

Parameter recommendations. The most recent systematic review is nearly a decade old (Monaghan et al 2010). Published randomized controlled trials (RCTs) use a wide range of parameters in the various studies,

and there is always a potential for bias (e.g. no blinding possible). Some studies have used Burst Mode AC. Despite this variability, there is a considerable weight of evidence that electrical muscle stimulation provides benefits for patients who have undergone total joint arthroplasty, and guidelines for appropriate parameters may be given.

Placement of electrodes is usually over the quadriceps, with large electrodes placed proximally and distally on the belly of the muscle/s, typically rectus femoris and vastus medialis. Electrodes should be positioned in line with the orientation of the muscle fibres, and the knee should be flexed to 60 degrees (or more) to maximize extensor muscle function. The waveform, where described, is biphasic pulsed current (both symmetric and asymmetric are reported) with a frequency generally in the range of 35–75 Hz (one study used 10 Hz and was able to show an increase in strength). Pulse duration is usually in the range of 250–400 μs. As usual, current amplitude needs to be the maximum tolerated (the use of large electrodes for increased comfort and to depolarize more motor units is recommended). On:Off ratios of 5–10:8–80 s are reported. Treatment should begin early, ideally on POD1 or POD2. Increased quadriceps activation was shown with sessions of 10–30 contractions/day, 3-7 days/week, for 6 weeks (Petterson et al 2009; Stevens et al 2004; Stevens-Lapsley et al 2012b). When the goal of treatment is to increase function, sessions are reported lasting 1–2 hours/day, 5 days/week, for 6 weeks (Avramidis et al 2011; Gotlin et al 1994).

Degenerative Arthritis and Osteoarthritis

Indications, rationale and literature support. Osteoarthritis (OA) is one of the ten most disabling diseases in developed countries (World Health Organization 2015). Osteoarthritis is associated with muscle weakness (e.g. arthrogenic muscle inhibition described in knee osteoarthritis) (Rice et al 2011). Any possible role of muscle weakness in the aetiology of OA is unclear (Slemenda et al 1997). The benefits of including NMES in a rehabilitation (or prehabilitation) programme have been shown to include strengthening of weak quadriceps muscles, endurance training, minimizing muscle atrophy, and increasing range of movement (ROM).

There is moderate evidence in favour of NMES alone or combined with isometric quadriceps exercises for strengthening; a large RCT (Bruce-Brand et al 2012) showed a significant effect of NMES on functional outcomes.

Benefits. Benefits that have been shown from the use of NMES for muscle strengthening in degenerative arthritis include: increased strength, improved self-reported function, objective functional measures, and reduction in pain (Durmuş et al 2007; Palmieri-Smith et al 2010; Rosemffet et al 2004; Talbot et al 2003).

Parameter recommendations. Published studies are uneven in description of methods, calculation of sample size and reporting of observed power. As well, there is the inherent risk of bias from inability to blind the participants in a study of ES of muscle contraction. A variety of parameters are reported, summarized below. A systematic review reports moderate evidence in favour of NMES alone or combined with exercise for isometric quadriceps muscle strengthening in OA of the knee (de Oliveira Melo et al 2013).

Large electrodes should be placed on the quadriceps proximally on rectus femoris and distally on vastus medialis, vastus lateralis, or both. Patient should be sitting, with hip flexed to 90 degrees, and knee flexed in the range 60–90 degrees to maximize muscle function. A biphasic pulsed current waveform is reported, either symmetrical or asymmetrical in shape. The frequency most often reported is 50 Hz, with pulse duration most often 300 µs. As usual, current intensity should be to the maximum tolerated by the patient. On:Off ratios are from 5:5 – 10:50 s. Treatment volume is often reported from 10–20 contractions per session, with outliers at 60 contractions and 180 contractions. Sessions are commonly delivered on 3–5 days/week for 4–8 weeks.

Patellofemoral Pain Syndrome

Indications, rationale and literature support. One of the main etiologic factors for the development of patellofemoral pain syndrome (PFPS) is believed to be weakness of the quadriceps femoris muscle, particularly the vastus medialis (Brown 2000; Dvir et al 1991) because of its function in patellar alignment during knee flexion (Peng et al 2017). Two recent systematic reviews determined that strengthening exercises for the hip external rotator and abductor muscles and knee extensor muscles were among the interventions with strongest supporting evidence for the management of PFPS (Alba-Martín et al 2015; Barton et al 2015).

Benefits. Benefits that have been shown from the use of NMES in the management of PFPS include: reduction in pain (VAS), increased force-generating capacity (EMG), and deactivation of vastus lateralis (Akarcali et al 2002; Callaghan et al 2001; Callaghan & Oldham 2004; Garcia et al 2010).

Parameter recommendations. The evidence supporting the use of NMES in the management of PFPS is not as strong as in some other orthopaedic conditions. A single older systematic review (evaluating 12 studies; three using NMES) concluded that NMES plus exercise was not more beneficial than exercise alone (Lake & Wofford 2011). However, the studies were reported as being of low to moderate quality. Additionally, there is a question of the effectiveness of the parameters used in the studies (e.g. low frequency, low

intensity, high number of daily contractions) as well as other issues.

Most studies placed electrodes over the quadriceps – over rectus femoris/vastus intermedius muscle bellies, and over vastus medialis. As usual, electrodes should be positioned in line with the orientation of the muscle fibres.

No standard limb position is reported in the literature, and at least one study was carried out in weight-bearing with the knee flexed. It would be advisable to avoid that portion of the range that is provocative of pain. The waveform is usually reported as asymmetric biphasic pulsed current, with a frequency in the range of 35–60 Hz. Pulse duration is generally in the range 200–300 µs. As always, current amplitude should be to individual maximum tolerated intensity. On:Off ratios from 6–10:10–50 s are reported, with shorter off times if endurance is the main goal, and longer off times (30–50 s) if the goal is muscle strengthening. Sessions usually consist of 12–15 contractions, on 3 days/week over 4–6 weeks.

Application in Neurological Conditions
Shoulder Subluxation Following Cerebrovascular Accident

Indications, rationale and literature support. Hemiplegic shoulder pain is a common complication of stroke. In broad terms, the complex pattern of changes found in patients with hemiplegic shoulder pain can be divided into 'flaccid' and 'spastic' presentations. During the flaccid stage, which may last from 24 hours to 12–18 months, the shoulder is prone to inferior subluxation and is vulnerable to soft-tissue damage, especially as a result of impingement of the rotator cuff. Additionally, the weight of the unsupported upper limb may cause traction damage to nerves including the axillary and suprascapular nerves, and the brachial plexus, which may further inhibit normal neuromuscular function (Turner-Stokes et al 2002). During the flaccid presentation, ES may reduce subluxation and enhance return of muscle activity.

During the spastic presentation, shoulder injury may occur as rotation may be impeded by increased tone in the latissimus dorsi, levator scapulae and the rhomboid muscles. Additionally, increased tone in the medial rotators may pull the humerus into internal rotation, increasing the risk of impingement during active and passive glenohumeral abduction (Turner-Stokes et al 2002). In this situation, ES may reduce shoulder girdle muscle imbalance, leading to a more normal glenohumeral alignment at rest and during movement. Nine RCTs investigating NMES in the management of shoulder subluxation post-stroke report significantly reduced glenohumeral displacement after NMES treatment when compared with control (Baker & Parker 1986; Chantraine et al 1999; Faghri et al 1994; Fil et al 2011; Kobayashi et al 1999; Koyuncu et al 2010; Linn et al 1999; Türkkan et al 2017; Wang et al 2000). Reduction in shoulder displacement after NMES treatment in patients following stroke is further supported by three meta-analyses (Ada & Foongchomcheay 2002; Lee et al 2017; Vafadar et al 2015) and three systematic reviews (Van Peppen et al 2004; Veerbeek et al 2014; Viana et al 2012). One large RCT (n=176) compared the addition of NMES or placebo to regular care in patients within 10 days of stroke onset with regard to upper limb function. This study found no difference between groups in arm function 3 months after stroke (Church et al 2006).

While the literature for reduced shoulder subluxation with the use of NMES post-stroke is supportive of this application, the literature concerning the effects of NMES post-stroke on arm function and shoulder pain is contradictory, with some studies showing benefit and others showing no benefit from the application of NMES. This diversity of results may be related to the multifactorial aetiology of shoulder pain post-stroke (orthopaedic versus neurological), or the duration of treatment (e.g. no benefit if less than 6 weeks), or proximity to onset (e.g. poorer outcomes in patient who did not start treatment soon after stroke onset).

Benefits. Benefits that have been shown from the use of NMES for strengthening in shoulder subluxation post stroke include: reduced subluxation on X-ray, increased muscle strength (shoulder abduction and external rotation), increased ROM, increased EMG activity, reduced pain at rest and with shoulder movement with either passive or active ROM, and improved arm function (Chantraine et al 1999; Faghri et al 1994; Fil et al 2011; Kobayashi et al 1999; Koyuncu et al 2010; Wang et al 2000).

Parameter recommendations. For the management of subluxation, electrodes should be placed over the muscle belly of supraspinatus and the posterior deltoid. Fibres of upper trapezius should be avoided, as this will promote excessive shoulder shrug. Applying a second channel to stimulate the long head of biceps can be beneficial in correcting deviations in humeral head alignment. The patient should be seated with the affected arm supported. Where reported, the NMES waveform is usually asymmetric biphasic pulsed current, with a frequency in the range 12–60 Hz, with the lower frequency being sufficient to cause tetany. The pulse duration is reported as between 100 and 350 μs. Intensity must be sufficient to produce a smooth, sustained muscle contraction and reduction of shoulder subluxation. On:Off ratios from 5:5 to 15:15 to 10:30 are reported. A longer ramp-up and down time may be required for patient comfort. Treatments tend to be long – 30 minutes three

to four times per day, or longer (up to 150 minutes per day in multiple sessions), mostly 5 days per week (some studies use 7 days per week). Treatment should be initiated as soon as shoulder flaccidity occurs and before pain has manifested, and should be applied in conjunction with other standard rehabilitation care. It is recommended that arm support be provided at the conclusion of NMES treatment to prevent further stretching of joint structures.

Loss of Hand and Upper Extremity (UE) Function

Indications, rationale and literature support. Distal from the shoulder, elbow flexion, forearm pronation and finger flexion are the most common patterns encountered in patients with hypertonicity following stroke (Marciniak et al 2011). Evidence suggests stimulation of the elbow and wrist extensors using NMES reduces spasticity and enhances muscle strength in the hemiparetic limb (Dimitrijevic and Soroker, 1994, Dimitrijevic et al 1996, Kraft, Fitts & Hammond, 1992). Evidence supports the use of NMES to improve upper limb function post-stroke by improving grip and wrist extensor strength (Powell et al 1999; Rosewilliam et al 2012), and increasing active ROM of the wrist (Heckmann et al 1997).

Benefits. Benefits that have been shown from the use of NMES for wrist and finger extension include: increased muscle recruitment, increased wrist and finger extension, increased grip strength, increased wrist ROM, reduced flexor spasticity and increased reach, increased cortical activation and improved function (Barker et al 2008; Lin & Yan 2011; Powell et al 1999; Rosewilliam et al 2012).

Parameter recommendations. The literature is generally supportive of the use of NMES (or EMG-NMES) to improve UE function following stroke. Electrodes are most commonly positioned on the wrist extensors, ensuring minimal radial or ulnar deviation during extension. The patient is usually seated, with elbow flexed to about 90 degrees and the forearm pronated. Where reported, the NMES waveform is biphasic pulsed current (symmetry usually not recorded), with frequency in the range 25–100 Hz, with most studies in the 30–50 Hz range. Pulse duration is mostly reported in the range of 200–300 μs. As usual, current amplitude should be to individual maximum tolerated intensity. On:Off ratios range from 1:1 to 1:5, with contractions in the range 5–15 s. Longer off periods will reduce muscle fatigue. Treatment sessions are usually of longer duration – ranging from 30–60 minutes per day, sometimes in divided sessions, with treatment occurring most commonly on 3–5 days per week.

Gait Impairments Resulting from Foot Drop and Impaired Control of Leg Muscles

Indications, rationale and literature support. The development of foot-drop (i.e. the decreased ability to dorsiflex the ankle during gait) frequently occurs in individuals following stroke. This gait impairment may result in compensatory movement patterns, a higher physiological cost of walking, slower walking speed and increased risk of stumbling and falls (Kluding et al 2013). The application of NMES to improve muscle strength of weakened ankle dorsiflexor muscles may reduce foot drop and decrease plantar muscle spasticity, leading to improvement in gait and reduced risk of falls.

Benefits. Benefits that have been shown from the use of NMES for footdrop and impaired control of leg muscles following stroke include: increase in muscle strength, increase in ankle dorsiflexion, increased EMG activity, decrease in ankle plantar flexor (gastrocnemius) spasticity, increase in gait speed, improved lower extremity function, improvement in gait kinematics and improved balance (Bogataj et al 1995; Burridge et al 1997; Chung et al 2014; Lin & Yan 2011; Merletti et al 1978; Sabut et al 2011).

Parameter recommendations. The literature is generally supportive of the use of NMES post stroke to improve functional gait, however there is little evidence supporting the benefits of electrical stimulation as greater than those obtained by using an ankle-foot orthosis (AFO) (although patients seem to prefer electrical stimulation to AFO) (Howlett et al 2015; Kafri & Läufer 2015). Where conflicting results have been reported, these might be explained by the heterogenous patient populations in the RCTs included in systematic reviews and meta-analyses, and the wide range of NMES protocols in use. Simple protocols seem to provide as much benefit as more sophisticated, multi-channel, computer-controlled devices.

In general, electrodes will be placed over the common peroneal nerve and over the motor point of tibialis anterior or both tibialis anterior and the peronei. An additional channel might be considered for gluteus medius stimulation. Stimulation is usually functional, so used for dorsiflexion during gait re-education. The waveform is frequently not described in studies, but expect symmetric or asymmetric biphasic pulsed current, with a frequency in the range of 30–50 Hz (some outliers use 80 or 100 Hz). Pulse duration is in the range 280–400 μs. Current amplitude should be to individual maximum tolerated. The On:Off ratio will depend on treatment protocol. During gait re-education, this will be controlled by a foot switch. For strengthening, ratios vary between 4–10:6–30 s. Treatment schedule is most often reported as 30 minutes/day on 3–5 days per week for 4–12 weeks.

Spinal Cord Injury

Indications, rationale and literature support. NMES has been used in rehabilitation for persons with spinal cord injury (SCI) for five therapeutic goals – increasing strength or reducing atrophy, reducing spasticity, increasing muscle endurance, improving cardiovascular health, and improving glucose metabolism and insulin sensitivity.

(a) Increasing muscle strength or reducing atrophy

Studies have shown benefit in increasing muscle strength or reducing muscle atrophy in persons with SCI, especially when using functional electrical stimulation (FES) cycling, or FES rowing (Bélanger 2000; Gibbons et al 2016; Sadowsky et al 2013; Wattchow et al 2018). A recent systematic review, including 10 studies using ES, concluded that there is consistent evidence of positive effects of early ES-assisted exercise on muscle hypertrophy in patients with spinal cord injury (Panisset et al 2016).

(b) Reducing spasticity

Spasticity is commonly found in individuals following SCI. Some estimates put the incidence as high as 65% (Sköld et al 1999). Spasticity may be managed pharmacologically or surgically or via non-pharmacological means, such as serial casting or botulinum toxin. Each of these approaches may have adverse effects. Electrical stimulation using surface electrodes has the potential to manage spasticity in a less invasive manner and with fewer side effects, with both TENS and electrical muscle stimulation having been shown to reduce spasticity. TENS is thought to reduce spasticity by modulating spinal inhibitory circuits and/or activating large diameter afferents, stimulation of plasticity of the CNS, unmasking or reorganization of somatosensory-motor cortical connections or some combination of these (Mills 2016; Sivaramakrishnan et al 2018). Electrical stimulation of spastic muscles is thought to reduce the excitability of motoneurons either by depressing the activity of propriospinal interneurons or promoting long-term changes in the synaptic connections of dorsal horn primary afferents; while stimulation of the antagonists to spastic muscles is thought to reduce spasticity by activating the Ia-reciprocal inhibition pathway, which ultimately leads to reduced motoneural excitability (Elbasiouny et al 2010).

(c) Increasing muscle endurance

Stimulation to increase muscle endurance generally requires a long duration of treatment – from 1 to 2 hours per day (Stein et al 2002). Erickson and co-workers (2017) published a trial involving 14 individuals with spinal cord injury who underwent 16 weeks of home-based electrically stimulated endurance training of knee extensor muscles. Stimulation parameters increased over the training period, based on the onset of muscle fatigue and evolved from 2 to 7 Hz, 10 mins to 75 mins, 3 to 5 sessions/week, for 16 weeks. Contractions increased from 1200/training session (i.e. 2400/week) to 31,500/training session and 157,000 per week. Skeletal muscle oxidative capacity increased significantly on average, but with a wide range from -14% to +387%.

An earlier case study published by Ryan and co-workers (2013) and involving a similar protocol, over 24 weeks, documented a three-fold increase in muscle oxidative capacity, measured by the increase in the rate of recovery of muscle oxygen consumption.

(d) Improving cardiovascular health

Three recent reviews cite evidence for improvement of cardiovascular health as a result of FES stimulation in patients with SCI (Davis et al 2008; Deley et al 2015; Dolbow 2016). While the cardiovascular benefits accrued are not to the same level as able-bodied exercisers, nonetheless, there is the opportunity for significant changes associated with an improved quality of life (Deley et al 2015; Hettinga & Andrews 2008). It is expected that the intensity and volume of exercise required in individuals with SCI to significantly lower the relative risk of chronic heart disease and to significantly improve the blood lipid profile will be similar to that required in able-bodied individuals (Andrews et al 2017).

(e) Improving glucose metabolism and insulin sensitivity

A recent review of the literature found that most studies report improvement in glucose metabolism, with the enhancement of insulin sensitivity being the major factor, following ES training of limbs in individuals with SCI (Gorgey et al 2015). Frequency of training ranged from 2 to 5 days/week. Most studies reported significant increases in muscle size, but without a significant reduction in adipose tissue. Muscle loading sufficient to evoke hypertrophy is thought to be a key component in ES-based training following SCI. However, the overall effects on lean muscle mass were modest, not exceeding 10%.

Application in Critical Illness
Critical Illness and Advanced Disease States

Indications, rationale and literature support. During critical illness skeletal muscle breaks down as inflammation reduces protein synthesis, and increases protein breakdown, despite enteral nutrition (Puthucheary et al 2013). In chronic lung disease, lung-derived inflammatory mediators (e.g. tumour necrosis factor) are associated with the muscle wasting seen in these conditions (Puthucheary

et al 2013). In mechanically ventilated patients, respiratory muscle weakness is correlated with limb muscle weakness and is associated with delayed extubation (De Jonghe et al 2007). Survivors of critical illness suffer long-term exercise limitation and concomitant reduction in physical quality of life (Herridge et al 2011; Iwashyna et al 2010). NMES has been shown to preserve muscle strength and muscle mass during critical illness and advanced disease states by reducing the rate of muscle degradation. Maintenance of limb muscle strength and mass may facilitate weaning from mechanical ventilation (Falavigna et al 2014; Maffiuletti et al 2013).

Benefits. Benefits from the use of NMES in patients with critical illness or advanced disease states have been established, and include decreased muscle protein degradation, increased thigh circumference and cross-sectional area, increased strength of lower extremity muscles and exercise capacity, prevention of muscle atrophy, increased levels of function, improved cardiopulmonary function and breathlessness, earlier weaning from ventilation, decreased intensive care unit (ICU) length of stay, and improved quality of life. Safety and feasibility have been demonstrated (Abdellaoui et al 2011; Bouletreau et al 1987; Chaplin et al 2013; Dirks et al 2015; Gruther et al 2010; Meesen et al 2010; Rodriguez et al 2012; Routsi et al 2010; Segers et al 2014; Sillen et al 2014; Vivodtzev et al 2012; Zanotti et al 2003).

Parameter recommendations. A recent review of 27 individual studies showed only three studies demonstrating no benefit in this patient population. Of the studies showing no benefit, two used an untreated limb as control, potentially leading to confounding, since there is a well-documented cross-transfer effect from NMES application to the non-treated limb (Nussbaum et al 2017).

Treatment usually involves lower extremity muscle groups bilaterally, most often quadriceps, but frequently also hamstrings and calf muscles. Studies report ICU patients usually in supine with the knee/s supported in 30–40 degrees flexion; chronic heart failure (CHF) patients sitting with knee flexion to 90 degrees; and with chronic obstructive pulmonary disease (COPD) patients sitting with knee flexion to 65–90 degrees. Waveform, where reported, is most frequently biphasic – symmetric or asymmetric, with a frequency most often reported at 50 Hz. Pulse duration is usually between 350–400 µs. Work–rest cycle depends on patient population: COPD patients, - On:Off 6–8:12–24 s (1:2 or 1:3 ratio; shorter ON times paired with shorter OFF times); ICU and CHF patients - On:Off 2–5:4–10 s (1:1 or 1:2 ratio; shorter ON times paired with shorter OFF times). Patients are usually treated daily (5/week) for between 4 and 10 weeks (ICU patients daily until extubation), with treatments lasting from 30–60 minutes (may be divided among muscle groups). As usual, current amplitude should be to individual maximum tolerated intensity (note: this may be difficult to determine in an ICU patient, and in ICU applications, muscle contraction is not always evident).

Application in the Genitourinary System
Urinary Incontinence

Indications, rationale and literature support. The use of NMES in the management of urinary incontinence is dependent on the type of incontinence diagnosed – stress incontinence, urge incontinence, detrusor instability or mixed incontinence. NMES may be used to induce hypertrophy of the striated muscles of the pelvic floor via tetanic contractions, or cause abolition of phasic detrusor contractions, or some combination of effects. Electrical stimulation may result recruitment of faster motor units and modification of the expression of myosin isoforms leading to conversion to type I muscle, which cannot be achieved by voluntary muscle contractions (Brubaker 2000). Additionally, the stimulation is able to activate the detrusor inhibitory reflex arc, as well as increase circulation to the muscles. The technique is variably described as being between 30% and 80% effective (Chêne et al 2013; Faiena et al 2015; Ghaderi et al 2014). The goals of treatment are to improve strength of the pelvic floor muscles (if strength grade 2/5), to promote sensory awareness due to sensory impairment, and to reduce pain (Ghaderi et al 2014).

The efficacy of ES in stress incontinence caused by pelvic floor insufficiency is similar to that of pelvic floor exercises, with up to 75% of patients referred for surgery for their stress incontinence becoming so improved by either intervention that surgery becomes unnecessary (Fall & Lindstrom 1994).

Treatment parameters vary depending on the type of incontinence diagnosed. Stress incontinence requires higher stimulation frequencies, generally in the range of 20–50 Hz. Urge incontinence treatment involves lower stimulation frequency ~10 Hz, causing the abolition of phasic detrusor contractions and an increase in bladder volume during stimulation (Fall & Lindstrom 1994). Mixed incontinence is usually treated at a recommended 10–20 Hz, if stress incontinence dominates, whereas if urge incontinence dominates, a slightly lower 10 Hz–12.5 Hz has been recommended.

Parameter recommendations. Electrode placement is generally intravaginal (anal for males post radical prostatectomy). Some studies use four surface electrodes (2 × suprapubic; 2 × medial to ischial tuberosity). Waveform is biphasic pulsed current with a frequency mostly in the range 20–100 Hz for stress incontinence and 10–12.5 Hz for urge incontinence. Pulse duration is quite variable 100–700 µs (a few studies up to 2 ms). On:Off ratio is generally 1:2 (e.g. 2:4 s; 4:8 s; 6:12 s). Treatment sessions usually last between 15–30 mins, on 2–3 days/week (some studies 1–2/days) for 6–12 weeks. Current intensity should be to a tolerable level (i.e. not maximum tolerated as for most strengthening applications) (Faiena et al 2015; Ghaderi et al 2014; Mariotti et al 2015; Moroni et al 2016; Richmond et al 2016; Stewart et al 2016, 2017; Wyndaele 2016).

Other Applications

Electrical muscle stimulation has also been used with beneficial effect in the management of patients with multiple sclerosis (Campbell et al 2016; Edwards & Pilutti 2017; Hammond et al 2015), in children with spastic cerebral palsy (Bosques et al 2016; Rose et al 2017; Yıldızgören et al 2014), in motor neuron disease and Parkinson's disease, among others.

NMES and the Central Nervous System

Strong sensory input from both the skin and muscle tissue in response to NMES has been shown to result in increased cortical activity in defined regions (Smith et al 2003), and (using specific parameters) recruitment of spinal motoneurons as a result of the evoked sensory volley (Collins 2007). Some authors have suggested that it is NMES-induced adaptations in the CNS that might explain observed strength gains in a time frame too short to be explained by muscle hypertrophy alone (Hortobágyi & Maffiuletti 2011; Vanderthommen & Duchateau 2007).

Application to Healthy Muscle

In healthy subjects, the use of NMES as part of a rigorous training programme may improve muscle function (Maffiuletti 2006). Generally, electrically stimulated contractions should be used in conjunction with voluntary contraction to achieve the best outcomes (Gondin et al 2011). However, it is worth noting that ES of muscle can cause damage similar to that seen in voluntary eccentric contractions. Damage from 40 or 50 electrically-stimulated isometric contractions leads to increased circulating levels of creatine kinase, a reduction in maximum voluntary contraction strength, and delayed-onset muscle soreness (Nosaka et al 2011). However, muscle damage may be avoided by modifying the NMES protocol to reduce the training volume.

Electrical Stimulation of Denervated Muscle

Indications, rationale and literature support. Denervation of muscles leads to loss of voluntary and reflex activity, muscle atrophy and changes in muscle excitability. Denervated muscles have some plasticity in regard to fibre-type, in that ES can alter muscle fibre type – from fast twitch to slow twitch. However, factors other than stimulation (muscle loading, circulating hormones, or blood flow) also affect denervated muscle. Consequently, denervation atrophy may not be prevented completely by ES (Eberstein & Eberstein 1996). In order to cause depolarization of muscle sarcolemma directly, a pulse of long duration is required. Rushton (1932) determined that pulses of 100 ms in duration were required. This means that special equipment will be needed, and this application is not really NMES *per se*.

Studies carried out in humans are sparsely reported in the literature. In general, stimulation at sufficient frequency and intensity to cause tetanic contraction, when applied frequently enough (up to 5 days per week), and for a sufficiently long time (5 to 18 months), has been shown to reduce (although not necessarily reverse) muscle atrophy, and preserve the normal properties of denervated muscle (Eberstein & Eberstein 1996; Kern et al 2004, 2005, 2010; Mödlin et al 2005). While some authors claim that ES of denervated muscle might interfere with collateral axon sprouting (Love et al 2003; Merletti & Pinelli 1980; Tam & Gordon 2003), others have found that reinnervation is unaffected, or may even proceed more quickly with the use of ES (Gordon et al 2010; Haastert-Talini et al 2011; Huang et al 2013; Kern et al 2005).

Rectangular or triangular pulses have been reported, but Pieber recommends a triangular waveform to reduce stimulation of innervated muscle nearby, and to reduce stimulation of sensory fibres (Pieber et al 2015). Pulse duration should be set to a minimum of 100 ms, Frequency is low, at least initially at 2 Hz. Current intensity needs to be high – taking care that the skin is not compromised by this (Kern et al 2005, 2010; Mödlin et al 2005). Dow and co-workers (2004) investigated the number of contractions required to maintain muscle mass and force in a denervated rat muscle. To maintain mass and fibre cross-sectional area required not fewer than 50 contractions per day, whereas to maintain force generated required between 200 and 800 contractions per day.

While ES of denervated muscle was historically the norm, and there is some evidence that a sufficient volume of stimulation (duration of treatment, number of treatments) may reduce muscle atrophy, there is also a suggestion of negative outcomes – interference with axon regeneration. On balance, it seems the published evidence of benefit cannot be said to outweigh the potential for negative outcomes at this stage.

THERAPEUTIC USES

In general, the therapeutic effects of NMES may include muscle strengthening, producing muscle twitch, increasing endurance, reducing spasticity, preventing loss of muscle mass from disuse, increasing joint ROM, preventing joint adhesions through ROM, and accelerating post-exercise performance recovery.

Muscle Strengthening

The use of ES to increase the load on skeletal muscle may stimulate an adaptive response within the muscle, causing muscle trophic changes (Gobbo et al 2011). NMES has been shown to stimulate muscle protein synthesis (Wall et al 2012) and, following disuse atrophy, to stimulate the recovery of muscle mass and function following disuse/immobilization (Snyder-Mackler et al 1994, 1995; Vanderthommen & Duchateau 2007)

In healthy subjects, the use of NMES in a rigorous training programme may improve muscle function (Maffiuletti 2006).

Muscle Twitch – Oedema Control

The muscle pumping effects of NMES – either as repeated tetanic contractions, or muscle twitch-like contractions (low frequency contractions, usually less than 10 Hz)– may be useful in the management of traumatic oedema. NMES has been shown in animal studies to increase the flow of lymphatic fluid out of the region being stimulated, and changes in venous blood flow have been observed following NMES stimulation. Stimulation of muscle by NMES increases microvascular perfusion of the muscle, and this effect may help to shift blood flow away from the site of injury and so facilitate reduction of oedema (Lake 1992). Intensity of stimulation needs to be sufficient to cause visible muscle contraction, but not so strong that the muscle contraction may impede lymphatic draining or blood flow.

Much of the work related to oedema control via ES uses the negative electrode of High Voltage Pulsed Current. See Chapter 4 for further details.

Muscle Endurance

NMES may be used to increase muscle endurance. Typical applications involve the use of short OFF times (Nussbaum et al 2017) and lower frequency stimulation (25 Hz) (Rosemffet et al 2004), or higher frequency stimulation (above 50 Hz) (Sillen et al 2014; Erickson et al 2017), and a high number of repetitions. Some authors advocate the use of twitch contractions without summation (e.g. 2–7 Hz) (Erickson et al 2017).

Spasticity Reduction

NMES may be used to reduce muscle spasticity. Two modes of action are commonly seen – fatiguing spastic muscles and strengthening antagonist muscles (Yıldızgören et al 2014).

Typical parameters involve short rest periods to fatigue the spastic agonist. If strengthening antagonists is the goal, parameters will be the same as those used for muscle strengthening.

Preservation of Muscle Mass During Prolonged Periods of Disuse/Immobilization

NMES use during periods of immobilization has been shown to reduce muscle atrophy and to decrease the reduction in muscle protein synthesis that usually occurs as a result of immobilization (Gibson et al 1988).

Increasing Joint ROM

Electrical stimulation of muscle contraction may be used to move a join through its range of motion where voluntary contraction is not possible. Such a movement would facilitate the mild joint compression that occurs with voluntary contraction of muscles to move joints through range – with all the attendant benefits to the joint articular cartilage, capsule and afferent nerve inputs.

Providing Active Movement to Prevent Adhesion

Emulating active movement of a joint by using stimulated muscle contractions may help prevent joint adhesions, in much the same way as passive ROM has been shown to do.

Post-Exercise Performance Recovery

NMES has been used as a recovery modality, using low stimulation frequencies, causing contractions of short duration and low intensity. There is evidence of some beneficial effects on lactate removal and creatine kinase activity. However, there is a paucity of evidence regarding the recovery of performance indicators, such as muscle strength (Babault et al 2011).

APPLICATION

Most frequently, the goal of treatment with electrical muscle stimulation will be to maximize muscle strength training. In this case, the aim of each application is to develop the greatest amount of torque with the least amount of nociceptive stimulation.

Current Frequency

Most applications for muscle strengthening use a frequency in the range 35–50 Hz (many studies use a lower frequency [down to 20 Hz] for endurance training, and a higher frequency – up to 100 Hz – when producing muscle fatigue is the therapeutic goal). The lower end of the range needs to be sufficient to cause tetany, which will depend on the individual properties of the muscle being stimulated. For other applications that do not require a tetanic response, frequencies in the range of 2–10 Hz are most commonly seen. However, it is well to remember that frequency is also important in terms of fatigue (see section on Minimizing Fatigue with NMES). The frequency of stimulation also has a bearing on patient comfort, with higher frequencies being perceived as more comfortable (Kramer et al 1984).

Current Intensity

In order to be most effective for muscle strengthening, NMES requires the intensity of stimulation to be at the maximum tolerable level. It is suggested that the therapist, or properly instructed patient, increase the intensity progressively throughout treatment to (i) depolarize muscle fibres at a greater distance from the electrodes and (ii) overcome fatigue in the superficial muscle fibres (Maffiuletti 2010, Vanderthommen 2000).

Current Density

Current density is responsible for stimulation of nociceptors. (Sha et al 1996) The maximum tolerable current density is in the range of 0.5 mA/cm^2 (see Prausnitz 1996 for further details), although some authors assert that this density is the maximum that should be delivered under the cathode, and that under the anode a current density of 1.0 mA/cm^2 is the limit that can be tolerated (Bélanger 2010). Current density is higher at the edges of electrodes. (Patriciu et al 2005).

Current density can be calculated based on the area of electrical contact with the skin – the area covered by electrode gel, or other conductor. However, it is well to be mindful that current density varies under electrodes, as discussed previously.

The presence of metal close to the skin surface may also affect local current density and this situation should be treated with caution (see contraindications and precautions in Chapter 22).

Pulse Duration

Most studies report pulse durations in the range of 100–400 µs; both longer and shorter pulses are said to be less comfortable (Benton et al 1981; Dreibati et al 2010). Pulses of duration longer than about 60 µs are more likely to stimulate pain fibres along with sensory and motor nerve fibres, as the separation of the strength-duration curves of each fibre type starts to decrease (Lake 1992).

Duration of Contraction

Bigland-Ritchie and co-workers (1979) evaluated muscle fatigue when stimulating at different frequencies and discovered that at 20 Hz the muscle remained free of fatigue for 30 s, but at higher frequencies, fatigue started to manifest more rapidly, so that at 50 Hz, fatigue became evident after 20 s of contraction and at 80 Hz, fatigue was evident after only 10 s of contraction. Hence the rate of fatigue is dependent on the frequency of the stimulation – the higher the frequency, the shorter the duration of contraction that will be possible before muscle fatigue is evident. For strengthening, the minimum reported duration of tetanic contraction seems to be 5 s, with many authors using contraction durations of between 5 and 20 s.

On:Off Ratio

The On:Off ratio is adjusted to allow muscle recovery between contractions. Weaker muscles require more rest between contractions, hence longer off periods. Consequently, determination of muscle strength is important in determining the On:Off ratio. Matheson and co-workers (1997) compared two On:Off ratios, 1:1 and 1:5, and found the shorter duty cycle produced more fatigue during stimulation, possibly due to increased intracellular acidosis and reduced availability of high-energy phosphate phosphocreatine. For weak muscles – Grades 1 and 2, an On:Off ratio of 1:5 is recommended. Some practitioners suggest that as the muscle gets stronger, the ratio may be reduced so that a Grade 3 muscle might be treated with a ratio of 1:3 or 1:2, progressing to 1:1 as the muscle strength increases.

Ramp – Amplitude Modulation

The ramp up allows the intensity of the stimulation to reach maximum over the period of the ramp – usually between 0.5 and 2 s. The purpose of the ramp is to make the application more comfortable. Suddenly increasing intensity from zero to maximum tolerated as the device switches from 'Off time' to 'On time' could be uncomfortable. Having the intensity ramp up can alleviate this discomfort.

Similarly, the ramp down allows the intensity to decrease over a short period of time, instead of just dropping off immediately. Again, this is for comfort. The down ramp is usually set automatically as a proportion of the up ramp (often 50%).

Duration of Application

NMES is fatiguing, therefore most treatments for strengthening atrophied muscle will be limited to between 12 and 15 contractions. If the treatment goal is to increase muscle endurance, then more contractions will be required, as will be the case if muscle fatigue is the goal, as in managing spasticity.

Electrode Size

Larger electrodes will be more comfortable (generally), due to lower current density and lower resistance at the electrode–skin interface. However, the size of area being treated is important, since electrodes that are too large may cause unwanted effects, such as the stimulation of muscles outside the therapeutic target. Two different sized electrodes used in one application will have different current densities – with the greater density at the smaller electrode. This greater current density may cause a stronger sensation, however small electrodes may be better at targeting specific motor nerves.

Electrode Placement

Marked differences in torque production in response to ES have been shown in relation to electrode placement. Electrodes positioned longitudinally along a muscle belly, close to either end, will stimulate more muscle fibres, and hence lead to the development of more torque, than electrodes positioned close together (Vieira et al 2016). Additionally, stimulation via the motoneuron supplying the muscle in question is more effective than stimulating either end of the muscle belly as a means to induce muscle contraction, meaning it may be more comfortable if the muscle is stimulated via the motor nerve and motor point (see later in this chapter) (Botter et al 2011; Forrester 2004; Gobbo et al 2011; Knaflitz et al 1990).

Electrode Types

Electrodes used for muscle stimulation will usually be carbon-impregnated silicon rubber, or self-adhesive carbon impregnated silicon rubber, although in some instances, flexible metal electrodes may be used (see Chapter 4, Fig. 4.20 and 4.22).

Carbon-Impregnated Silicone Rubber

This type of electrode is commonly encountered. Impedance has been shown to be fairly even across these electrodes, leading to fairly uniform current distribution under the electrodes, provided the electrodes are not worn (Petrofsky et al 2006). Reusable carbon rubber electrodes have been shown to be the most effective for torque production (Lieber & Kelly 1991). They require conductive gel or wet sponge coupling and require strapping in place. These electrodes should not be rubbed during cleaning, as this can damage the conducting surface.

Carbon-Impregnated Silicone Rubber with Self-Adhesive Conductive Layer

The conductive layer could be, for example, hydrogel, a synthetic electrolyte. These electrodes may appear as fabric or mesh bonded to the outside, with a thin layer of conductive carbon between the fabric and the adhesive. Previous work with self-adhesive electrodes has shown them to require more stimulation to produce the same degree of muscle contraction. Petrofsky et al (2006) tested self-adhesive electrodes and observed uneven current distribution across the electrode surface; current density was highest in the centre of the electrode, resulting in a different pattern of muscle stimulation. Self-adhesive electrodes are the simplest and quickest to apply as they do not require tape or strapping. However, they are a more expensive option. In addition, self-adhesive electrodes have a limited shelf life: as they sit in storage, the gel tends to dry out and this will affect conductivity, and consequently current density, as well as adhesion.

Metal Foil

Lastly, metal foil electrodes are still available. These are usually an alloy of lead, tin and zinc. Metal foil electrodes are cheap and reusable. They require the use of wet sponge pockets or pads (0.5–1 cm thick) to make contact with the skin, and need to be strapped in place.

Electrode Resistance

Nolan (1991) undertook a study to measure impedance of 25 different commercially available electrodes of the carbon-impregnated silicon rubber and self-adhesive types. The author found variability up to 7.8-fold, indicating that electrodes differ greatly in impedance.

Beyond these differences due to manufacturing (or perhaps storage conditions or duration), it is recommended that carbon rubber electrodes in use be tested yearly, at a minimum, to ensure that conductivity is adequate to permit effective and safe application of ES. Using an ohm meter, test each electrode by placing one probe at one point on the electrode and the second probe at a point about 1 cm away from the first. You should test at least three different places on each electrode. If the resistance reads greater than 500 ohms between any two points, the electrode should be discarded and replaced.

Electrode Position

The inter-electrode distance will affect the depth and density of current flow between electrodes. Electrodes positioned closer together cause the current to pass more superficially in the tissues, with increased current density. Electrodes positioned further apart cause the current to pass more deeply in the tissues (Forrester 2004). Vieira and colleagues (2016) investigated the effect on torque of four different electrode positions on the quadriceps muscle – from close together to further apart – and noted that the greatest knee torque was generated when stimulation electrodes were positioned further apart. Brooks and colleagues (1990) studied the effect of electrode position perpendicular to the direction of muscle fibres versus

parallel. Electrodes positioned along the muscle belly, that is, parallel to the direction of muscle fibres, generated 64% more torque than electrodes positioned transversely (see Chapter 4, Fig. 4.20 and 4.22).

Three potential applications are described for stimulating *innervated* muscle:

(i) The most effective stimulation (greatest torque for least current applied) is achieved by ensuring the nerve supplying the muscle is in the path of the electric current. To do this, electrodes are placed over the nerve trunk (nerve supplying the muscle in question) and over the motor point of the muscle to be stimulated (e.g. one electrode positioned over the radial nerve as it crosses the humerus in the radial groove, and the second electrode on the motor point of the extensor carpi radialis longus). See the following discussion of motor points.

(ii) If the nerve trunk is inaccessible, the next most effective electrode placement is over the motor point and somewhere more distal on the belly of the muscle to be stimulated.

(iii) Lastly, if the motor point–muscle belly placement cannot be achieved, position the electrodes at either end of the belly of the muscle to be stimulated.

Motor Point

The motor point is defined as the skin area showing the lowest motor threshold for a given electrical current intensity (Botter et al 2011; Gobbo et al 2011). In the past, it was thought that the motor point corresponds to a point at the entry of a peripheral nerve into a muscle. However, recent work has shown that this is not always anatomically correct (Franz et al 2018). The approximate location of motor points is given in charts shown in Figs 16.1 to 16.10 and may also be estimated as being located near the junction of the proximal third and the distal two-thirds of the muscle belly (Botter et al 2011). However, because of anatomical variability, the exact location should be determined for each application, using one of the following techniques described. The skin over the motor point has reduced impedance, allowing current to transverse more readily, requiring less current to achieve a muscle contraction (Forrester 2004; Robinson & Snyder-Mackler 1995).

Current applied at motor points affects the greatest number of motor nerve fibres using the lowest current intensity, leading to a muscle contraction with correspondingly greater patient comfort. Gobbo et al (2011), using a biphasic square wave of 100 µs duration, determined that stimulation with the cathode over the motor point was the most comfortable and allowed development of the most torque. Clinicians should be prepared to move the position of the electrodes after initial set-up to (a) increase comfort and (b) maximize the amount of torque generated.

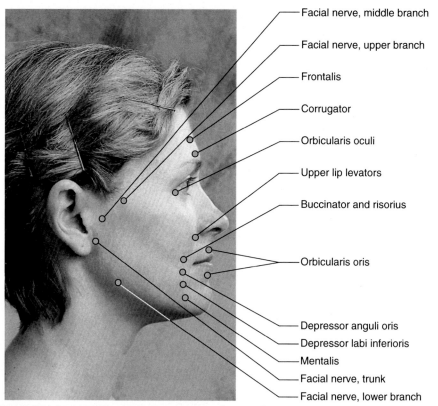

Facial nerve, middle branch

Facial nerve, upper branch

Frontalis

Corrugator

Orbicularis oculi

Upper lip levators

Buccinator and risorius

Orbicularis oris

Depressor anguli oris

Depressor labi inferioris

Mentalis

Facial nerve, trunk

Facial nerve, lower branch

Fig. 16.1 Approximate position of the motor points of some of the muscles supplied by the facial nerve.

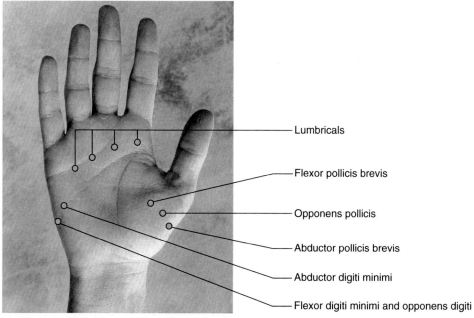

Lumbricals

Flexor pollicis brevis

Opponens pollicis

Abductor pollicis brevis

Abductor digiti minimi

Flexor digiti minimi and opponens digiti

Fig. 16.2 Approximate positions of some of the motor points on the anterior aspect of the hand.

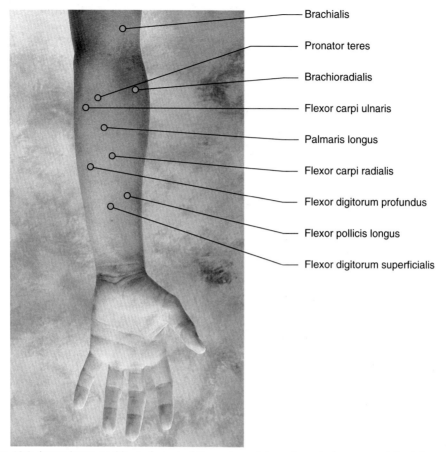

Brachialis

Pronator teres

Brachioradialis

Flexor carpi ulnaris

Palmaris longus

Flexor carpi radialis

Flexor digitorum profundus

Flexor pollicis longus

Flexor digitorum superficialis

Fig. 16.3 Approximate positions of some of the motor points on the anterior aspect of the right arm.

Locating the motor point: using a point localizer or 'surfing'. Motor points can be located by moving an impedance probe over the muscle. Many mains-power-operated muscle stimulators have the option of an impedance probe, or these may be purchased separately as small, battery-operated portable devices. The point where the motor point enters the muscle can be easily located as the point that is associated with the lowest skin impedance.

This technique can also be accomplished by using the therapist's hand in circuit with the patient, as follows. Attach the indifferent electrode to the patient as you would for the treatment application (i.e. over the nerve trunk or the muscle belly of the muscle to be stimulated). Take the active electrode, with gel applied, and hold it against the palm of your dominant hand, with the medial three fingers curled to hold the electrode in place. Apply a small amount of gel to your index finger tip. Using a chart, or the one-third–two-thirds rule, estimate the location of the motor point for the muscle to be stimulated. Place your index finger with gel over the approximate location of the motor point. Carefully increase the intensity of the NMES stimulator until you (the therapist) feel a definite tingle. Without removing your index finger from the patient's skin, slowly glide your finger around the area. The motor point will be at the point where you feel the strongest intensity of current – the strongest tingling sensation. Take note of that point. Turn down the stimulation intensity to zero and remove your finger. Apply the electrode that had been in your palm over the motor point to begin the treatment.

Electrode Gel Versus Ultrasound Gel

The recommendation has long been to use electrode gel rather than ultrasound gel for the application of ES. The reasons for this are twofold: (i) electrode gel has better electrical conductivity than ultrasound gel, and (ii) because many formulations are free of sodium or potassium chloride, these gels may be left in place for long periods of time without causing skin irritation. It is also possible to use wet sponge or lint pad, which is particularly recommended if the electrode is very large.

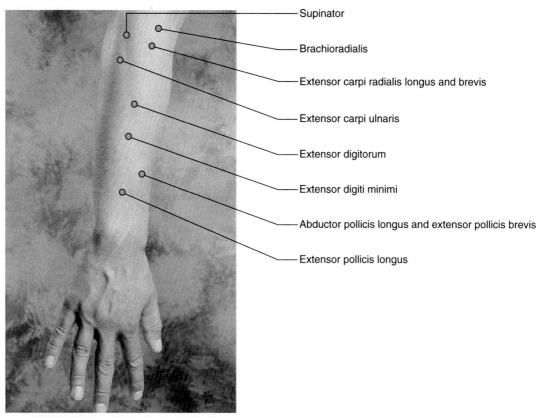

Supinator

Brachioradialis

Extensor carpi radialis longus and brevis

Extensor carpi ulnaris

Extensor digitorum

Extensor digiti minimi

Abductor pollicis longus and extensor pollicis brevis

Extensor pollicis longus

Fig. 16.4 Approximate positions of some of the motor points on the posterior aspect of the right arm.

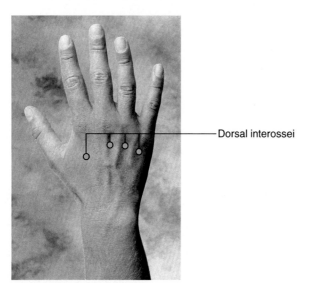

Dorsal interossei

Fig. 16.5 Approximate positions of some of the motor points on the posterior aspect of the hand.

Electrode Sponges

Sponge sheet a few millimetres thick may be cut to size to fit electrodes and moistened with tap water to couple carbon rubber electrodes to the skin. Sponges should be completely saturated with water and then gently wrung out so as to be damp – that is, a small amount of water should remain within the sponge to allow conduction of the current.

Sponges should be cleaned between uses, and allowed to dry completely before the next use to limit the growth of water-borne bacteria, such as *Pseudomonas aeruginosa* (Lambert et al 2000).

Skin Preparation

Several aspects of the treatment application can have a role to play in reducing discomfort: frequency, waveform, electrode size, electrode placement and skin preparation (wet and warm). In order to reduce skin resistance, pulse width can be reduced. See Chapter 22 for further recommendations.

Skin resistance will be lower than usual over cuts or skin abrasions and higher than usual over scars or over skin oils,

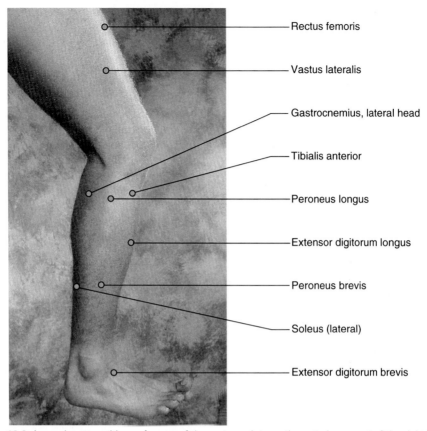

Rectus femoris

Vastus lateralis

Gastrocnemius, lateral head

Tibialis anterior

Peroneus longus

Extensor digitorum longus

Peroneus brevis

Soleus (lateral)

Extensor digitorum brevis

Fig. 16.6 Approximate positions of some of the motor points on the anterior aspect of the right leg.

grease from ointment, etc. and electrode placement in these cases should be modified or appropriate alterations made to current intensity. Additionally, it is critical to use a conductive electrode gel. In the absence of a conductive electrode gel, skin has been shown to break down, with current being shunted at high density through regions of lower resistance, causing localized heating and damage (Prausnitz 1996).

Subcutaneous fat has a high resistivity to current; consequently the stimulation of motor nerves in this case requires a higher intensity of stimulating current, which may lead to patient discomfort. Using very large electrodes may overcome this issue.

Securing Electrodes

Failure to secure electrodes may not only lead to ineffective treatment, but may result in regions of high current density, leading to discomfort or skin injury: see Chapter 22.

Monopolar Versus Bipolar Application

These terms are used to describe a situation in which the stimulating effect (and sensation) is perceived more under

one electrode than the other, or, perceived fairly equally under both electrodes. The term monopolar is really a misnomer, since one always needs at least two electrodes (i.e. two poles) to create a circuit. The term monopolar refers to having one 'active' electrode, that is, one electrode with a much smaller area than the other, causing greater current density and consequently greater motor effects at the smaller electrode (and greater sensation). The second electrode is the 'inactive' electrode (sometimes termed 'indifferent' or 'dispersive'), which has an area at least two times that of the active electrode and consequently lower current density and motor and sensory effects (Merletti et al 1992). A monopolar set-up is used to stimulate a specific muscle belly, or a small, targeted muscle group, and electrode placement would be nerve trunk and motor point, or motor point and muscle belly. (see Chapter 4, Fig. 4.20 and 4.22).

A bipolar set-up will consist of two equal (or almost equal) sized electrodes (Merletti et al 1992). In this case, current density will be equal or almost equal. A bipolar set-up may be used when a muscle belly–muscle belly

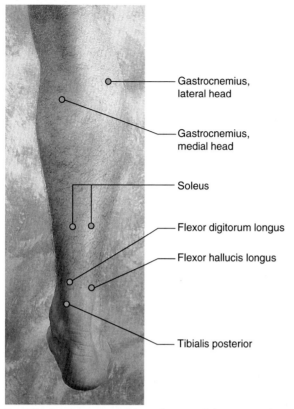

Gastrocnemius, lateral head

Gastrocnemius, medial head

Soleus

Flexor digitorum longus

Flexor hallucis longus

Tibialis posterior

Fig. 16.7 Approximate positions of some of the motor points on the posterior aspect of the right leg.

application is chosen, or when it is necessary to cover a greater area (e.g. for stimulating large muscle groups) (See Chapter 4, Fig. 4.20 and 4.22).

Multiple Electrodes

It is possible to stimulate a large muscle or muscle group by applying multiple electrodes to different points on the muscle. For example, using lead splitters or commercial multi-electrode sets, it is possible to have two electrodes from one lead of the stimulator and another two electrodes from the second lead of the stimulator, allowing four electrodes to complete the circuit, and covering a greater area of muscle (Fig. 16.11).

Because stimulation recruits the same group of motor units throughout treatment – supplied by nerves closest to the stimulating electrodes – increased fatigue may occur. It may be possible to reduce fatigue and increase the total amount of muscle stimulated by moving the electrodes during treatment. After a certain number of contractions, the intensity would be reduced to zero, the electrodes moved elsewhere on the muscle, and a new group of motor units activated. In this way it may be possible to stimulate more of the muscle than could be achieved if the electrodes remain in one position throughout the treatment (Maffiuletti 2010).

Two Channels

Most NMES devices provide two separate channels, with two intensity controls, to allow more muscle groups to be stimulated, or allow the placing of more electrodes over a single large muscle. In the case of the former, the muscle

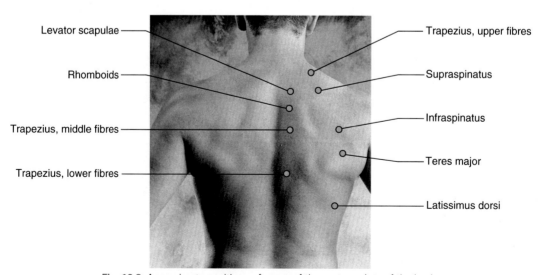

Levator scapulae

Rhomboids

Trapezius, middle fibres

Trapezius, lower fibres

Trapezius, upper fibres

Supraspinatus

Infraspinatus

Teres major

Latissimus dorsi

Fig. 16.8 Approximate positions of some of the motor points of the back.

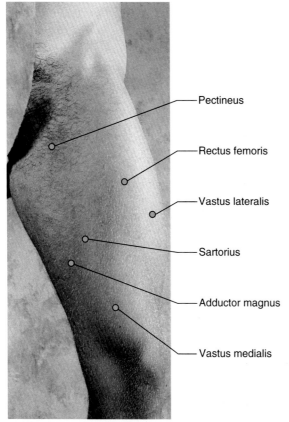

Pectineus

Rectus femoris

Vastus lateralis

Sartorius

Adductor magnus

Vastus medialis

Fig. 16.9 Approximate positions of some of the motor points of the left anterior thigh.

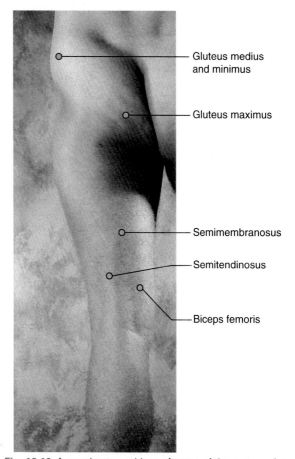

Gluteus medius and minimus

Gluteus maximus

Semimembranosus

Semitendinosus

Biceps femoris

Fig. 16.10 Approximate positions of some of the motor points of the posterior thigh.

groups can be stimulated at the same time by both channels – called 'synchronous' or 'co-contraction' – or the muscle groups may be stimulated alternately, in which case the channels would operate in 'reciprocal' mode (e.g. stimulating the quadriceps and hamstring muscles).

Some devices additionally will allow a Channel 2 delay, in which case Channel 2 will switch 'on' at some defined time after Channel 1 switches to the 'on' cycle. This can allow a partial overlap between contractions, or the muscles may be made to contract in sequence, all to achieve a desired therapeutic effect. This approach is commonly found when using ES to simultaneously strengthen and retrain normal motor patterning. Examples might include activating vastus medialis on Channel 1 followed by vastus lateralis and rectus femoris on Channel 2 in order to focus on medial quadriceps activation. In order to strengthen shoulder girdle muscles and retrain scapulohumeral rhythm, activating external rotators-depressors of the shoulder girdle before supraspinatus and medial deltoid.

Simply stimulating one muscle (group) and then giving it a period of rest is the most simplistic approach to NMES and may not be especially functional, nor reflect how advanced NMES applications may be employed.

Patient Position

In many applications it is important for the patient to be able to participate with voluntary muscle contractions to augment the stimulated contractions, where appropriate. If the joint is positioned so that the muscle is in its mid-length range, this will optimize the contraction force (e.g. quadriceps stimulation with knee flexion at about 65 degrees). In some situations, the patient will need to be positioned with gravity eliminated. Additionally, there may be circumstances in which there is an advantage to generating isometric contractions – in which case the recommendation is to stabilize the joint at the optimal angle.

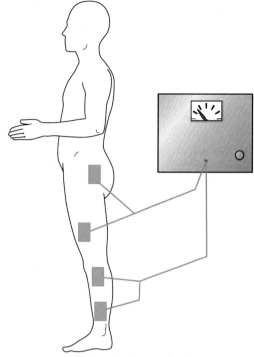

Fig. 16.11 Bifurcated leads.

Device Settings and Features
Constant Stimulation Mode

It is imperative that clinicians be aware of the On and Off cycles of the NMES application, and that current intensity only be adjusted during the On cycle. Some devices will default to continuously On until the clinician has finished setting the current intensity – usually determined by no increase in set amplitude for one second or longer. Other devices default to cycling On and Off, and in this case the clinician must use the 'Constant stim' button while setting the current amplitude. After release of the 'Constant stim' button, the device will start cycling On and Off.

Protocol Saving

Many modern devices will allow the clinician the option of saving a protocol associated with a particular patient. This is a time-saving feature, although clinicians should always be prepared to modify the parameter settings based on patient response.

System Lock

It is usually possible to lock a device so that settings can no longer be changed. This is a safety feature to ensure that

patients or others do not change treatment parameters (apart from current intensity). This may be particularly useful if the patient is to take the NMES device home for use.

Compliance Monitoring

Some NMES devices permit tracking of use. In this case it is possible for the clinician to monitor patient use of the device at home.

Adverse Effects

As with any electrophysical modality, an improper application, application in the presence of contraindications or without due regard to precautions, or using faulty equipment, may lead to adverse effects. Muscle contraction can cause injury in some circumstances (e.g. post-tendon repair or muscle transfer, over an area of recent surgery and over a fracture). In addition, injury has been reported by inappropriate self-application of NMES (e.g. to lower abdominal muscles). Further details of potential adverse effects of NMES are covered in Chapter 22.

SUMMARY

The application of electrical current to stimulate muscle contraction has been used therapeutically since the mid-18th century. The nature of any stimulated muscle contraction will depend on the frequency, intensity and pulse duration of the stimulating current, as well as the location and size of the electrodes. Stimulated contractions are different from physiological contractions in four important ways: both temporal and spatial recruitment of motor units, fibre firing order during recruitment and metabolic demand. The result of these differences is increased fatigue from stimulated contractions compared with physiological contractions. Therapeutic uses may include muscle strengthening, muscle twitch, increasing muscle endurance, reduction of muscle spasticity, increasing joint range of motion, providing active movement to reduce joint adhesions, and enhancing post-exercise performance recovery. There is a substantial body of clinical evidence to suggest that NMES may assist patients with a wide variety of orthopaedic, neurological and critical illness conditions to achieve their clinical goals, or to do so more effectively. Parameters vary somewhat within defined ranges, depending on the main therapeutic objective. Contraindications and precautions are similar to those encountered with other electrical modalities, with the addition of specific precautions where muscle contraction might cause injury. Evidence suggests that NMES is both safe and effective when used appropriately.

REFERENCES

Abdellaoui, A., Préfaut, C., Gouzi, F., et al. (2011). Skeletal muscle effects of electrostimulation after COPD exacerbation: A pilot study. *European Respiratory Journal, 38*(4), 781–788.

Ada, L., & Foongchomcheay, A. (2002). Efficacy of electrical stimulation in preventing or reducing subluxation of the shoulder after stroke: A meta-analysis. *Australian Journal of Physiotherapy, 48*(4), 257–267.

Adams, G. R., Harris, R. T., Woodard, D., & Dudley, G. A. (1993). Mapping of electrical muscle stimulation using MRI. *Journal of Applied Physiology, 74*(2), 532–537.

Akarcali, I., Tugay, N., Kaya, D., Atay, A., & Doral, M. N. (2002). The role of high voltage electrical stimulation in the rehabilitation of patellofemoral pain. *The Pain Clinic, 14*(3), 207–212.

Alba-Martín, P., Gallego-Izquierdo, T., Plaza-Manzano, G., Romero-Franco, N., Núñez-Nagy, S., & Pecos-Martín, D. (2015). Effectiveness of therapeutic physical exercise in the treatment of patellofemoral pain syndrome: A systematic review. *Journal of Physical Therapy Science, 27*(7), 2387–2390.

Alon, G., Kantor, G., & Ho, H. S. (1994). Effects of electrode size on basic excitatory responses and on selected stimulus parameters. *Journal of Orthopaedic & Sports Physical Therapy, 20*(1), 29–35.

Andrews, B., Gibbons, R., & Wheeler, G. (2017). Development of functional electrical stimulation rowing: The rowstim series. *Artificial Organs, 41*(11), E212.

Avramidis, K., Karachalios, T., Popotonasios, K., Sacorafas, D., Papathanasiades, A. A., & Malizos, K. N. (2011). Does electric stimulation of the vastus medialis muscle influence rehabilitation after total knee replacement? *Orthopedics, 34*(3), 175.

Babault, N., Cometti, C., Maffiuletti, N. A., & Deley, G. (2011). Does electrical stimulation enhance post-exercise performance recovery? *European Journal of Applied Physiology, 111*(10), 2501.

Bade, M. J., Kohrt, W. M., & Stevens-Lapsley, J. E. (2010). Outcomes before and after total knee arthroplasty compared to healthy adults. *Journal of Orthopaedic & Sports Physical Therapy, 40*(9), 559–567.

Baker, L. L., Bowman, B. R., & McNeal, D. R. (1988). Effects of waveform on comfort during neuromuscular electrical stimulation. *Clinical Orthopaedics and Related Research* (233), 75–85.

Baker, L. L., & Parker, K. (1986). Neuromuscular electrical stimulation of the muscles surrounding the shoulder. *Physical Therapy, 66*(12), 1930–1937.

Barker, R. N., Brauer, S. G., & Carson, R. G. (2008). Training of reaching in stroke survivors with severe and chronic upper limb paresis using a novel nonrobotic device: A randomized clinical trial. *Stroke, 39*(6), 1800–1807.

Barton, C. J., Lack, S., Hemmings, S., Tufail, S., & Morrissey, D. (2015). The 'best practice guide to conservative management of patellofemoral pain': Incorporating level 1 evidence with expert clinical reasoning. *British Journal of Sports Medicine, 49*(14), 923–934.

Bélanger, A. (2010). *Therapeutic electrophysical agents: Evidence behind practice*. Philadelphia: Wolters Kluwer Health/ Lippincott Williams & Wilkins.

Bélanger, M., Stein, R. B., Wheeler, G. D., Gordon, T., & Leduc, B. (2000). Electrical stimulation: Can it increase muscle strength and reverse osteopenia in spinal cord injured individuals? *Archives of Physical Medicine and Rehabilitation, 81*(8), 1090–1098.

Bellew, J. W., Sanders, K., Schuman, K., & Barton, M. (2014). Muscle force production with low and medium frequency burst modulated biphasic pulsed currents. *Physiotherapy Theory and Practice, 30*(2), 105–109.

Benton, L. A., Baker, L. L., Bowman, B. R., & Waters, R. L. (1981). *Functional electrical stimulation – a practical clinical guide (revised)*. Downey, CA: Rancho Los Amigos Rehabilitation Engineering Center.

Bickel, C. S., Gregory, C. M., & Dean, J. C. (2011). Motor unit recruitment during neuromuscular electrical stimulation: A critical appraisal. *European Journal of Applied Physiology, 111*(10), 2399.

Bigland-Ritchie, B., Jones, D. A., & Woods, J. J. (1979). Excitation frequency and muscle fatigue: Electrical responses during human voluntary and stimulated contractions. *Experimental Neurology, 64*(2), 414–427.

Binder-Macleod, S. A., & Snyder-Mackler, L. (1993). Muscle fatigue: Clinical implications for fatigue assessment and neuromuscular electrical stimulation. *Physical Therapy, 73*(12), 902–910.

Bistolfi, A., Zanovello, J., Ferracini, R., Allisiardi, F., Lioce, E., Magistroni, E., et al. (2018). Evaluation of the effectiveness of neuromuscular electrical stimulation after total knee arthroplasty: A meta-analysis. *American Journal of Physical Medicine & Rehabilitation, 97*(2), 123–130.

Blair, E. A., & Erlanger, J. (1933). A comparison of the characteristics of axons through their individual electrical responses. *American Journal of Physiology-Legacy Content, 106*(3), 524–564.

Bogataj, U., Gros, N., Kljajić, M., Aćimović, R., & Maležič, M. (1995). The rehabilitation of gait in patients with hemiplegia: A comparison between conventional therapy and multichannel functional electrical stimulation therapy. *Physical Therapy, 75*(6), 490–502.

Bosques, G., Martin, R., McGee, L., & Sadowsky, C. (2016). Does therapeutic electrical stimulation improve function in children with disabilities? A comprehensive literature review. *Journal of Pediatric Rehabilitation Medicine, 9*(2), 83–99.

Botter, A., Oprandi, G., Lanfranco, F., Allasia, S., Maffiuletti, N. A., & Minetto, M. A. (2011). Atlas of the muscle motor points for the lower limb: Implications for electrical stimulation procedures and electrode positioning. *European Journal of Applied Physiology, 111*(10), 2461.

Bouletreau, P., Patricot, M. C., Saudin, F., Guiraud, M., & Mathian, B. (1987). Effects of intermittent electrical stimulations on muscle catabolism in intensive care patients. *Journal of Parenteral and Enteral Nutrition, 11*(6), 552–555.

Bowman, B. R., & Baker, L. L. (1985). Effects of waveform parameters on comfort during transcutaneous neuromuscular electrical stimulation. *Annals of Biomedical Engineering, 13*(1), 59–74.

Brooks, M. E., Smith, E. M., & Currier, D. P. (1990). Effect of longitudinal versus transverse electrode placement on torque production by the quadriceps femoris muscle during neuromuscular electrical stimulation. *Journal of Orthopaedic & Sports Physical Therapy, 11*(11), 530–534.

Brown, J. (2000). Physiotherapists' knowledge of patello-femoral pain syndrome. *British Journal of Therapy and Rehabilitation, 7*(8), 346–354.

Bruce-Brand, R. A., Walls, R. J., Ong, J. C., Emerson, B. S., O'Byrne, J. M., & Moyna, N. M. (2012). Effects of home-based resistance training and neuromuscular electrical stimulation in knee osteoarthritis: A randomized controlled trial. *BMC Musculoskeletal Disorders, 13*(1), 118.

Brubaker, L. (2000) May. Electrical stimulation in overactive bladder. *Urology, 55*(5), 17–23.

Burridge, J. H., Taylor, P. N., Hagan, S. A., Wood, D. E., & Swain, I. D. (1997). The effects of common peroneal stimulation on the effort and speed of walking: A randomized controlled trial with chronic hemiplegic patients. *Clinical Rehabilitation, 11*(3), 201–210.

Callaghan, M. J., & Oldham, J. A. (2004). Electric muscle stimulation of the quadriceps in the treatment of patellofemoral pain. *Archives of Physical Medicine and Rehabilitation, 85*(6), 956–962.

Callaghan, M. J., Oldham, J. A., & Winstanley, J. (2001). A comparison of two types of electrical stimulation of the quadriceps in the treatment of patellofemoral pain syndrome. A pilot study. *Clinical Rehabilitation, 15*(6), 637–646.

Cambridge, N. A. (1977). Electrical apparatus used in medicine before 1900. *Journal of the Royal Society of Medicine, 70.*

Campbell, E., Coulter, E. H., Mattison, P. G., Miller, L., McFadyen, A., & Paul, L. (2016). Physiotherapy rehabilitation for people with progressive multiple sclerosis: A systematic review. *Archives of Physical Medicine and Rehabilitation, 97*(1), 151.e3.

Chantraine, A., Baribeault, A., Uebelhart, D., & Gremion, G. (1999). Shoulder pain and dysfunction in hemiplegia: Effects of functional electrical stimulation. *Archives of Physical Medicine and Rehabilitation, 80*(3), 328–331.

Chaplin, E. J. L., Houchen, L., Greening, N. J., et al. (2013). Neuromuscular stimulation of quadriceps in patients hospitalised during an exacerbation of COPD: A comparison of low (35 Hz) and high (50 Hz) frequencies. *Physiotherapy Research International, 18*(3), 148–156.

Chêne, G., Mansoor, A., Jacquetin, B., et al. (2013). Female urinary incontinence and intravaginal electrical stimulation: An observational prospective study. *European Journal of Obstetrics & Gynecology and Reproductive Biology, 170*(1), 275–280.

Chizmadzhev, Y. A., Indenbom, A. V., Kuzmin, P. I., Galichenko, S. V., Weaver, J. C., & Potts, R. O. (1998a). Electrical properties of skin at moderate voltages: Contribution of appendageal macropores. *Biophysical Journal, 74*(2), 843–856.

Chung, Y., Kim, J., Cha, Y., & Hwang, S. (2014). Therapeutic effect of functional electrical stimulation-triggered gait training corresponding gait cycle for stroke. *Gait & Posture, 40*(3), 471–475.

Church, C., Price, C., Pandyan, A. D., Huntley, S., Curless, R., & Rodgers, H. (2006). Randomized controlled trial to evaluate the effect of surface neuromuscular electrical stimulation to the shoulder after acute stroke. *Stroke, 37*(12), 2995–3001.

Collins, D. F. (2007). Central contributions to contractions evoked by tetanic neuromuscular electrical stimulation. *Exercise and Sport Sciences Reviews, 35*(3), 102–109.

Davis, G. M., Hamzaid, N. A., & Fornusek, C. (2008). Cardiorespiratory, metabolic, and biomechanical responses during functional electrical stimulation leg exercise: Health and fitness benefits. *Artificial Organs, 32*(8), 625–629.

De Jonghe, B., Bastuji-Garin, S., Durand, M., et al. (2007). Respiratory weakness is associated with limb weakness and delayed weaning in critical illness. *Critical Care Medicine, 35*(9), 2007–2015.

De Oliveira Melo, M., Aragão, F. A., & Vaz, M. A. (2013). Neuromuscular electrical stimulation for muscle strengthening in elderly with knee osteoarthritis–a systematic review. *Complementary Therapies in Clinical Practice, 19*(1), 27–31.

Deley, G., Denuziller, J., & Babault, N. (2015). Functional electrical stimulation: Cardiorespiratory adaptations and applications for training in paraplegia. *Sports Medicine, 45*(1), 71–82.

Delitto, A., & Rose, S. J. (1986). Comparative comfort of three waveforms used in electrically eliciting quadriceps femoris muscle contractions. *Physical Therapy, 66*(11), 1704–1707.

Dimitrijević, M. M., & Soroker, N. (1994). Mesh-glove. 2. Modulation of residual upper limb motor control after stroke with whole-hand electric stimulation. *Scandinavian Journal of Rehabilitation Medicine, 26*(4), 187–190.

Dimitrijevic, M. M., Stokié, D. S., Wawro, A. W., & Wun, C. C. (1996). Modification of motor control of wrist extension by mesh-glove electrical afferent stimulation in stroke patients. *Archives of Physical Medicine and Rehabilitation, 77*(3), 252–258.

Dirks, M. L., Hansen, D., Van Assche, A., Dendale, P., & Van Loon, L. J. (2015). Neuromuscular electrical stimulation prevents muscle wasting in critically ill comatose patients. *Clinical Science, 128*(6), 357–365.

Dolbow, D. R., & Gorgey, A. S. (2016). Effects of use and disuse on non-paralyzed and paralyzed skeletal muscles. *Aging and Disease, 7*(1), 68.

Doucet, B. M., Lam, A., & Griffin, L. (2012). Neuromuscular electrical stimulation for skeletal muscle function. *Yale Journal of Biology & Medicine, 85*(2), 201.

Dow, D. E., Cederna, P. S., Hassett, C. A., Kostrominova, T. Y., Faulkner, J. A., & Dennis, R. G. (2004). Number of contractions to maintain mass and force of a denervated rat muscle. *Muscle & Nerve: Official Journal of the American Association of Electrodiagnostic Medicine, 30*(1), 77–86.

Dreibati, B., Lavet, C., Pinti, A., & Poumarat, G. (2010). Influence of electrical stimulation frequency on skeletal muscle force and fatigue. *Annals of Physical and Rehabilitation Medicine, 53*(4), 266–277.

Duchenne, G. (1871). *A treatise on localized electrization, and its applications to pathology and therapeutics* (3rd ed.). Philadelphia: Lindsay & Blakiston.

Durigan, J. L., Delfino, G. B., Peviani, S. M., et al. (2014). Neuromuscular electrical stimulation alters gene expression and delays quadriceps muscle atrophy of rats after anterior cruciate ligament transection. *Muscle & Nerve, 49*(1), 120–128.

Durmuş, D., Alayli, G., & Cantürk, F. (2007). Effects of quadriceps electrical stimulation program on clinical parameters in the patients with knee osteoarthritis. *Clinical Rheumatology, 26*(5), 674–678.

Dvir, Z., Halperin, N., Shklar, A., & Robinson, D. (1991). Quadriceps function and patellofemoral pain syndrome. Part I: Pain provocation during concentric and eccentric isokinetic activity. *Isokinetics and Exercise Science, 1*(1), 26–30.

Eberstein, A., & Eberstein, S. (1996). Electrical stimulation of denervated muscle: Is it worthwhile? *Medicine & Science in Sports & Exercise, 28*(12), 1463–1469.

Ediz, L., Ceylan, M. F., Turktas, U., Yanmis, I., & Hiz, O. (2012). A randomized controlled trial of electrostimulation effects on effusion, swelling and pain recovery after anterior cruciate ligament reconstruction: A pilot study. *Clinical Rehabilitation, 26*(5), 413–422.

Edwards, T., & Pilutti, L. A. (2017). The effect of exercise training in adults with multiple sclerosis with severe mobility disability: A systematic review and future research directions. *Multiple Sclerosis and Related Disorders, 16*, 31–39.

Edwards, R., Young, A., Hosking, G. P., & Jones, D. A. (1977). Human skeletal muscle function: Description of tests and normal values. *Clinical Science, 52*(3), 283–290.

Elbasiouny, S. M., Moroz, D., Bakr, M. M., & Mushahwar, V. K. (2010). Management of spasticity after spinal cord injury: Current techniques and future directions. *Neurorehabilitation and Neural Repair, 24*(1), 23–33.

Enoka, R. M. (2002a). Activation order of motor axons in electrically evoked contractions. *Muscle & Nerve, 25*(6), 763–764.

Erickson, M. L., Ryan, T. E., Backus, D., & McCully, K. K. (2017). Endurance neuromuscular electrical stimulation training improves skeletal muscle oxidative capacity in individuals with motor-complete spinal cord injury. *Muscle & Nerve, 55*(5), 669–675.

Faghri, P. D., Rodgers, M. M., Glaser, R. M., Bors, J. G., Ho, C., & Akuthota, P. (1994). The effects of functional electrical stimulation on shoulder subluxation, arm function recovery, and shoulder pain in hemiplegic stroke patients. *Archives of Physical Medicine and Rehabilitation, 75*(1), 73–79.

Faiena, I., Patel, N., Parihar, J. S., Calabrese, M., & Tunuguntla, H. (2015). Conservative management of urinary incontinence in women. *Reviews in Urology, 17*(3), 129.

Falavigna, L. F., Silva, M. G., Freitas, A. L., et al. (2014). Effects of electrical muscle stimulation early in the quadriceps and tibialis anterior muscle of critically ill patients. *Physiotherapy Theory and Practice, 30*(4), 223–228.

Fall, M., & Lindström, S. (1994). Functional electrical stimulation: Physiological basis and clinical principles. *International Urogynecology Journal, 5*(5), 296–304.

Feiereisen, P., Duchateau, J., & Hainaut, K. (1997). Motor unit recruitment order during voluntary and electrically induced contractions in the tibialis anterior. *Experimental Brain Research, 114*(1), 117–123.

Fil, A., Armutlu, K., Atay, A. O., Kerimoglu, U., & Elibol, B. (2011). The effect of electrical stimulation in combination with Bobath techniques in the prevention of shoulder subluxation in acute stroke patients. *Clinical Rehabilitation, 25*(1), 51–59.

Fitzgerald, G. K., Piva, S. R., & Irrgang, J. J. (2003). A modified neuromuscular electrical stimulation protocol for quadriceps strength training following anterior cruciate ligament reconstruction. *Journal of Orthopaedic & Sports Physical Therapy, 33*(9), 492–501.

Forrester, B. J., & Petrofsky, J. S. (2004). Effect of electrode size, shape, and placement during electrical stimulation. *Journal of Applied Research, 4*(2), 346–354.

Franz, A., Klaas, J., Schumann, M., Frankewitsch, T., Filler, T. J., & Behringer, M. (2018). Anatomical versus functional motor points of selected upper body muscles. *Muscle & Nerve, 57*(3), 460–465.

Fuglevand, A. J., Winter, D. A., Patla, A. E., & Stashuk, D. (1992). Detection of motor unit action potentials with surface electrodes: Influence of electrode size and spacing. *Biological Cybernetics, 67*(2), 143–153.

Garcia, F. R., Azevedo, F. M., Alves, N., Carvalho, A. C., Padovani, C. R., & Negrão Filho, R. F. (2010). Effects of electrical stimulation of vastus medialis obliquus muscle in patients with patellofemoral pain syndrome: An electromyographic analysis. *Brazilian Journal of Physical Therapy, 14*(6), 477–482.

Garland, S. J., Garner, S. H., & McComas, A. J. (1988). Relationship between numbers and frequencies of stimuli in human muscle fatigue. *Journal of Applied Physiology, 65*(1), 89–93.

Garnett, R., & Stephens, J. A. (1981). Changes in the recruitment threshold of motor units produced by cutaneous stimulation in man. *The Journal of Physiology, 311*(1), 463–473.

Gersh, M. R. (1992). *Electrotherapy in rehabilitation*. FA Davis Company.

Ghaderi, F., & Oskouei, A. E. (2014). Physiotherapy for women with stress urinary incontinence: A review article. *Journal of Physical Therapy Science, 26*(9), 1493–1499.

Gibbons, R. S., Beaupre, G. S., & Kazakia, G. J. (2016). FES-rowing attenuates bone loss following spinal cord injury as assessed by HR-pQCT. *Spinal Cord Series and Cases, 2*(1), 15041.

Gibson, J. N. A., Smith, K., & Rennie, M. J. (1988). Prevention of disuse muscle atrophy by means of electrical stimulation: Maintenance of protein synthesis. *The Lancet, 332*(8614), 767–770.

Gobbo, M., Gaffurini, P., Bissolotti, L., Esposito, F., & Orizio, C. (2011). Transcutaneous neuromuscular electrical stimulation: Influence of electrode positioning and stimulus amplitude settings on muscle response. *European Journal of Applied Physiology, 111*(10), 2451–2459.

Gondin, J., Cozzone, P. J., & Bendahan, D. (2011). Is high-frequency neuromuscular electrical stimulation a suitable tool for muscle performance improvement in both healthy humans and athletes? *European Journal of Applied Physiology, 111*(10), 2473.

Gordon, T., Amirjani, N., Edwards, D. C., & Chan, K. M. (2010). Brief post-surgical electrical stimulation accelerates axon regeneration and muscle reinnervation without affecting the functional measures in carpal tunnel syndrome patients. *Experimental Neurology*, *223*(1), 192–202.

Gorgey, A. S., Dolbow, D. R., Dolbow, J. D., Khalil, R. K., & Gater, D. R. (2015). The effects of electrical stimulation on body composition and metabolic profile after spinal cord injury–Part II. *The Journal of Spinal Cord Medicine*, *38*(1), 23–37.

Gorgey, A. S., Mahoney, E., Kendall, T., & Dudley, G. A. (2006). Effects of neuromuscular electrical stimulation parameters on specific tension. *European Journal of Applied Physiology*, *97*(6), 737–744.

Gotlin, R. S., Hershkowitz, S., Juris, P. M., Gonzalez, E. G., Scott, W. N., & Insall, J. N. (1994). Electrical stimulation effect on extensor lag and length of hospital stay after total knee arthroplasty. *Archives of Physical Medicine and Rehabilitation*, *75*(9), 957–959.

Gregory, C. M., & Bickel, C. S. (2005). Recruitment patterns in human skeletal muscle during electrical stimulation. *Physical Therapy*, *85*(4), 358–364.

Gruther, W., Kainberger, F., Fialka-Moser, V., et al. (2010). Effects of neuromuscular electrical stimulation on muscle layer thickness of knee extensor muscles in intensive care unit patients: A pilot study. *Journal of Rehabilitation Medicine*, *42*(6), 593–597.

Guyton, A. C. (1976). *Textbook of medical physiology* (5th ed.). Philadelphia: Saunders, 242.

Haastert-Talini, K., Schmitte, R., Korte, N., Klode, D., Ratzka, A., & Grothe, C. (2011). Electrical stimulation accelerates axonal and functional peripheral nerve regeneration across long gaps. *Journal of Neurotrauma*, *28*(4), 661–674.

Hainaut, K., & Duchateau, J. (1992). Neuromuscular electrical stimulation and voluntary exercise. *Sports Medicine*, *14*(2), 100–113.

Hammond, E. R., Recio, A. C., Sadowsky, C. L., & Becker, D. (2015). Functional electrical stimulation as a component of activity-based restorative therapy may preserve function in persons with multiple sclerosis. *The Journal of Spinal Cord Medicine*, *38*(1), 68–75.

Hasegawa, S., Kobayashi, M., Arai, R., Tamaki, A., Nakamura, T., & Moritani, T. (2011). Effect of early implementation of electrical muscle stimulation to prevent muscle atrophy and weakness in patients after anterior cruciate ligament reconstruction. *Journal of Electromyography and Kinesiology*, *21*(4), 622–630.

Hauger, A., Reiman, M., Bjordal, J., Sheets, C., Ledbetter, L., & Goode, A. (2018). Neuromuscular electrical stimulation is effective in strengthening the quadriceps muscle after anterior cruciate ligament surgery. *Knee Surgery, Sports Traumatology, Arthroscopy*, *26*(2), 399–410.

Heckmann, J., Mokrusch, T., Kröckel, A., Warnke, S., Von Stockert, T., & Neundörfer, B. (1997). EMG-triggered electrical muscle stimulation in the treatment of central hemiparesis after a stroke. *European Journal of Physical Medicine and Rehabilitation*, *7*(5), 138–141.

Henneman, E. (1957). Relation between size of neurons and their susceptibility to discharge. *Science*, *126*(3287), 1345–1347.

Henneman, E., Somjen, G., & Carpenter, D. O. (1965). Functional Significance of Cell Size In Spinal Motoneurons. *Journal of Neurophysiology*, *28*(3), 560–580.

Herridge, M. S., Tansey, C. M., Matté, A., et al. (2011). Functional disability 5 years after acute respiratory distress syndrome. *New England Journal of Medicine*, *364*(14), 1293–1304.

Hettinga, D. M., & Andrews, B. J. (2008). Oxygen consumption during functional electrical stimulation-assisted exercise in persons with spinal cord injury. *Sports Medicine*, *38*(10), 825–838.

Hortobágyi, T., & Maffiuletti, N. A. (2011). Neural adaptations to electrical stimulation strength training. *European Journal of Applied Physiology*, *111*(10), 2439–2449.

Howlett, O. A., Lannin, N. A., Ada, L., & McKinstry, C. (2015). Functional electrical stimulation improves activity after stroke: A systematic review with meta-analysis. *Archives of Physical Medicine and Rehabilitation*, *96*(5), 934–943.

Huang, J., Zhang, Y., Lu, L., Hu, X., & Luo, Z. (2013). Electrical stimulation accelerates nerve regeneration and functional recovery in delayed peripheral nerve injury in rats. *European Journal of Neuroscience*, *38*(12), 3691–3701.

Hultman, E., Sjöholm, H., Jäderholm-Ek, I., & Krynicki, J. (1983). Evaluation of methods for electrical stimulation of human skeletal muscle in situ. *Pflügers Archiv*, *398*(2), 139–141.

Iwashyna, T. J., Ely, E. W., Smith, D. M., & Langa, K. M. (2010). Long-term cognitive impairment and functional disability among survivors of severe sepsis. *Journal of the American Medical Association*, *304*(16), 1787–1794.

Jackson, E., & Seddon, H. J. (1945). Influence of galvanic stimulation on muscle atrophy resulting from denervation. *British Medical Journal*, 485–486.

Jones, D. A., Bigland-Ritchie, B., & Edwards, R. (1979). Excitation frequency and muscle fatigue: Mechanical responses during voluntary and stimulated contractions. *Experimental Neurology*, *64*(2), 401–413.

Jubeau, M., Gondin, J., Martin, A., Sartorio, A., & Maffiuletti, N. A. (2007). Random motor unit activation by electrostimulation. *International Journal of Sports Medicine*, *28*(11), 901–904.

Kafri, M., & Laufer, Y. (2015). Therapeutic effects of functional electrical stimulation on gait in individuals post-stroke. *Annals of Biomedical Engineering*, *43*(2), 451–466.

Kantor, G., Alon, G., & Ho, H. S. (1994). The effects of selected stimulus waveforms on pulse and phase characteristics at sensory and motor thresholds. *Physical Therapy*, *74*(10), 951–962.

Keller, T., & Kuhn, A. (2008). Electrodes for transcutaneous (surface) electrical stimulation. *Journal of Automatic Control*, *18*(2), 35–45.

Kern, H., Boncompagni, S., Rossini, K., et al. (2004). Long-term denervation in humans causes degeneration of both contractile and excitation-contraction coupling apparatus, which is reversible by functional electrical stimulation (FES): A role for myofiber regeneration? *Journal of Neuropathology & Experimental Neurology*, *63*(9), 919–931.

Kern, H., Carraro, U., Adami, N., et al. (2010). Home-based functional electrical stimulation rescues permanently denervated muscles in paraplegic patients with complete lower motor neuron lesion. *Neurorehabilitation and Neural Repair*, 24(8), 709–721.

Kern, H., Salmons, S., Mayr, W., Rossini, K., & Carraro, U. (2005). Recovery of long–term denervated human muscles induced by electrical stimulation. *Muscle & Nerve: Official Journal of the American Association of Electrodiagnostic Medicine*, 31(1), 98–101.

Kim, K., Croy, T., Hertel, J., & Saliba, S. (2010). Effects of neuromuscular electrical stimulation after anterior cruciate ligament reconstruction on quadriceps strength, function, and patient-oriented outcomes: A systematic review. *Journal of Orthopaedic & Sports Physical Therapy*, 40(7), 383–391.

Kluding, P. M., Dunning, K., O'Dell, M. W., et al. (2013). Foot drop stimulation versus ankle foot orthosis after stroke: 30-week outcomes. *Stroke*, 44(6), 1660–1669.

Knaflitz, M., Merletti, R., & De Luca, C. J. (1990). Inference of motor unit recruitment order in voluntary and electrically elicited contractions. *Journal of Applied Physiology*, 68(4), 1657–1667.

Kobayashi, H., Onishi, H., Ihashi, K., Yagi, R., & Handa, Y. (1999). Reduction in subluxation and improved muscle function of the hemiplegic shoulder joint after therapeutic electrical stimulation. *Journal of Electromyography and Kinesiology*, 9(5), 327–336.

Konishi, Y., Fukubayashi, T., & Takeshita, D. (2002). Mechanism of quadriceps femoris muscle weakness in patients with anterior cruciate ligament reconstruction. *Scandinavian Journal of Medicine & Science in Sports*, 12(6), 371–375.

Koyuncu, E., Nakipoğlu-Yüzer, G. F., Doğan, A., & Özgirgin, N. (2010). The effectiveness of functional electrical stimulation for the treatment of shoulder subluxation and shoulder pain in hemiplegic patients: A randomized controlled trial. *Disability & Rehabilitation*, 32(7), 560–566.

Kraft, G. H., Fitts, S. S., & Hammond, M. C. (1992). Techniques to improve function of the arm and hand in chronic hemiplegia. *Archives of Physical Medicine and Rehabilitation*, 73(3), 220–227.

Kramer, J. F. (1987). Effect of electrical stimulation current frequencies on isometric knee extension torque. *Physical Therapy*, 67(1), 31–38.

Kramer, J. F., Lindsay, D. M., Magee, D., Wall, T., & Mendryk, S. W. (1984). Comparison of voluntary and electrical stimulation contraction torques. *Journal of Orthopaedic & Sports Physical Therapy*, 5(6), 324–331.

Lake, D. A. (1992). Neuromuscular electrical stimulation. *Sports Medicine*, 13(5), 320–336.

Lake, D. A., & Wofford, N. H. (2011). Effect of therapeutic modalities on patients with patellofemoral pain syndrome: A systematic review. *Sports Health*, 3(2), 182–189.

Lambert, I., Tebbs, S. E., Hill, D., Moss, H. A., Davies, A. J., & Elliott, T. (2000). Interferential therapy machines as possible vehicles for cross-infection. *Journal of Hospital Infection*, 44(1), 59–64.

Lee, J., Baker, L. L., Johnson, R. E., & Tilson, J. K. (2017). Effectiveness of neuromuscular electrical stimulation for management of shoulder subluxation post-stroke: A systematic review with meta-analysis. *Clinical Rehabilitation*, 31(11), 1431–1444.

Lepley, L. K., Wojtys, E. M., & Palmieri-Smith, R. M. (2015). Combination of eccentric exercise and neuromuscular electrical stimulation to improve quadriceps function post-ACL reconstruction. *The Knee*, 22(3), 270–277.

Levine, M., McElroy, K., Stakich, V., & Cicco, J. (2013). Comparing conventional physical therapy rehabilitation with neuromuscular electrical stimulation after TKA. *Orthopedics*, 36(3), e324.

Liberson, W. T. (1961). Functional electrotherapy: Stimulation of the peroneal nerve synchronized with the swing phase of the gait of hemiplegic patients. *Archives of Physical Medicine*, 42, 101–105.

Licht, S. (1967). *Therapeutic electricity and ultraviolet radiation* (2nd ed.). New Haven, CT: Licht.

Lieber, R. L., & Kelly, M. J. (1991). Factors influencing quadriceps femoris muscle torque using transcutaneous neuromuscular electrical stimulation. *Physical Therapy*, 71(10), 715–721.

Lieber, R. L., & Kelly, M. J. (1993). Torque history of electrically stimulated human quadriceps: Implications for stimulation therapy. *Journal of Orthopaedic Research*, 11(1), 131–141.

Lindemans, F. W., & Zimmerman, A. N. (1979). Acute voltage, charge, and energy thresholds as functions of electrode size for electrical stimulation of the canine heart. *Cardiovascular Research*, 13(7), 383–391.

Linn, S. L., Granat, M. H., & Lees, K. R. (1999). Prevention of shoulder subluxation after stroke with electrical stimulation. *Stroke*, 30(5), 963–968.

Lin, Z., & Yan, T. (2011). Long-term effectiveness of neuromuscular electrical stimulation for promoting motor recovery of the upper extremity after stroke. *Journal of Rehabilitation Medicine*, 43(6), 506–510.

Love, F. M., Son, Y., & Thompson, W. J. (2003). Activity alters muscle reinnervation and terminal sprouting by reducing the number of Schwann cell pathways that grow to link synaptic sites. *Journal of Neurobiology*, 54(4), 566–576.

Maffiuletti, N. A. (2006). The use of electrostimulation exercise in competitive sport. *International Journal of Sports Physiology and Performance*, 1(4), 406–407.

Maffiuletti, N. A. (2010). Physiological and methodological considerations for the use of neuromuscular electrical stimulation. *European Journal of Applied Physiology*, 110(2), 223–234.

Maffiuletti, N. A., Roig, M., Karatzanos, E., & Nanas, S. (2013). Neuromuscular electrical stimulation for preventing skeletal-muscle weakness and wasting in critically ill patients: A systematic review. *BMC Medicine*, 11(1), 137.

Marciniak, C. (2011). Poststroke hypertonicity: Upper limb assessment and treatment. *Topics in Stroke Rehabilitation*, 18(3), 179–194.

Mariotti, G., Salciccia, S., Innocenzi, M., et al. (2015). Recovery of urinary continence after radical prostatectomy using early vs late pelvic floor electrical stimulation and biofeedback-associated treatment. *Urology, 86*(1), 115–121.

Matheson, G. O., Dunlop, R. J., McKenzie, D. C., Smith, C. F., & Allen, P. S. (1997). Force output and energy metabolism during neuromuscular electrical stimulation: A 31P-NMR study. *Scandinavian Journal of Rehabilitation Medicine, 29*(3), 175–180.

McNeal, D. R., & Baker, L. L. (1988). Effects of joint angle, electrodes and waveform on electrical stimulation of the quadriceps and hamstrings. *Annals of Biomedical Engineering, 16*(3), 299–310.

Meesen, R. L., Dendale, P., Cuypers, K., et al. (2010). Neuromuscular electrical stimulation as a possible means to prevent muscle tissue wasting in artificially ventilated and sedated patients in the intensive care unit: A pilot study. *Neuromodulation: Technology at the Neural Interface, 13*(4), 315–321.

Merletti, R., Knaflitz, M., & De Luca, C. J. (1992). Electrically evoked myoelectric signals. *Critical Reviews in Biomedical Engineering, 19*(4), 293–340.

Merletti, R., & Pinelli, P. (1980). A critical appraisal of neuromuscular stimulation and electrotherapy in neurorehabilitation. *European Neurology, 19*(1), 30–32.

Merletti, R., Zelaschi, F., Latella, D., Galli, M., Angeli, S., & Sessa, M. B. (1978). A control study of muscle force recovery in hemiparetic patients during treatment with functional electrical stimulation. *Scandinavian Journal of Rehabilitation Medicine, 10*(3), 147–154.

Mills, P. B., & Dossa, F. (2016). Transcutaneous electrical nerve stimulation for management of limb spasticity: A systematic review. *American Journal of Physical Medicine & Rehabilitation, 95*(4), 309–318.

Mizner, R. L., Stevens, J. E., & Snyder-Mackler, L. (2003). Voluntary activation and decreased force production of the quadriceps femoris muscle after total knee arthroplasty. *Physical Therapy, 83*(4), 359–365.

Mödlin, M., Forstner, C., Hofer, C., et al. (2005). Electrical stimulation of denervated muscles: First results of a clinical study. *Artificial Organs, 29*(3), 203–206.

Monaghan, B., Caulfield, B., & O'Mathúna, D. P. (2010). Surface neuromuscular electrical stimulation for quadriceps strengthening pre and post total knee replacement. *Cochrane Database of Systematic Reviews* (1), CD007177.

Moroni, R., Magnani, P., Haddad, J., Castro, R., & Brito, L. (2016). Conservative treatment of stress urinary incontinence: A systematic review with meta-analysis of randomized controlled trials. *Revista Brasileira de Ginecologia e Obstetrícia, 38*(2), 97.

Nolan, M. F. (1991). Conductive differences in electrodes used with transcutaneous electrical nerve stimulation devices. *Physical Therapy, 71*(10), 746–751.

Nosaka, K., Aldayel, A., Jubeau, M., & Chen, T. C. (2011). Muscle damage induced by electrical stimulation. *European Journal of Applied Physiology, 111*(10), 2427.

Nussbaum, E. L., Houghton, P., Anthony, J., Rennie, S., Shay, B. L., & Hoens, A. M. (2017). Neuromuscular electrical stimulation for treatment of muscle impairment: Critical review and recommendations for clinical practice. *Physiotherapy Canada/Physiothérapie Canada, 69*(5), 1–76.

Nyland, J., Mattocks, A., Kibbe, S., Kalloub, A., Greene, J. W., & Caborn, D. N. (2016). Anterior cruciate ligament reconstruction, rehabilitation, and return to play: 2015 update. *Open Access Journal of Sports Medicine, 7*, 21.

Paillard, T. (2008). Combined application of neuromuscular electrical stimulation and voluntary muscular contractions. *Sports Medicine, 38*(2), 161–177.

Palmieri-Smith, R. M., Thomas, A. C., Karvonen-Gutierrez, C., & Sowers, M. (2010). A clinical trial of neuromuscular electrical stimulation in improving quadriceps muscle strength and activation among women with mild and moderate osteoarthritis. *Physical Therapy, 90*(10), 1441–1452.

Panisset, M. G., Galea, M. P., & El-Ansary, D. (2016). Does early exercise attenuate muscle atrophy or bone loss after spinal cord injury? *Spinal Cord, 54*(2), 84.

Patriciu, A., Yoshida, K., Struijk, J. J., Demonte, T. P., Joy, M. L., & Stodkilde-Jorgensen, H. (2005). Current density imaging and electrically induced skin burns under surface electrodes. *IEEE Transactions on Bio-Medical Engineering, 52*(12), 2024–2031.

Peng, Y., Tenan, M. S., & Griffin, L. (2017). Recruitment properties in vastus medialis and vastus medialis Oblique in individuals with patellofemoral pain syndrome: 3627 Board #74 June 3 9. *Medicine & Science in Sports & Exercise, 49*(5S), 1035.

Petrofsky, J. S. (2004). Electrical stimulation: Neurophysiological basis and application. *Basic and Applied Myology, 14*(4), 205–213.

Petrofsky, J., Schwab, E., Cuneo, M., et al. (2006). Current distribution under electrodes in relation to stimulation current and skin blood flow: Are modern electrodes really providing the current distribution during stimulation we believe they are? *Journal of Medical Engineering & Technology, 30*(6), 368–381.

Petterson, S. C., Mizner, R. L., Stevens, J. E., et al. (2009). Improved function from progressive strengthening interventions after total knee arthroplasty: A randomized clinical trial with an imbedded prospective cohort. *Arthritis Care & Research, 61*(2), 174–183.

Pieber, K., Herceg, M., Paternostro-Sluga, T., & Schuhfried, O. (2015). Optimizing stimulation parameters in functional electrical stimulation of denervated muscles: A cross-sectional study. *Journal of NeuroEngineering and Rehabilitation, 12*(1), 51.

Poore, G. V. (1883). *Selections from the Clinical Works of Dr. Duchenne (de Boulogne)*. Translated, edited and condensed by G. V. Poore. London: New Sydenham Society.

Powell, J., Pandyan, A. D., Granat, M., Cameron, M., & Stott, D. J. (1999). Electrical stimulation of wrist extensors in poststroke hemiplegia. *Stroke, 30*(7), 1384–1389.

Prausnitz, M. R. (1996). The effects of electric current applied to skin: A review for transdermal drug delivery. *Advanced Drug Delivery Reviews, 18*(3), 395–425.

Puthucheary, Z. A., Rawal, J., McPhail, M., et al. (2013). Acute skeletal muscle wasting in critical illness. *Journal of the American Medical Association*, 310(15), 1591–1600.

Rebai, H., Barra, V., Laborde, A., Bonny, J., Poumarat, G., & Coudert, J. (2002). Effects of two electrical stimulation frequencies in thigh muscle after knee surgery. *International Journal of Sports Medicine*, 23(8), 604–609.

Rice, D. A., McNair, P. J., & Lewis, G. N. (2011). Mechanisms of quadriceps muscle weakness in knee joint osteoarthritis: The effects of prolonged vibration on torque and muscle activation in osteoarthritic and healthy control subjects. *Arthritis Research and Therapy*, 13(5), R151.

Richmond, C., Martin, D., Yip, S., Dick, M., & Erekson, E. (2016). Effect of supervised pelvic floor biofeedback and electrical stimulation in women with mixed and stress urinary incontinence. *Female Pelvic Medicine & Reconstructive Surgery*, 22(5), 324–327.

Robinson, A. J., & Snyder-Mackler, L. (1995). *Clinical electrophysiology: electrotherapy and Electrophysiological testing* (2nd ed.). Philadelphia My copy states: Baltimore, Maryland: Williams & Wilkins.

Rodriguez, P. O., Setten, M., Maskin, L. P., et al. (2012). Muscle weakness in septic patients requiring mechanical ventilation: Protective effect of transcutaneous neuromuscular electrical stimulation. *Journal of Critical Care*, 27(3), 319. e1-8.

Rose, J., Cahill-Rowley, K., & Butler, E. E. (2017). Artificial walking technologies to improve gait in cerebral palsy: Multichannel neuromuscular stimulation. *Artificial Organs*, 41(11), E239.

Rosemffet, M. G., Schneeberger, E. E., Citera, G., et al. (2004). Effects of functional electrostimulation on pain, muscular strength, and functional capacity in patients with osteoarthritis of the knee. *Journal of Clinical Rheumatology*, 10(5), 246–249.

Rosewilliam, S., Malhotra, S., Roffe, C., Jones, P., & Pandyan, A. D. (2012). Can surface neuromuscular electrical stimulation of the wrist and hand combined with routine therapy facilitate recovery of arm function in patients with stroke? *Archives of Physical Medicine and Rehabilitation*, 93(10), 17–21. e1.

Routsi, C., Gerovasili, V., Vasileiadis, I., et al. (2010). Electrical muscle stimulation prevents critical illness polyneuromyopathy: A randomized parallel intervention trial. *Critical Care*, 14(2), R74.

Rushton, W. (1932). Identification of Lucas's α excitability. *The Journal of Physiology*, 75(4), 445–470.

Ryan, T. E., Erickson, M. L., Young, H., & McCully, K. K. (2013). Case report: Endurance electrical stimulation training improves skeletal muscle oxidative capacity in chronic spinal cord injury. *Archives of Physical Medicine and Rehabilitation*, 94(12), 2559–2561.

Sabut, S. K., Sikdar, C., Kumar, R., & Mahadevappa, M. (2011). Functional electrical stimulation of dorsiflexor muscle: Effects on dorsiflexor strength, plantarflexor spasticity, and motor recovery in stroke patients. *NeuroRehabilitation*, 29(4), 393–400.

Sadowsky, C. L., Hammond, E. R., Strohl, A. B., et al. (2013). Lower extremity functional electrical stimulation cycling promotes physical and functional recovery in chronic spinal cord injury. *The Journal of Spinal Cord Medicine*, 36(6), 623–631.

Scott, W. B., Causey, J. B., & Marshall, T. L. (2009). Comparison of maximum tolerated muscle torques produced by 2 pulse durations. *Physical Therapy*, 89(8), 851–857.

Segers, J., Hermans, G., Bruyninckx, F., Meyfroidt, G., Langer, D., & Gosselink, R. (2014). Feasibility of neuromuscular electrical stimulation in critically ill patients. *Journal of Critical Care*, 29(6), 1082–1088.

Selkowitz, D. M. (1985). Improvement in isometric strength of the quadriceps femoris muscle after training with electrical stimulation. *Physical Therapy*, 65(2), 186–196.

Sillen, M. J., Franssen, F. M., Delbressine, J. M., Vaes, A. W., Wouters, E. F., & Spruit, M. A. (2014). Efficacy of lower-limb muscle training modalities in severely dyspnoeic individuals with COPD and quadriceps muscle weakness: Results from the DICES trial. *Thorax*, 69(6), 525–531.

Sivaramakrishnan, A., Solomon, J. M., & Manikandan, N. (2018). Comparison of transcutaneous electrical nerve stimulation (TENS) and functional electrical stimulation (FES) for spasticity in spinal cord injury - A pilot randomized cross-over trial. *The Journal of Spinal Cord Medicine*, 41(4), 397–406.

Sköld, C., Levi, R., & Seiger, Å. (1999). Spasticity after traumatic spinal cord injury: Nature, severity, and location. *Archives of Physical Medicine and Rehabilitation*, 80(12), 1548–1557.

Slemenda, C., Brandt, K. D., Heilman, D. K., et al. (1997). Quadriceps weakness and osteoarthritis of the knee. *Annals of Internal Medicine*, 127(2), 97–104.

Smith, G. V., Alon, G., Roys, S. R., & Gullapalli, R. P. (2003). Functional MRI determination of a dose-response relationship to lower extremity neuromuscular electrical stimulation in healthy subjects. *Experimental Brain Research*, 150(1), 33–39.

Snyder-Mackler, L., Delitto, A., Bailey, S. L., & Stralka, S. W. (1995). Strength of the quadriceps femoris muscle and functional recovery after reconstruction of the anterior cruciate ligament. A prospective, randomized clinical trial of electrical stimulation. *The Journal of Bone & Joint Surgery*, 77(8), 1166–1173.

Snyder-Mackler, L., Delitto, A., Stralka, S. W., & Bailey, S. L. (1994). Use of electrical stimulation to enhance recovery of quadriceps femoris muscle force production in patients following anterior cruciate ligament reconstruction. *Physical Therapy*, 74(10), 901–907.

Snyder-Mackler, L., Garrett, M., & Roberts, M. (1989). A comparison of torque generating capabilities of three different electrical stimulating currents. *Journal of Orthopaedic & Sports Physical Therapy*, 10(8), 297–301.

Solomonow, M. (1984). External control of the neuromuscular system. *IEEE Transactions on Biomedical Engineering*, 31(12), 752–763.

Stein, R. B., Chong, S. L., James, K. B., et al. (2002). Electrical stimulation for therapy and mobility after spinal cord injury. *Progress in Brain Research*, 137, 27–34.

Stevens-Lapsley, J. E., Balter, J. E., Wolfe, P., Eckhoff, D. G., & Kohrt, W. M. (2012a). Early neuromuscular electrical stimulation to improve quadriceps muscle strength after total knee arthroplasty: A randomized controlled trial. *Physical Therapy*, 92(2), 210–226.

Stevens-Lapsley, J. E., Balter, J. E., Wolfe, P., et al. (2012b). Relationship between intensity of quadriceps muscle neuromuscular electrical stimulation and strength recovery after total knee arthroplasty. *Physical Therapy*, 92(9), 1187–1196.

Stevens, J. E., Mizner, R. L., & Snyder-Mackler, L. (2004). Neuromuscular electrical stimulation for quadriceps muscle strengthening after bilateral total knee arthroplasty: A case series. *Journal of Orthopaedic & Sports Physical Therapy*, *34*(1), 21–29.

Stewart, F., Berghmans, B., Bø, K., & Glazener, C. M. (2017). Electrical stimulation with non-implanted devices for stress urinary incontinence in women. *Cochrane Database of Systematic Reviews* (*12*), CD012390.

Stewart, F., Gameiro, L. F., El Dib, R., Gameiro, M. O., Kapoor, A., & Amaro, J. L. (2016). Electrical stimulation with non-implanted electrodes for overactive bladder in adults. *Cochrane Database of Systematic Reviews* (*12*), CD010098.

Talbot, L. A., Gaines, J. M., Ling, S. M., & Metter, E. J. (2003). A home-based protocol of electrical muscle stimulation for quadriceps muscle strength in older adults with osteoarthritis of the knee. *Journal of Rheumatology*, *30*(7), 1571–1578.

Tam, S. L., & Gordon, T. (2003). Neuromuscular activity impairs axonal sprouting in partially denervated muscles by inhibiting bridge formation of perisynaptic Schwann cells. *Journal of Neurobiology*, *57*(2), 221–234.

Taradaj, J., Halski, T., Kucharzewski, M., et al. (2013). The effect of neuromuscular electrical stimulation on quadriceps strength and knee function in professional soccer players: Return to sport after ACL reconstruction. *BioMed Research International*, *2013*.

Türkkan, C., Öztürk, G. T., Uğurlu, F. G., & Ersöz, M. (2017). Ultrasonographic assessment of neuromuscular electrical stimulation efficacy on glenohumeral subluxation in patients with hemiplegia: A randomized-controlled study. *Turkish Journal of Physical Medicine and Rehabilitation*, *63*(4), 287–293.

Turner-Stokes, L., & Jackson, D. (2002). Shoulder pain after stroke: A review of the evidence base to inform the development of an integrated care pathway. *Clinical Rehabilitation*, *16*(3), 276–298.

Tyerman, L. (1890). *The life and times of the Rev. John Wesley, M.A.: Founder of the Methodists.* (Vol. 2). Hodder and Stoughton.

Vafadar, A. K., Côté, J. N., & Archambault, P. S. (2015). Effectiveness of functional electrical stimulation in improving clinical outcomes in the upper arm following stroke: A systematic review and meta-analysis. *BioMed Research International*, *2015*.

Valenti, F. (1964). Neuromuscular electrostimulation in clinical practice. *Acta Anaesthesiologica Italica*, *15*, 227–245.

Van Peppen, R. P., Kwakkel, G., Wood-Dauphinee, S., Hendriks, H. J., Van Der Wees, P. J., et al. (2004). The impact of physical therapy on functional outcomes after stroke: What's the evidence? *Clinical Rehabilitation*, *18*(8), 833–862.

Vanderthommen, M., Depresseux, J., Dauchat, L., Degueldre, C., Croisier, J., & Crielaard, J. (2000). Spatial distribution of blood flow in electrically stimulated human muscle: A positron emission tomography study. *Muscle & Nerve*, *23*(4), 482–489.

Vanderthommen, M., & Duchateau, J. (2007). Electrical stimulation as a modality to improve performance of the neuromuscular system. *Exercise and Sport Sciences Reviews*, *35*(4), 180–185.

Veerbeek, J. M., Van Wegen, E., Van Peppen, R., et al. (2014). What is the evidence for physical therapy poststroke? A systematic review and meta-analysis. *PLoS One*, *9*(2), e87987.

Viana, R., Pereira, S., Mehta, S., Miller, T., & Teasell, R. (2012). Evidence for therapeutic interventions for hemiplegic shoulder pain during the chronic stage of stroke: A review. *Topics in Stroke Rehabilitation*, *19*(6), 514–522.

Vieira, T. M., Potenza, P., Gastaldi, L., & Botter, A. (2016). Electrode position markedly affects knee torque in tetanic, stimulated contractions. *European Journal of Applied Physiology*, *116*(2), 335–342.

Vivodtzev, I., Debigaré, R., Gagnon, P., et al. (2012). Functional and muscular effects of neuromuscular electrical stimulation in patients with severe COPD: A randomized clinical trial. *Chest*, *141*(3), 716–725.

Wall, B. T., Dirks, M. L., Verdijk, L. B., et al. (2012). Neuromuscular electrical stimulation increases muscle protein synthesis in elderly type 2 diabetic men. *American Journal of Physiology-Endocrinology and Metabolism*, *303*(5), E614–E623.

Walls, R. J., McHugh, G., O'Gorman, D. J., Moyna, N. M., & O'Byrne, J. M. (2010). Effects of preoperative neuromuscular electrical stimulation on quadriceps strength and functional recovery in total knee arthroplasty. A pilot study. *BMC Musculoskeletal Disorders*, *11*(1), 119.

Walmsley, R. P., Letts, G., & Vooys, J. (1984). A comparison of torque generated by knee extension with a maximal voluntary muscle contraction vis-a-vis electrical stimulation. *Journal of Orthopaedic & Sports Physical Therapy*, *6*(1), 10–17.

Wang, R., Chan, R., & Tsai, M. (2000). Functional electrical stimulation on chronic and acute hemiplegic shoulder subluxation. *American Journal of Physical Medicine & Rehabilitation*, *79*(4), 385–394.

Watanabe, S., Fukuhara, S., Fujinaga, T., & Oka, H. (2017). Estimating the minimum stimulation frequency necessary to evoke tetanic progression based on muscle twitch parameters. *Physiological Measurement*, *38*(3), 466.

Wattchow, K. A., McDonnell, M. N., & Hillier, S. L. (2018). Rehabilitation interventions for upper limb function in the first four weeks following stroke: A systematic review and meta-analysis of the evidence. *Archives of Physical Medicine and Rehabilitation*, *99*(2), 367–382.

Wilk, K. E., Macrina, L. C., Cain, E. L., Dugas, J. R., & Andrews, J. R. (2012). Recent advances in the rehabilitation of anterior cruciate ligament injuries. *Journal of Orthopaedic & Sports Physical Therapy*, *42*(3), 153–171.

Williams, J. G., & Street, M. (1976). Sequential faradism in quadriceps rehabilitation. *Physiotherapy*, *62*(8), 252.

World Health Organization. (2015). Chronic rheumatic conditions. Online. Available: http://www.who.int/chp/topics/rheumatic/en/.

Wyndaele, J. (2016). Study on the influence of the type of current and the frequency of impulses used for electrical stimulation on the contraction of pelvic muscles with different fibre content. *Scandinavian Journal of Urology*, *50*(3), 228–233.

Yildizgören, M. T., Yüzer, G. F. N., Ekiz, T., & Özgirgin, N. (2014). Effects of neuromuscular electrical stimulation on the wrist and finger flexor spasticity and hand functions in cerebral palsy. *Pediatric Neurology*, *51*(3), 360–364.

Yue, C., Zhang, X., Zhu, Y., Jia, Y., Wang, H., & Liu, Y. (2018). Systematic review of three electrical stimulation techniques for rehabilitation after total knee arthroplasty. *The Journal of Arthroplasty*, 33(7), 2330–2337.

Zanotti, E., Felicetti, G., Maini, M., & Fracchia, C. (2003). Peripheral muscle strength training in bed-bound patients with COPD receiving mechanical ventilation: Effect of electrical stimulation. *Chest*, 124(1), 292–296.

Zhou, B., Baratta, R., & Solomonow, M. (1987). Manipulation of muscle force with various firing rate and recruitment control strategies. *IEEE Transactions on Biomedical Engineering* (2), 128–139.

17

Functional Electrical Stimulation (FES)

Sally Durham, Sarah Taylor

CHAPTER OUTLINE

INTRODUCTION

Functional electrical stimulation (FES) is the application of electrical impulses to produce a muscle contraction that mimics voluntary movement, in order to restore lost or impaired function. One of the earliest published examples of FES was as a gait assist for patients with flaccid foot drop (Liberson et al 1961). Simple one-channel stimulation to the ankle dorsiflexors during swing phase of gait is still the most widely used clinical application of FES, though with the development of more sophisticated equipment and mechanisms for the triggering and timing of stimulation, functional applications are expanding.

PHYSICAL PRINCIPLES

In most reported applications of FES, electrical impulses are applied to innervated muscles such that impulses result in nerve depolarization and then subsequent muscle contraction. Stimulation parameters for innervated muscles range from frequencies of 10–100 Hz and pulse duration of 100–1000 μs. The amplitude of the stimulus varies with application and the impedance characteristics of the patient; for surface stimulation values up to 120 mA are not uncommon. Direct stimulation of denervated muscles requires much higher pulse durations in order to directly depolarize muscle fibres and therefore requires different stimulation

equipment. Although this is an interesting application of electrical stimulation, the rest of this chapter will focus upon the application of FES to innervated muscles.

The electrical impulses may be applied using skin surface electrodes, percutaneous electrodes (e.g. through the skin and into the muscle belly, near the motor point), or totally implanted electrodes (e.g. peripheral nerve cuffs or spinal roots, receiving power and control through radio frequency link from an external unit), with skin electrodes being the most common in routine clinical practice.

The use of a triggering mechanism that allows stimulation to replicate a lost movement at the correct time, for example ankle dorsiflexion in swing phase of gait, or wrist and finger extension to allow grasp of an object, is what differentiates FES from neuromuscular electrical stimulation (NMES).

BIOPHYSICAL EFFECTS

Use of FES in upper motor neuron lesions (UMNLs) is accompanied by biophysical changes at both peripheral (nerve and muscle) and 'central' (cortical) levels (Rushton 2003). At the peripheral level, FES, like NMES, has the potential to improve both muscle strength and length as well as modulate spasticity.

Muscles affected by UMNL have an altered ratio of fibre types with a higher proportion of fast twitch, fatigable fibres.

FES has been shown to induce both muscle hypertrophy and to increase the force of muscle contraction (Newsam & Baker 2004). Following FES to the ankle dorsiflexors in patients post stroke, Kottink et al (2008) reported significant improvements in the RMSmax during a maximal voluntary contraction of the muscles; and Shendkar et al (2015) report an increase in tibialis anterior (TA) muscle activity during gait measured by surface EMG activity. These results are indicative of both improved motor strength and the velocity of nerve fibre conduction. Regular use of FES in children with Cerebral Palsy resulted in use-dependent muscle plasticity, with increases in muscle cross-sectional area and muscle thickness, together with improvement in the active range of ankle dorsiflexion (Damiano et al 2012). However, improvements in muscle properties in patients with UMNLs do not necessarily translate into improvements in function. For example, Hazlewood et al (1995) demonstrated an increase in range of motion at the ankle joint in children with hemiplegic cerebral palsy following NMES, but this was not accompanied by improvement in walking.

There are varying approaches to the use of stimulation to modify muscle activation patterns during gait. Stimulation of the agonist muscles is thought to reduce spasticity in the antagonist by reciprocal inhibition. For example, stimulation of the anterior tibial muscle group has been shown to reduce spasticity in the ankle plantar flexors; Yan (2005) reported a reduction in calf spasticity and an improvement in DF activity following reciprocal stimulation of both during walking.

In order to promote motor re-learning and recovery of function, neuroplastic changes must occur at the central level. Kafri and Laufer (2015) summarize evidence that FES has the potential to enhance brain plasticity. They conclude from functional Magnetic Resonance Imaging studies that FES-induced movement concurrent with voluntary movement/effort can alter cortical excitability and promote neuronal plasticity at different levels of the nervous system. When used together, FES and active movement were associated with multiple effects that included increased brain activity in the primary motor cortex, the primary and secondary somatosensory cortices, the sensorimotor cortex and the cerebellum, as well as increased coupling between specific brain regions.

FES combined with voluntary movement and user 'ownership' of the movement is reported to give better results in terms of changes in brain activity than FES alone in patients following stroke (Nudo 2003) and in patients with spinal cord injury (SCI) (Gater et al 2011). These neuroplastic changes are not seen with passive movement alone. Rushton (2003) describes enhanced synchronization between pre- and post-synaptic activation when FES is coupled with voluntary movement.

Furthermore, Damiano et al (2012) suggested that it is possible that the user could become dependent on FES

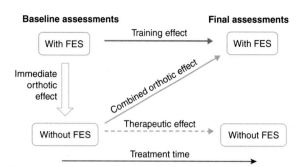

Fig. 17.1 Representation of the different effects that can be described for a period of use of FES. (Adapted from Kluding PM et al 2013.)

unless voluntary movement is incorporated at the same time. As a result of the movement being generated externally by the device and not internally through voluntary effort, it cannot be considered task-specific practice.

In summary, the biophysical effect of physiological changes at peripheral and central levels may be to achieve long-term therapeutic benefit, which must be a major goal of rehabilitation therapy.

CLINICAL EVIDENCE

The most common clinical application of FES is for the correction of foot drop resulting from UMNL and is where the majority of evidence relating to FES lies. FES for foot drop involves stimulation of the common peroneal nerve such that contraction of the dorsiflexor muscles occurs during the swing phase of gait. Whilst research tends to be focused on the adult population, there is evidence to support its use in children with UMNL (Moll et al 2017).

In this section, the evidence for the orthotic (immediate and combined) effect of FES. The definitions provided by Prenton (2016) are helpful (Fig. 17.1):

- **Immediate orthotic effect** – a same day comparison of the unassisted (without device) walking to the assisted walking (with device).
- **Therapeutic effects** – the effects of the device on the patient's unaided walking; a comparison of baseline unassisted walking with the patient's unassisted walking some time later following a period of use of the device.
- **Training effects** – a comparison of the patient's assisted walking at baseline with their assisted walking some time later.
- **Combined orthotic effect** – a comparison of the unassisted walking at baseline to the assisted walking following a period of use of the device. This effect will include any therapeutic and training effects.

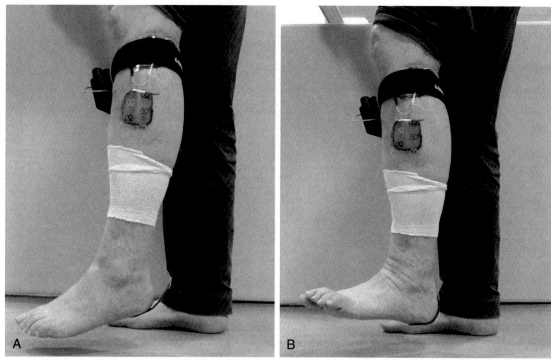

Fig. 17.2 FES applied to correct foot drop in a patient following stroke. (A) FES switched off showing plantar-flexed foot in swing. (B) FES switched on (triggered through a foot switch) showing a dorsiflexed foot in swing.

Orthotic Effects – Foot Drop

Foot drop results in toe catch and tripping, which impacts on walking safety, endurance and speed. FES applied to the dorsiflexors (Figs 17.2 and 17.3) during swing phase using a simple one-channel system has been repeatedly shown to have an immediate positive orthotic effect on ankle DF, clinically meaningful increases in walking speed, reduction of trips and falls and reduction of energy costs (Bethoux et al 2014; O'Dell et al 2014; Springer and Khamis 2017; Taylor et al 1999b). Improvements in swing knee flexion have also been achieved as a result of the withdrawal reflex, which might be initiated by common peroneal nerve stimulation (Scott et al 2013).

Gervasoni et al (2017) examined the combined orthotic effect on foot clearance and found that, on average, participants' swing-phase foot clearance increased by 5 mm with FES following 4 weeks of use, together with a reduction in the number of reported falls, supporting earlier work by Esnouf et al (2010). This could explain an increase in confidence in walking as reported in an audit of FES users (Taylor et al 2004).

A reduction in effort of walking has been cited as a primary reason to use FES for gait assist (Taylor et al 2004). The reduction in effort described here is supported by changes in Borg RPE Scale (Khurana et al 2017) along with a reduction in physiological cost index (PCI) (Paul et al 2008). There are, however, other contradictory studies that do not support this (Barrett et al 2009; Miller et al 2015). In each of these studies comparing effort with and without FES, the subjects were walking in optimal conditions, indoors on flat surfaces. Burridge et al (2007), however, found that PCI only reduced with stimulation when subjects were walking on more challenging surfaces. Miller et al (2016) also found that changes in energy expenditure were dependent upon the patient's initial walking speed; those with slower speeds saw a positive improvement in energy expenditure with FES.

Esnouf et al (2010) showed a clinically meaningful improvement in user-reported quality of life as measured by the Canadian Occupational Performance Measure (COPM), alongside a reduction in falls, a perception of reduced trips and an increase in walking distance in the FES group. Laufer et al (2009) described a significant combined orthotic effect of increased participation over a 1-year period of using FES demonstrated by the Stroke Impact Scale (SIS). However, in this study there was no control group. Examining participation is difficult, particularly when rehabilitation is ongoing or patients are adapting to a newly acquired disability.

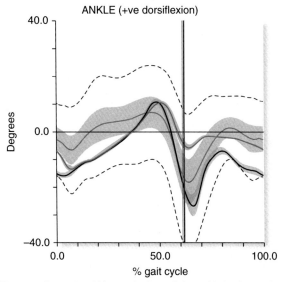

Fig. 17.3 Example of kinematic data of the ankle in the sagittal plane during gait. *Thin black line with grey band*— local normative adult mean ±1.5 stdev; *dotted lines = ±4.5 stdev; bold black line* – FES off ±1 stdev; *Green line*– FES on ±1 stdev. FES corrects the reduced dorsiflexion in swing and initial contact. It also negatively reduces the plantarflexion at toe off; this is to be expected as the device used here (PACE, Odstock Medical) was triggered via a heel switch. FES therefore ramps on during pre-swing ready for toe off. (Data source: Queen Mary's Hospital, Roehampton.)

The cost of use of an ODFS PACE (Odstock Medical Ltd, wired foot switch) over a 5-year period is, on average, estimated at £3,320, compared to an ankle foot orthosis (AFO), which is, on average, estimated at £615 over a 5-year period (NICE 2016). The evidence available suggests that FES provides a comparable immediate and combined orthotic effect to that of an AFO in terms of gait speed, physiological cost index (PCI) and perceived safety (Bethoux et al 2015; Everaert et al 2013; Kluding et al 2013; Prenton et al 2016; Sheffler et al 2006, 2009).

FES shows no superior orthotic effect across users with a range of diagnoses. However there is strong evidence that some patients prefer FES, having rejected an AFO (Everaert et al 2013; Kafri & Laufer 2015; Sheffler et al 2006). In our clinical experience, many patients with MS or stroke show a clear preference for FES, finding it lighter, less restrictive, less hot to wear and/or find it more effective in assisting walking. Reasons cited for rejecting AFOs include discomfort, activity restriction (e.g. stairs or getting up from the floor), restrictions on footwear, weight of the AFO and the perception that gait was 'non normal' (Bulley et al 2011). Barriers to use of FES include difficulties with set up, restrictions in clothing (cosmetically) and fear of device failure. For this reason, some patients decide to use both an

AFO and FES, choosing one or the other depending on the circumstances, clothing/footwear choice or time available to get ready on any particular day. Evidence comparing the therapeutic effects of using FES versus an AFO is inconclusive and is discussed in the following section.

Multichannel Systems

Use of FES for assistance in walking is not limited to foot drop. Dual and multichannel systems allow additional muscle groups to be stimulated; for example, the calf to enhance push off (Kesar et al 2009), or proximal muscles to improve hip or knee control (Kim et al 2012; Springer et al 2012, 2013). Each channel of stimulation may be timed differently in order to coincide with the appropriate phase of gait. For example, stimulation of the quadriceps during terminal swing and loading response to aid knee extension and stability (Springer et al 2012, 2013).

There is limited published literature on the additional orthotic benefits of these additional stimulation channels. Springer et al (2012) attempted to examine the effect of quadriceps or hamstring stimulation (timing and group dependent on gait dysfunction) and found that there was a further significant improvement in overground and obstacle course walking speed on top of that provided by dorsiflexion stimulation alone; on average, between 0.02 and 0.04 m/s additional improvement. An additional channel of stimulation for the gluteus medius during stance in addition to stimulation for foot drop has also been shown to improve gait symmetry and temporal spatial parameters (Kim et al 2012). Further research is required to understand how much these changes impact participation and quality of life over and above that offered by stimulation for foot drop.

The Bioness L300 Go (and L300, Ottobock) offers a practical method of applying an additional channel to the thigh (hamstrings or quadriceps) through the use of a cuff and wireless sensing technology (Fig. 17.4); without this, dual-channel stimulation can become cumbersome to use and set up due to the number of wires and switches that may be needed.

Multichannel FES devices that stimulate many lower extremity muscle groups are used for gait training and cycle training, particularly for patients with SCI; however, these systems are not widely available outside specialist rehabilitation units at present. The Xcite (Restorative Therapies) multichannel FES system has been reportedly used for gait training in children with CP with positive changes in some cases (Rose et al 2017). This device, however, has no triggering input and therefore the timing of stimulation of each muscle group can only be adjusted manually – the system does not adapt to the user's pace of walking without input. As a result of this, it can be described as a therapeutic device only.

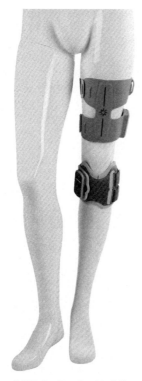

Fig. 17.4 Bioness L300 Go (Ottobock). Offers both a dorsiflexor and thigh cuff to give a practical method of donning and doffing a dual-channel system. (Source Ottobock (2019).)

For higher-level injuries or those with complete spinal cord injury, stimulation of the lower limb for standing, walking or cycling has been reported, but requires significantly more channels of stimulation to be effective. Eight channels of electrical stimulation can be used to power the sit-to-stand transition and standing for, on average, 10 minutes (Triolo et al 2012), which may enable greater participation in social, leisure or household activities. Use of the stimulation reduced the requirements on the upper limb for support with up to 90% of weight bearing through the lower legs.

Stepping of 369 m has also been achieved in some cases, using pre-programmed stimulation of 8- and 16-channel implanted electrodes (Hardin et al 2007; Kobetic et al 1999). Kobetic et al (1999) reported limitations as a result of ineffective recruitment of the required muscles and muscular fatigue on the single patient it was tried on. Hardin et al (2007) found a significant training effect but no therapeutic effect over a 12-week period of use.

One of the main current uses of FES in the spinal cord population is for cycling, and there are commercial systems available (Restorative Therapies) (Fig. 17.5). Multiple channels of stimulation are used to allow the patient to cycle a static bike, and this is used to provide cardiovascular exercise. There is an indication that this has a potential to increase muscle mass and quality of life of individuals using it long term (3 sessions of 45–60 minutes per week) (Sadowsky et al 2013).

Some studies have attempted to look at the additional therapeutic changes offered by multiple channels of stimulation in the acute phases of stroke rehabilitation; however,

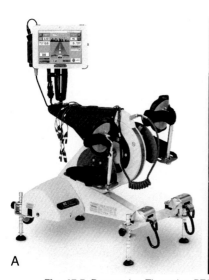

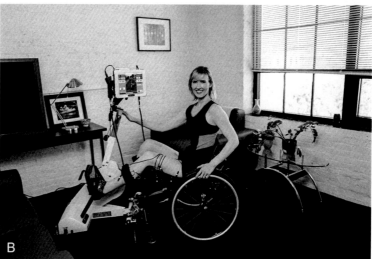

A   B

Fig. 17.5 Restorative Therapies RT300-SL allows 6 to 16 channels of stimulation for pedalling a static bike without having to transfer from the wheelchair. (Source Cyclone website (2019).)

it is difficult to draw conclusions owing to the large variation in muscle groups stimulated, study design and treatment periods.

Guidelines

The Royal College of Physicians' Stroke Rehabilitation (RCP 2016) Guidelines (United Kingdom) recommend the use of FES in stroke patients who have foot drop; the National Institute for Health and Care Excellence interventional procedure guidelines also support the use of FES for foot drop caused by UMNL (NICE 2009). The National Health Service (United Kingdom) funding arrangements are in place but may differ between local commissioning groups. The RCP guidelines indicate that any additional (non-foot drop) therapeutic use of FES for the lower limb should be in the context of a clinical trial.

Recommendations for the use of FES for gait assist are included in other national guidelines, including the Australian Clinical Guidelines for Stroke Management 2017, the American Heart Association/American Stroke Association Guidelines for adult stroke rehabilitation and recovery (2016) and the Canadian stroke best practice recommendations: Stroke rehabilitation practice guidelines, update 2015. Medicare (USA) will consider coverage of FES for SCI patients to enable walking provided certain conditions are met. Examples of FDA approved products included were the Parastep, RT300, NESS L300, Walkaide and PACE.

THERAPEUTIC EFFECTS AND USES

While there is strong evidence for the use of FES as an orthotic device, the evidence for therapeutic changes ('carry over') or motor learning is less clear. Use of FES has consistently been shown to have therapeutic effects on various outcome measures related to mobility (Kafri & Laufer 2015). However, improvements are also reported following use of AFOs.

Studies (Everaert et al 2013; Kluding et al 2013; Sheffler et al 2013, 2015) have shown therapeutic improvements in unaided walking over various treatment periods ranging from 6 to 30 weeks following either FES or AFO use. Kottink et al (2008), on the other hand, did not find a significant therapeutic effect for AFOs or FES for walking speed over a 6-month treatment period. Despite this, from the evidence available, one can conclude that AFOs and FES offer comparable therapeutic benefits on functional mobility and quality of life in the stroke population (Prenton et al 2018).

It could be argued that changes in gait speed and kinetic parameters are not as a result of motor recovery but rather from improvements in overall mobility. In fact,

those studies that do report on swing phase dorsiflexion and tibilis anterior activation during gait do not demonstrate an improvement, and some indicate a reduction in peak swing dorsiflexion (Kottink et al 2008; Sheffler et al 2015). The improvements in mobility may be attributable to the orthotic effects that these interventions allow, such as increased confidence and safety, and increased walking distance and speed, which in turn may facilitate task-specific repetitive practice, which is widely accepted as leading to therapeutic improvement (Langhorne et al 2009). Further research is needed to identify the origin of these therapeutic changes, for example using kinematics, kinetics, EMG and activity monitoring in the home environment.

Kafri and Laufer (2015) concluded that although FES resulted in clinically significant therapeutic improvements, there was not enough evidence to draw a conclusion over its superiority compared to other standard rehabilitation interventions. Furthermore, they conclude that the therapeutic changes achieved by using FES generally were not of a magnitude that meant patients no longer needed to use the FES to assist with their walking.

Several studies have indicated that use of an AFO or FES may have the potential to reduce the activity/recruitment of the dorsiflexor muscles over a period of 6 months (Kottink et al 2008; Sheffler et al 2015). This mirrors the suggestion made by Damiano et al (2012) that users may become dependent on orthoses/FES as there is no voluntary effort involved.

The lack of evidence to support a therapeutic effect greater than other standard treatments is surprising given the evidence that FES has the potential to promote neural plasticity and enhance motor learning. One explanation may be that as Gandolla (2016) observed, only certain individuals experience carry over, specifically those with the ability to plan the movement and perceive stimulation as part of their own control loop. Systems utilizing biosignals (EMG) to trigger FES during walking may therefore be beneficial as this would encourage voluntary effort from users, tapping into this control loop.

Upper Limb Systems

To date, much of the focus on upper limb electrical stimulation has been on its therapeutic benefits rather than as an orthosis to achieve function. The primary reason for this is the difficulty with triggering a reliable and useful movement for upper limb activities of daily living that do not follow a repeatable cyclic movement in the way the lower limb does during gait. Difficulties recruiting the required muscles can also be problematic as a result of the anatomy of the arm. Achieving a practical functional aid, therefore, is difficult. The Bioness H200 (Fig.

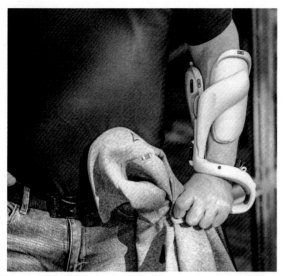

Fig. 17.6 The Bioness H200 (Ottobock) can be used for functional tasks through the use of a button on the device or remote control. (Source: Ottobock.)

17.6) is the most recent commercial device that has both therapeutic and functional modes. Functional tasks are triggered through the use of a control unit that has been pre-programmed with specific tasks, such as grasp and release. Several studies indicate possible additional therapeutic benefits over and above typical therapy; none have looked at the orthotic functional changes seen in activities of daily living whilst using the device (Alon et al 2007; Ring & Rosenthal 2005). ETHZ-paracare is another functional system that has been reported upon (Popovic et al 2002); it consists of four channels of stimulation that can be interfaced with various control inputs. Popovic et al (2006) found that SCI patients were able to use the device to improve their ability to conduct ADLs.

The Second Generation Freehand system (Kilgore et al 2008) involves transfer of tendons together with the implantation of electrodes in the muscles of the forearm and hand of patients with tetraplegia. The electrode wires go up the arm to a control box located under the skin in the pectoral region. Two EMG channels on the ipsilateral upper limb are used to control the system. One channel, usually on the most distal muscle that has voluntary control, is used to control the grasp opening and closing. A second channel is used to provide system commands such as on/off or selection of the grasp pattern; this channel is usually placed on a proximal muscle, such as the trapezius. The use of the ipsilateral limb is to allow bilateral systems to be implanted. Improvements in ADLs have been reported (Kilgore et al 2008) both with this system and with the first-generation design (Mulcahey et al 2004; Taylor et al

2002). This system does not appear to be commercially available, however.

APPLICATION

FES is used to restore or reproduce function. The initial step before the application of FES must be a comprehensive assessment of the potential user to establish the issues to be addressed. From this, the decision on which muscles to target and the timing of stimulation should be clear. This will also enable clear and measurable goal setting.

There are a variety of commercially available devices designed to deliver FES to assist walking (Table 17.1). The DMO flexitrode sock/cuff system is also available in Europe and is designed to provide physical orthotic support with built in electrodes to form a hybrid of traditional orthotic and FES systems (DM Orthotics). The technology of each system varies, but they all include a stimulation unit, which allows the user to set stimulation parameters, and an event detection device to trigger the stimulation. It is the use of a triggering mechanism allowing precise timing of stimulation appropriate to the functional task that differentiates a machine designed for FES from one designed to deliver NMES.

Skin surface electrodes are the most commonly used in routine clinical practice. Self-adhesive electrodes come in various shapes and sizes and with various types of gel. Alternatives include fabric and silicone electrodes. These may be particularly useful as an alternative should skin irritation arise when using gel electrodes. Recent innovations in electrode design include the development of wearable electronic textiles (Yang et al 2018) and multipad electrode arrays (Malešević et al 2017). Electrode size and positioning are selected using the same criteria as discussed for NMES in Chapter 16. In some cases, for gait assist, rather than direct stimulation of the motor nerve, stimulation may be used to target a reflex action. The classic example is that of stimulation of the common peroneal nerve withdrawal reflex, which, if successful, can lead to a combination of hip and knee flexion as well ankle dorsiflexion to assist foot clearance during walking.

Historically, gait assist devices with implantable electrodes have been commercially available; currently, however, these are only being used in a research capacity.

At the most basic level a simple switch is used to trigger the stimulation at the correct time, for example for the upper limb a hand-held switch may be used to time the muscular contractions correctly or alternatively an EMG signal. The simplest (and least expensive) option for gait assist applications is to use a wired system where timing of stimulation is controlled by a force sensitive foot switch (FSR) inside the shoe. The site of the switch (ipsilateral

TABLE 17.1   A Summary of Some Commercially Available Stimulators for Functional Use in the Lower Limb, Their Features and Regional Approval for Sale

Stimulator	Manufacturer	Target	Trigger Mechanism	Number of Channels/ Muscle Groups	FDA Approved	CE Marked
PACE	Odstock Medical Limited	Gait assist	Wired foot switch	1	✓	✓
PACE XL	Odstock Medical Limited	Gait assist	Wireless foot switch	1	✓	✓
O2CHS	Odstock Medical Limited	Gait assist	Wired foot switch (1 or 2)	2	✓	✓
Walkaide	Trulife	Gait assist	Tilt sensor	1	✓	✓
Parastep	Sigmedics INC	Gait assist	Hand activated switches	6	✓	
XFT-2001D G3	Shenzhen XFT Medical Limited	Gait assist	Motion sensor	1	✓	✓
Ness L300	Bioness Inc	Gait assist	Wireless foot switch	1	✓	✓
Ness L300 Plus	Bioness Inc	Gait assist	Wireless foot switch	2	✓	✓
Ness L300 Go	Bioness Inc	Gait assist	Motion sensor (gyroscope and accelerometer) or optional wireless foot switch	2	✓	✓

FDA, Food and Drug Administration.

or contralateral foot–heel or under the metatarsal heads) can be changed to accommodate altered foot contact patterns, or to optimize timing of stimulation. For example, the FSR may have to be placed under the metatarsal heads or the contralateral leg if there is no heel contact on the affected side. Wireless versions of this simple mechanism exist through the use of radio frequency signals (Figs 17.4 and 17.7).

The challenge for any trigger is to be able to adapt to real-time variations in walking, changes in speed, direction of progression (side stepping or stepping backwards) and foot contact patterns (toe contact instead of heel contact). Increasingly more sophisticated methods of triggering, such as tilt sensors (Walkaide, Innovative Neurotronics), 3-axis gyroscopes and accelerometers (Bioness L300 Go, Bioness) are being used. In each case the sensors are used to determine the timing of stimulation during gait by sensing the position of the leg in space. From clinical experience, accurate timing of stimulation using foot switches is difficult for muscle groups other

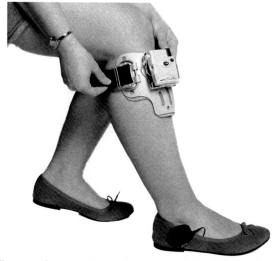

Fig. 17.7 Odstock Medical PACE XL; wireless foot switch and optional cuff.

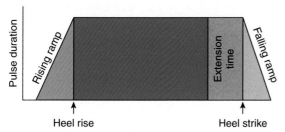

Fig. 17.8 Stimulation envelope for drop foot stimulation triggered by a heel switch.

than the dorsiflexors, which are stimulated throughout swing phase; this is also reported by Kesar et al (2009). The use of some of these more advanced sensing methods, such as in the Bioness L300 Go, or the use of multiple sensors, including EMG, as reported by Kojović et al (2009) may offer better timing control for more complex timing requirements.

Myoelectric signals from muscles that still have voluntary control are also being utilized along with EEG for creation of brain computer interfaces (BCI). The development of FES systems in which the electrical stimulation is elicited when the EMG signal from the target muscle reaches a predetermined threshold might provide a mechanism to promote involvement of voluntary movement when it is possible. As previously discussed this is particularly relevant as FES in combination with voluntary effort has been shown to promote motor learning and might therefore enable therapeutic effects. There are currently no commercially available walking systems which utilize such a mechanism.

Typically, stimulation is applied at a frequency that achieves a tetanic contraction i.e. between 30 and 50 Hz, with ramped intensity and on and off periods. These can be adjusted by changing ramp durations and adjusting the extension time. A slower rising ramp may be preferable to minimize stretch reflex activity in the calf muscle. A longer falling edge ramp with an extension added will help lower the foot after heel contact, minimizing 'foot slap' for drop foot applications. However, attention must be paid to the self-selected walking speed of the user – faster walkers will need ramp times and extensions minimized or stimulation will be on for too long. The stimulation window for

drop foot stimulation triggered using a foot switch is shown in Fig. 17.8.

Stimulation parameters should be adjusted to achieve the desirable response within levels of tolerance of sensation. Amplitude and pulse duration are adjusted to achieve muscle contraction at a comfortable level. Most devices offer both biphasic symmetrical or asymmetrical waveforms. Odstock Medical recommend the use of symmetrical waveform for those patients at higher risk of, or those who have experienced, skin irritation as it gives a charge-balanced waveform, which may prevent the build up of ions and therefore minimize changes in pH in the skin (Green 2011).

Apart from the sensory effects, which can be a problem for some patients, a limitation of surface-electrode FES systems is electrode placement. In a review of use of the Odstock dropped-foot stimulator, Taylor et al (1999a) noted that one of the principal reasons for discontinuing use was electrode positioning difficulties. User education is key – ensuring users know the correct response to aim for, how to use the 'test' procedure to ensure the electrode position is correct and how to adjust the electrode position if necessary. Providing a photograph of the electrode placement and marking electrode position on the skin (with a skin marker pen) may be helpful. Many of the current FES systems use a leg cuff to house the electrodes, which may facilitate the placing of the electrodes more consistently.

Regular follow up and technical support are necessary to ensure success in the initial stages of use. Timely repairs or replacement of equipment and consumables must be available.

Treatment Intensity

Where FES is used as an orthosis, for example to correct foot drop, the advice would be to use it for all walking activities where achievable; use should be built up slowly to the required level.

It is difficult to determine optimal protocols for therapeutic use from published literature because of the inconsistency in subjects' time since lesion, outcome measures, FES parameters and varying time usage reported between the studies. However, what evidence there is, supports the concept that FES combined with voluntary effort gives the best chance of carry over or motor learning.

REFERENCES

Alon, G., Levitt, A. F., & McCarthy, P. A. (2007). Functional electrical stimulation enhancement of upper extremity functional recovery during stroke rehabilitation: A pilot study. *Neurorehabilitation and Neural Repair, 21*, 207–215.

Barrett, C. L., Mann, G. E., Taylor, P. N., & Strike, P. (2009). A randomized trial to investigate the effects of functional electrical stimulation and therapeutic exercise on walking performance for people with multiple sclerosis. *Multiple Sclerosis, 15*, 493–504.

Bethoux, F., Rogers, H. L., Nolan, K. J., et al. (2014). The effects of peroneal nerve functional electrical stimulation versus ankle-foot orthosis in patients with chronic stroke: A randomized controlled trial. *Neurorehabilitation and Neural Repair, 28* (7), 688–697. https://doi.org/10.1177/1545968314521007.

Bethoux, F., Rogers, H. L., Nolan, K. J., et al. (2015). Long-term follow-up to a randomized controlled trial comparing peroneal nerve functional electrical stimulation to an ankle foot orthosis for patients with chronic stroke. *Neurorehabilitation and Neural Repair, 29*, 911–922. https://doi.org/10.1177/1545968315570325.

Bulley, C., Shiels, J., Wilkie, K., & Salisbury, L. (2011). User experiences, preferences and choices relating to functional electrical stimulation and ankle foot orthoses for foot-drop after stroke. *Physiotherapy, 97*, 226–233.

Burridge, J. H., Elessi, K., Pickering, R. M., & Taylor, P. N. (2007). Walking on an uneven surface: The effect of common peroneal stimulation on gait parameters and relationship between perceived and measured benefits in a sample of participants with a drop-foot. *Neuromodulation, 10*, 59–67.

Damiano, D. L., Prosser, L. A., Curatalo, L. A., & Alter, K. E. (2012). Muscle plasticity and ankle control after repetitive use of a functional electrical stimulation device for foot drop in cerebral palsy. *Neurorehabilitation and Neural Repair, 27*(3), 200–207.

Esnouf, J. E., Taylor, P. N., Mann, G. E., & Barrett, C. L. (2010). Impact on activities of daily living using a functional electrical stimulation device to improve dropped foot in people with multiple sclerosis, measured by the Canadian Occupational Performance Measure. *Multiple Sclerosis, 16*, 1141–1147.

Everaert, D. G., Stein, R. B., Abrams, G. M., et al. (2013). Effect of a foot-drop stimulator and ankle-foot orthosis on walking performance after stroke: A multicenter randomized controlled trial. *Neurorehabilitation and Neural Repair, 27*, 579–591. https://doi.org/10.1177/1545968313481278.

Gandolla, M., Ward, N.S., Molteni, F., Guanziroli, E., Ferrigno, G., Pedrocchi, A., 2016. The neural correlates of long-term carryover following functional electrical stimulation for stroke. *Neural Plasticity, 2016*, 1–13. https://doi.org/10.1155/2016/4192718.

Gater, J. D. R., David, D., Britney, T., & S, G. A. (2011). Functional electrical stimulation therapies after spinal cord injury. *NeuroRehabilitation, 28*(3), 231–248. https://doi.org/10.3233/NRE-2011-0652.

Gervasoni, E., Parelli, R., Uszynski, M., et al. (2017). Effects of functional electrical stimulation on reducing falls and improving gait parameters in multiple sclerosis and stroke. *PM&R, 9*, 339–347.e1. https://doi.org/10.1016/j.pmrj.2016.10.019.

Green, J. (2011). Newsletter Article: Winter 2011. FES skin irritation Information Sheet (Clinicians).

Hardin, E., Kobetic, R., Murray, L., et al. (2007). Walking after incomplete spinal cord injury using an implanted FES system: A case report. *Journal of Rehabilitation Research and Development, 44*, 333. https://doi.org/10.1682/JRRD.2007.03.0333.

Hazlewood, L., Brown, J. K., Rowe, P. J., & Salter, P. M. (1995). The use of therapeutic electrical stimulation in the treatment of hemiplegic cerebral palsy. *Physiotherapy, 81* 743–743.

Kafri, M., & Laufer, Y. (2015). Therapeutic effects of functional electrical stimulation on gait in individuals post-stroke. *Annals of Biomedical Engineering, 43*, 451–466. https://doi.org/10.1007/s10439-014-1148-8.

Kesar, T. M., Perumal, R., Reisman, D. S., et al. (2009). Functional electrical stimulation of ankle plantarflexor and dorsiflexor muscles: Effects on poststroke gait. *Stroke, 40*, 3821–3827.

Khurana, S. R., Beranger, A. G., & Felix, E. R. (2017). Perceived exertion is lower when using a functional electrical stimulation neuroprosthesis compared with an ankle-foot orthosis in persons with multiple sclerosis: A preliminary study. *American Journal of Physical Medicine & Rehabilitation, 96*, 133–139. https://doi.org/10.1097/PHM.0000000000000626.

Kilgore, K. L., Hoyen, H. A., Bryden, A. M., Hart, R. L., Keith, M. W., & Peckham, P. H. (2008). An implanted upper-extremity neuroprosthesis using myoelectric control. *The Journal of Hand Surgery, 33*, 539–550. https://doi.org/10.1016/j.jhsa.2008.01.007.

Kim, J.-H., Chung, Y., Kim, Y., & Hwang, S. (2012). Functional electrical stimulation applied to gluteus medius and tibialis anterior corresponding gait cycle for stroke. *Gait & Posture, 36*, 65–67. https://doi.org/10.1016/j.gaitpost.2012.01.006.

Kluding, P. M., Dunning, K., O'Dell, M. W., Wu, S. S., Ginosian, J., Feld, J., et al. (2013). Foot drop stimulation versus ankle foot orthosis after stroke: 30-week outcomes. *Stroke, 44*, 1660–1669. https://doi.org/10.1161/STROKEAHA.111.000334.

Kobetic, R., Triolo, R. J., Uhlir, J. P., et al. (1999). Implanted functional electrical stimulation system for mobility in paraplegia: A follow-up case report. *IEEE Transactions on Rehabilitation Engineering, 7*, 390–398. https://doi.org/10.1109/86.808942.

Kojović, J., Djurić-Jovičić, M., Došen, S., Popović, M. B., & Popović, D. B. (2009). Sensor-driven four-channel stimulation of paretic leg: Functional electrical walking therapy. *Journal of Neuroscience Methods, 181*, 100–105. https://doi.org/10.1016/j.jneumeth.2009.04.005.

Kottink, A. I., Hermens, H. J., Nene, A. V., Tenniglo, M. J., Groothuis-Oudshoorn, C. G., & IJzerman, M. J. (2008). Therapeutic effect of an implantable peroneal nerve stimulator in subjects with chronic stroke and footdrop: A randomized controlled trial. *Physical Therapy, 88*, 437–448. https://doi.org/10.2522/ptj.20070035.

Langhorne, P., Coupar, F., & Pollock, A. (2009). Motor recovery after stroke: A systematic review. *The Lancet Neurology, 8*, 741–754. https://doi.org/10.1016/S1474-4422(09)70150-4.

Laufer, Y., Hausdorff, J. M., & Ring, H. (2009). Effects of a foot drop neuroprosthesis on functional abilities, social participation, and gait velocity. *American Journal of Physical Medicine & Rehabilitation, 88*, 14–20. https://doi.org/10.1097/PHM.0b013e3181911246.

Liberson, W. T., Holmquest, H. J., Scot, D., & Dow, M. (1961). Functional electrotherapy: Stimulation of the peroneal nerve synchronized with the swing phase of the gait of hemiplegic patients. *Archives of Physical Medicine and Rehabilitation, 42*, 101–105.

Malešević, J., Dedijer Dujović, S., Savić, A. M., Konstantinović, L., Vidaković, A., Bijelić, G., et al. (2017). A decision support system for electrode shaping in multi-pad FES foot drop correction. *Journal of NeuroEngineering and Rehabilitation, 14.* https://doi.org/10.1186/s12984-017-0275-5.

Miller, L., Rafferty, D., Paul, L., & Mattison, P. (2015). A comparison of the orthotic effect of the Odstock Dropped Foot Stimulator and the Walkaide functional electrical stimulation systems on energy cost and speed of walking in multiple sclerosis. *Disability and Rehabilitation: Assistive Technology, 10*, 482–485. https://doi.org/10.3109/17483107.2014.898340.

Miller, L., Rafferty, D., Paul, L., & Mattison, P. (2016). The impact of walking speed on the effects of functional electrical stimulation for foot drop in people with multiple sclerosis. *Disability and Rehabilitation: Assistive Technology, 11*, 478–483. https://doi.org/10.3109/17483107.2015.1027296.

Moll, I., Vles, J. S. H., Soudant, D. L. H. M., et al. (2017). Functional electrical stimulation of the ankle dorsiflexors during walking in spastic cerebral palsy: A systematic review. *Developmental Medicine and Child Neurology, 59*, 1230–1236. https://doi.org/10.1111/dmcn.13501.

Mulcahey, M. J., Betz, R. R., Kozin, S. H., Smith, B. T., Hutchinson, D., & Lutz, C. (2004). Implantation of the freehand system during initial rehabilitation using minimally invasive techniques. *Spinal Cord, 42*, 146–155. https://doi.org/10.1038/sj.sc.3101573.

Newsam, C. J., & Baker, L. L. (2004). Effect of an electric stimulation facilitation program on quadriceps motor unit recruitment after stroke. *Archives of Physical Medicine and Rehabilitation, 85*, 2040–2045. https://doi.org/10.1016/j.apmr.2004.02.029.

NICE. (2009). Functional electrical stimulation for drop foot of central neurological origin. Interventional procedure guidance, 278.

NICE. (2016). ODFS Pace and Pace XL functional electrical stimulation devices for treating drop foot, guidance and guidelines (Med tech briefing).

Nudo, RJ. (2003). Functional and structural plasticity in motor cortex: Implications for stroke recovery. *Physical Medicine and Rehabilitation Clinics of North America, 14*(Suppl. 1):S57-S76.

O'Dell, M. W., Dunning, K., Kluding, P., Wu, S. S., Feld, J., Ginosian, J., et al. (2014). Response and prediction of improvement in gait speed from functional electrical stimulation in persons with poststroke drop foot. *PM&R, 6*, 587–601. https://doi.org/10.1016/j.pmrj.2014.01.001.

Paul, L., Rafferty, D., Young, S., Miller, L., Mattison, P., & McFadyen, A. (2008). The effect of functional electrical stimulation on the physiological cost of gait in people with multiple sclerosis. *Multiple Sclerosis, 14*, 954–961.

Popovic, M. R., Popovic, D. B., & Keller, T. (2002). Neuroprostheses for grasping. *Neurological Research, 24*, 443–452.

Popovic, M. R., Thrasher, T. A., Adams, M. E., Takes, V., Zivanovic, V., & Tonack, M. I. (2006). Functional electrical therapy: Retraining grasping in spinal cord injury. *Spinal Cord, 44*, 143–151.

Prenton, S., Hollands, K., & Kenney, L. (2016). Functional electrical stimulation versus ankle foot orthoses for foot-drop: A meta-analysis of orthotic effects. *Journal of Rehabilitation Medicine, 48*, 646–656. https://doi.org/10.2340/16501977-2136.

Prenton, S., Hollands, K., Kenney, L., & Onmanee, P. (2018). Functional electrical stimulation and ankle foot orthoses provide equivalent therapeutic effects on foot drop: A meta-analysis providing direction for future research. *Journal of Rehabilitation Medicine, 50*, 129–139. https://doi.org/10.2340/16501977-2289.

RCP. (2016). National clinical guidelines for stroke.

Ring, H., & Rosenthal, N. (2005). Controlled study of neuroprosthetic functional electrical stimulation in sub-acute post-stroke rehabilitation. *Journal of Rehabilitation Medicine, 37*, 32–36.

Rose, J., Cahill-Rowley, K., & Butler, E. E. (2017). Artificial walking technologies to improve gait in cerebral palsy: Multichannel neuromuscular stimulation: NMES-assisted gait for cerebral palsy. *Artificial Organs, 41*, E233–E239. https://doi.org/10.1111/aor.13058.

Rushton, D. N. (2003). Functional electrical stimulation and rehabilitation–an hypothesis. *Medical Engineering & Physics, 25*, 75–78.

Sadowsky, C. L., Hammond, E. R., Strohl, A. B., et al. (2013). Lower extremity functional electrical stimulation cycling promotes physical and functional recovery in chronic spinal cord injury. *The Journal of Spinal Cord Medicine, 36*, 623–631. https://doi.org/10.1179/2045772313Y.0000000101.

Scott, S. M., van der Linden, M. L., Hooper, J. E., Cowan, P., & Mercer, T. H. (2013). Quantification of gait kinematics and walking ability of people with multiple sclerosis who are new users of functional electrical stimulation. *Journal of Rehabilitation Medicine, 45*, 364–369.

Sheffler, L. R., Bailey, S. N., & Chae, J. (2009). Spatiotemporal and kinematic effect of peroneal nerve stimulation versus an ankle-foot orthosis in patients with multiple sclerosis: A case series. *Pharmacy Management R, 1*, 604–611. https://doi.org/10.1016/j.pmrj.2009.04.002.

Sheffler, L. R., Hennessey, M. T., Naples, G. G., & Chae, J. (2006). Peroneal nerve stimulation versus an ankle foot orthosis for correction of footdrop in stroke: Impact on functional ambulation. *Neurorehabilitation and Neural Repair, 20*, 355–360. https://doi.org/10.1177/1545968306287925.

Sheffler, L. R., Taylor, P. N., Bailey, et al. (2015). Surface peroneal nerve stimulation in lower limb hemiparesis: Effect on quantitative gait parameters. *American Journal of Physical Medicine & Rehabilitation, 94*, 341–357. https://doi.org/10.1097/PHM.0000000000000269.

Sheffler, L. R., Taylor, P. N., Gunzler, D. D., Buurke, J. H., IJzerman, M. J., & Chae, J. (2013). Randomized controlled trial of surface peroneal nerve stimulation for motor relearning in lower limb hemiparesis. *Archives of Physical Medicine and Rehabilitation, 94*, 1007–1014. https://doi.org/10.1016/j.apmr.2013.01.024.

Shendkar, C. V., Lenka, P. K., Biswas, A., Kumar, R., & Mahadevappa, M. (2015). Therapeutic effects of functional electrical stimulation on gait, motor recovery, and motor cortex in stroke survivors. *Hong Kong Physiotherapy Journal, 33*, 10–20. https://doi.org/10.1016/j.hkpj.2014.10.003.

Springer, S., Vatine, J.-J., Lipson, R., Wolf, A., Laufer, Y., 2012. Effects of dual-channel functional electrical stimulation on gait performance in patients with hemiparesis. *The Scientific World Journal, 2012*, 1–8. https://doi.org/10.1100/2012/530906

Springer, S., & Khamis, S. (2017). Effects of functional electrical stimulation on gait in people with multiple sclerosis – a systematic review. *Multiple Sclerosis and Related Disorders, 13*, 4–12. https://doi.org/10.1016/j.msard.2017.01.010.

Springer, S., Laufer, Y., & Becher, V. (2013). Dual-channel functional electrical stimulation improvements in speed-based gait classifications. *Clinical Interventions in Aging, 271*. https://doi.org/10.2147/CIA.S41141.

Taylor, P., Burridge, J., Dunkerley, A., Lamb, A., Wood, D., Norton, J., & Swain, I. (1999a). Patients' perceptions of the Odstock dropped foot stimulator (ODFS). *Clinical Rehabilitation, 13*, 439–446.

Taylor, P., Burridge, J., Dunkerley, A., Wood, D., Norton, J., Singleton, C., & Swain, I. (1999b). Clinical audit of 5 years provision of the Odstock dropped foot stimulator. *Artificial Organs, 23*, 440–442.

Taylor, P., Esnouf, J., & Hobby, J. (2002). The functional impact of the Freehand System on tetraplegic hand function. Clinical Results. *Spinal Cord, 40*, 560–566. https://doi.org/10.1038/sj.sc.3101373.

Taylor, P., Johnson, M., Mann, G., & Swain, I. (2004). *Patterns of use and users' perceptions of the Odstock Dropped Foot Stimulator following stroke and multiple sclerosis. Presented at the 9th Annual Conference of the International FES Society.* Bournemouth: UK.

Triolo, R. J., Bailey, S. N., Miller, M. E., et al. (2012). Longitudinal performance of a surgically implanted neuroprosthesis for lower-extremity exercise, standing, and transfers after spinal cord injury. *Archives of Physical Medicine and Rehabilitation, 93*, 896–904. https://doi.org/10.1016/j.apmr.2012.01.001.

Yang, K., Meadmore, K., Freeman, C., et al. (2018). Development of user-friendly wearable electronic textiles for healthcare applications. *Sensors, 18*, 2410. https://doi.org/10.3390/s18082410.

Yan, T., Hui-Chan, C. W. Y., & Li, L. S. W. (2005). Functional electrical stimulation improves motor recovery of the lower extremity and walking ability of subjects with first acute stroke: A randomized placebo-controlled trial. *Stroke, 36*, 80–85. https://doi.org/10.1161/01.STR.0000149623.24906.63.

18

Alternating Currents: Interferential Therapy, Russian Stimulation and Burst-Modulated Low-Frequency Stimulation

Jorge Fuentes C.

CHAPTER OUTLINE

INTRODUCTION

Medium-frequency alternating currents, defined as currents in the frequency range of 1 to 10 kHz, represent a common therapeutic approach used in rehabilitation. The two most commonly used frequencies are 4 kHz (interferential currents) and 2.5 kHz (Russian currents) for the main purpose of pain relief and muscle strengthening, respectively. Interferential current (IFC) is the transcutaneous application of alternating current (AC) usually in the range 1000–5000 Hz, amplitude modulated at low frequency (0 to 250 Hz). Originally developed by Hans Nemec in Europe in the 1950s, today IFC is considered one of the most common electrophysical modalities in the management of pain. Surveys confirm its high availability and widespread use in different countries. For example, 74.7% of physical therapists in Quebec, Canada, reported using IFC at least once during an episode of care for patients with low back pain (Poitras et al 2005). Similarly, IFC was the most widely used modality for this condition in the UK and Northern

Ireland (Foster et al 1999; Gracey et al 2002), although a review of the literature about the availability and usage of IFC from 1990 to 2010 showed a slightly declining trend in its availability and use (Shah & Farrow 2012). In Chile, a recent national survey showed that IFC is available in 69% of workplaces and is used daily by 61% of physiotherapists (Cid et al 2016). Similar results were shown in Israel where the reported availability was 85% with a frequency of use of 48% (Springer et al 2015). These data accord with previous surveys in the field (Lindsay et al 1990; Pope et al 1995).

Another type of current is the burst-modulated alternating current (BMAC), which is based on a kilohertz-frequency alternating current primarily used to produce muscle force gains. One of the most common and most researched forms of BMAC is the Russian current (RC). RC is a medium frequency sinusoidal alternating current, traditionally applied at a frequency of 2.5 kHz that is burst modulated at a frequency of 50 Hz with a 50% duty cycle. This form of current was introduced in 1977 by Dr Yavor

Kots, a Russian coach for the Olympic weightlifting team, who claimed force gains of up to 40% in elite athletes as a result of RC (Ward & Shkuratova 2002). During the last decade its superiority over low-frequency pulsed current has been challenged (da Silva et al 2015; Vaz et al 2012). In addition, recent evidence has shown that variations on the traditional pattern for RC produce greater muscle force (Iijima et al 2018; Vaz & Frasson 2018).

Information about the availability and physiotherapists' use of BMAC is seldom reported in the literature. For example, a review based on published studies describing trends in the availability and usage of electrophysical agents in physiotherapy practices from 1990 to 2010 does not include BMAC (Shah & Farrow 2012). From the available data, RC was present in 9% of workplaces and used only by 2.2 % of Australian physiotherapists (Chipchase et al 2009). An Israeli survey showed that neuromuscular electrical stimulation (NMES) was available in 80% of workplaces and was used by 30% of physiotherapists; however, there was no mention of the specific types of current used (Springer et al 2015). Russian current was reported to be available in 59% of workplaces and used by 41% of Chilean respondents (Cid et al 2016).

PHYSICAL PRINCIPLES

It is well known that skin impedance to electrical current is inversely proportional to the pulse frequency and capacitance of the skin. Direct current and low-frequency biphasic pulsed currents encounter high electrical resistance in the outer layers of the skin. This makes the treatment of deep structures difficult and painful (Goats 1990). Although this claim has been widely reported in the literature, some authors contradict this assertion because skin impedance to low-frequency pulsed currents would depend on the phase duration rather than the pulse frequency (Pantaleão et al 2011; Ward 2009).

A claimed advantage of IFC is its capacity to be more comfortable than transcutaneous electrical nerve stimulation (TENS) currents and to be able to penetrate more deeply than TENS (Low & Reed 2000).

IFC and the Principle of Interference

To produce IFC, two constant-intensity sinusoidal currents of slightly differing medium frequency (in the range of 2000–5000 Hz) are applied simultaneously; these are referred to as the carrier frequencies. When the currents are 'in sync' the two sine waves will superimpose and the current amplitude will increase. When the sine waves are 'out of sync' the currents will cancel each other out and the current amplitude will reduce. The resultant current rhythmically increases and decreases in amplitude (see Fig. 18.1) giving the appearance of bursts of current referred to as 'beats'.

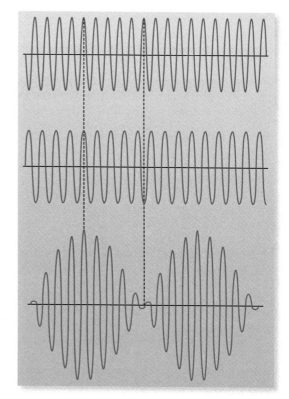

Fig. 18.1 The simultaneous application of two constant-intensity sinusoidal currents of slightly differing medium frequency results in a combined current which has a sinusoidal wave envelope. This oval-shaped field of pulses or burst is referred to as 'beats'. (From: Ozcan, J, Ward, AR & Robertson, VJ (2004) A comparison of true and premodulated interferential currents, *Archives of Physical Medicine & Rehabilitation* **85**(3) 409–415.)

The beat frequency has the value of the difference between the two original alternating medium frequencies. For example, if 4000 and 4080 Hz medium-frequency currents are superimposed in the body, the resultant beat frequency will be 80 Hz. This beat frequency current with a variable intensity is also known as the amplitude-modulated frequency (AMF) parameter when using IFC (Goats 1990; Nikolova 1987).

Classically, the intersection of the current between two sets of electrodes arranged in a crossfire pattern is reported to produce a three-dimensional 'clover-leaf' shaped electric field within the tissues. Theoretically, this would produce the maximum interference within the central portion of the field (Goats 1990; Nikolova 1987). However, this classical representation has not been supported by the literature. The formation of the classic clover-leaf pattern requires that the electrical impedance of the tissues is uniform. Even in water such a pattern has only partially been reproduced (Treffene 1983). When this pattern was tested in biological tissues, the interference pattern was found to be complex and unpredictable. More recently, an interesting study has shed light on the penetration and spread of IFC in cutaneous, subcutaneous and muscle tissue (Beatti et al 2011). In this investigation, 12 healthy subjects received premodulated (two electrodes) IFC at 90 Hz (AMF) and 'true' IFC via four electrodes in the distal medial thigh applied at a 'strong but comfortable sensation' level of intensity. The main outcome included the voltage measured by Teflon-coated needle electrodes at three locations (centred between the four electrodes, in line with one circuit and outside the four circuits) (see Fig. 18.2) and at three depths (skin, subcutaneous and muscle). The results showed that for true IFC, the lowest voltages of all currents were recorded in the centre of the four electrodes (theoretically this should have been the area of maximum interference), with the highest voltage being recorded 5 cm outside of the electrodes. For the premodulated IFC, the highest voltage was registered in line with one circuit.

In light of these results the authors highlighted that first, IFC was able to reach muscle tissue without producing discomfort in the participants; second, surprisingly, and in contrast to classical literature theory, the lowest voltages were present in the intersection of the four electrodes; third, no differences in voltages were obtained when applying different beat frequencies; and finally, true IFC was more efficient in terms of higher recorded voltages than the premodulated IFC when targeting deeper tissue. Then, a simple recommendation would be to arrange the electrodes so that the area of maximum perceived intensity by the patient is over or around the target area.

Although additional evidence is needed to confirm the work of Beatti et al (2011), the results of this study support the fact that the interaction of medium-frequency electrical currents with biological and heterogeneous tissues is complex. Far from a simple distribution pattern, the different impedance and nerve fibre orientation will affect the areas of interference in a way that is not always central or uniform.

Traditional Russian Current and BMAC

A justification for using Russian and BMAC in rehabilitation is the capacity to activate multiple nerve fibre action potentials per burst, producing firing rates that are multiples of the burst frequency (Ward & Shkuratova 2002). These long-duration bursts are thought to maximize muscle torque through twitch summation while minimizing discomfort due to the lower skin impedance offered to medium frequency currents (da Silva et al 2015; Ward et al 2006) (See Fig. 18.3).

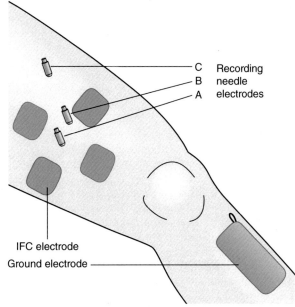

Fig. 18.2 Recording, ground and IFC electrode attachment. Recording electrodes were situated in different locations relative to the IFC electrodes: (*A*) in the centre of the IFC electrodes for the true IFC application, (*B*) in line with one circuit close to the electrode for the premodulated IFC application, and (*C*) outside (5 cm) of the four IFC electrodes. (From: Beatti A, Rayner A, Chipchase L et al (2011). Penetration and Spread of Interferential Current in Cutaneous, Subcutaneous and Muscle Tissues. *Physiotherapy* **97**:319–326.)

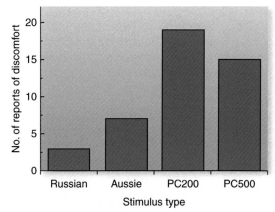

Fig. 18.3 The number of reports of discomfort for each of the four currents assessed. Alternating current, AC stimuli (Russian and Aussie), Low-frequency pulsed current at 200 μs (PC-200), Low-frequency pulsed current at 500 μs (PC-500). The difference was significant (n=32, z=2.83, p=0.005), with the AC stimuli more comfortable than the PC stimuli. (From: Ward AR, Oliver WG, Buccella D (2006) Wrist extensor torque production and discomfort associated with low-frequency and burst- modulated kilohertz-frequency currents. *Physical therapy* **86**(10):1360–1367.)

BIOPHYSICAL INTERACTIONS

A variety of effects have been associated with the application of IFC and BMAC/Russian. This section discusses experimental evidence supporting their benefits, including laboratory-based studies involving healthy participants.

Interferential Current

Pain Mechanisms

Although the exact pain relief mechanism for IFC is not well understood, it is believed that innocuous stimulation and noxious stimulation play a relevant role. The gate control theory of pain is most commonly utilized as pain theory to explain the pain-relieving effects of IFC. The activation of non-nociceptor, Aβ fibres can inhibit the transmission of nociceptive stimuli from the spinal cord to the brain (Melzack & Wall 1965). Studies involving healthy volunteers confirm the hypoalgesic effects of IFC (Bueno et al 2017; Rocha et al 2012; Venancio et al 2013). The stimulation of peripheral nociceptive fibres (Aδ and C) by the application of noxious stimuli has been presented as an opioid-mediated mechanism to explain the hypoalgesic effects of IFC (Goats 1990; Low & Reed 2000). Although there appears to be no research to verify this assertion, some indirect clinical evidence supports the hypoalgesic effect of IFC when noxious stimulation is applied (Defrin et al 2005).

Recent brain research using functional magnetic resonance imaging reveals that low-frequency electrical stimulation modulates the functional connectivity of the periaqueductal grey matter with other brain areas activating the descending pain-inhibitory pathway (Choi et al 2016; Kocyigit et al 2012). However, studies of this nature have not been performed using medium-frequency currents.

The effectiveness of IFC in reducing inflammatory pain and oedema was assessed in an animal model (Jorge et al 2006). IFC was able to reduce the formalin-evoked nociceptive response when applied to the paw immediately after but not before the formalin injection. Also, in the same study, primary mechanical hyperalgesia induced by carrageenan was reduced. Interestingly, the pain-reducing effect does not appear to be the result of an anti-inflammatory action, since IFC did not significantly reduce the oedema induced by either formalin or carrageenan. Based on the stimulation parameters used in this study (140-Hz beat frequency, sensory level of intensity), it is plausible that this antinociceptive effect could have been the result of the activation of large-diameter afferent nerves (i.e. a pain gate mechanism). However, the clinical relevance of this work is yet to be supported by clinical research.

Experimental Pain

1. *Ischaemic pain*
   A recent study compared the analgesic effects of TENS and IFC on induced ischaemic pain in pain-free healthy volunteers (Bae et al 2014). Subjects were allocated to receive each 50 Hz TENS, 50 Hz IFC, 100 Hz TENS and 100 Hz IFC. No differences among groups were found on pain intensity; however, the 50 Hz IFC treatment was more comfortable than the other treatments. Previous studies also reported no differences in the magnitude of analgesia between IFC and TENS, but IFC reduced pain intensity to a greater extent than sham electrotherapy (Johnson & Tabasam 2003c) and control/no intervention (Johnson & Tabasam 2002).

2. *Mechanical pain*
   Early evidence on the effects of IFC on mechanical pain presents conflicting results (Alves-Guerreiro et al 2001); however, more recent literature supports its effects on either raising pressure pain thresholds (PPT) or reducing pain intensity. One study examined PPT achieved over the lumbar area when a beat (100 Hz AMF) was present and absent (0 Hz). Both treatments produced a comparable decrease in pain sensitivity (Fuentes et al 2010). Also, when compared to a sham IFC intervention and a control condition, active IFC was able to significantly raise the PPT (Fuentes et al 2011). In addition, the use of a carrier frequency of 1 kHz has been shown to promote a higher hypoalgesic response during and after stimulation when compared with carrier frequencies of 8 kHz and 10 kHz (Venancio et al 2013).

   Dounavi et al (2012) assessed the segmental and extra-segmental hypoalgesic effects of different IFC parameter combinations upon muscle pain sensitivity. The results showed that IFC delivered at high to tolerance intensity and high AMF did not produce significant segmental and extra-segmental hypoalgesia in healthy participants compared with a control or placebo group. Interestingly, the findings of the Dounavi et al study disagree with previous clinical trials in which IFC was applied with similar parameters (i.e. high AMF and high to tolerance intensity) and produced hypoalgesic effects (Cheing et al 2008; Tugay et al 2007).

3. *Cold-induced pain*
   Some studies have demonstrated that IFC is able to reduce cold pain perception (Johnson & Tabasam 1999, 2003b; Johnson & Wilson 1997) while others have found no effect of IFC on cold pain threshold, intensity or unpleasantness (Johnson & Tabasam 2003a), or the absence of hypoalgesic effect of IFC when compared with sham stimulation or a control/no intervention condition (Stephenson & Walker 2003). In addition, a rise in pain thresholds was not influenced by the different swing patterns of IFC

(Johnson & Tabasam 2003b). New evidence using this model of pain is lacking, therefore the hypoalgesic effects of IFC on cold-induced pain still remain equivocal.

Placebo Effects

The placebo effect is acknowledged as an important phenomenon in modern medicine. The placebo effect represents the psychosocial aspect of every treatment, including the psychosocial context surrounding the patient (Rossettini et al 2018). Few studies have directly measured the placebo effect of IFC by comparing placebo IFC (i.e. sham) with no intervention (i.e. control). Roche et al (2002), in a study of induced ischemic pain in 12 healthy volunteers, compared subjects' reports of pain threshold, pain tolerance and pain endurance under three conditions: control, placebo IFC and placebo TENS. Both the placebo conditions significantly delayed time to reach pain threshold. Placebo IFC also delayed time to reach pain tolerance. Later, Fuentes et al (2011), in a randomized placebo-controlled cross-over trial in which 40 volunteers received active IFC, placebo IFC and no treatment/control over the lumbar area, also tested the effect of placebo and active IFC. In this study, muscle pain sensitivity, measured using pressure pain threshold, was not significantly different under placebo IFC treatment compared with the control condition (see Fig. 18.4). Finally, Defrin et al (2005), in a randomized controlled trial (RCT) about the effect of IFC on osteoarthritis (OA) knee pain, concluded that both control and placebo IFC treatments did not significantly affect pain intensity, ROM, morning stiffness and pain thresholds compared with active IFC treatment. Thus, there appears to be contradictory evidence about the placebo effect when applying IFC in different conditions. To reach definitive conclusions, additional research is clearly needed. However, this imposes a difficulty, particularly in clinical settings, where the use of placebo and the no treatment/control groups generates an intense debate and an ethical dilemma.

Increased Blood Flow

Authors of the 1970s claimed that IFC improved circulation (Belcher 1974; Nikolova-Troeva 1968). However, studies in the field have presented contradictory evidence. Some authors have demonstrated a positive effect on vasodilatation of the hand when IFC was applied across the

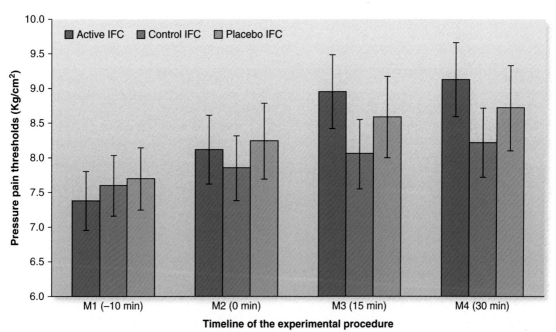

Fig. 18.4 Average pressure pain thresholds (PPT) (kg/cm^2/seconds) during the timeline of the experimental procedure for the three conditions (active IFC, placebo IFC and control). *M1*, PPT taken 10 minutes pre-treatment; *M2*, PPT taken at time 0; *M3*, PPT taken 15 minutes into treatment; *M4*, PPT taken at the end of treatment. Results are shown as mean ± SEM. (Fuentes C J, Armijo-Olivo SL, Gross D et al (2011) A preliminary investigation into the effects of active interferential current therapy and placebo on pressure pain sensitivity: a random crossover placebo-controlled study. *Physiotherapy* **97**:291–301.)

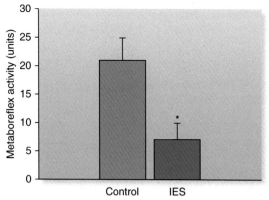

Fig. 18.5 Estimated muscle metaboreflex (vasoconstrictor tone) control of calf vascular resistance in young and older individuals during IFC stimulation (IES) or placebo condition (control). This suggests that IES may attenuate sympathetic nervous system activity. *Significant (p< 0.01). (From: Santos FV, Chiappa GR, Vieira PJ et al (2013) Interferential electrical stimulation improves peripheral vasodilatation in healthy individuals. *Brazilian Journal of Physical Therapy* **17**(3):281–288.)

brachial plexus (Ganne 1976) or when various IFC frequencies targeted the tibial artery (Lamb & Mani 1994). Others, however, concluded that there is no effect of IFC on peripheral blood flow when IFC was applied over the cervical sympathetic chain and stellate ganglion, the dorso-lumbar sympathetic outflow, and the peripheral sympathetic nerves (Nussbaum et al 1990).

Noble et al (2000) investigated the effect of various IFC frequencies on cutaneous blood flow. The results showed a significant increase in blood flow, along with an increase in skin temperature for IFC at 10–20 Hz beat frequency. The increase in skin temperature has been previously suggested to be indicative of vasodilatation due to decreased sympathetic nerve activity (Wong & Jette 1984). This effective range of frequencies (AMF 10-20 Hz) is in agreement with a previous study (Lamb & Mani 1994) where beat frequencies of 0–30 Hz produced the optimal effect; however, it differs from the frequencies (AMF 40–100 Hz) suggested by classical authors (De Domenico 1987; Goats 1990). In addition, Santos et al (2013) applied active IFC and placebo IFC to the stellate ganglion region in healthy subjects. Active IFC was able to reduce mean blood pressure (vasoconstrictor tone), promoting higher calf blood flow, lower calf vascular resistance and a reduction in the muscle metaboreflex activity (see Fig. 18.5). These results suggest that IFC may attenuate sympathetic nervous system activity and thereby induce vasodilatation.

Very recent evidence confirms that IFC alters blood flow velocity and vessel size. Jin et al (2017) investigated

the changes in the autonomic nervous system produced by different intensity levels of stimulation. IFC using a bipolar approach was used to stimulate the autonomic nervous system at the thoracic vertebrae 1–4 levels for 20 minutes. Subjects were assigned into three groups: sensory level stimulation, muscle contraction level stimulation group and pain level stimulation group. The results showed that the group experiencing muscle contractions (AMF beat frequency 5 Hz + 45–50 mA) displayed the greatest effect on both the blood flow velocity of the carotid artery and the vessel size. This study confirms the importance of selecting adequate stimulation parameters to increase blood flow when applying IFC.

In summary, recent evidence supports the positive effect of IFC on blood flow. These physiological changes may vary depending on the stimulation parameters used. Thus, low beat frequencies (AMF 0–20 Hz) and a high level of intensity (motor level stimulation) showed the most significant increase in blood flow. Finally, it is worth noting that these studies involved mainly healthy volunteers. Since the autonomic nervous system may respond differently in patients suffering from a clinical condition (e.g. focal ischaemia), future research is necessary to verify these findings in clinical populations.

BMAC/Russian Currents
Muscle Strength

The burst-modulated alternating current (BMAC) is based on a kilohertz-frequency alternating current used to produce muscle force gains. It is believed that by delivering BMAC, additional APs would be generated during the burst of AC cycles than when using a low-frequency pulsed current (PC); therefore, summation occurs, which generates stronger muscle contractions without producing pain. Several studies have investigated the effects of BMAC in healthy volunteers (Bellew et al 2014; Laufer & Elboim 2008; Vaz et al 2012; Ward et al 2006); most of these investigations compared RC with other medium frequency currents (IFC, Aussie) or low-frequency PC on muscle force production and perceived discomfort. For example, Ward et al (2006) reported that RC elicited lower mean torque for wrist extensors but was more comfortable than Aussie currents and low-frequency PC. A later study (Laufer & Elboim 2008) demonstrated that both RC and low-frequency PC applied to the wrist extensors produced strong muscle contractions, but the PC was less fatiguing. In addition, Vaz et al (2012) showed that low-frequency PC was more effective than RC for achieving 10% of the maximal isometric voluntary contraction. More recently, Bellew et al (2014) concluded that greater quadriceps force was elicited by IFC and burst modulated biphasic PC when compared with RC. Finally, Dantas et al (2015) reported that in healthy women, despite comparable levels of discomfort, the RC evoked lower isometric knee torque than Aussie currents and low-frequency PC. Also, it has been demonstrated that after 6 weeks of training, BMAC and low-frequency PC showed the same results regarding architectural adaptations and voluntary neuromuscular performance in the quadriceps muscle of athletes (Oliveira 2018).

More recent papers have extended these concepts and evidence further. For example, findings of different reviews comparing lower kHz frequency to BMAC for maximum force production question the advantage of BMAC currents (Iijima et al 2018; Vaz & Frasson 2018).

In summary, the mixed results to date challenge the beliefs of a theoretical superiority attributed to Russian currents compared with other currents when eliciting isometric force.

CLINICAL EVIDENCE

This section covers the clinical evidence supporting the common uses of IFC and BMAC/Russian currents. As per the evidence-based focus of this book, a comprehensive analysis of influential articles, and most importantly, the recently published literature will be presented and discussed. RCTs represent the best design to demonstrate effectiveness; appropriately conducted RCTs minimize confounding and bias and thus allow causal inferences regarding the effects of interventions, such as IFC and BMAC/Russian currents (Armijo-Olivo et al 2015).

Clinical Evidence for Interferential Current

During previous decades, IFC was widely used for the management of several conditions, including asthma (Emberson 1996), fractures (Fourie & Bowerbank 1997), palmar psoriasis (Philipp et al 2000), swelling (Christie & Willoughby 1990) and for accelerating tissue healing (Ganne et al 1979; Nikolova 1987). However, most of the supporting studies lacked methodological rigour. Current evidence of IFC focuses on the management of painful musculoskeletal conditions, and the reduction of urinary stress incontinence. Thus, this section will concentrate on the recent high-quality evidence (i.e. RCTs and systematic reviews) of IFC for the management of these conditions.

Musculoskeletal Painful Conditions

Compared with modalities such as TENS, few systematic reviews/meta-analyses have been published on the efficacy of IFC in musculoskeletal (MSK) pain. Fuentes et al (2010) included a range of MSK conditions, whilst other authors reviewed the literature related to one specific condition, such as spinal pain (Resende et al 2018), fibromyalgia (Tavares da Silva et al 2018) and knee OA (Zeng et al

2015). A recent review contrasted the pain-relieving effects of IFC and TENS in acute and chronic pain (de Almeida et al 2018) (see Table 18.1).

The Fuentes review (2010) included 20 RCTs and comprised acute and chronic low back pain, OA knee pain, shoulder pain, fibromyalgia and bicipital tendonitis pain. The authors concluded that IFC combined with another intervention, such as exercise, education or reassurance seems to be more effective for reducing pain at discharge than a control treatment (pooled mean difference (MD) in visual analogue scale (VAS) 2.45 (95% confidence interval [CI] 1.69–3.2, p<.0001)) for acute and chronic low back pain, frozen shoulder and OA knee pain. Also, it was found that IFC combined with other treatments was more effective than a placebo treatment at the 3-month follow-up (pooled MD in VAS 1.85 (95% CI 1.47–2.23, p<.0001)). IFC alone was not significantly better than placebo or other therapy (e.g. manual therapy, traction and massage) at discharge or follow-up for chronic low back pain, OA knee pain and jaw pain.

More recently, de Almeida et al (2018) summarized trials comparing the pain-relieving effects of TENS and IFC on acute and chronic pain. Eight studies with a pooled sample of 825 patients were included. In five studies, the impact of TENS and IFC were assessed as isolated therapies. When applied alone, both TENS and IFC improved pain and functional outcomes in knee OA pain, chronic low back pain, menstrual pain, neck pain, carpal tunnel syndrome pain, with no difference between TENS and IFC (MD in VAS 0.36 (95% CI -0.56–1.27, p = 0.45)). Only one study included a placebo group, which showed no significant differences between active and placebo IFC on pain (Atamaz et al 2012). In three studies, IFC or TENS were applied in combination with exercise as part of a multimodal treatment plan. In these, IFC or TENS combined with exercises seemed to be equally effective when compared with exercises alone. These findings contrast with previous evidence, which suggests that IFC should be included as part of a multimodal treatment plan to be effective (Fuentes 2010).

Chronic Low Back Pain (LBP) and Neck Pain

Resende et al (2018) conducted a systematic review and meta-analysis analysing the evidence on TENS or IFC for chronic LBP and/or neck pain function and disability. Nine RCTs were selected (eight LBP; one neck pain), and seven studies with complete data sets were included for meta-analysis (655 participants). They found that TENS or IFC intervention was significantly better than placebo/control (MD in VAS -0.92 (95% CI -1.73 to -0.12; p<0.02)). Sensitivity analyses demonstrated that when only those studies with adequate stimulation parameters (intensity strong but

TABLE 18.1   Evidence for IFC on Pain

Author	Type of Review	Pain Condition	Number of Studies (Total N)	Quality of Included Studies	Results
Fuentes et al 2010	Systematic review/ meta-analysis	A variety of acute and chronic musculoskeletal conditions	20 (1748)	Three of high methodological quality, 14 of moderate, and three of poor quality (Delphi List, PEDro Scale, Maastricht, Maastricht-Amsterdam List, Bizzini, van Tulder, and Jadad scale)	IFC as a supplement to another intervention seems to be more effective for reducing pain than a control treatment at discharge and more effective than placebo at the 3-month follow-up. IFC alone was not significantly better than placebo or other therapy at discharge or follow-up.
Zang et al 2015	Systematic review/ meta-analysis	Knee osteoarthritis	27 (1233)	Eight low-quality studies (Modified Oxford score ≤ 3), ten medium-quality studies (scored 4 or 5), and nine high-quality studies (scored 6 or 7)	Contrasted to other electrical modalities, such as h-TENS, l-TENS, NMES, PES, NIN, and control condition, IFC is the only significantly effective treatment in terms of both pain intensity and change pain score at last follow-up time point when compared with the control group.
Tavares da Silva et al 2018	Systematic review	Fibromyalgia	1 (17)	The study presented a high risk of bias (Cochrane Collaboration tool)	The combination of ultrasound and IFC improved pain relief and the sleep quality of patients with fibromyalgia. However, the validity of this assertion is questioned for the lack of RCTs in the field and the poor quality of the published evidence.
Rosende et al 2018	Systematic review/ meta analysis	Spinal pain (low back pain and neck pain)	9 (655)	All studies presented a high risk of bias (Cochrane Collaboration tool)	There is inconclusive evidence of TENS/IFC benefits in spinal pain patients because the quality of the studies was low and adequate parameters and timing of assessment were not uniformly used or reported.
de Almeida et al 2018	Systematic review/ meta-analysis	A variety of acute and chronic painful conditions	8 (825)	Moderate (an average of 6 on the 0–10 PEDro scale)	Both TENS and IFC improved pain and functional outcomes with no statistical difference between them.

PEDro, h-TENS, high-frequency TENS; *IFC,* interferential current therapy; *l-TENS,* low-frequency TENS; *NIN,* non-invasive interactive neurostimulation; *NMES,* neuromuscular electrical stimulation; *PES,* pulsed electrical stimulation; *US,* ultrasound.

comfortable or greater, frequency 1–150 Hz, and pulse duration 50–350 µs) were analysed, there was no significant effect for changes in pain intensity (MD in VAS -0.99; 95% CI -2.52-0.54; p = 0.21). In the same way, in studies with inadequate or unknown stimulation parameters, there was also no effect (MD in VAS -0.95; 95% C -2.36 to 0.47, p = 0.19). The authors suggest that this disagreement in effects between the whole sample and the sub-sample analysis could be explained by the lower power based on the inclusion of few studies with small sample sizes for each analysis.

Thus, the benefits of TENS or IFC intervention remain debatable because of the poor quality of the studies and inadequacy or non-reporting of stimulation parameters.

Lara-Palomo et al (2012), in a single-blinded randomized controlled trial, showed that the combined effect of massage and electrical stimulation with IFC obtained statistically and clinically significant results in several outcomes, such as the VAS (p = 0.001), Oswestry Disability Index (ODI) (p = 0.019), Roland Morris Disability Questionnaire (RMDQ) (p = 0.006), quality of life (physical function p = 0.001), physical role (p = 0.001) and body pain (p = 0.001). Clinically meaningful differences using IFC were reached for the ODI (d = 0.53), the RMDQ (d = 0.75) and the VAS (d = 1.06). These results are in agreement with two recent investigations. Fuentes et al (2014) used IFC to assess the impact of contextual factors when delivering therapy in LBP patients. In this study 117 individuals received a single session of active or sham IFC. The authors concluded that IFC (4 kHz, sensory level of intensity) applied for 30 minutes in an enhanced therapeutic alliance (i.e. being supportive, including active listening, showing empathy and encouragement (Kaptchuk 2008)) was able to reduce pain intensity compared with sham IFC accompanied by an enhanced therapeutic alliance (p< 0.01). The magnitude of this change (d = 1.0) reached clinically meaningful levels. More recently, Albornoz-Cabello et al (2017) confirmed the efficacy of IFC on pain perception and disability in subjects with chronic LBP. In this study, 64 patients were allocated to IFC (4 kHz, AMF beat frequency 65 Hz and sweep frequency of 95 Hz, quadripolar technique, and sensory intensity level) or a control group (usual care treatment). Significant between-group differences were found for IFC on pain perception (p = 0.032) and disability level (p = 0.002).

Recent evidence also assessed the combined effect of Pilates and IFC on LBP (Moura et al 2017). In this RCT, 148 patients were assigned to receive active IFC plus Pilates or placebo IFC plus Pilates for 6 weeks. Both groups showed reduced pain and disability at discharge and 6-month follow-up with no differences between them. These findings suggest that active IFC plus Pilates exercise is not more effective than placebo IFC.

Finally, a recent study evaluated the effect of IFC on both subjective and objective outcomes with respect to other types of electrotherapies (Rajfur et al 2017). In this study 127 patients were randomized to six groups (conventional TENS, acupuncture-like TENS, high-voltage electrical stimulation (HVPC), diadynamic current, IFC and control). Outcomes included pain measurements and functional testing. In addition, stabilometric platform measurement was used as an objective measurement tool for evaluating postural stability. The results pointed out the comparative superiority of IFC over other modalities

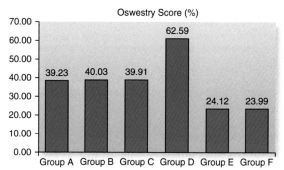

Fig. 18.6 Intergroup comparisons of reduction in Oswestry disability score (%). *Group A* = conventional TENS; *Group B* = acupuncture-like TENS; *Group C* = high-voltage electrical stimulation; *Group D* = IFC; *Group E* = diadynamic current; *Group F* = control. (From: Rajfur J, Pasternok M, Rajfur K et al (2017) Efficacy of selected electrical therapies on chronic low back pain: a comparative clinical pilot study. *Med Sci Monit* **23**:85–100.)

for functional ability and pain reduction (see Fig. 18.6). The authors concluded that although other types of current (i.e. TENS, HVPC) were helpful, the use of IFC led to greater remission of symptoms.

Knee Osteoarthritis

The effect of IFC on knee OA pain has been widely investigated. Quality of early studies (Ní Chiosoig et al 1994; Young et al 1991) is poor and equivocal. Adedoyin et al (2002) showed a positive effect of IFC and placebo IFC stimulation on pain; although both interventions reduced pain, the change was significantly better for the active IFC. Defrin et al (2005) assessed the difference between innocuous and noxious stimulus on pain intensity, morning stiffness, range of motion (ROM), pain threshold and pain reduction. When compared with sham and control groups, both noxious and innocuous stimulation significantly decreased chronic pain (p<0.001), morning stiffness (p<0.01) and significantly increased pain threshold (p<0.001) and ROM (p<0.001), but noxious stimulation was more effective in reducing pain intensity (p< 0.05) and increasing pain thresholds (p< 0.001).

One RCT compared the effectiveness of different AMF beat frequencies of IFC and sham IFC (Gundog et al 2012). The results showed a superior effect of active IFC over sham IFC on pain and disability outcomes with no differences in effectiveness for the different beat frequencies (40, 100 and 180 Hz). In a double-blind, RCT multicentre trial (n=203), Atamaz et al (2012) evaluated the differences in pain, function and paracetamol intake (in grams) for active and sham TENS, active and sham IFC and active and sham shortwave diathermy (SWD) accompanied by exercise training and education. The authors found a significant decrease in all variables assessed (p<0.05), without a significant difference among groups, except in analgesic use between the IFC groups: the active IFC group used a lower amount of paracetamol at 6 months (p< 0.05) when compared with the IFC sham group.

Finally, a recent systematic review and network meta-analysis of RCTs was conducted to compare six treatment regimens (high-frequency TENS, low-frequency TENS, NMES, IFC, pulsed electrical stimulation and non-invasive interactive neurostimulation) with the control group (sham or no intervention) for pain relief in patients with knee OA (Zeng et al 2015). In this study, 27 trials were included and the authors concluded that IFC was the only effective treatment for pain when compared with the control group (standardized MD VAS 2.06, 95% CI: 1.1–3.19). When low methodological quality and small sample size trials were excluded, the sensitivity analysis demonstrated that IFC still achieved significantly more pain reduction when compared with control and low-frequency TENS.

Overall, there appears to be conflicting evidence regarding the clinical effects of IFC in reducing pain in patients with knee OA.

Urinary Incontinence

Some evidence supports the benefits of IFC in the reduction of stress urinary incontinence in different populations. Early literature suggested that inclusion of IFC along with exercises would be a simple, inexpensive and conservative alternative for the management of postpartum genuine stress incontinence (Dumoulin et al 1995a). Several studies have confirmed that IFC can be used to stimulate pelvic floor musculature and can be helpful in retraining these muscles in adults (Alves et al 2011; Demirtürk et al 2008; Oh-Oka 2008; Vahtera et al 1997) and children (Kajbafzadeh et al 2009, 2015, 2016; Ladi-Seyedian et al 2018).

Common outcomes in these studies used to determine the effect of IFC included the severity of symptoms and signs, assessed subjectively using a VAS (Alves et al 2011) and questionnaires (Ladi-Seyedian et al 2017; Oh-Oka 2008; Demirtürk et al 2008; Vahtera et al 1997) and objectively by using a 1-hour pad test (Alves et al 2011, Oh-Oka 2008), surface EMG (Vahtera et al 1997), biofeedback (Demirtürk et al 2008), mean maximal detrusor pressure, maximum bladder capacity, mean detrusor compliance, detrusor sphincter dyssynergia (Kajbafzadeh et al 2009), the mean number of wet nights per week (Kajbafzadeh et al 2015), uroflowmetry with EMG (Ladi-Seyedian et al 2018), bladder capacity (Kajbafzadeh et al 2016), maximum urine flow (Alves et al 2011; Kajbafzadeh et al 2016) and voiding time (Kajbafzadeh et al 2016).

For example, one study compared two electrical stimulation therapy interventions for stress urinary incontinence (Alves et al 2011). Twenty volunteers were randomly allocated into two groups: medium-frequency current and low-frequency current. Both treatments significantly reduced the amount of urine lost, the discomfort and perineal pressure with no differences between them. In addition, in elderly overactive bladder patients with urinary incontinence for whom anticholinergic drugs had not been effective, IFC was safe and had better effects than anticholinergics in quality of life and incontinence symptoms (Oh-Oka 2008). More recently, a series of prospective trials assessed the safety and efficacy of IFC in children with urinary incontinence (Kajbafzadeh et al 2015, 2016; Ladi-Seyedian et al 2018). In these studies, the application of IFC plus standard urotherapy was better than standard urotherapy alone (Kajbafzadeh et al 2015, 2016), and IFC combined with training through biofeedback was more effective than in improving symptoms after 1 year. These results suggest that IFC can be applied as a safe, effective and well tolerated therapy in the management of children with urinary incontinence. (Ladi-Seyedian et al 2018).

The definition of optimal protocols for treating incontinence has always attracted the attention of investigators. For example, Dumoulin et al (1995b) explored the effect of different bipolar electrode placements during IFC stimulation of the pelvic-floor musculature. Today, although there is still a lack of full consensus over the best electrical parameters for IFC, some consistent protocols associated with positive effects are found in the literature. For example, when treating incontinence in children, IFC is commonly applied daily for 20 minutes, for a two-week period, with a carrier frequency of 4kHz and a beat frequency sweep of 1–25 Hz, with an intensity until the child reports a strong but comfortable level of sensory awareness below pain threshold (Kajbafzadeh et al 2009, 2015, 2016; Ladi-Seyedian et al 2018). For this specific purpose, IFC was delivered by two channels using rectangular self-adhesive electrodes; two electrodes placed bilaterally on the skin of the symphysis pubis and two other electrodes from each channel placed crosswise on the skin under the ischial tuberosity (Kajbafzadeh et al 2009, 2015, 2016; Ladi-Seyedian et al 2018). The number of sessions ranged from 10 (Ladi-Seyedian et al 2018) to 18 (Kajbafzadeh et al 2009).

Compared with the literature on children, the IFC protocol for the management of adults with incontinence seems less consistent. Some authors did not provide information about the carrier frequency and level of intensity used (Demirtürk et al 2008; Oh-Oka 2008). In addition, a discrepancy exists in the type of electrodes and the beat frequency used. For example, protocols included either intravaginal (Alves et al 2011; Vahtera et al 1997), intra-anal (Vahtera et al 1997), or surface electrodes (Demirtürk et al 2008; Oh-Ka 2008). For the surface electrodes, two were applied over the suprapubic region and the corresponding electrodes were positioned near to the medial side of the ischial tuberosity (Demirtürk et al 2008) or lower buttocks (Oh-Ka 2008). Regarding the beat frequency, this is reported to be fixed at 50 Hz (Alves et al 2011), fixed at 20 Hz (Oh-Ka 2008) or using a sweep frequency between 1–100 Hz (Demirtürk et al 2008), or 5–50 Hz (Vahtera et al 1997). The treatment time ranged from 10 to 20 minutes. Points of agreement included the level of intensity and the treatment duration. Most of the studies used the maximum tolerance level of intensity (Alves et al 2011; Vahtera et al 1997) and the treatment was applied for 2 to 3 weeks (Alves et al 2011; Demirtürk et al 2008; Vahtera et al 1997).

Thus, in the light of this, there is still a lack of consensus among authors about optimal IFC protocol when treating stress urinary incontinence in adults.

Besides stress urinary incontinence, little evidence is found for the effect of IFC in other forms of incontinence, such as urge and mixed presentations (Gopalakrishnan 2017; Lo et al 2003; Switzer & Hendriks 1988). Overall, these studies show that IFC applied alone (Switzer & Hendriks 1988), combined with pelvic floor muscle strengthening exercises (Lo et al 2003) or in addition to Acu-TENS and exercises, is effective in reducing the symptoms and improving the quality of life in women with urge and mixed urinary incontinence. Finally, much attention has been focused on the effects of IFC for the management of chronic constipation in children. The evidence is overall weak, but growing. Early studies have shown beneficial results in children with slow transit constipation (Clarke et al 2009; Leong et al 2012; Yik et al 2012).

Other recent papers have extended these concepts and evidence further. For example, Ladi-Seyedian et al (2017) demonstrated that IFC plus behavioural therapy (high fibre diet, hydration, toilet training) was better than just behavioural therapy in constipation symptoms and pain scores in Hirschsprung's disease patients. In addition, six months of home-based IFC (applied daily for 1 hour) was able to increase the defecation frequency, decrease of abdominal pain and improve the quality of life for children with intractable slow transit constipation (Yik et al 2018).

Together these studies suggest that IFC stimulation is an effective, cheap and low-risk intervention to treat chronic constipation, emerging as a promising option for this population before surgery is considered.

Soft-Tissue Pain

Evidence has emerged recently about the effect of IFC in soft-tissue painful conditions. A systematic review assessed the impact of IFC in fibromyalgia (de Almeida et al 2018). However, due to the lack of good quality trials, its effects remain inconclusive.

In carpal tunnel syndrome, a three-arm parallel trial comparing the effects on pain of splinting alone, TENS alone and IFC alone, showed that IFC was more effective than a splinting regimen and more effective than TENS ($p < 0.01$) at 6-weeks follow-up (Koca et al 2014).

In chronic neck and shoulder pain, the combination of ultrasound, together with IFC plus exercise, applied to thoracic spine area trigger points, reported greater improvements in pain intensity and size of the pain area compared with IFC plus exercise (Waschl et al 2014). In contrast, positive effects were reported for IFC alone for treating depression and pain in chronic myofascial pain syndrome ($p < 0.05$) (Ofluoğlu et al 2013). In addition, IFC has been found to be more effective than TENS in inducing upper trapezius muscle relaxation (assessed by electromyography) in patients with chronic non-specific neck discomfort. Although both therapies reduced the pain, clinically important differences were found only in the IFC group (minimally clinically important difference (MCID); 2.2 for IFC and 1.3 for TENS) (Acedo et al 2015).

Finally, IFC plus conventional therapy (e.g. continuous ultrasound, contrast baths, stretching and strengthening exercises) was shown to be more effective than conventional therapy alone in decreasing pain ($p = 0.00$) and improving functional ability in plantar fasciitis ($p = 0.00$) (Das & Dutta 2015).

Shoulder Pain

Limited evidence exists for the management of hemiplegic shoulder pain. In one study, IFC was no more effective than laser in decreasing pain and increasing the patient level of satisfaction with the shoulder function. No treatment control or placebo group was included in this study (Jan 2017). In contrast, Suriya-Amarit et al (2014) concluded that active IFC improved pain-free passive ROM of the shoulder post stroke ($p < 0.01$) compared to placebo IFC.

In patients with unilateral shoulder impingement syndrome, adding IFC to exercise or manual therapy did not produce any superior effect in pain, disability and catastrophizing compared with only exercise and with an exercise and placebo ultrasound (de Paula Gomes et al 2018). These results contrast with a similar study where the application of active ultrasound, active IFC and active TENS as a supplement to exercise all displayed similar improvements in terms of pain, function and physical component of quality of life (Gunay Ucurum et al 2018). However, IFC showed significantly better outcomes for the mental component of the quality of life scale.

In summary, there seems to be an increase in the number of RCTs and systematic reviews/meta-analyses about the efficacy of IFC for a variety of painful conditions. However, the report of the clinical significance (effect size, MCID) is still lacking among the published RCTs. The evidence tends to support its use for chronic pain, such as chronic LBP and knee OA. However, more high-quality trials are necessary to confirm this. In addition, emerging evidence exists from RCTs to support the use of IFC in myofascial pain and chronic neck pain. Finally, conflicting and insufficient evidence exists for the role of IFC in conditions such as hemiplegic shoulder pain, shoulder impingement syndrome and fibromyalgia.

Clinical Evidence for BMAC/ Russian Currents

In contrast to the amount of literature on BMAC/Russian currents in healthy volunteers, little evidence is found for these currents in clinical populations. Most of the published literature has assessed the effect of Russian stimulation in knee OA. For example, a recent study investigated the combined application of progressive resistance training and Russian electrical stimulation on quadriceps muscle strength in elderly women with knee OA (Park & Hwangbo 2015). Thirty women were randomly assigned to a control group (n=10), a progressive resistance training group (n=10), or a Russian stimulation group plus resistance training (n=10). The peak torque was assessed at baseline and at 4 and 8 weeks. There were significant intergroup differences between the Russian stimulation group and the other groups. The authors concluded that the combined protocol was effective in strengthening the quadriceps femoris muscle in this population. In addition, Heggannavar et al (2014) compared the application of short wave therapy (SWT) and exercises to the application of SWT, exercises and Russian stimulation. Patients allocated to the group receiving the Russian stimulation showed significant benefits in quadriceps muscle strength and functional ability.

Even more recently, Omole et al (2018) assessed the effects of Russian current and isometric resisted exercises on quadriceps angle and joint space width amongst patients with primary knee OA. Forty-seven patients were randomly assigned to an exercise only group or exercise plus Russian current group. Each participant received treatment twice a week for a total of 8 weeks. Both groups showed a significant mean change in quadriceps angle score with no significant mean change in joint space width. There were no significant differences for these outcomes between groups. Therefore, in this study Russian currents did not show additional effects.

However, positive effects of Russian currents, plus conventional physical therapy (splinting, massage, stretching, ROM exercise, functional training) compared with conventional therapy alone was found for quadriceps muscle peak torque and ambulation speed in patients with anterior thigh burn (Abdel-aziem & Ahmed 2013).

And in a further study, Abd-Elmonem et al (2015) showed that children with knee hemarthrosis who had received 8 weeks of Russian current stimulation in addition to a physical therapy programme (strengthening, stretching and gait training) showed better results in peak torque of knee flexors, power of knee flexors and power of knee extensors when compared with the physical therapy programme alone. However, no differences between groups were found for functional walking.

Even more recently, Ganesh et al (2018) assessed the effect of Russian stimulation on the level of spasticity and motor recovery in adult patients post stroke. Eighty-three patients were randomly assigned to one of three groups: task-oriented exercises, Faradic current for 10 minutes in addition to task-oriented exercises and Russian current for 10 minutes in addition to task-oriented exercises for a period of 5 sessions per week for 6 weeks. All groups improved in passive and active ankle ROM (p< 0.05) and soleus and gastrocnemius muscle spasticity (p< 0.05). Thus, adding Russian stimulation to exercises did not show superiority compared to other groups.

Finally, Russian currents together with conventional therapy (ventilation with pursed lips, vibrocompression and huffing) improved the respiratory abdominal muscle strength in patients with chronic obstructive pulmonary disease during hospitalization (Dall Acqua et al 2012).

THERAPEUTIC USES

IFC is a safe non-invasive treatment with relatively few contraindications. It is usually applied as part of a full rehabilitation plan and can be therapist-administered or self-administered with the recent development of small portable units. IFC is often used on patients to provide pain relief in a variety of acute and chronic painful conditions including muscle pain, joint problems, postoperative pain and soft-tissue pain.

Russian current (RC) has commonly been applied to increase or to prevent loss of muscle strength in a variety of conditions including musculoskeletal (Omole et al 2018; Park & Hwangbo 2015), neurological (Ganesh et al 2018) and respiratory (Dall Acqua et al 2012). In all of these, RC is applied as part of a multimodal plan. Common co-interventions for RC are exercises, massage and functional training.

TREATMENT PARAMETERS AND METHODS OF APPLICATION

A typical IFC unit allows the parameters of carrier frequency, intensity and AMF to be manipulated by the clinician. The description and relevance of these parameters are presented here.

The Carrier Frequency

Classic electrotherapy literature suggests that the frequency of 2 kHz would be more appropriate to elicit muscle contractions for strengthening, whereas the frequency of 4 kHz is optimal for pain control (Goats 1990; Hogenkamp et al 2005). A randomized study assessed the effect of the carrier frequency of IFC (AMF 100 Hz at sensory level of stimulation) on pressure pain threshold (PPT) in healthy humans (Venancio et al 2013). They found a significant increase in PPT in the 1 kHz group when compared with the 8k Hz and 10 kHz groups. However, carrier frequencies of 1 kHz and 2 kHz are perceived as more uncomfortable than carrier frequencies of 4 kHz, 8 kHz and 10 kHz. Correa et al (2016) compared the effects of 1 kHz, 4 kHz and placebo in pain intensity, disability, use of analgesics and physiological measures of pain in patients with chronic LBP. They concluded that consumption of analgesics was significantly decreased in the active groups and that temporal summation of pain due to repeated pressure stimuli was reduced in the 1 kHz group compared with the other groups. Taken together, these studies suggest that lower carrier frequencies (1 kHz) would be preferred over higher carrier (4–8 kHz) frequencies to elicit a pain-relieving effect.

The Amplitude-Modulated Frequency (AMF)

The selection of AMF or 'beat frequency' has been claimed in the past to play an important role in the physiological effects and therapeutic response to IFC treatment, differentially stimulating nerve and other tissues at different AMF settings. However, as discussed, the evidence from laboratory and clinical studies casts doubt on this classical theory. A modification of AMF has been shown to have little effect on the threshold activation of nerve responses (Kinnunen & Alasaarela 2004; Palmer et al 1999). The absence of any differential analgesic and physiological effects for the AMF has also been confirmed in clinical pain when IFC was delivered at strong but comfortable amplitude level (Gundog et al 2012). AMF is therefore unlikely to have a clinical or physiological hypoalgesic effect beyond that achieved with the medium carrier frequency. However, more research is needed before definite conclusions can be drawn on this matter.

Intensity of Stimulation

Pulse amplitude refers to the strength of the output and is commonly measured in mA. In general, the current could be administered at sensory, motor or noxious levels. Review of the clinical literature shows that the most commonly used intensity is associated with a sensory (Aβ fibre) level of stimulation (Acedo et al 2015; Albornoz-Cabello et al 2017; Fuentes et al 2014; Gundog et al 2012; Suriya-Amarit 2014). Stimulation at the highest tolerable sub-motor level (Waschl et al 2014), motor (Aα fibre) (Lara-Palomo et al 2012) and noxious levels (Aδ–C fibre) are less common (Defrin et al 2005). Despite the fact that hypoalgesia induced by activation of noxious fibres (Aδ and C) is stronger and of longer duration than that of Aβ fibres (Defrin et al 2005; Liu et al 1998), most of the clinical researchers appear to select the sensory level of stimulation when investigating the effect of IFC (Fuentes 2010). It is important to note that most of the evidence on stimulation intensity relates to chronic painful conditions, thus under this scenario, the use of a 'strong but comfortable' level of intensity is debatable. The use of a motor level or noxious level of intensity could likely produce significantly greater clinical benefit (Defrin et al 2005; Liu et al 1998).

Treatment Duration

Recommendations for treatment time seem not to be based on scientific rationale. An analysis of the treatment time in two recent systematic reviews on IFC and musculoskeletal pain revealed that 15–20 minutes of application is effective for pain relief (de Almeida et al 2018; Fuentes 2010); this is also the most frequently reported time in the included trials. This treatment time could be related to the type of equipment used. The application of IFC has been traditionally confined to physiotherapy rooms using large and bulky stimulators. Today, small, portable IFC units have emerged. The portability will allow IFC to be delivered for longer periods; however, the real benefits of longer treatment durations for IFC remains unknown.

True IFC and Premodulated IFC

IFC may be produced either by applying the two medium-frequency currents via four electrodes (true IFC or quadripolar method) so that they intersect in the tissues, or alternatively by mixing the two currents within the generator prior to the application, via two electrodes (premodulated IFC or bipolar method) (see Fig. 18.7). As noted previously, there is doubt with true IFC that the maximal stimulation occurs within the tissues around the geometric centre between the four electrodes. Available data suggest that both methods seem to be accepted and applied by physiotherapists with no clear preference for one or another (Tabasam & Johnson 2000; Gracey et al 2001).

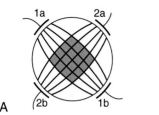
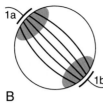

Fig. 18.7 Regions of maximum stimulation (*shaded*), which are predicted with the application of (A) true and (B) premodulated IFC. (From: Ozcan, J, Ward, AR & Robertson, VJ (2004) A comparison of true and premodulated interferential currents. *Archives of Physical Medicine & Rehabilitation* **85**(3):409–415.)

Evidence for differences in the effectiveness of true and premodulated IFC is still insufficient; therefore, no conclusive recommendations about the superiority of one method over another can be made. Although either method could be used when applying IFC, laboratory evidence is clear showing a depth advantage of true IFC over the premodulated method (Beatti et al 2011).

In addition, the latest evidence which shows the penetration efficiency of true IFC when compared with TENS in chronic back patients clearly demonstrates that true IFC is more effective than TENS in reaching deeper tissues (Ariel et al 2019).

In summary, new findings suggest that the mechanism of action of IFC for pain relief might not depend on the AMF. Thus, it seems pointless to recommend specific AMF settings when delivering IFC for treating pain. Some claim that actual stimulation intensity and site of stimulation may be more relevant than the actual depth of penetration. However, there is still controversy about the impact of both the intensity level and the selected carrier frequency. Therefore, further studies should focus on these parameters to elucidate their contribution to the hypoalgesic effects of IFC. Similarly, recent evidence challenges the traditional theory about the interference pattern when a 'true' IFC is applied. Although with some level of controversy, the quadripolar method should be selected when targeting deeper tissues. If this is not the case, the premodulated IFC is the option based on its simplicity, popularity and effectiveness.

TREATMENT PARAMETERS FOR BMAC AND RUSSIAN CURRENTS

The response of skeletal muscle to therapeutic electrical current is dependent upon the specific parameters of the electrical stimulus. Pulse duration, pulse frequency and intensity all play a role in skeletal muscle excitation. Based on the current evidence, optimal dosage when using RC is not clear.

It seems, however, that regardless of the condition being treated, the stimulation parameters have some similarities. These include a treatment time between 10–30 minutes, 3–5 sessions/week during a period of 6–8 weeks. The intensity level should be adjusted to tolerance level and the electrodes placed over the muscle belly. Regarding carrier frequency, most studies used a 2.5 kHz frequency, burst-modulated at 50 Hz with a 25–50% duty cycle. The latter contrasts with a review of some clinical and laboratory-based evidence, which suggests that when selecting BMAC, a carrier frequency of 1 kHz, burst durations of 2 or 4 ms and burst duty cycles of 10–20% should be used, as opposed to the 2.5 kHz, 10 ms burst duration and 50% burst duty cycle of traditional RC to increase or prevent loss of strength (Bellew et al 2014; Ward 2009; Ward et al 2004).

SUMMARY

This chapter has covered the main physical aspects, theoretical mechanisms of action, and relevant laboratory and clinical investigations for IFC and BMAC in the form of Russian stimulation. An overview of the treatment parameters and methods of application has also been presented.

Recent evidence has challenged both the classic interference pattern when 'true' IFC is applied, and the real impact of the AMF parameter as contributor in the hypoalgesic effect of IFC. In addition, most of the trials still use the 'strong but comfortable' level of intensity, thus, little is known about the effects of motor level or noxious level of intensity in pain modulation. This warrants further research. Also, both, the premodulated and the quadripolar methods seem to be equally effective when delivering IFC. It is suggested, however, to select the quadripolar method when targeting deeper tissues.

In recent years significant efforts have been made to determine the clinical effectiveness of IFC in chronic musculoskeletal conditions and urinary incontinence. Based on several randomized clinical trials and systematic reviews, there seems to be some positive effects on pain and functional outcomes, especially when IFC is applied as complement to other interventions, such as exercise or other modalities. For stress urinary incontinence, although there is lack of consensus about the optimal IFC protocol, the literature tends to support its application for the management of symptoms and signs. Additional research is needed to confirm its effects on other forms of incontinence (e.g. urge and mixed). Finally, growing evidence exists for its use in the management of chronic constipation in children.

Russian stimulation combined with exercises has been shown to be effective in increasing muscle strength in different clinical conditions. However, very recent findings challenge the beliefs of a theoretical superiority attributed to RC compared to other currents when eliciting isometric force. Moreover, evidence suggests that modification of the traditional RC parameters would be more effective and would produce less discomfort.

REFERENCES

Abdel-aziem, A. A., & Ahmed Emad, T. (2013). Effect of Russian current stimulation on quadriceps strength of patients with burn. *International Journal of Health and Rehabilitation Sciences, 2*(2), 123–130.

Acedo, A. A., Antunes, A. C., Barros dos Santos, A., et al. (2015). Upper trapezius relaxation induced by TENS and interferential current in computer users with chronic nonspecific neck discomfort: An electromyographic analysis. *Journal of Back and Musculoskeletal Rehabilitation, 28,* 19–24.

Adedoyin, R. A., Olaogun, M. O. B., & Fabeja, O. O. (2002). Effect of interferential current stimulation in the management of osteoarthritic knee pain. *Physiotherapy, 88*(8), 493–499.

Albornoz-Cabello, M., Maya-Martín, J., Domínguez-Maldonado, G., Espejo-Antúnez, l, & Heredia-Rizo, A. (2017). Effect of interferential current therapy on pain perception and disability level in subjects with chronic low back pain: A randomized controlled trial. *Clinical Rehabilitation, 31*(2), 242–249.

Alves, P. G. J., Nunes, M., Fabiana, R., et al. (2011). Comparison between two different neuromuscular electrical stimulation protocols for the treatment of female stress urinary incontinence: A randomized controlled trial. *Revista Brasileira De Fisioterapia, 15*(5) 393–339.

Alves-Guerreiro, J., Noble, J. G., Lowe, A. S., & Walsh, D. M. (2001). The effect of three electrotherapeutic modalities upon peripheral nerve conduction and mechanical pain threshold. *Clinical Physiology, 21*(6), 704–711.

Amira Mahmoud, A.-E., Reham, H. D., & Hazem Atyea, A. A. (2015). Alteration of muscle function and mobility after Russian current stimulation in children with knee hemarthrosis. *Trends in Applied Sciences Research, 10,* 183–194.

Ariel, E., Ratmansky, M., Levkovitz, Y., & Goor-Arveh, I. (2019). Efficiency of tissue penetration by currents induced by three electrotherapeutic techniques: A comparative study using a novel deep-tissue measuring technique. *Physical Therapy, 99*(5), 540–548.

Armijo-Olivo, S., da Costa, B., Cummings, G., et al. (2015). PEDro or Cochrane to assess the quality of clinical trials? A meta-epidemiological study. *PLoS One, 10*(7), 1–14.

Atamaz, F. C., Durmaz, B., Baydar, M., et al. (2012). Comparison of the efficacy of transcutaneous electrical nerve stimulation, interferential currents, and shortwave diathermy in knee osteoarthritis: A double-blind, randomized, controlled, multicenter study. *Archives of Physical Medicine and Rehabilitation, 93,* 748–756.

Bae, Y., & Lee, S. M. (2014). Analgesic effects of transcutaneous electrical nerve stimulation and interferential current on experimental ischemic pain models: Frequencies of 50 Hz and 100 Hz. *Journal of Physical Therapy Science, 26,* 1945–1948.

Beatti, A., Rayner, A., Chipchase, L., et al. (2011). Penetration and spread of interferential current in cutaneous, subcutaneous and muscle tissues. *Physiotherapy, 97,* 319–326.

Belcher, J. F. (1974). Interferential therapy. *New Zealand Journal of Physiotherapy, 6,* 29–34.

Bellew, J. W., Sanders, K., Schuman, K., & Bart, M. (2014). Muscle force production with low and medium frequency burst modulated biphasic pulsed currents. *Physiotherapy Theory and Practice, 30*(2), 105–109.

Bueno, K. S., Dallacorte, D. A., Silva Sprizon, G., et al. (2017). Comparison of the effects of interferential current between male and female healthy adults. *Sci Med, 3,* 1–6.

Cheing, G. L., So, E. M., & Chao, C. Y. (2008). Effectiveness of electroacupuncture and interferential electrotherapy in the management of frozen shoulder. *Journal of Rehabilitation Medicine, 40,* 166–170.

Chipchase, L., Williams, M., & Robertson, V. (2009). A national study of the availability and use of electrophysical agents by Australian physiotherapists. *Physiotherapy Theory and Practice, 25*(4), 279–296.

Choi, J. C., Kim, J., Kang, E., et al. (2016). Brain mechanisms of pain relief by transcutaneous electrical nerve stimulation: A functional magnetic resonance imaging study. *European Journal of Pain, 20,* 92–105.

Christie, A. D., & Willoughby, G. L. (1990). The effect of interferential therapy on swelling following open reduction and internal fixation of ankle fractures. *Physiotherapy Theory and Practice, 6*(1), 3–7.

Cid, J., Escárate, S., Mardones, P., Villegas, D., & Fuentes, J. (2016). *Availability, the frequency of use, and treatment objective of the electrophysical agents in the clinical practice. A national survey of the registered physiotherapists in Chile. Bachelor's thesis.* Concepcion, Chile: University Andres Bello.

Clarke, M. C., Chase, J. W., Gibb, S., et al. (2009). Decreased colonic transit time after transcutaneous interferential electrical stimulation in children with slow transit constipation. *Journal of Pediatric Surgery, 44,* 408–412.

Correa, J. B., Costa, L. O. P., & Oliveira, N. T. B. (2016). Effects of the carrier frequency of interferential current on pain modulation and central hypersensitivity in people with chronic nonspecific low back pain: A randomized placebo-controlled trial. *European Journal of Pain, 20,* 1653–1666.

Dall Acqua, A. M., Döhnert, M. P., & Dos Santos, L. J. (2012). Neuromuscular electrical stimulation with Russian current for expiratory muscle training in patients with chronic obstructive pulmonary disease. *Journal of Physical Therapy Science, 24,* 955–959.

Dantas, L. O., Vieira, A., Siqueira Junior, A., et al. (2015). Comparison between the effects of 4 different electrical stimulation current waveforms on isometric knee extension torque and perceived discomfort in healthy women. *Muscle & Nerve, 51,* 76–82.

Das, H., & Dutta, A. (2015). The effects of interferential therapy for industrial workers in case of plantar fasciitis. *International Journal of Physiotherapy, 2*(5), 772–777.

de Almeida, C., Maldaner da Silva, V. Z., Cipriano Júnior, G., Liebano, R. E., & Quagliotti Duriganc, J. L. (2018). Transcutaneous electrical nerve stimulation and interferential current demonstrate similar effects in relieving acute and chronic pain: A systematic review with meta-analysis. *Brazilian Journal of Physical Therapy*, 22(5), 347–354.

De Domenico, G. (1987). *New dimensions in interferential therapy: A theoretical and clinical guide*. Lindfield, Australia: Reid Medical Books.

Defrin, R., Ariel, E., & Peretz, C. (2005). Segmental noxious versus innocuous electrical stimulation for chronic pain relief and the effect of fading sensation during treatment. *Pain*, 115(1-2), 152–160.

Demirtürk, F., Akbayrak, T., Karakaya, I. C., et al. (2008). Interferential current versus biofeedback results in urinary stress incontinence. *Swiss Medical Weekly*, 138(21–22), 317–321.

Demmink, J. H. (1995). *The effect of a biological conducting medium on the pattern of modulation and distribution in a two-circuit static interferential field*. In *Proceedings of the 12th International Conference of the World Confederation for Physical Therapy*, 583. Washington DC.

Dounavi, M. D., Chesterton, L. S., & Sim, J. (2012). Effects of interferential therapy parameter combinations upon experimentally induced pain in pain-free participants: A randomized controlled trial. *Physical Therapy*, 92(7), 911–923.

de Paula Gomes, C. A., Vieira Dibai-Filho, A., Arruda Moreira, W., et al. (2018). Effect of adding interferential current in an exercise and manual therapy program for patients with unilateral shoulder impingement syndrome: A randomized clinical trial. *Journal of Manipulative and Physiological Therapeutics*, 41(3), 218–226.

da Silva, V. Z., Quaglioti Durigan, J. L., Arena, R., et al. (2015). Current evidence demonstrates similar effects of kilohertz-frequency and low-frequency current on quadriceps evoked torque and discomfort in healthy individuals: A systematic review with meta-analysis. *Physiotherapy Theory and Practice*, 31(8), 533–539.

Dumoulin, C., Seaborne, D. E., & Quirion-DeGirardi, C. (1995a). Pelvic-floor rehabilitation part 1: Comparison of two surface electrode placements during stimulation of the pelvic-floor musculature in women who are continent using bipolar interferential currents. *Physical Therapy*, 75(12), 1067–1074.

Dumoulin, C., Seaborne, D. E., & Quirion-DeGirardi, C. (1995b). Pelvic-floor rehabilitation, part 2: Pelvic-floor reeducation with interferential currents and exercise in the treatment of genuine stress incontinence in postpartum women—a cohort study. *Physical Therapy*, 75(12), 1075–1081.

Emberson, W. (1996). Asthma and interferential therapy (IFT). *In Touch*, 79, 2–8.

Figen, K., Elif, A., Gezer Naciye, S., et al. (2012). Functional magnetic resonance imaging of the effects of low-frequency transcutaneous electrical nerve stimulation on central pain modulation a double-blind, placebo-controlled trial. *The Clinical Journal of Pain*, 28, 581–588.

Foster, N. E., Thompson, K. A., Baxter, G., & Allen, J. M. (1999). Management of nonspecific low back pain by physiotherapists in Britain and Ireland: A descriptive questionnaire of current clinical practice. *Spine*, 24, 1332–1342.

Fourie, J. A., & Bowerbank, P. (1997). Stimulation of bone healing in new fractures of the tibial shaft using interferential currents. *Physiotherapy Research International*, 2(4), 255–268.

Fuentes, C. J. (2010). Effectiveness of interferential current therapy in the management of musculoskeletal pain: Systematic review and meta-analysis. *Physical Therapy*, 90(9), 1219–1238.

Fuentes, J., Armijo-Olivo, S., Funabashi, M., et al. (2014). Enhanced therapeutic alliance modulates pain intensity and muscle pain sensitivity in patients with chronic low back pain: A randomized controlled study. *Physical Therapy Journal*, 94(4), 477–489.

Fuentes, C. J., Armijo-Olivo, S. L., Gross, D., & Magee, D. J. (2011). A preliminary investigation into the effects of active interferential current therapy and placebo on pressure pain sensitivity: A random crossover placebo-controlled study. *Physiotherapy*, 97, 291–301.

Fuentes, J., Armijo-Olivo, S., Magee, D. J., & Gross, D. (2010). Does amplitude-modulated frequency have a role in the hypoalgesic response of interferential current on pressure pain sensitivity in healthy subjects? A randomized crossover study. *Physiotherapy*, 96, 22–29.

Ganesh, G. S., Kumari, R., Pattnaik, M., et al. (2018). Effectiveness of Faradic and Russian currents on plantar flexor muscle spasticity, ankle motor recovery, and functional gait in stroke patients. *Physiot Res Int*, 23, 1–8.

Ganne, J. M. (1976). Interferential therapy. *Australian Journal of Physiotherapy*, 22, 101–110.

Ganne, J M., Speculand, B., Mayne, L. H., et al. (1979). Interferential therapy to promote union of mandibular fractures. *Australian and New Zealand Journal of Surgery*, 49(1), 81–83.

Goats, G. C. (1990). Interferential current therapy. *British Journal of Sports Medicine*, 24(2), 87–92.

Gopalakrishnan. (2017). *Effects of Acu-TENS, interferential therapy and exercises on the quality of life in women with mixed urinary incontinence: An experimental study*. Unpublished Master's thesis, College of Physiotherapy, Sri Ramakrishna Institute of Paramedical Sciences. Coimbatore, India.

Gracey, J. H., Mc Donough, S. M., & Bater, G. D. (2002). Physiotherapy management of low back pain: A survey of current practice in Northern Ireland. *Spine*, 27, 406–411.

Gracey, J. H., Noble, W. H., & Noble, J. G. (2001). *Clinical use of interferential therapy in the management of low back pain. A survey of current practice in Northern Ireland. The Physiotherapy Research Society*. University of Ulster.

Gunay Ucurum, S., Ozer Kaya, D., Kayali, Y., & Askin, A. (2018). Agah Tekindal. Comparison of different electrotherapy methods and exercise therapy in shoulder impingement syndrome: A prospective randomized controlled trial. *Acta Orthopaedica et Traumatologica Turcica*, 52, 249–255.

Gundog, M., Atamaz, F., Kanyilmaz, S., Kirazli, Y., & Celepoglu, G. (2012). Interferential current therapy in patients with knee osteoarthritis. Comparison of the effectiveness of different amplitude-modulated frequencies. *American Journal of Physical Medicine & Rehabilitation, 91,* 107–113.

Heggannavar, A. B., Dharmayat, S. R., Nerurkar, S. S., & Akambe, S. (2014). Effect of Russian current on quadriceps muscle strength in subjects with primary osteoarthritis of knee: A randomized control trial. *International Journal of Physiotherapy and Research, 2*(3), 555–560.

Hogenkamp, M., Mittelmeijer, E., Smits, I., & Stralen, C. V. (2005). *Interferential therapy.* Rotterdam, Netherlands: Enraf-Nonius B.V.

Iijima, H., Takahashi, M., Tashiro, Y., & Aoyama, T. (2018). Comparison of the effects of kilohertz- and low-frequency electric stimulations: A systematic review with meta-analysis. *PLoS One, 13*(4), 1–19.

Jan, F., Naeem, A., Nawaz Maik, A., Amjad, I., & Mailk, T. (2017). Comparison of low level laser therapy and interferential current on post stroke shoulder pain. *Journal of Pakistan Medical Association, 67*(5), 788–789.

Jin, H.-K., Hwang, T.-Y., & Cho, S.-H. (2017). Sung-Hyoun Cho. Effect of electrical stimulation on blood flow velocity and vessel size. *Open Medicine, 12,* 5–11.

Johnson, M. I., & Tabasam, G. (1999). A double blind placebo controlled investigation into the analgesic effects of inter-ferential currents (IFC) and transcutaneous electrical nerve stimulation (TENS) on cold-induced pain in healthy subjects. *Physiotherapy Theory and Practice, 15,* 217–233.

Johnson, M. I., & Tabasam, G. (2002). A single-blind place-bo-controlled investigation into the analgesic effects of interferential currents on experimentally induced ischaemic pain in healthy subjects. *Clinical Physiology and Functional Imaging, 22,* 187–196.

Johnson, M. I., & Tabasam, G. (2003a). An investigation into the analgesic effects of different frequencies of the ampli-tude-modulated wave of interferential current therapy on cold-induced pain in normal subjects. *Archives of Physical Medicine and Rehabilitation, 84*(9), 1387–1394.

Johnson, M. I., & Tabasam, G. (2003b). A single-blind investigation into the hypoalgesic effects of different swing patterns of inter-ferential currents on cold-induced pain in healthy volunteers. *Archives of Physical Medicine and Rehabilitation, 84*(3), 350–357.

Johnson, M. I., & Tabasam, G. (2003c). An investigation into the analgesic effects of interferential currents and transcutaneous electrical nerve stimulation on experimentally induced isch-emic pain in otherwise pain-free volunteers. *Physical Therapy, 83*(3), 208–223.

Johnson, M. I., & Wilson, H. (1997). The analgesic effects of different swing patterns of interferential currents on cold-in-duced pain. *Physiotherapy, 83*(9), 461–467.

Jorge, S., Parada, C., Ferreira, S., & Tambeli, C. (2006). Interferential therapy produces antinociception during application in various models of inflammatory pain. *Physical Therapy, 86*(6), 800–808.

Kajbafzadeh, A. M., Sharifi-Rad, L., Baradaran, N., et al. (2009). Effect of pelvic floor interferential electrostimulation on urodynamic parameters and incontinency of children with myelomeningocele and detrusor overactivity. *Urology, 74,* 324–331.

Kajbafzadeh, A. M., Sharifi-Rad, L., Mozafarpour, S., et al. (2015). Efficacy of transcutaneous interferential electrical stimulation in treatment of children with primary nocturnal enuresis: A randomized clinical trial. *Pediatric Nephrology, 30,* 1139–1145.

Kajbafzadeh, A. M., Sharifi-Rad, L., Ladi-Seyedian, S., & Mozafarpour, S. (2016). Transcutaneous interferential elec-trical stimulation for the management of non-neuropathic underactive bladder in children: A randomized clinical trial. *BJU International, 117,* 793–800.

Kaptchuk, T. J., KelleyJ.M., ConboyL.A., et al. (2008). Components of placebo effect: randomised controlled trial in patients with irritable bowel syndrome. *BMJ, 336* (7651), 999–1003.

Kinnunen, M., & Alasaarela, E. (2004). Registering the response of tissues exposed to an interferential electric current stimulation. *Acupuncture & Electro-Therapeutics Research, 29,* 213–226.

Koca, I., Boyaci, A., Tutoglu, A., Ucar, M., & Kocaturk, O. (2014). Assessment of the effectiveness of interferential cur-rent therapy and TENS in the management of carpal tunnel syndrome: A randomized controlled study. *Rheumatology International, 34,* 1639–1645.

Ladi-Seyedian, S. S., Sharifi-Rad, L., & Kajbafzadeh, A. M. (2019). Pelvic floor electrical stimulation and muscles train-ing: A combined rehabilitative approach for management of non-neuropathic urinary incontinence in children. *Journal of Pediatric Surgery, 54*(4), 825–830.

Ladi-Seyedian, S. S., Sharifi-Rad, L., Manouchehri, N., & Ashjaei, B. (2017). A comparative study of transcutaneous inter-ferential electrical stimulation plus behavioral therapy and behavioral therapy alone on constipation in postoperative Hirschsprung disease children. *Journal of Pediatric Surgery, 52*(1), 177–183.

Lamb, S., & Mani, R. (1994). Does interferential therapy affect blood flow? *Clinical Rehabilitation, 8,* 213–218.

Lara-Palomo, I. C., Aguilar-Ferrándiz, M. E., Matarán-Peñarrocha, G. A., et al. (2012). Short-term effects of interferential current electro-massage in adults with chronic non-specific low back pain: A randomized controlled trial. *Clinical Rehabilitation, 27*(5), 439–449.

Laufer, Y., & Elboim, M. (2008). Effect of burst frequency and duration of kilohertz-frequency alternating currents and of low- frequency pulsed currents on strength of contraction, muscle fatigue, and perceived discomfort. *Physical Therapy, 88*(10), 1167–1176.

Leong, L. C., Yik, Y. I., Catto-Smith, A. G., et al. (2012). Long-term effects of transabdominal electrical stimulation in treating children with slow-transit constipation. *Journal of Pediatric Surgery, 46*(12), 2309–2312.

Lindsay, D., Dearness, J., Richardson, C., et al. (1990). A survey of electromodality usage in private physiotherapy practices. *Australian Journal of Physiotherapy, 36*(4), 249–256.

Liu, X. G., Morton, C. R., Azkue, J. J., Zimmermann, M., & Sandkuhler, J. (1998). Long-term depression of c-fi-bre-evoked spinal field potentials by stimulation of primary afferent Ad-fibres in the adult rat. *European Journal of Neuroscience, 10,* 3069–3076.

Lo, S. K., Naidu, J., & Cao, Y. (2003). Additive effect of interferential therapy over pelvic floor exercise alone in the treatment of female urinary stress and urge incontinence: A randomized controlled trial. *Hong kong Physiotherapy Journal, 21*, 37–42.

Low, J., & Reed, A. (2000). Electrical stimulation of nerve and muscle. In J. Low & A. Reed (Eds.), *Electrotherapy explained. Principles and practice* (3rd ed.) (Vol. 3) (pp. 43–140). Oxford: Butterworth-Heinemann.

Melzack, R., & Wall, P. (1965). Pain mechanisms: A new theory. *Science, 150*(3699), 971–979.

Moura Franco, K., dos Santos Franco, Y., Bastos de Oliveira, N., et al. (2017). Is interferential current before Pilates exercises more effective than placebo in patients with chronic nonspecific low back pain? A randomized controlled trial. *Archives of Physical Medicine and Rehabilitation, 98*, 320–328.

Ní Chiosoig, F., Hendriks, O., & Malone, J. (1994). A pilot study of the therapeutic effects of bipolar and quadripolar interferential therapy, using bilateral osteoarthritis as a model. *Physiotherapy Ireland, 15*(1), 3–7.

Nikolova, L. (1987). Introduction to interferential therapy. In L. Nikolova (Ed.), *Treatment with interferential therapy* (pp. 3–16). Singapore: Churchill Livingstone.

Nikolova-Troeva, L. (1968). The modem electrotherapeutic methods in the therapy of endarteritis obliterans. *Ther Gegenw, 102*, 190–198.

Noble, J. G., Henderson, G., Cramp, A. F. L., Walsh, D. M., & Lowe, A. S. (2000). The effect of interferential therapy upon cutaneous blood flow in humans. *Clinical Physiology, 20*(1), 2–7.

Nussbaum, E., Rush, P., & Disenhaus, L. (1990). The effect of interferential therapy on peripheral blood flow. *Physiotherapy, 76*, 803–807.

Ofluoğlu, D., Bulak, E. A., Kablan, N., & Akyüz, G. (2013). Short-term effects of interferential currents on chronic myofascial pain syndrome. *Turk J Phys Med Rehab, 59*, 209–213.

Oh-Oka, H. (2008). Efficacy of interferential low-frequency therapy for elderly wet overactive bladder patients. *Indian Journal of Urology, 24*(2), 178–181.

Oliveira, P., Guida, K, A., Bottaro, M., et al. (2018). Training effects of alternated and pulsed currents on the quadriceps muscles of athletes. *Int J Sports Med, 39*(7), 535–540.

Omole, J. O., Egwu, M. O., Ojoawo, A. O., & Ogundele, A. O. (2018). Comparative effects of Russian current and isometric resisted exercise on quadriceps angle and joint space width among patients with primary knee osteoarthritis. *International Journal of Advanced Research and Publications, 2*(2), 92–99.

Ozcan, J., Ward, A. R., & Robertson, V. J. (2004). A comparison of true and premodulated interferential currents. *Archives of Physical Medicine and Rehabilitation, 85*(3), 409–415.

Palmer, S. T., Martin, D. J., Steedman, W. M., & Ravey, J. (1999). Alteration of interferential current and transcutaneous electrical nerve stimulation frequency: Effects on nerve excitation. *Archives of Physical Medicine and Rehabilitation, 80*, 1065–1071.

Pantaleão, M. A., Laurino, M. F., Gallego, N. L., et al. (2011). Adjusting pulse amplitude during transcutaneous electrical nerve stimulation (TENS) application produces greater hypoalgesia. *The Journal of Pain, 12*, 581–590.

Park, S. H., & Hwangbo, G. P. (2015). Effects of combined application of progressive resistance training and Russian electrical stimulation on quadriceps femoris muscle strength in elderly women with knee osteoarthritis. *Journal of Physical Therapy Science, 27*, 729–731.

Philipp, A., Wolf, G. K., Rzany, B., Dertinger, H., & Jung, E. G. (2000). Interferential current is effective in palmar psoriaris: An open prospective trial. *European Journal of Dermatology, 10*(3), 195–198.

Poitras, S., Blais, R., Swaine, B., & Rossignol, M. (2005). Management of work-related low back pain: A population-based survey of physical therapists. *Physical Therapy, 85*(11), 1168–1181.

Pope, G. D., Mockett, S. P., & Wright, J. P. (1995). A survey of electrotherapeutic modalities: Ownership and use in the NHS in England. *Physiotherapy, 81*(2), 82–91.

Rajfur, J., Pasternok, M., Rajfur, K., et al. (2017). Efficacy of selected electrical therapies on chronic low back pain: A comparative clinical pilot study. *Medical Science Monitor, 23*, 85–100.

Resende, L., Merriwether, D. D., et al. (2018). Meta-analysis of transcutaneous electrical nerve stimulation for relief of spinal pain. *European Journal of Pain, 22*(4), 663–678.

Robertson, V., Ward, A., Low, J., & Reed, A. (2006). *Electrotherapy explained: Principles and practice* (4th ed.). Edinburgh: Butterworth Heinemann Elsevier.

Rocha, C. S., Lanferdini, F. J., Kolberg, C., et al. (2012). Interferential therapy effect on mechanical pain threshold and isometric torque after delayed onset muscle soreness induction in human hamstrings. *Journal of Sports Sciences, 30*(8), 733–742.

Roche, P. A., Tan, H. Y., & Stanton, W. R. (2002). Modification of induced ischaemic pain by placebo electrotherapy. *Physiotherapy Theory and Practice, 18*(3), 131–139.

Rossettini, G., Carlino, E., Testa, M. (2018). Clinical relevance of contextual factors as triggers of placebo and nocebo effects in musculoskeletal pain. *BMC Musculoskeletal Disorders, 19*(1), 1–15.

Santos, F. V., Chiappa, G R., Vieira, P. J., et al. (2013). Interferential electrical stimulation improves peripheral vasodilatation in healthy individuals. *Brazilian Journal of Physical Therapy, 17*(3), 281–288.

Schmitz, R. J., Martin, D. E., Perrin, D. H., et al. (1997). Effect of interferential current on perceived pain and serum cortisol associated with delayed onset muscle soreness. *Journal of Sport Rehabilitation, 6*(1), 30–37.

Shah, S. G. S., & Farrow, A. (2012). Trends in the availability and usage of electrophysical agents in physiotherapy practices from 1990 to 2010: A review. *Physical Therapy Reviews, 17*(4), 207–226.

Rocha, C. S., Lanferdini, F. J., Kolberg, C., Silva, M. F., Vaz, M. A., Partata, W. A., et al. Interferential therapy effect on mechanical pain threshold and isometric torque after delayed onset muscle soreness induction in human. *Journal of Sports Sciences, 30*(8):733–742

Springer, S., Laufer, Y., & Elboim-Gabyzon, M. (2015). Clinical decision making for using electro-physical agents by physiotherapists, an Israeli survey. *Israel Journal of Health Policy Research, 4*(1), 14.

Stephenson, R., & Walker, E. M. (2003). The analgesic effects of interferential (IF) current on cold-pressor pain in healthy subjects: A single-blind trial of three IF currents against sham IF and control. *Physiotherapy: Theory and Practice, 19*(2), 99–107.

Suriya-Amarit, D., Gaogasigam, C., Siriphorn, A., & Boonyong, S. (2014). Effect of interferential current stimulation in management of hemiplegic shoulder pain. *Archives of Physical Medicine and Rehabilitation, 95*, 1441–1446.

Switzer, D., & Hendriks, O. (1988). Interferential therapy for the treatment of stress and urge incontinence. *Irish Medical Journal, 81*(1), 30–31.

Tabasam, G., & Johnson, M. I. (2000). A survey of the procedures used to administer interferential currents (IFC) by physiotherapists. Pain Society Annual Scientific Meeting. *Warwick, 3–5*, 90.

Tavares da Silva, M., Mendonça Araújo, F., Ferreira Araújo, M., & Melo DeSantana, J. (2018). Effect of interferential current in patients with fibromyalgia: A systematic review. *Fisioter Pesqui, 25*(1), 107–114.

Treffene, R. J. (1983). Interferential fields in a fluid medium. *Australian Journal of Physiotherapy, 29*, 209–216.

Tugay, N., Akbayrak, T., Demirtürk, F., et al. (2007). Effectiveness of transcutaneous electrical nerve stimulation and interferential current in primary dysmenorrhea. *Pain Medicine, 8*, 295–300.

Ucurum, S. G., Ozer Kaya, D., Kayali, Y., Askin, A., & Tekinda, M. A. (2018). Comparison of different electrotherapy methods and exercise therapy in shoulder impingement syndrome: A prospective randomized controlled trial. *Acta Orthopaedica et Traumatologica Turcica, 52*, 249–255.

Vahtera, T., Haaranen, M., Viramo-Koskela, A. L., et al. (1997). Pelvic floor rehabilitation is effective in patients with multiple sclerosis. *Clinical Rehabilitation, 11*, 211–219.

Vaz, M. A., Aragao, F. A., Boschi, E. S., et al. (2012). Effects of Russian current and low-frequency pulsed current on discomfort level and current amplitude at 10% maximal knee extensor torque. *Physiotherapy Theory and Practice, 28*(8), 617–623.

Vaz, M. A., & Frasson, V. B. (2018). low-frequency pulsed current versus kilohertz-frequency alternating current: a scoping literature review. *Archives of Physical Medicine and Rehabilitation, 99*(4), 792–805.

Venancio, R. C., Pelegrini, S., Queiroz Gomes, D., Yoshio Nakano, E., & Liebano, R. (2013). Effects of carrier frequency of interferential current on pressure pain threshold and sensory comfort in humans. *Archives of Physical Medicine and Rehabilitation, 94*, 95–102.

Ward, A. R. (2009). Electrical stimulation using kilohertz-frequency alternating current. *Physical Therapy, 89*, 181–190.

Ward, A. R., Oliver, W. G., & Buccella, D. (2006). Wrist extensor torque production and discomfort associated with low-frequency and burst-modulated kilohertz-frequency currents. *Physical Therapy, 86*(10), 1360–1367.

Ward, A., Robertson, V., & Ioannou, H. (2004). The effect of duty cycle and frequency on muscle torque production using kHz frequency range alternating current. *Medical Engineering & Physics, 26*, 569–579.

Ward, A. R., & Shkuratova, N. (2002). Russian electrical stimulation: The early experiments. *Physical Therapy, 82*, 1019–1030.

Waschl, S., Morrissey, M. C., & Rugelj, D. (2014). The efficacy of ultrasound-facilitated electrical stimulation as an adjunct to exercise in treating chronic neck and shoulder pain. *Journal of Musculoskeletal Pain, 22*(1), 78–88.

Watson, T. (2000). The role of electrotherapy in contemporary physiotherapy practice. *Manual Therapy, 5*, 132–141.

Wong, R. A., & Jette, D. U. (1984). Changes in sympathetic tone associated with different forms of transcutaneous electrical nerve stimulation in healthy subjects. *Physical Therapy, 64*, 478–482.

Yik, Y. I., Hutson, J., & Southwell, B. (2018). Home-based transabdominal interferential electrical stimulation for six months improves paediatric slow transit constipation (STC). *Neuromodulation, 21*(7), 676–681.

Yik, Y. I., Ismail, K. A., Hutson, J. M., et al. (2012). Home transcutaneous electrical stimulation to treat children with slow-transit constipation. *Journal of Pediatric Surgery, 47*(6), 1285–1290.

Young, S. L., Woodbury, M. G., Fryday-Field, K., et al. (1991). Efficacy of interferential current stimulation alone for pain reduction in patients with osteoarthritis of the knee: A randomized placebo control clinical trial. *Physical Therapy, 71*(6), S52.

Zeng, C., Li, H., Yang, T., Deng, Z. H., Yang, Y., Zhang, Y., et al. (2015). Electrical stimulation for pain relief in knee osteoarthritis: Systematic review and network meta-analysis. *Osteoarthritis and Cartilage, 23*, 189–202.

19

Electrical Stimulation for Wounds

Luther Kloth, Anna Polak, Tim Watson

BRIEF HISTORY

The first documented use of electric energy for enhancement of wound healing was published in 1688 by Sir Kenelm Digby in Digby's 'Receipts'. In a 1925 review of Digby's work, Robertson (1925) found that Digby reported the application of charged gold leaf to smallpox lesions that were observed to heal without scarring. However, other clinical research with gold leaf reported inconsistent healing outcomes (Kanof 1964; Risbrook et al 1973; Smith et al 1967; Wolf et al 1966). Between 1969 and 1991 clinical researchers evaluated the effects of low-voltage, constant micro-amperage (200–1000 µA), direct current (DC) on chronic wounds, reporting positive healing outcomes (Carley & Wainapel 1985; Gault & Gatens 1976; Walcott et al 1969; Wood et al 1991). In clinical trials conducted between the 1990s and 2018, pulsed currents (PCs) rather than direct currents were mainly used to treat chronic wounds.

PHYSICAL PRINCIPLES

Types of Electrical Currents Used to Treat Wounds

Human wounds are treated with electrical stimulation (ES) utilizing subsensory amplitudes of DC and PCs (Adunsky & Ohry 2005; Baker et al 1996, 1997; Hampton & Collis 2006; Hampton & King 2005; Karba et al 1997; Katelaris et al 1987; Ullah 2007), as well as sensory ES below muscle contraction threshold. Sensory ES utilizes monophasic, high-voltage pulsed current (HVPC) (Ahmad 2008; Franek et al 2000, 2012; Griffin et al 1991; Houghton et al 2003; Kloth 1988; Peters et al 2001; Polak et al 2016a, 2016b, 2017, 2018), monophasic, low-voltage pulsed current (LVPC) (Weiss et al 1989; Feedar et al 1991; Gentzkow et al 1991, 1993; Junger et al 1997; Barczak et al 2001), or biphasic LVPC (Baker et al 1996, 1997; Karba et al 1990; Lawson & Petrofsky 2007; Lundeberg et al 1992; Petrofsky et al 2010; Stefanowska et al 1987; Suh et al 2009). These current waveforms are illustrated in Chapter 4 Fig 4.4 (DC), Fig 4.16 (PCs), and Fig 4.9 (HVPC waveform). LVPC is also used at an intensity above the threshold of skeletal muscle excitability (Foulds & Barker 1983; Jercinovic et al 1994; Karba et al 1991, 1995; Sebastian et al 2011; Stefanowska et al 1993). Alternating current (AC) seldom appears in the wound healing literature (Sebastian et al 2011).

Research has confirmed the existence of endogenous biophysical currents in healthy moist wound and peri-wound tissues (Foulds & Barker 1983; Reid & Zhao 2014). Thus, clinical wound healing with ES is best enhanced by maintaining wound moisture with 0.9% physiological saline that also enhances ES signal conductivity. The inherent biophysical current that influences wound healing is the transepithelial 'skin battery' that generates an endogenous 'current of injury' within the wound tissues. The skin surface has an average negative potential of -23.4 mV relative to the dermis (Foulds & Barker 1983). This transepithelial potential contributes to normal skin function by stimulating cell migration, division and proliferation that enhance wound healing (Foulds and Barker 1983).

Preclinical studies report that exogenous ES can also promote multiple signalling pathways essential for wound healing and provides a directional signal for cell migration to the wound. In vitro (Fukushima Gruler 1953; Orida & Feldman 1982) and in vivo (Eberhardt et al 1986) studies have revealed that anodal stimulation facilitates electro-taxis of macrophages (Orida & Feldman 1982) and neutrophils (Eberhardt et al 1986; Erickson & Nuccitelli 1984) for autolysis and reactivation of the inflammatory phase of healing. In vitro studies (Erickson & Nuccitelli 1984; Nishimura et al 1996; Yang et al 1984; Zhao et al 2006) have demonstrated that fibroblasts (Erickson & Nuccitelli 1984; Yang et al 1984), keratinocytes (Nishimura et al 1996) and epithelial cells (Zhao et al 2006) migrate towards the cathode, suggesting that cathodal ES may promote cellular proliferation. Both anode and cathode can stimulate cellular processes that enhance growth of blood vessels (Bai et al 2004). An in vitro study revealed that an electrical field (75–200 mV/mm) induced by DC, comparable in amplitude to the current of wound injury, induced directional migration, orientation and elongation of vascular endothelial cells, fibroblasts and smooth muscle cells (Bai et al 2004). Vascular endothelial cells migrated towards the cathode, whereas vascular fibroblasts and smooth muscle cells migrated towards the anode (Bai et al 2004).

A common factor that delays wound healing is compromised perfusion of the wound and peri-wound tissues. Preclinical (Bai et al 2004; Petrofsky et al 2007; Zhao et al 2003) and clinical (Asadi et al 2017; Mohajeri-Tehrani et al 2014) studies have demonstrated that DC (Asadi et al 2017; Bai et al 2004; Mohajeri-Tehrani et al 2014) and biphasic LVPC (Petrofsky et al 2007) increases the release of nitric oxide, a blood vessel dilator (Mohajeri-Tehrani et al 2014; Petrofsky et al 2007) and stimulates release of angiogenic factors (vascular endothelial growth factor (VEGF) (Asadi et al 2017; Mohajeri-Tehrani et al 2014; Zhao et al 2003) and hypoxic inducible factor-1α (Asadi et al 2017).

Chronic wounds are characterized by increased activity of pro-inflammatory cytokines as well as reduced expression of anti-inflammatory cytokines and growth factors (Goldberg et al 2007; Jiang et al 2014; Kurose et al 2015; Mirza & Koh 2015). ES inhibits pro-inflammatory cytokines (Kanno et al 1999), increases the synthesis of factors that stimulate angiogenesis (Asadi et al 2011, 2013; 2017; Bai et al 2011; Görgen et al 2014; Rouabhia et al 2013; Sebastian et al 2011; Ud-Din et al 2015; Zhao et al 2003), cellular proliferation (Asadi et al 2011, 2013; 2017; Bai et al 2011; Rouabhia et al 2013; Sebastian et al 2011; Ud-Din et al 2015; Zhao et al 2003), maturation and remodelling of wounds (Görgen et al 2014; Sebastian et al 2011). These effects were observed in preclinical studies in vitro (Ud-Din et al 2015), in vivo in animals (Asadi et al 2013; Bai et al 2011), in vivo in healthy people (Rouabhia et al 2013; Sebastian et al 2011) and in a clinical trial in patients with diabetic ulcers (Asadi et al 2017).

The impact of electrical energy on cellular processes in wound healing has been observed in humans (Asadi et al 2017; Rouabhia et al 2013; Sebastian et al 2011). In experimental wounds in healthy volunteers, an increase in platelet derived growth factor (PDGF) was noted after ES with low amplitude AC (0.005 mA, 20–80 V, 60 Hz, 60 ms) (Rouabhia et al 2013).[70] Also observed was an increase in gene expression of anti-inflammatory factors (including macrophage migration inhibitory factor and interleukin-10), angiogenic factors (including connective tissue growth factor, transforming growth factor (TGF-β1) and metalloproteinase (MMP-2)) and factors responsible for wound proliferation and remodelling (type IV collagen, fibronectin and interferon-γ) (Sebastian et al 2011). In a clinical study by Asadi et al (2017), cathodal ES using DC (3.36 mA) increased the concentration of VEGF in fluid obtained from diabetic foot ulcers.

CLINICAL EVIDENCE

Low Intensity Direct Current (LIDC)

Results of LIDC (50–1000 μA) in the treatment of venous leg ulcers (VLUs) (Assimacopoulos 1968), pressure ulcers (PUs) (Barron et al 1985) and ulcers of mixed aetiologies (Gault & Gatens 1976; Walcott et al 1969) were reported between 1968 and 1985 in one randomized clinical trial (Carley & Wainapel 1985) and four case series (Assimacopoulos 1968; Barron et al 1985; Gault & Gatens 1976; Walcott et al 1969). Current was applied at sensory level for 20–168 hours per week (Assimacopoulos 1968; Carley & Wainapel 1985; Gault & Gatens 1976; Walcott et al 1969). Treatments were usually performed for 2 hours, 2–3 times/day (Carley & Wainapel 1985; Gault & Gatens 1976; Walcott et al 1969), five (Carley & Wainapel 1985) or seven (Gault & Gatens 1976; Walcott et al 1969) days per week for 3–5 weeks (Barron et al 1985; Carley & Wainapel 1985) or until wound closure (Walcott et al 1969).

Results of these early studies were promising, but LIDC is currently not widely used to treat wounds because possible pH changes at the electrode–skin interfaces may cause tissue damage. Fortunately, studies conducted in subsequent years provided evidence that chronic wounds can be effectively treated with high- and low-voltage pulsed currents (monophasic and biphasic), that are delivered just above sensory perception without pH changes that harm tissues.

Monophasic High-Voltage Pulsed Current (HVPC)

The use of monophasic HVPC for treatment of chronic wounds, delivered just below skeletal muscle excitability threshold, is supported by numerous randomized clinical trials (RCTs) (Ahmad 2008; Franek et al 2000, 2012; Griffin et al 1991; Houghton et al 2003, 2010; Kloth & Feedar 1988; Peters et al 2001; Polak et al 2016a, 2016b, 2017, 2018). It has been used to treat chronic VLUs, PUs and diabetic foot ulcers (DFUs). Clinical studies (Ahmad 2008; Franek et al 2000, 2012; Griffin et al 1991; Houghton et al 2003, 2010; Kloth & Feedar 1988; Peters et al 2001; Polak et al 2016a, 2016b, 2017, 2018) have revealed that wound area decreased more in ES groups (standard wound care (SWC) plus HVPC) than in controls (SWC alone) (Franek et al 2012; Houghton et al 2010; Polak et al 2016a) or SWC plus sham HVPC (Ahmad 2008; Griffin et al 1991; Houghton et al 2003; Kloth & Feedar 1988; Polak et al 2016b, 2017, 2019). HVPC can also stimulate peri-wound skin blood flow (Polak et al 2018). HVPC was used in eight RCTs to treat stage II–IV PUs occurring in people with neurological injuries (Griffin et al 1991; Houghton et al 2003; Polak et al 2018), elderly persons (Kloth & Feedar 1988; Polak et al 2016a, 2016b, 2017), and in people with orthopaedic injuries (Franek et al 2012). Examples of portable stimulators that deliver HVPC are shown in Fig. 19.1.

In an early study Kloth and Feedar (1988) found that stage IV PUs of nine elderly patients in the ES group (SWC plus monophasic HVPC) closed in a mean of 7.3 weeks at 45% per week. In the control group of seven patients (SWC plus sham HVPC), PU size increased a mean of 29% during a mean of 7.4 weeks. HVPC (100 μs, 105 pps; 342 μC/s) was delivered for 45 minutes, 5 days weekly directly into the wounds. Wounds were treated with anode in five patients. In four patients, the treatment electrode polarity was changed to cathode when wound healing stalled. In a 1991 RCT, Griffin et al (1991) noted that in people with spinal cord injury (SCI), after 20 consecutive days of SWC plus cathodal HVPC treatment (100 pps, 200 V, 500 μC/s), the median reduction in area of eight stage II–IV PUs was 80% compared with 52% for nine PUs in the placebo group (SWC plus sham HVPC, p<0.05).

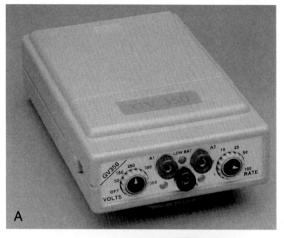

A

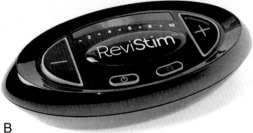

B

Fig. 19.1 A and B. Examples of portable stimulators which can generate HVPC stimulation.

The results of these early clinical trials involving a small number of patients with PUs were validated in RCTs conducted between 2010 and 2018 (Franek et al 2012; Houghton et al 2010; Polak et al 2016a, 2016b, 2017, 2018). Houghton et al (2010), in a single-blind RCT, noted that after 12 weeks of treatment, the average percentage decrease in stage II–IV PU surface area in people with SCI was greater (p = 0.048) in the SWC plus HVPC group (70%, 16 PUs) than in the control group (SWC plus sham ES) (36%, 18 PUs). During nocturnal hours, HVPC (50 μs) was applied for 20 minutes at 100 pps, followed by 20 minutes at 10 pps, followed by a 20-minute break. The total duration of nocturnal ES was 5.35 hours. The polarity of the treatment electrode was negative for the first week then alternated weekly.

In an RCT Franek et al (2012) used monophasic HVPC (100 μs, 100 pps) to treat 26 stage II–III PUs in patients with orthopaedic conditions for 50 minutes/day, 5 days/week. Cathodal stimulation was applied to wounds for the first 1–2 weeks to stimulate granulation, followed by anodal stimulation for the remaining treatment period. At 6 weeks, granulation tissue growth had increased in both groups, but the difference was significant only in the SWC plus HVPC group (p<0.001, p = 0.845 in the control

SWC-alone group). A mean decrease in wound surface area (WSA) was 88.9% in the HVPC group compared with 44.4% in the SWC control group (p<0.001). In a blinded clinical trial, Polak et al (2016b) treated 25 stage II–III PUs in elderly patients using cathodal HVPC (154 µs, 100 pps, 250 µC/s) for 50 minutes/day, 5 days/week for 6 weeks. The results were similar to the findings of Franek et al (2012). At 6 weeks, the surface area of PUs in the HVPC group had decreased by 80.31%, versus 54.65% in the control group (SWC plus sham HVPC, 24 PUs, p = 0.046). The healing outcome was confirmed by Gilman's parameter of 0.95 and 0.57 in the ES and control groups, respectively (p = 0.015) (Polak et al 2016b).

In each of the three studies cited above (Franek et al 2012; Houghton et al 2010; Polak et al 2016b), the authors used different wound treatment electrode polarities. In two subsequent blinded RCTs, Polak et al (2017, 2018) evaluated the effect of monophasic HVPC (154 µs, 100 pps, 250–360 µC/s) on healing of stage II–IV PUs using different treatment electrode polarities in the two studies. Patients' wounds were treated with SWC 23 hours/day in addition to HVPC applied 50 minutes/day, 5 days/week, for 6 weeks in the elderly persons (Polak et al 2017) and 8 weeks in patients with neurological injuries (Polak et al 2018). In both studies control groups received SWC plus sham HVPC (Polak et al 2017, 2018). The first study (Polak et al 2017) involved 63 patients with PUs: 23 PUs were treated with cathodal HVPC, 20 PUs were treated in the first week with cathodal HVPC and for the next 5 weeks with anodal HVPC, while 20 PUs in the control group received sham HVPC. At week 6, the WSA in the cathodal-ES group had decreased from baseline by 82.34% and in cathodal plus anodal ES group by 70.77%. The between-group differences were insignificant (p = 0.99). The results obtained in both ES groups were significantly greater (p<0.001 and p = 0.012, respectively) than in the control group, in which WSA decreased by 40.53%. Authors noted that for cathodal HVPC to decrease WSA by 50%, 1.92 weeks of treatment were required (95% CI 1.62–2.23), and for cathodal plus anodal HVPC, 2.6 weeks were required (95% CI 2.08–3.13). The differences between both ES groups were insignificant (p>0.05), but in both, the time necessary for PUs to decrease by 50% was significantly shorter than in the control group (10.6 weeks, 95% CI 7.25–13.95). Kaplan-Meier analysis showed that the probability of wounds treated with cathodal or cathodal plus anodal HVPC not closing was significantly smaller than with treatment using SWC plus sham HVPC (p<0.01 in both cases).

In the second study by Polak et al (2018) investigating relevance of polarity, 61 patients with stage II–IV PUs were randomized to anodal HVPC (n = 20), cathodal HVPC (n = 21) or placebo ES (n = 20). After 8 weeks of anodal HVPC, surface area decreased by 64.10%, and after cathodal HVPC by 74.06%. The difference between the ES groups was insignificant (p = 0.99). However, in both ES groups the results were significantly greater (p = 0.04 and p = 0.002, respectively) than in the control group where PUs decreased by 41.42%. The authors calculated that to decrease WSA by 50% would require 4.3 weeks using anodal HVPC (95% CI 0.20–0.26), whereas 3.86 weeks would be required using cathodal HVPC (95% CI 0.23–0.28). Differences between ES groups were not significant (p>0.05), while in both ES groups treatment time was significantly shorter than in the control group (9.86 weeks, 95% CI 0.08–0.11, p<0.05). Polak et al (2018) also observed that after 2 weeks treatment with both anodal and cathodal HVPC, peri-wound skin blood flow was significantly greater than in the control group (anodal ES group increased 109.52% from baseline versus 131.54% in the cathodal-ES group, and by 35.83% in the control group). The differences were significant between both ES groups and the control group (p = 0.047 and p = 0.015, respectively).

With regard to selecting polarity, since enhanced blood perfusion is very desirable for chronic wounds that have variable degrees of ischaemia, the recommendation is to commence ES using the cathode in the wound.

Monophasic HVPC has also been used successfully in RCTs to treat VLUs (Franek et al 2000) and mixed aetiology leg ulcers (Houghton et al 2003). Franek et al (2000) in an RCT found that the rate of VLU area reduction was similar at 6 weeks among three groups of patients treated with either HVPC plus SWC (33 patients), SWC alone (32 patients), or Unna's boot (14 patients). However, they observed that after 2 weeks of treatment the amount of granulation tissue in the HVPC group (84.9%) was greater than in the other groups (53.9% and 63.0% respectively, p<0.003 in both cases). HVPC (100µs; 100 Hz) was applied for 50 minutes/day, 6 days/week, for 6 weeks. For the first 1–3 weeks, ulcers were treated with the cathode to stimulate granulation, followed by anodal treatment. In a blinded RCT, Houghton et al (2003) observed positive effects of treatment of leg ulcers of various aetiology despite a short cathodal HVPC treatment (45 minutes/day, 3 days/week, 2.25 hours/week). By the 4th week WSA in the HVPC group had decreased 44.3% compared with 16% in the sham HVPC group (p<0.05).

An RCT by Peters et al (2001) provides the basis for use of monophasic HVPC in the treatment of DFUs. HVPC (100 µs) was delivered to 20 ulcers via a Dacron-mesh silver nylon stocking worn nightly for 8 hours. An 8-hour cycle consisted of 20 minutes on, 40 minutes off, 160 min total treatment/night, 7 nights/week (total treatment time

18.7 hours/week). For the first 10 minutes, current was delivered at 80 pps followed by 10 minutes at 8 pps. After 12 weeks of treatment authors noted that 65% of DFUs closed in the HVPC group, versus 35% closed in sham HVPC control group, but the difference was not significant (p = 0.058).

Systematic Reviews and Meta-Analyses

In recent years (2014–2019), several systematic (Liu et al 2014 and Polak et al 2014) and comprehensive (Houghton 2017) reviews of clinical trials and meta-analyses (Barnes, et al 2014 and Lala et al 2016)on the impact of electrical energy on the healing of chronic wounds have been published. The authors of all studies have made extensive reviews of various scientific databases (including Scopus, Medline, EBSCO, PubMed, CINHAL, Embase) (Liu et al 2014; Polak et al 2014; Houghton 2017; Barnes et al 2014 and Lala et al 2014). The authors of two study reviews focused exclusively on the treatment of PUs in patients with SCI (Liu et al 2014; Lala et al 2015).Other reviews included wounds of various aetiologies (including PUs, VLUs, diabetic and arterial wounds, wounds of mixed aetiology) (Polak et al 2014; Houghton 2014; Barnes et al 2014).Randomized controlled clinical trials, controlled clinical trials and non-controlled studies and case reports were included in the reviews. In all reviews, the quality of the test methods used in the individual studies was evaluated (Houghton 2014). Many of these studies were rated as medium and good quality controlled and randomized controlled clinical trials. The results of all five reviews favoured the use of electrical currents in the treatment of various types of chronic wounds (Liu et al 2014; Polak et al 2014; Houghton 2014; Barnes et al 2014; Lala et al 2016)

In studies included in the reviews, currents with different waveforms were used, including monophasic and biphasic LVPCs and monophasic HVPCs applied at the sensory level below the threshold of skeletal muscle excitability, and DCs and PCs applied below the threshold of excitability of sensory receptors. In a systematic review concerning monophasic HVPCs, Polak et al (2014) emphasized the existence of scientific evidence of the positive impact of this current on the healing of PUs and VLUs. In a comprehensive 2014 review of clinical trials, Houghton (2014) drew attention to the positive impact of monophasic and biphasic LVPCs applied at the sensory level in the treatment of chronic wounds of various aetiologies. However, she stated that there is no unambiguous evidence of the effects of currents applied at the subsensory level on wound healing.

Houghton (2017), based on a review of reviews of clinical trials, concluded that there is clear and consistent research evidence to support the use of electrical currents for wound treatment when the results from 22 well-designed RCTs and 11 systematic reviews with PRISMA ('Preferred Reporting Items for Systematic Reviews and Meta-Analysis') scores

above 5 out of 11 are considered (*PRISMA scores of 5 or greater indicate well-conducted systematic reviews and meta-analyses*).

According to Houghton (2017), pooled results from well-constructed reviews provide strong support for the use of electrical energy on all types of chronic wounds in general, and PUs in particular. There is only one well-designed systematic review that supports the use of electrical currents on DFUs, and no good review that has compiled the research that is known to exist for electrical stimulation of VLUs (Houghton 2017).

The authors of the research reviews stated that there is still a need to conduct high-quality RCTs that allow development of the most effective methods of ES for chronic wounds of various aetiologies (Houghton 2014, Liu et al 2014; Polak et al 2014; Houghton 2017; Barnes et al 2014; Lala et al 2016). According to Houghton (2017), common recommendations for future research in this field include performing more robust clinical research that has greater sample sizes and longer treatment times so that complete wound closure is achieved. Additional research that evaluates the effect of electrical energy on PU may not be needed. Properly designed clinical trials with randomization, valid healing outcomes and intention-to-treat analysis are needed to determine if electrical current can accelerate healing of diabetic foot wounds and ischaemic ulcers. Well-conducted and comprehensive reviews that pool results across all the available research regarding the effects of electrical currents on healing of VLUs are also needed (Houghton 2017).

THERAPEUTIC EFFECTS

Physical therapy involvement in the treatment of human wounds with ES has a history of over 30 years. Wounds typically selected for treatment are those that have been recalcitrant to standard wound care methods (e.g. dressings, topical agents). Such wounds include superficial and deep pressure ulcers, and leg ulcers caused by venous and arterial insufficiency and diabetes. All of these wounds significantly contribute to patients' declining function. Delivery of ES into viable, non-healing wound tissue is preceded by debridement of overlying necrotic eschar and yellow slough tissue.

APPLICATION

Wound Treatment Using Monophasic HVPC

High-quality RCTs indicate that HVPC can effectively promote healing of chronic human wounds. Similar methodology is used by different authors.

Treatment with HVPC can be achieved using adhesive or carbon rubber electrodes, the latter of which are separated from wound tissue by sterile gauze pads moistened

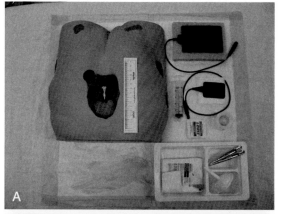

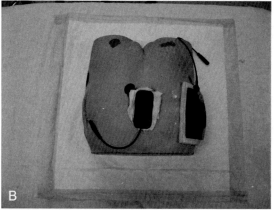

Fig. 19.2 Illustration of electrical stimulation application to a wound (using a wound model). (A) Gathering equipment. (B) Showing the wound filled with gauze moistened in a hydrogel-saline mix and electrodes in situ.

with 0.9% physiological saline to improve electrical conductivity and maintain a moist wound environment.

Following debridement of necrotic tissue, the treatment electrode is placed directly on wound tissue and the return (dispersive) electrode on intact peri-wound skin, ideally 15 cm from wound edge (see Fig. 19.2). Studies reviewed in this chapter show that both anode and cathode are effective as treatment electrodes in treating chronic human wounds. The anode may be used to stimulate autolysis in wounds partially or completely covered with fibrous material or slough, to reduce wound inflammation in cases of infected wounds and to increase blood perfusion to wound and peri-wound tissues. If weekly measurable wound healing occurs (10–15% reduction in WSA or visible progress of healing in the form of slough removal, increased percentage granulation, etc.) the anode may be used throughout the course of treatment. If the wound makes little or no measurable progress towards healing, the cathode can be

used to stimulate granulation and epithelialization and, like the anode, to increase peri-wound blood perfusion. If wound healing occurs, cathodal stimulation may be continued throughout the remaining treatment period.

HVPC with twin-peaked pulses (50–154 µs, 100 pps, 250–500 µC/s) applied at sensory level (dosage of 0.89–1.78 µC/day) enhances wound healing and should be applied for 45–60 minutes, once a day, 3–7 days a week (2.25–7 hours per week) while healing progresses and preferably until wound closure. Changing the polarity of the treatment electrode from cathode to anode or vice versa, every 3 or 7 days is recommended if healing of wounds is slowed or stalls.

Wound Treatment Using Monophasic Rectangular Low-Voltage Pulsed Current (LVPC)

Between 2007 and 2009, several clinical trials were published (Barczak et al 2001; Feedar et al 1991; Gentzkow et al 1991, 1993; Junger et al 1997; Weiss et al 1989) in which monophasic rectangular LVPC was used for the treatment of human wounds, all using the same device named Varipulse (Staodyn Inc., Logmont, CO), later named Dermapulse and, most recently, WoundEL (GerroMed GMBH, Germany). In all studies, current was applied at sensory level for 30 minutes, twice daily, 7 days/week, for 4 or 7 weeks. The accumulated pulse charge 250–500 µC/s (0.89–1.78 C/day) was delivered to wounds with a single-use electrode placed over stage II wounds or into stage III and IV wounds. The return electrode was placed at least 15–30 cm away from the wound.

In two blinded, placebo-controlled RCTs (Feedar et al 1991; Gentzkow et al 1991) and one prospective, baseline-controlled study (Gentzkow et al 1993), PUs were treated starting with cathodal stimulation for debridement and then alternating the cathode and anode every third day. Initially, pulses of 140 µs and frequency of 128 pps were used, and when the wound decreased to 44% of its original size (Feedar et al 1991), pulses of 132 µs with a frequency of 64 pps were delivered. Feedar et al (1991) reported that after 4 weeks the WSA of 26 mixed aetiology wounds (PUs, surgical, vascular, traumatic) subjected to LVPC decreased 67% compared to the previous SWC rate (14%/week). This result was significantly greater (p<0.02) than in the control group, in which surface area of 24 wounds decreased an average of 44% (8.24%/week). Gentzkow et al (1993) treated stage III–IV PUs over a mean of 8.4 weeks. A cohort of 61 PUs served as their own control. The first 4 weeks were a controlled phase, during which all wounds received SWC. Only wounds that did not demonstrate measurable progress toward closure or regressed during the control period were enrolled in the second phase of the study. After 4 weeks all wounds met the inclusion criteria for phase-two enrolment in which patients received the same SWC plus LVPC. In the last week of the study (mean 7.3 weeks), 50 of 61 wounds (82%) had improved two or more wound characters and 45 of 61 wounds (73.8%) had improved one or more stages toward wound closure.

Wound Treatment Using Biphasic LVPC

Several clinical studies, including a pre-post study (Stefanowska et al 1987), case series (Karba et al 1990, 1991) and prospective control trials (Jercinovic et al 1994; Karba et al 1995; Stefanowska et al 1993), for treatment of PUs (Jercinovic et al 1994; Karba et al 1991, 1995; Stefanowska et al 1987, 1993), and wounds of various aetiologies (Karba et al 1990) (PUs, VLUs, postsurgical or post-trauma wounds) have been published by researchers in Slovenia (1987–1993) (Jercinovic et al 1994; Karba et al 1990, 1991, 1995; Stefanowska et al 1987, 1993). In all studies, wounds were treated successfully with biphasic LVPC applied to the wound edge at a current amplitude that produced visible muscle contractions. The ES parameters were set to deliver 250 µs pulses at 40 pps, in a 4-second pulse train with a 50:50 on-off-ratio. Treatments were given 2 hours/day at least 5 days weekly until complete closure occurred. In a review of ES in chronic wounds, Houghton (2014) recommends that the muscle contraction methodology be replicated by other investigators in order to establish the validity of this treatment method.

Several other research groups applied biphasic LVPC at sensory level to peri-ulcer skin to treat PUs (Baker et al 1996) and DFUs (Baker et al 1997; Lundeberg et al 1992). The following studies using this sensory approach were all prospective RCTs that included appropriate control groups in which patients were treated with SWC plus sham ES (Baker et al 1996, 1997; Lundeberg et al 1992).

Lundeberg et al (1992) conducted an RCT using LVPC. After 12 weeks of treatment, 42% of the 32 DFUs treated with LVPC closed versus 15% of 32 DFUs in the control group (SWC alone). During ES, 1 ms pulses at 80 pps were delivered to the peri-ulcer skin at sensory level for 20 minutes, twice daily, 7 days/week.

Baker et al (1996, 1997) published two large RCTs that involved patients with PUs (Baker et al 1996) and DFUs (Baker et al 1997). Both reports indicated faster healing rates when biphasic LVPC was applied using rectangular asymmetrical pulses (100 µs, 50 pps, 7:7 on: off ratio), possibly due to pH effects, rather than rectangular symmetrical pulses (300 µs, 50 pps, 7:7 on: off ratio) or subsensory, microcurrent (<1 mA) DC. In all groups ES was applied for 30 minutes, repeated 3 times/day, 5 days/week until wound closure. (Lawson & Petrofsky 2007; Petrofsky et al 2010; Suh et al 2009).

Three clinical studies (Lawson & Petrofsky 2007; Petrofsky et al 2010; Suh et al 2009) on PUs and DFUs found that biphasic LVPC increased peri-wound skin blood perfusion and reduced wound area. In all three studies, balanced sine wave LVPC (30 pps, 250 µs) was applied at sensory level, 30 minutes/day, 3 times/week, for 4 weeks. Current was delivered via electrodes placed on opposite wound edges. In two studies (Lawson & Petrofsky 2007; Petrofsky et al 2010), researchers used a unique electrode arrangement that included three electrodes placed around the wound, and the ES device automatically alternated current flow between two electrodes every second throughout the treatment. According to the authors, this three-electrode set up produced a more uniform electric field in the wound base and at the wound edge (Petrofsky et al 2010). In an RCT by Lawson and Petrofsky (2007), biphasic LVPC was applied to two groups of 10 patients with stage III–IV wounds of mixed aetiology. The first group of patients had type 2 diabetes, and the second group was non-diabetic. Peri-wound skin blood flow in patients with diabetes measured during ES was significantly greater than in non-diabetic patients measured at 2 weeks (215% from baseline and no change respectively, $p < 0.003$) and at 4 weeks (87% and 6% respectively, $p < 0.003$) of treatment. In both groups, authors noted a significant wound area reduction after 4 weeks of treatment with LVPC ($p < 0.05$).

Petrofsky et al (2010) conducted an RCT involving 20 patients with DFUs in which they compared the effect of biphasic LVPC when combined with infrared radiation (IR) versus a control group that received SWC plus IR and found significantly greater wound size reduction in ES and IR-treated wounds. Unfortunately, the effects of LVPC were confounded by concurrent treatment with IR.

Summary of Treatment Using Monophasic and Biphasic LVPC

Based on results of the cited studies, healing of chronic human wounds can be enhanced using monophasic LVPC with rectangular pulses, duration 132 µs, frequency 64 pps, duration 140 µs and frequency 128 pps, applied for 60 minutes, 7 days/week. Cathodal ES may be used to stimulate wound debridement and granulation tissue growth. During the proliferative phase of healing, polarity of the treatment electrode may be changed every three days. When treating an infected wound, the anode is recommended. Daeschlein et al (2007) showed that LVPC has an antibacterial effect that is greater with anode than cathode and that bacterial reduction differed significantly between anode and control, and cathode and control, with the highest log 10 reduction factor achieved with anode.

Cited clinical studies suggest that symmetrical and asymmetrical biphasic LVPC (0.1–1 ms, 30–80 pps) applied to the wound edges can stimulate wound healing. ES should be applied for 20–30 minutes, 2–3 times/day, 3–7 days/week.

Subsensory ES Stimulation

Subsensory ES using DC (Adunsky & Ohry 2005; Karba et al 1997; Katelaris et al 1987) or PC (Ullah 2007) has been used in clinical trials to treat VLUs (Katelaris et al 1987), stage III–IV PUs (Adunsky & Ohry 2005; Karba et al 1997; Katelaris et al 1987; Ullah 2007), and DFUs (Baker et al 1997). Generally, an intensity not exceeding 1 mA (20 µA–600 µA) has been used.

Katelaris et al (1987) treated VLUs using electrodes mounted in wound dressings. The cathode was placed on the wound surface, and anode on the wound edge. The treatments were performed 24 hours/day, every day until the wound closed. Baker et al (1996, 1997) applied subsensory ES to PUs (Baker et al 1996) and DFUs (Baker et al 1997) for 30 minutes, 3 times/day, 5 days/week until healing. Neither of these two studies showed accelerated healing of wounds under the influence of micro-amperage current. In contrast, a positive effect of subsensory ES was found by Karba et al (1997) in the treatment of PUs, but only when the wound was stimulated with the anode or cathode placed in the wound did the area of wounds decrease at a rate of 7.4% per day. Anode and cathode placed on opposite wound edges did not produce better healing outcomes than occurred in the control group subjected to sham ES (4.8% per day in the ES group, and 4.2% in the control group, respectively).

There are also scientific reports describing the promising results of wound healing using ES applied at subsensory level, obtained with the use of mini-electrostimulators inserted into wound dressings adhered to wounds (Hampton & Collis 2006; Hampton & King 2005). Results of clinical trials are contradictory; thus, it is difficult to determine its effectiveness in chronic human wounds.

SUMMARY

Electrical stimulation should be combined with prevention and treatment of wounds based on the principles of the best clinical practice. ES should be carried out at least once a day for 45–60 minutes, 3–7 times a week. In clinical trials, the treatment electrode is usually placed on the surface of the wound and the return electrode is located at least 15 cm from the wound. Sometimes (especially when using biphasic currents) electrodes are placed on opposite wound edges. The electrodes are separated from the skin by means of 0.9% physiological saline wet gauze pads.

Strong evidence from clinical research studies shows that monophasic HVPC and LVPC, as well as biphasic LVPC, can be used to enhance healing of chronic wounds. These currents should be applied at levels above the threshold of excitability of sensory receptors and below skeletal muscle excitability. The use of subsensory ES for wound healing still needs to be confirmed in scientific research.

During ES, an electrical charge in the range of 250–500 µC/seconds should be delivered to the tissues. Clinical studies confirm that monophasic HVPC with twin-peaked pulses with a duration of 50–154 µs, applied at 100 pps are effective in the treatment of chronic wounds. The monophasic rectangular LVPC with a duration of 132 µs and frequency 64 pps can also be successfully used, as well as with pulse duration of 140 µs and frequency 128 pps.

The largest number of clinical trials, study reviews and meta-analyses highlights the high efficiency of electric currents in the treatment of PUs. Electrotherapy is recommended in the treatment of stage II–IV pressure ulcers in clinical guidelines published in 2014 by the National Pressure Ulcer Advisory Panel, the European Pressure Ulcer Advisory Panel and the Pan Pacific Pressure Injury Alliance 2014. These recommendations are based on reviews of clinical trials.

Ideally, physiotherapists should be directly involved in the treatment of chronic wounds. The physiotherapist's task should be to develop a methodology and conduct electrostimulation treatments. Therapists should also be able to assess the progress of wound healing and choose the method of electrostimulation (including the polarity of the treatment electrode) in such a way as to obtain the best effects of improving blood perfusion and wound healing.

REFERENCES

Adunsky, A., & Ohry, A. (2005). Decubitus direct current treatment (DDCT) of pressure ulcers: Results of a randomized double-blinded placebo controlled study. *Archives of Gerontology and Geriatrics, 41,* 261–269.

Ahmad, E. T. (2008). High-voltage pulsed galvanic stimulation: Effect of treatment duration on healing of chronic pressure ulcers. *Annals of Burns and Fire Disasters, 21*(3), 124–128.

Asadi, M. R., Torkaman, G., & Hedayati, M. (2011). Effect of sensory and motor electrical stimulation in vascular endothelial growth factor expression of muscle and skin in full-thickness wound. *Journal of Rehabilitation Research and Development, 48,* 195–202.

Asadi, M. R., Torkaman, G., Hedayati, M., et al. (2013). Role of sensory and motor intensity of electrical stimulation on fibroblastic growth factor-2 expression, inflammation, vascularization, and mechanical strength of full-thickness wounds. *Journal of Rehabilitation Research and Development, 50*(4), 489–498.

Asadi, M. R., Torkaman, G., Hedayati, M., et al. (2017). Angiogenic effects of low-intensity cathodal direct current on ischemic diabetic foot ulcers: A randomized controlled trial. *DRCP, 127,* 47–155.

Assimacopoulos, D. (1968). Low intensity negative electric current in treatment of ulcers of leg due to chronic venous insufficiency: Preliminary report of three cases. *American Journal of Surgery, 115,* 683–687.

Bai, H., Forrester, J. V., & Zhao, M. (2011). DC electric stimulation upregulates angiogenic factors in endothelial cells through activation of VEGF receptors. *Cytokine, 55,* 110–115.

Bai, H., McCaig, C. D., Forrester, J. V., & Zhao, M. (2004). DC electrical fields induce distinct preangiogenic responses in microvascular and macrovascular cells. *Arteriosclerosis, Thrombosis, and Vascular Biology, 24,* 1234–1239.

Baker, L., Chambers, R., DeMuth, S., et al. (1997). Effects of electrical stimulation on wound healing in patients with diabetic ulcers. *Diabetes Care, 20,* 405–412.

Baker, L., Rubayi, S., Villar, F., et al. (1996). Effect of electrical stimulation waveform on healing of ulcers in human beings with spinal cord injury. *Wound Repair and Regeneration, 4,* 21–28.

Barnes, R., Shahin, Y., Gohil, R., et al. (2014). "Electrical stimulation vs. standard care for chronic ulcer healing: a systematic review and meta-analysis of randomised controlled trials." *Eur J Clin Invest, 44*(4): 429-440.

Barczak, M., Kluger, P., Kluger, I., et al. (2001). *Therapeutic effectiveness of electric stimulation in paraplegic patients with pressure sores [dissertation of M. Barczak].* Medical School of the University of Ulm, Germany.

Barron, J., Jacobson, W., & Tidd, G. (1985). Treatment of decubitus ulcers: A new approach. *Minnesota Medicine, 68,* 103–106.

Carley, P. J., & Wainapel, S. F. (1985). Electrotherapy for acceleration of wound healing: Low intensity direct current. *Archives of Physical Medicine and Rehabilitation, 66,* 443.

Daeschlein, G., Assadian, G., Kloth, L. C., et al. (2007). Antibacterial activity of positive and negative polarity low-voltage pulsed current (LVPC) on six typical gram-positive and gram-negative bacterial pathogens of chronic wounds. *Wound Repair and Regeneration, 15,* 399–409.

Eberhardt, A., Szczypiorowski, P., & Korytowski, G. (1986). Effect of transcutaneous electrostimulation on the cell composition of skin exudates. *Acta Physiologica Polonica, 37,* 41–46.

Erickson, C. A., & Nuccitelli, R. (1984). Embryonic fibroblast motility and orientation can be influenced by physiological electric fields. *The Journal of Cell Biology, 98,* 296–307.

Feedar, J. A., Kloth, L. C., & Gentzkow, G. D. (1991). Chronic dermal ulcer healing enhanced with monophasic pulsed electrical stimulation. *Physical Therapy, 71,* 639–649.

Foulds, I. S., & Barker, A. T. (1983). Human skin battery potentials and their possible role in wound healing. *British Journal of Dermatology, 109,* 515–522.

Franek, A., Kostur, R., Polak, A., et al. (2012). Using high-voltage electrical stimulation in the treatment of recalcitrant pressure ulcers: Results of a randomized, controlled trial. *Ostomy/ Wound Management, 58*(3), 30–44.

Franek, A., Polak, A., & Kucharzewski, M. (2000). Modern application of high-voltage for enhanced healing of venous crural ulceration. *Medical Engineering & Physics, 22,* 647–655.

Fukushima Gruler, K. H. (1953). Studies of galvanotaxis of leukocytes. *Medical Journal of Osaka University, 4,* 195–208.

Gault, W. R., & Gatens, P. F., Jr. (1976). Use of low intensity direct current in management of ischemic skin ulcers. *Physical Therapy, 56,* 265–269.

Gentzkow, G. D., Alon, G., Taler, G. A., et al. (1993). Healing of refractory stage III and IV pressure ulcers by a new electrical stimulation device. *Wounds, 5,* 160–172.

Gentzkow, G. D., Pollack, S. V., Kloth, L. C., et al. (1991). Improved healing of pressure ulcers using Dermapulse, a new electrical stimulation device. *Wounds, 3,* 158–170.

Goldberg, M. T., Han, Y.-P., Yan, C., et al. (2007). TNF-α suppresses α-smooth muscle actin expression in human dermal fibroblasts: An implication for abnormal wound healing. *The Journal of Investigative Dermatology, 127*(11), 2645–2655.

Griffin, J., Tooms, R., Mendius, R., et al. (1991). Efficacy of high-voltage pulsed current for healing of pressure ulcers in patients with spinal cord injury. *Physical Therapy, 71,* 433–442.

Görgen, S. G., Saym, O., Cetin, F., & Yücel, A. T. (2014). Transcutaneous electrical nerve stimulation (TENS) accelerates cutaneous wound healing and inhibits pro-inflammatory cytokines. *Inflammation, 37*(3), 775–784.

Hampton, S., & Collis, F. (2006). Treating a pressure ulcer with bio-electric stimulation therapy. *British Journal of Nursing, 15,* 14–18.

Hampton, S., & King, L. (2005). Healing an intractable wound using bio-electrical stimulation therapy. *British Journal of Nursing, 14,* 30–32.

Houghton, PE. (2017). Electrical stimulation therapy to promote healing of chronic wounds: a review of reviews. *Chronic Wound Care Manage Res, 4,* 25–44.

Houghton, P. (2014). Clinical trials involving biphasic pulsed current, microcurrent, and/or low-intensity direct current. *Advances in Wound Care, 3*(2), 166–183.

Houghton, P. E., Campbell, K. E., Fraser, C. H., et al. (2010). Electrical stimulation therapy increases rate of healing of pressure ulcers in community-dwelling people with spinal cord injury. *Archives of Physical Medicine and Rehabilitation, 91,* 669–678.

Houghton, P. E., Kincaid, C. B., Lovell, M., et al. (2003). Effect of electrical stimulation on chronic leg ulcer size and appearance. *Physical Therapy, 831,* 17–28.

Jercinovic, A., Karba, R., Vodovnik, L., et al. (1994). Low frequency pulsed current and pressure ulcer healing. *IEEE Transactions on Rehabilitation Engineering, 2*(4), 225–233.

Jiang, I., Dai, Y., Cui, F., Pan, Y., et al. (2014). Expression of cytokines, growth factors and apoptosis-related signal molecules in chronic pressure ulcer wounds healing. *Spinal Cord, 52,* 145–151.

Jünger, M., Zuder, D., Steins, A., et al. (1997). Treatment of venous ulcers with low frequency pulsed current (Dermapulse): Effects on cutaneous microcirculation. *Hautarzt, 48,* 879–903.

Kanno, S., Oda, N., Abe, M., et al. (1999). Establishment of a simple and practical procedure applicable to therapeutic angiogenesis. *Circulation, 99,* 2682–2687.

Kanof, N. (1964). Gold leaf in the treatment of cutaneous ulcers. *The Journal of Investigative Dermatology, 43,* 441.

Karba, R., Benko, H., Savrin, R., & Vodovnik, L. (1995). Combination of occlusive dressings and electrical stimulation in pressure ulcer treatment. *Medical Science Research, 23*, 671–673.

Karba, R., Presern-Strukeij, M., Vodovnik, B. L., et al. (1990). Accelerated wound healing of lower extremities by means of electrical stimulation. *Advances in External Control of Human Extremities, 8*, 509–517.

Karba, R., Semrov, D., Vodovnik, L., et al. (1997). DC electrical stimulation for chronic wound healing enhancement. Part 1. Clinical study and determination of electrical field distribution in the numerical wound model. *Bioelectrochemistry and Bioenergetics, 43*, 265–270.

Karba, R., Vodovnik, B. L., Presern-Strukeij, M., & Klesnik, M. (1991). Promoted healing of chronic wounds due to electrical stimulation. *Wounds, 3*, 16–23.

Katelaris, P., Fletcher, J., Little, J., et al. (1987). Electrical stimulation in the treatment of chronic venous ulceration. *Australian and New Zealand Journal of Surgery, 57*, 605–607.

Kloth, L. C., & Feedar, J. A. (1988). Acceleration of wound healing with high-voltage monophasic, pulsed current. *Physical Therapy, 68*, 503–508.

Kurose, T., Hashimoto, M., Ozawa, J., et al. (2015). Analysis of gene expression in experimental pressure ulcers in the rat with special reference to inflammatory cytokines. *PLoS One, 10*(7), 1–13.

Lala, D., Spaulding, S. J., Burke, S. M., et al. (2016). "Electrical stimulation therapy for the treatment of pressure ulcers in individuals with spinal cord injury: a systematic review and meta-analysis." *Int Wound J, 13*(6): 1214-1226.

Lawson, D., & Petrofsky, J. S. (2007). A randomized control study on the effect of biphasic electrical stimulation in a warm room on skin blood flow and healing rates in chronic wounds of patients with and without diabetes. *Medical Science Monitor, 13*(6), CR258–263.

Liu, L. Q., Moody, J., Traynor M., et al. (2014). "A systematic review of electrical stimulation for pressure ulcer prevention and treatment in people with spinal cord injuries." *J Spinal Cord Med* 37(6): 703-718.

Lundeberg, T. C., Eriksson, S. V., & Malm, M. (1992). Electrical nerve stimulation improves healing of diabetic ulcers. *Annals of Plastic Surgery, 29*(4), 28–331.

Mirza, R. E., & Koh, T. J. (2015). Contributions of cell subsets to cytokine production during normal and impaired wound healing. *Cytokine, 71*(2), 409–412.

Mohajeri-Tehrani, M. R., Nasiripoor, F., Torkaman, G., et al. (2014). Effect of low-intensity direct current on expression of vascular endothelial growth factor and nitric oxide in diabetic foot ulcers. *Journal of Rehabilitation Research and Development, 51*(5), 815–824.

National Pressure Ulcer Advisory Panel, European Pressure Advisory Panel and Pan Pacific Pressure Injury Alliance. Prevention and Treatment of Pressure Ulcers: Clinical Practice Guideline. Emily Haesler (ed.) Cambridge Media: Perth, Australia; 2014.

Nishimura, K. Y., Isseroff, R. R., & Nuccitelli, R. (1996). Human keratinocytes migrate to the negative pole in direct current electric fields comparable to those measured in mammalian wounds. *Journal of Cell Science, 109*(1), 199–207.

Orida, N., & Feldman, J. (1982). Directional protrusive pseudopodial activity and motility in macrophages induced by extra-cellular electric fields. *Cell Motility, 2*, 243–255.

Peters, E. J., Lavery, L. A., Armstrong, D. G., et al. (2001). Electric stimulation as an adjunct to heal diabetic foot ulcers: A randomized clinical trial. *Archives of Physical Medicine and Rehabilitation, 82*, 721–725.

Petrofsky, J., Hinds, C. M., Batt, J., et al. (2007). The interrelationships between electrical stimulation, the environment surrounding the vascular endothelial cells of the skin, and the role of nitric oxide in mediating the blood flow response to electrical stimulation. *Medical Science Monitor, 13*(9), CR391–397.

Petrofsky, J., Lawson, D., Berk, L., et al. (2010). Enhanced healing of diabetic foot ulcers using local heat and electrical stimulation for 30 min three times per week. *Journal of Diabetes, 2*, 41–46.

Polak, A., Franek, A., Taradaj, J. (2014). High-voltage pulsed current electrical stimulation in wound treatment. *Adv Wound Care, 3*(2), 104–117.

Polak, A., Kloth, L. C., Blaszczak, E., et al. (2016). Evaluation of the healing progress of pressure ulcers treated with cathodal high-voltage monophasic pulsed current. The results of a prospective, double blind, randomized clinical trial. *Advances in Skin & Wound Care, 29*(10), 447–459.

Polak, A., Kloth, L. C., Blaszczak, E., et al. (2017). The efficacy of pressure ulcer treatment with cathodal and cathodal-anodal high-voltage monophasic pulsed current: A prospective, randomized, controlled clinical trial. *Physical Therapy, 97*(8), 777–789.

Polak, A., Kucio, C., Kloth, L. C., et al. (2018). A randomized, controlled clinical study to assess the effect of anodal and cathodal electrical stimulation on periwound skin blood flow and pressure ulcer size reduction in persons with neurological injuries. *Ostomy/Wound Management, 64*(2), 10–29.

Polak, A., Kloth, L.C., Paczula, M., et al. (2019). "Pressure injuries treated with anodal and cathodal high-voltage electrical stimulation: the effect on blood serum concentration of cytokines and growth factors in patients with neurological injuries. A randomized clinical study." *Wound Manag Prev* 65(11): 19-32.

Polak, A., Taradaj, J., Nawrat-Szoltysik, A., et al. (2016). Reduction of pressure ulcer size with high-voltage pulsed current and high-frequency ultrasound: A randomised trial. *Journal of Wound Care, 25*(12), 742–754.

Reid, B., & Zhao, M. (2014). The electrical response to injury: Molecular mechanisms and wound healing. *Advances in Wound Care, 3*, 184–201.

Risbrook, A. T., Goodfriend, S. S., & Reiter, J. M. (1973). Gold leaf in the treatment of leg ulcers. *Journal of the American Geriatrics Society, 21*, 325.

Robertson, W. S. (1925). Digby's receipts. *Annals of Medical History, 7*(3), 216.

Rouabhia, M., Park, H., Meng, S., et al. (2013). Electrical stimulation promotes wound healing by enhancing dermal fibroblast activity and promoting myofibroblast transdifferentiation. *PLoS One, 8*(8), e71660.

Sebastian, A., Syed, F., Perry, D., et al. (2011). Acceleration of cutaneous healing by electrical stimulation: Degenerative electrical waveform down-regulates inflammation, up-regulates angiogenesis and advances remodeling in temporal punch biopsies in a human volunteer study. *Wound Repair and Regeneration, 19*, 693–708.

Smith, K. W., Oden, P. W., & Blaulock, W. K. (1967). A comparison of gold leaf and other occlusive therapy. *Archives of Dermatology, 96*, 703.

Stefanowska, A., Vodovnik, L., Benko, H., et al. (1987). *Enhancement of ulcerated tissue healing by electrical stimulation.* Proceedings of the RESNA 10th Annual Conference, San Jose, CA.

Stefanowska, A., Vodovnik, L., Benko, H., et al. (1993). Treatment of chronic wounds by means of electric and electromagnetic fields. Part 2. Value of FES parameters for pressure sore treatment. *Medical & Biological Engineering & Computing, 31*, 213–220.

Suh, H., Petrofsky, J. S., Lo, T., et al. (2009). The combined effect of a three-channel electrode delivery system with local heat on the healing of chronic wounds. *Diabetes Technology & Therapeutics, 11*(10), 681–688.

Ud-Din, S., Sebastian, A., Giddings, P., et al. (2015). Angiogenesis is induced and wound size is reduced by electrical stimulation in an acute wound healing model in human skin. *PLoS One, 10*(4), 1–22.e0124502.

Ullah, M. (2007). A study to detect the efficacy of microcurrent electrical therapy on decubitus wound. *Journal of Medical Science, 7*(8), 1320–1324.

Weiss, D. S., Eaglstein, W. H., & Falanga, V. (1989). Exogenous electric current can reduce the formation of hypertrophic scars. *Journal of Dermatologic Surgery & Oncology, 15*, 1272–1275.

Wolcott, L. E., Wheeler, P. C., Hardwick, H. M., et al. (1969). Accelerated healing of skin ulcers by electrotherapy: Preliminary clinical results. *Southern Medical Journal, 62*, 795–801.

Wolf, M., Wheeler, P. C., & Wolcott, L. E. (1966). Gold leaf treatment of ischemic ulcers. *Journal of the American Medical Association, 196*, 105.

Wood, J. M., Evans, P. E., Schallreuter, K. U., et al. (1991). A multi-center study on the use of pulsed low intensity direct current for healing chronic stage II and III decubitus ulcers. *Archives of Dermatology, 129*, 999–1009.

Yang, W. P., Onuma, E. K., & Hui, S. W. (1984). Response of C3H/10T1/2 fibroblasts to an external steady electric field stimulation: Reorientation, shape change, cona receptor and intramembranous particle distribution and cytoskeleton reorganization. *Experimental Cell Research, 155*, 92–104.

Zhao, M., Bai, H., Wang, E., et al. (2003). Electrical stimulation directly induces pre-angiogenic responses in vascular endothelial cells by signalling through VEGF receptors. *Journal of Cell Science, 117*(3), 397–405.

Zhao, M., Song, B., Pu, J., et al. (2006). Electrical signals control wound healing through phosphatidylinositol-3-OH kinase-gamma and PTEN. *Nature, 442*, 457–460.

Diagnostics

Electrodiagnosis

Michael C. Lescallette

INTRODUCTION AND HISTORY

Electrodiagnosis involves the stimulation and recording of bioelectric potentials from excitable tissues such as nerves and muscles (Mallik & Weir 2005). The intent of this type of testing is to assess the physiological health of these tissues to contribute to a medical diagnosis (Mallik & Weir 2005). Electrodiagnostic testing is not a new discovery. In fact, not long after the introduction and harnessing of electricity in the late 1700s scientists started to explore the electrical properties of animal and human muscle tissue (Kazamel et al 2017). Improvements in recording of electrical responses greatly increased the clinical utility of testing and development of test algorithms used to detect nerve and/or muscle impairment (Kazamel et al 2017). Modern day electrodiagnostic testing is built upon the work of the pioneers from centuries ago. The chief advantage in the present day is the advent of solid-state recording devices and computer processing speed.

PHYSICAL PRINCIPLES

A clinical electrodiagnostic test involves two separate tests preferably done in the same evaluation: nerve conduction studies (NCS) and needle electromyography (EMG). Each test has specific strengths and weaknesses that are complementary and when combined can provide an accurate assessment of nerve and muscle tissue health. The combination of these two tests is considered an extension of the physical examination (Fuller 2005). Nerve conduction tests are able to assess the status of the myelin sheath of each nerve fibre, as well as the number of functioning axons in the nerve trunk. Motor axons and sensory axons can be tested separately to further define the extent of potential nerve impairment. Needle electromyography is used to detect motor axon and/or muscle tissue damage by recording electrical instability that emanates from corresponding denervated muscle cell membranes (Coster et al 2010). The electrical activity generated from individual motor units can also be displayed and quantitatively analysed for signs of motor axon reinnervation on a time continuum (Coster et al 2010). The majority of electrodiagnostic tests are performed in a clinical setting and are used to assess the peripheral nervous system. There are other types of electrodiagnostic tests often performed in specialized laboratories and academic centres (Fig. 20.1). Although these tests are different and are capable of assessing specific areas of the nervous system, the same underlying principles are utilized.

BIOPHYSICAL EFFECTS/RESPONSES

Nerve conduction tests involve the application of an electrical current to a target nerve with the goal of creating an

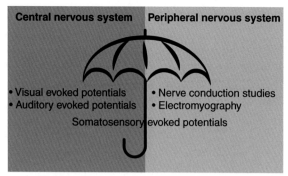

Fig. 20.1 Types of Electrodiagnostic Testing

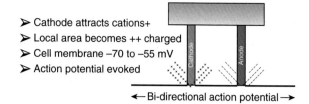

- Cathode attracts cations+
- Local area becomes ++ charged
- Cell membrane −70 to −55 mV
- Action potential evoked

←— Bi-directional action potential —→

Fig. 20.2 Initiation of an Evoked Potential The goal is to produce an electrical circuit in proximity to a nerve cell membrane.

action potential at the site of stimulation (Mallik & Weir 2005). The stimulator consists of a cathode and anode that is placed on the skin or subcutaneously in the vicinity of a target nerve. The stimulation is activated by a button which generates an 'instant on' rectangular wave. There are two ways to increase the amount of electrical stimulation applied to the target nerve: increase the stimulus intensity as measured in mA and/or increase the stimulus duration measured in ms. The minimum stimulus duration is 0.1 ms, which correlates with the average chronaxie of muscle and nerve tissue as determined through strength–duration curve research (Schuhfried et al 2005). The stimulator intensity is increased until the desired nerve and muscle response is achieved (Mallik & Weir 2005). The cathode attracts positively charged ions within the local vicinity including positively charged ions at and about the nerve cell membrane (Fig. 20.2) (Preston & Shapiro 2013). This changes the resting membrane potential from a resting value of −70 mV to −55 mV, at which point sodium gates open and the action potential flows, bidirectionally (Preston & Shapiro 2013). Each action potential represents reversals of membrane potential from −55 mV to +20 mV to −90 mV with a return to the resting value of −70 mV (Preston & Shapiro 2013). At the same time stimulation is applied, receiver electrodes are placed upon target nerves or muscles with the ability to detect the passage of action potential reversals as they travel along the nerve fibres or evoke a muscle contraction (Tapadia et al 2010). Each receiver electrode is differentially amplified so that the detection of a subcutaneous action potential hits the electrode closest to the stimulator and a deflection from a neutral baseline is created. The second electrode detects the moving action potential after the first electrode has already registered a deflection. The second electrode also creates a deflection from baseline in the opposite direction as it is differentially amplified (Tapadia et al 2010). The end product is a waveform that is distinct from a neutral baseline with a return to a neutral baseline (Fig. 20.3).

The waveform and resultant nerve conduction data that is gathered by recording electrodes can be analysed to answer two basic questions: 'how long?' and 'how strong?'. Each nerve stimulus will create a waveform that is placed on gridlines with time on the X axis and amplitude on the Y axis (Fig. 20.4). The gridlines allow the computer to demarcate the important parts of the waveform used in data collection. 'How long?' refers to the speed of action potential propagation. Often referred to as a latency or conduction velocity, it represents the length of time from the applied stimulation to when the waveform was recorded (Tapadia et al 2010). 'How strong?' refers to the amplitude or size of the resulting waveform. The numbers are then compared to normative data that has been gathered by peer reviewed studies or from normative data produced in the electromyographer's laboratory. Normative data for most nerve tests are published in textbooks as well as lab manuals. To establish normative data, test subjects are all tested using the exact same body positions and similar limb temperatures. A mean time and amplitude is established with the assumption of a normal bell curve distribution (Dorfman & Robinson 1997). Latencies and conduction velocities that are more than two standard deviations above or slower than the mean are considered abnormal (Dorfman & Robinson 1997). Amplitudes that are less than 50% of the mean amplitude are considered abnormal (Dorfman & Robinson 1997). Normative data has also been established that compares contralateral nerve data as well as similar ipsilateral nerve fibre types. The speed of conduction is affected by myelin thickness, health and type. Thickly myelinated nerve fibres with nodes of Ranvier interspersed at up to 1.5 mm distances are the fastest conducting fibres as the action potentials jump in a saltatory fashion from node to node (Fig. 20.5) (Belin et al 2017). Nerve conduction testing is designed to capture data from this type of nerve fibre (i.e. type 1A sensory and alpha motor neurons) (Tapadia et al 2010). A disruption in myelin structure will affect the propagation speed of action potentials and result in slowing. Both intrinsic factors and extrinsic factors can affect the health of the myelin sheath through anoxia, mechanical compression, autoimmune attack and

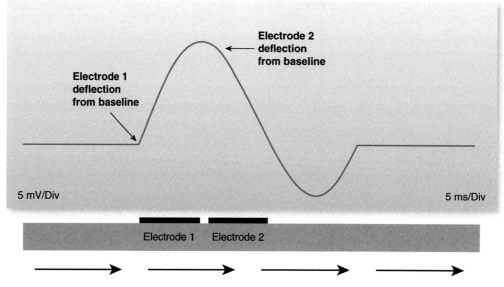

Electrode 2 deflection from baseline

Electrode 1 deflection from baseline

5 mV/Div

5 ms/Div

Electrode 1   Electrode 2

Direction of action potential under skin

Fig. 20.3 Evoked potential produces a waveform through differential amplification.

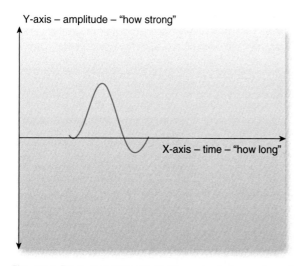

Y-axis – amplitude – "how strong"

X-axis – time – "how long"

Fig. 20.4 Recorded Waveform The recorded waveform is placed on gridlines for numerical and visual analysis.

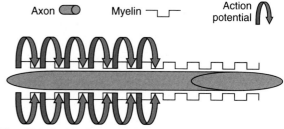

Axon   Myelin   Action potential

Fig. 20.5 Action Potential Propagation by Saltatory Conduction

nutritional deficits (Belin et al 2017). The Schwann cells that produce myelin are independent entities, therefore the damage that occurs in one location does not necessarily mean that the damage will proceed distally (Tapadia et al 2010). In summary, slowing of action potentials as detected during nerve conduction testing is indicative of damage to nerve fibre myelin. This is in contrast to axonal damage when the principles of Wallerian degeneration dictate that the nerve fibres will degenerate from the site of the lesion distally to the ends of the fibres (Tapadia et al 2010). Nerve conduction tests can utilize data regarding the strength of the recorded action potentials and assumptions can be made that assess axonal damage. For example, if the median sensory nerve fibres produce a waveform that is 12 µV in strength on the right and 3 µV on the left, it can be assumed that 75% of the axons on the left are not functioning. Pure axonal damage will result in a recording that is not slow but is weak compared to norms.

Sensory nerves can be tested by placing the recording electrodes on subcutaneous nerve fibres distal or proximal to the stimulating cathode, preferably on areas where the sensory nerve is superficial just under the skin (Fig. 20.6) (Tapadia et al 2010). The dose of stimulation can be altered by changing intensity, which is measured in mA, and duration of current flow, which is measured in ms.

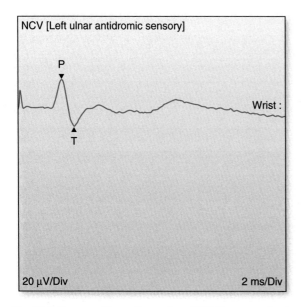

Fig. 20.6 Sensory Nerve Recording *NCV*, Nerve conduction velocity; *P*, Peak; *T*, Trough.

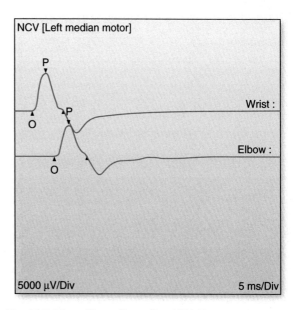

Fig. 20.7 Motor Nerve Recording *NCV*, Nerve conduction velocity; *O*, onset; *P*, Peak.

Sensory nerves tend to have a lower threshold for stimulation and are more superficial to the skin than motor fibres. Therefore, low stimulation doses are able to trigger action potentials from just sensory nerve fibres and recording methods can be tailored to detect just sensory nerve fibres. Action potential recordings from sensory nerves are measured in the μV range. It is important in these types of tests that all sources of ambient electrical noise are dampened to the point that they do not enter into nerve conduction results.

Motor nerve testing also involves the initiation of action potentials on a target nerve trunk. However, the recording electrodes are placed on the motor point of a target muscle that is innervated by the nerve being tested (Tapadia et al 2010). For instance, a supramaximal stimulation of the ulnar nerve trunk at the elbow would create action potential flow to every ulnar innervated muscle in the forearm/hand. Recording electrodes could be placed on any one of these muscles and data would be collected. Each motor axon that is stimulated will carry action potentials to all of the individual muscle fibres that are part of its motor unit (Tapadia et al 2010). The 'all or none' principle dictates that all of the muscle fibres in the target muscle will be stimulated to contract, thus creating one large waveform that is measured in mV (Fig. 20.7) (Preston & Shapiro 2013). The large waveform is referred to as a compound muscle action potential or a CMAP. It is not that sensory nerve axons were not also stimulated, but the settings for detection are 1000 times less sensitive and sensory nerve data is not

collected (Preston & Shapiro 2013). Motor nerve testing requires supramaximal stimulation intensity. The goal is to activate every available motor axon in the trunk to ensure the fastest conducting fibres are stimulated.

Nerve conduction testing is not able to directly measure motor or sensory nerve axonal damage. Assumptions can be made regarding the number of functioning axons, but the true extent of axonal damage cannot be assessed. Needle EMG is capable of directly assessing motor axon damage and muscle tissue damage (Tapadia et al 2010). In the clinical setting, EMG testing involves inserting a needle electrode into muscle tissue. The needle acts in much the same manner as a radio antenna as it is able to detect electrical charges and action potentials as they propagate along the sarcolemma membrane of individual muscle fibres (Tapadia et al 2010). If a motor axon has been damaged (i.e. neurotmesis or axonotmesis), all of the muscle fibres that belong to its corresponding motor unit will be denervated (Tapadia et al 2010). When the needle slips by these denervated fibres, they become mechanically stimulated and individual action potentials within approximately 0.5 mm of the needle tip can be detected both visually on a computer screen and audibly on the EMG machine speakers. These sights and sounds referred to as spontaneous potentials (Fig. 20.8A) fit a very distinctive pattern and are indicators of acute nerve damage that has occurred within the past 2–3 months (Robinson 2015). A damaged axon in the peripheral nervous system has the capability of regeneration. This process can also be detected by the EMG needle

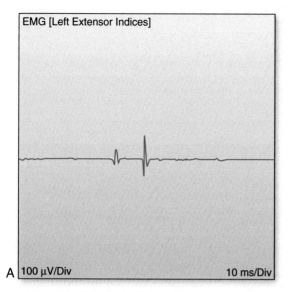

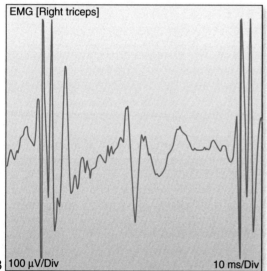

Fig. 20.8 Electromyography (EMG) (A) Sign of acute motor axon denervation: spontaneous potentials. (B) Reinnervation of motor units by collateral sprouting.

through the analysis of motor unit potential size, shape and duration (Coster et al 2010). The motor unit potential represents the firing of all of the muscle fibres that belong to one motor axon (Tapadia et al 2010). The morphology of a motor unit potential under regeneration will change in a predictable manner through time in a process that can take up to a year. Regenerative motor unit changes are considered chronic due to the length of time it takes for this process to occur. Based on these changes, the regeneration

can be classified as direct or through collateral sprouting (Fig. 20.8B) (Tapadia et al 2010). There are other ways the EMG needle can be utilized. It can be used as the cathode during nerve conduction tests with stimulation of axons well below the skin surface. The needle can also be used to record the action potentials of target nerves and muscles in what is known as a 'near nerve technique' (Mallik & Weir 2005).

There are alternative ways physical therapists are able to determine the status of motor axons and muscle fibres. Strength-duration curves (SDC) can be used to assess motor axon denervation, partial reinnervation, and normal innervation (Russo et al 2007). Equipment needed is a device capable of generating a rectangular, constant current or voltage impulse and settings that can adjust the duration of the impulse from 0.01 to 300 ms (Stillman 1967). The key elements are to determine: the rheobase or minimal current required to establish a muscle twitch contraction at a long duration of at least 300 ms, the chronaxie or time it takes to establish a muscle twitch contraction at twice the rheobase intensity, and a plotted curve that reflects the various intensities and durations to elicit a contraction (Fig. 20.9A) (Schuhfried et al 2005). The curve for a normally innervated muscle will take on a characteristic shape that demonstrates an inverse relationship between intensity and duration (Schuhfried et al 2005). A denervated muscle will demonstrate an SDC that is also curvilinear shape but will be shifted to the right of a normal nerve (Schuhfried et al 2005). With denervation, the first SDC should be plotted at between 14 and 21 days post injury (Stillman 1967). Then successive SDCs should be determined at weekly intervals. If regeneration has started to occur, a 'kink' will develop in the curve that reflects detection of reinnervated and denervated fibres at the same time (Fig. 20.9B) (Schuhfried et al 2005). The kink in the curve will move downwards and to the right as newly innervated fibres begin to dominate the curve with new sodium channels that are more responsive to electrical stimulation. The final SDC will regain a smooth shape similar to the contralateral muscle. The chronaxie provides direction for various forms of electrotherapies such as functional electrical stimulation (FES) (Schuhfried et al 2005). There is research to support use of FES on denervated muscle tissue as it has been shown to down regulate the expression of myoD, a myogenic regulatory factor and atrogin-1, a ubiquitin-ligase that promotes proteolysis of muscle proteins (Russo et al 2007). Both of these factors are expressed within denervated muscle tissue. In a study that utilized a denervated tibialis anterior muscle from a rat, electrical stimulation was applied to the muscle on alternate days for 28 days. The chronaxie was calculated at each session as it changed based on the amount of reinnervation and 20 maximal muscle contractions were elicited

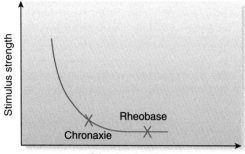

Rheobase

Chronaxie

Stimulus strength

Stimulus duration

Rheobase - minimal current required to establish a muscle twitch contraction at a long duration of at least 300 ms

Chronaxie - time it takes to establish a muscle
A   twitch contraction at twice the rheobase intensity

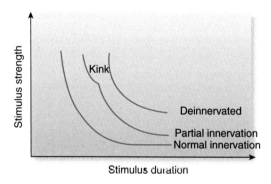

Kink

Deinnervated

Partial innervation
Normal innervation

Stimulus strength

Stimulus duration

B **Curves shift from right to left as muscle reinnervates**

Fig. 20.9 Strength-Duration Curves (A) From a normal muscle. (B) From a denervated muscle.

TABLE 20.1 Uses of Clinical EMG/NCS Testing	
Major Classifications of Impairment	**Conditions Detected by EMG/NCS**
Entrapment neuropathies	• Carpal tunnel syndrome • Ulnar neuropathy at the elbow • Tarsal tunnel syndrome • Brachial plexopathies
Radiculopathies	• Cervical • Thoracic • Lumbar
Peripheral neuropathies	• Axonal • Demyelinating
Myopathies	• Duchenne's muscular dystrophy • Polymyositis
Neuromuscular junction disorders	• Myasthenia gravis • Lambert Eaton myasthenic syndrome

EMG, Electromyography; *NCS*, nerve conduction studies.

(Russo et al 2007). The results did indicate the treatment was able to down regulate the expression of myo-D and atrogin-1; however, muscle atrophy still occurred (Russo et al 2007). Other studies that have elicited up to 500 muscle contractions have shown that muscle atrophy was prevented (Russo et al 2007). It is prudent for the therapist to periodically assess muscle excitability through plotting of strength–duration data and identifying chronaxie prior to treatment. These values must be plotted periodically as the chronaxie may change with reinnervation or continued denervation. Adjustments to FES treatment protocols will change as new research emerges.

CLINICAL EVIDENCE

Using established normative data, clinical electrodiagnostic testing is utilized throughout the world to help rule in or rule out a multitude of conditions (Table 20.1) (Tapadia et al 2010). Entrapment neuropathies, such as carpal tunnel syndrome, tarsal tunnel syndrome and ulnar neuropathy at the elbow, encompass the majority of tests performed on patients. Patients with these conditions often report symptoms such as pain, numbness, tingling, pins and needles sensations and, on occasion, muscle weakness in the regions distal to these entrapment sites (Tapadia et al 2010). Research has shown that focal entrapment neuropathies typically involve myelin structures at the site of the entrapment. If the myelin has become compressed or anoxic, it will become less efficient at conduction of action potentials (i.e., action potentials slow down) (Fig. 20.10) (Tapadia et al 2010). Less often, and in more substantial entrapments, the axons are also affected. That is what makes the nerve conduction test powerful as it is able to detect these entrapments. The basic idea is to provide an electrical stimulus to the nerve tissue below and above the site of the suspected entrapment. The waveforms gathered from the gridlines produce data that is compared to normative data.

Entrapment Neuropathies

Carpal tunnel syndrome is by far the most common reason patients are referred to electrodiagnostic laboratories. Approximately 7.8% of the general population has this

Site	NR	Onset (ms)	Norm onset (ms)	O-P amp (mV)	Norm O-P amp	Site 1	Site 2	Delta-o (ms)	Dist (cm)	Vel m/s	Norm vel (ms)
Right median motor (Abd poll brev) 31.6°C											
Wrist		3.6	<4.2	12	>5	Elbow	Wrist	4.3	22.0	51	>50
Elbow		7.9		11.8							
Right radial motor (ExtIndProp) 31.5°C											
Mid FA		2.9	<3.2	3.8	>3	AElbow	Mid FA	3.0	18.0	60	>50
AElbow		5.9		3.6		AElbow	BElbow	2.1	12.0	57	>50
SpirGrv		8.0		3.5							
Right ulnar motor (ADM) 31.8°C											
Wrist		4.1	<4.5	11.1	>5	BElbow	Wrist	3.2	18.0	53	>50
BElbow		7.3		10.5		AElbow	BElbow	2.0	8.0	40	>50
AElbow		9.3		10.4							

Fig. 20.10 A Typical Nerve Conduction Data Table This data table shows ulnar motor slowing across the elbow due to myelin impairment. *NR*, no response; *ms*, milliseconds; *mv*, millivolts; *spirGrv*, spiral groove; *ADM*, abductor digiti minimi; *ExtIndProp*, extensor indicis proprius; *Abd poll brev*, abductor pollicis brevis; *O-P*, onset-peak; *Delta-O*, change in onset.

condition, whether symptomatic or asymptomatic (Dale et al 2013). A great deal of research has been conducted over the years to develop accurate testing protocols and severity grading systems. Standard carpal tunnel testing protocols have sensitivities that vary from 49% to 84% (Emad et al 2016). The specificities are much better at about 95% (Lee et al 2016). Testing protocols that utilize comparison tests between median, ulnar and radial nerves have much better sensitivities up to −72% while still maintaining excellent 92% specificity (Emad et al 2016). Carpal tunnel syndrome refers to a focal entrapment at or about the transcarpal ligament of the wrist (Lee et al 2016). The sensory nerves at this location tend to be more superficial, which places them in a position to sustain more damage from an entrapment compression. The nerve conduction test is able to detect sensory and/or motor nerve myelin impairment and sensory nerve axon impairment. A needle EMG electrode is then inserted into the abductor pollicis brevis muscle and/or the opponens pollicis muscle as these are median innervated and distal to the entrapment site. The distal degeneration of motor axons dictates that the only denervated muscle fibres would be distal to the wrist and other median innervated muscles proximal to the wrist, such as the flexor carpi radialis and pronator teres muscles, would be normal. Several grading systems have been devised to allow referring physicians to quickly assess the severity of nerve impairment that was observed.

A mild rating generally means that the sensory nerve myelin has been affected as that relates to median sensory or motor nerve slowing. A moderate rating means that both the median motor and sensory nerve fibres demonstrated slowing. A severe rating means that both median motor and sensory nerve fibres have demonstrated slowing, plus there are signs of median motor axonal damage, as seen with the needle EMG electrode. Other entrapment neuropathies follow a similar pattern to testing the carpal tunnel, although the grading systems vary greatly and there is not a great deal of agreement among electromyographers worldwide.

Nerve Root Impairment

A patient who presents with radicular pain and/or muscle weakness will often present with symptoms that are similar to an entrapment neuropathy. However, due to the position of the dorsal root ganglion (DRG) and the fact that root-level impairment normally occurs proximal to the DRG, all sensory nerve tests will be essentially normal (Fuller 2005). Even motor nerve conduction tests will often be normal owing to multi-segmental innervations of muscles. The needle EMG evaluation, however, will be abnormal when motor axons have been damaged to the point that distal muscle fibres are denervated (Coster et al 2010). For instance, if the right C7 nerve root was damaged by a protruding disc 6 weeks ago, a few, many, or all of the muscles innervated by that root will

Side	Muscle	Nerve	Root	Ins act	Fibs	Psw	Amp	Dur	Poly	Rec pat	Inter pat
Right	Biceps	Musculo	C5-6	Nml			Nml	Nml	Nml	Nml	Full
Right	Deltoid	Axillary	C5-6	Nml	Nml	Nml	Nml	Nml	Nml	Nml	Full
Right	Triceps	Radial	C6-7-8	Nml	1+	1+	Nml	Nml	Nml	Nml	Full
Right	FlexCarRad	Median	C6-7	Nml	2+	1+	Nml	Nml	Nml	Nml	Full
Right	ExtDigCom	Radial	C7-8	Nml	Nml	Nml	Nml	Nml	Nml	Nml	Full
Right	Abd poll brev	Median	C8-T1	Nml	Nml	Nml	Nml	Nml	Nml	Nml	Full
Right	1stDorInt	Ulnar	C8-T1	Nml	Nml	Nml	Nml	Nml	Nml	Nml	Full

Fig. 20.11 Typical EMG data chart for an acute C7 nerve root impairment. *Ins act*, Insertional Activity; *Fibs*, Fibrillation Potentials; *PSW*, Positive sharp waves; *Amp*, Amplitude; *Dur*, Duration; *Poly*, Polyphasics; *Rec Pat*, Recruitment Pattern; *Inter Pat*, Interference Pattern.

demonstrate excessive acute, spontaneous potentials. The needle EMG test may show excessive spontaneous potentials in the median innervated flexor carpi radialis and the radial innervated triceps muscle. These muscles share commonality at the C7 root level at the cervical spine (Fig. 20.11) (Fuller 2005). The needle would then be inserted into the cervical paraspinal muscles at the C6–7 vertebral interspace and similar findings may be seen. The dorsal rami branches of that root that run to the paraspinal muscles at that level are mono-segmentally innervated, which adds strength to using the needle EMG to pinpoint root-level lesions (Fuller 2005). There is a window of time to capture abnormalities that are detected by the needle EMG electrode. Tests that are done within 3 weeks of the initial insult to the nerve root are too early as the effects of Wallerian degeneration have not fully developed in distal musculature (Coster et al 2010). The optimum window is from approximately 6 weeks to 6 months for the upper extremities. The window for the lower extremities is from 6 weeks to 12 months. Ongoing nerve root damage will often demonstrate acute spontaneous findings and signs of chronic motor axon reinnervation in the same muscles. The nerve root has the ability to heal and reinnervate. This is often reflected in EMG tests that show signs of chronic reinnervation in muscles within its respective myotome without the acute findings.

Peripheral Neuropathies

Electrodiagnostic testing is often used to evaluate the extent and pattern of nerve damage from acquired disease processes such as diabetes, vitamin deficiencies, exposure to toxins and Guillain Barré syndrome (GBS) to inherited diseases such as Charcot-Marie-Tooth (Fuller 2005). These different disease pathologies will cause nerve damage in predictable ways, locations, patterns and nerve structures. The nerve damage that occurs from many of these conditions is often seen distally in the feet and hands due to the small calibre of the arteries, compressive pressures from body weight, and repetitive use of the limb (Fuller 2005). The nerve conduction data will often show a pattern of multiple nerves with low amplitudes, slow latencies and slow conduction velocities. The needle EMG electrode will often detect motor axon denervation and/or reinnervation in distal muscles more than proximal muscles (Fuller 2005). The description of the pattern of abnormalities can often be used by referring physicians to pinpoint the exact cause of the patient's symptoms to expedite a treatment regime. There are certain conditions that have an affinity for damaging proximal nerve myelin. GBS results from an auto-immune attack against the body's own myelin structures (Pithadia & Kakadia 2010). The exact trigger is unknown but it often follows an infection or even an influenza vaccine (Pithadia & Kakadia 2010). Traditional nerve conduction testing is not able to assess proximal nerve myelin owing to an inability to easily stimulate deep nerves from the surface. Therefore, a person with GBS would likely have a normal nerve conduction test (Mallik & Weir 2005). However, there is a test that can be used to capture proximal nerve conduction: the F-wave test (Mallik & Weir 2005). When a motor nerve is stimulated, action potentials flow bidirectionally. The action potentials that flow proximally will travel proximally to the anterior horn cells (Mallik & Weir 2005). An eddy of current flows around each axon hillock to the point that approximately 2%–3% of the axons 'back-fire' or are stimulated enough to send a volley of action potentials distally to the muscle fibres (Mallik & Weir 2005). This return firing can be amplified and displayed on the computer screen. The time for this whole process is compared to norms and compared to the contralateral side. This specialized test can detect a slow time, which implicates diffuse, proximal myelin impairment.

APPLICATION

Electrodiagnostic testing is typically in the purview of medical doctors such as neurologists and physiatrists. The number of physical therapists who can perform and interpret the results of electrodiagnostic tests is very small compared to the overall number of physical therapists throughout the world. In most of the United States, for instance, physical therapists can perform and interpret electrodiagnostic tests as long as a referral for testing is provided by a medical doctor. Obviously, specialized training is required, as well as long-term mentorship from established electrodiagnosticians. However, the majority of physical therapists are exposed to electrodiagnostic reports that often are part of the medical record for their patients. It is essential that all physical therapists are trained in how to read test data and make sense of the final impression. There is a great deal of variability among electrodiagnostic tests in both technique and accuracy of the final impression. The essential elements of a quality study include a medical history, physical examination, data tables that include normative data, summary of results, an impression/conclusion and waveforms (Feinberg 2006). Analysis of these elements can reveal details that affect the accuracy of the final impression. The following essential elements to be included in every electrodiagnostic test provide a quick reference to allow the treating therapist to judge the quality of the data:

Skin temperature As a general rule, the temperature of a nerve will affect the speed of action potential propagation. The mechanical opening/closing of sodium gates on the nerve cell membrane is slower in a cold nerve versus a warm nerve (Feinberg 2006). That translates into a slower flow of action potentials and consequently a slower time from stimulus to electrode detection. The normative data that is used to determine whether the conduction across the suspected site of entrapment was normal is based on subjects that were in a target range (upper extremity temperatures should be above 32°C and lower extremity temperatures above 30°C) (Feinberg 2006). On occasion, the patient temperature is below this number. Therefore, if the conduction across the entrapment is slow, it is unclear if that was due to temperature or true myelin impairment. The patient temperature for each nerve stimulation should be included in the data chart.

Conduction velocities The fastest conducting nerve fibres in the upper extremities conduct between 50 and 70 m/s with nerve conduction testing (Chen et al 2016). In the lower extremities, the conduction velocities are a bit slower with a range between 39 to 70 m/s (Chen et al 2016). A good quality nerve conduction study will list the conduction velocities for each nerve tested. The determination of a conduction velocity requires a physical measurement by the electromyographer. Errors in this measurement will have a direct effect on the accuracy of the results. Confounding factors include morbid obesity and areas of swelling. If these factors exist, the factor needs to be documented in the report. If conduction velocities are entered into the report above 80 m/s the technical quality is called into question and brings about other possible errors in the study produced by sloppy technique (Mallik & Weir 2005).

Waveforms Waveforms should be included for every nerve that was tested. The data that reside in the data charts are derived from the recorded waveforms. Errors in marking this waveform will translate directly to errant data used to determine the final impression. The nerve conduction study works by amplifying the reversal of action potentials (Mallik & Weir 2005). In order to accomplish this task, the recording electrodes are connected to an amplifier that can display recordings in the microvolt to millivolt range. The inherent danger with such amplification is that other sources of ambient electrical signals can enter into the recordings. Technical factors include poor electrical grounding, oils on the patient skin and using old recording electrodes. Recorded waveforms in the electrodiagnostic report divulge technical errors and the final impression can be incorrect. Modern day electrodiagnostic computers are programmed to automatically mark the important points of each of the recorded waveforms. The important points (cursors) such as 'O' for onset and 'P' for peak will automatically be entered into the resultant data charts to be compared to normative data. However, the automatic placement is not a perfect process, and the computer does not always mark the correct spot. Whether it be due to ambient noise that was recorded or possibly cross-talk from adjacent muscles, the cursors need to be moved manually by the astute electromyographer (Fig. 20.12) (Mallik & Weir 2005).

EMG data The data that is generated during the EMG needle examination is subjective to some extent, but pictures of abnormal EMG findings can also be taken and inserted into the section with the waveforms. EMG data is displayed in tables that list the side tested, muscle tested, corresponding myotomes and innervating nerve. Beyond this, there are columns with headings. Normally, the first three columns list insertional activity, fibrillation potentials and positive sharp waves. The grading scale runs from normal to 1+ to 4+. The higher the number the more dense or profuse the findings. This is subjective to the point that one person may see a run of fibrillation potentials and call it 1+ where another may call it 3+. Both are correct and some of that has to do with training. But the more important fact is that there were signs of acute denervation of motor axons and/or muscle tissue damage. Acute is considered to be from time of axon damage to about 4 months (Feinberg 2006). The next three column headings are amplitude, duration and polyphasic. These are descriptors of entire motor unit waveforms that were observed during light isometric muscle contraction. This process involves capturing a single motor unit for morphologic analysis. Amplitude is listed as either large or small compared to normative data. Duration is listed as short or long compared to normative data, and it refers

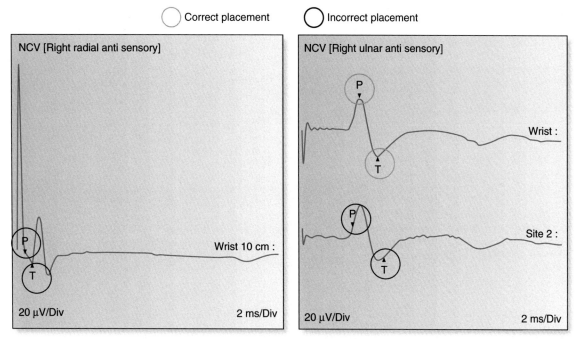

Fig. 20.12 The Electromyography Report Can you trust the data? Waveforms: correct or incorrect cursor placement? *NCV,* Nerve conduction velocity; *P,* Peak; *T,* Trough; *Anti,* Antidromic.

to the time it took the motor unit to completely discharge (Feinberg 2006). Polyphasic is documented from normal to 1+ to 4+. This refers to the number of times a single captured motor unit waveform crossed the baseline of the recording graph (Feinberg 2006). Some EMG data charts also include descriptors of recruitment and interference pattern. These refer to what was observed when the patient isometrically contracted the target muscle from very light to full contraction. Both of these headings use descriptors such as decreased, increased, full, discrete or normal.

Each section of the electrodiagnostic report should provide evidence that feeds into the final impression. For instance, a patient with a cervical nerve root impairment at the C7 nerve root will often report issues with activities of daily living (ADLs) that involve cervical spine extension or flexion. The physical examination may show a decreased triceps muscle reflex compared to the contralateral reflex. The nerve conduction test data should essentially be normal and the needle EMG will likely show acute and/or chronic changes in several muscles that share the C7 myotome. The final statement, the impression, should make clinical sense of this information to the consumer and help guide a treatment plan and eventual prognosis. An impression that does not make sense requires going back over the data charts and waveforms to look for technical errors.

REFERENCES

Belin, S., Zuloaga, K., & Poitelon, Y. (2017). Influence of mechanical stimuli on Schwann cell biology. *Frontiers in Cellular Neuroscience, 1,* 1–11.

Chen, S., Andary, M., Buschbacher, R., et al. (2016). Electrodiagnostic reference values for upper and lower limb nerve conduction studies in adult populations. *Muscle & Nerve, 54,* 71–377.

Coster, S., De Bruijn, S. F., & Tavy, D. L. (2010). Diagnostic value of history, physical examination and needle electromyography in diagnosing lumbosacral radiculopathy. *Journal of Neurology, 257,* 332–337.

Dale, A., Harris-Adamson, C., Rempel, D., et al. (2013). Prevalence and incidence of carpal tunnel syndrome in US working populations: Pooled analysis of six prospective studies. *Scandinavian Journal of Work, Environment & Health, 39*(5), 495–505.

Dorfman, L., & Robinson, L. (1997). AAEM minimonograph #47: Normative data in electrodiagnostic medicine. *Muscle & Nerve, 20,* 4–14.

Emad, M., Jahani, N., Azadeh, A., & Bemana, G. (2016). Is the difference between median sensory and ulnar motor latencies better than combined sensory index in carpal tunnel syndrome diagnosis? *Turkish Journal of Physical Medicine Rehabilitation, 62*(3), 229–233.

Feinberg, J. (2006). EMG: Myths and facts. *The Musculoskeletal Journal of Hospital for Special Surgery, 2,* 19–21.

Fuller, G. (2005). How to get the most out of nerve conduction studies and electromyography. *Journal of Neurology, Neurosurgery, and Psychiatry, 76*(Suppl. II), ii41–ii46.

Kazamel, M., & Warren, P. (2017). History of electromyography and nerve conduction studies: A tribute to the founding fathers. *Journal of Clinical Neuroscience, 43*, 54–60.

Lee, S., Kim, D., Cho, H., Nam, H., & Park, D. (2016). Diagnostic value of the second lumbrical-interosseous distal motor latency comparison test in severe carpal tunnel syndrome. *Annuals of Rehabilitation Medicine, 40*(1), 50–55.

Mallik, A., & Weir, A. (2005). Nerve conduction studies: Essentials and pitfalls in practice. *Journal of Neurology, Neurosurgery, and Psychiatry, 76*(Suppl. II), ii23–ii31.

Pithadia, A., & Kakadia, N. (2010). Guillain-Barré syndrome (GBS). *Pharmacological Reports, 62*(2), 220–232.

Preston, D. C., & Shapiro, B. (2013). *Electromyography and neuromuscular disorders: Clinical-electrophysiologic correlations.* New York, NY: Elsevier Saunders.

Robinson, L. (2015). How electrodiagnosis predicts clinical outcome of focal peripheral nerve lesions. *Muscle & Nerve, 52*(3), 321–333.

Russo, T. L., Peviani, S., Freria, C., Gigo-Benato, D., Geuna, S., & Salvini, T. (2007). Electrical stimulation based on chronaxie reduces atrogin-1 and myoD gene expressions in denervated rat muscle. *Muscle & Nerve, 35*, 87–97.

Schuhfried, O., Kollman, C., & Paternostro-Shuga, T. (2005). Excitability of chronic hemiparetic muscles: Determination of chronaxie values and strength-duration curves and its implication in functional electrical stimulation. *IEEE Transactions on Neural Systems and Rehabilitation Engineering, 13*(1), 105–109.

Stillman, B. (1967). Some aspects of the theory, performance, and interpretation of the strength-duration test. *Australian Journal of Physiotherapy, XIII*(2), 62–71.

Tapadia, J. D., Mozaffar, T., & Gupta, R. (2010). Compressive neuropathies of the upper extremity: Update on pathophysiology, classification, and electrodiagnostic findings. *Journal of Hand Surgery, 35A*, 668–677.

Ultrasound Imaging

John Leddy, Mark Maybury

INTRODUCTION

Ultrasound is an extraordinary tool, which enables the soft tissues of the body to be dynamically visualized and examined in incredible detail as part of a clinical examination. The prohibitive cost of equipment and the lack of availability of training has long been a bar to the use of ultrasound in physiotherapy; however in recent years the cost of scanners has fallen steadily and training programmes are now far more accessible. Consequently, ultrasound imaging is integrating into fields as diverse as women's health, respiratory, neurology and musculoskeletal physiotherapy, enhancing the accuracy of practitioners' assessment and enabling them to deliver treatments with more precision and confidence.

PRINCIPLES

GREY SCALE

When a sound wave passes through the body, a small percentage of the wave's energy (typically less than 1%) is reflected at each boundary that is encountered. The

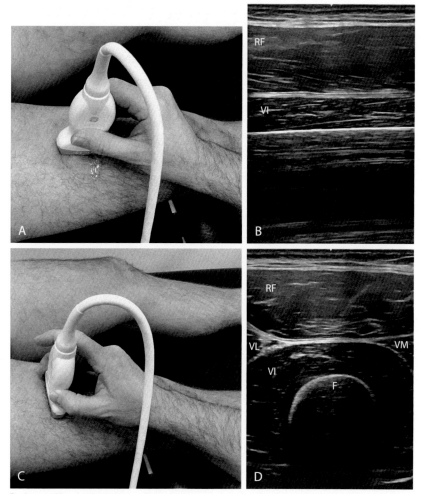

Fig. 21.1 Probe position and corresponding ultrasound appearance of normal right thigh. Longitudinal section (A) and (B), and cross or transverse section (C) and (D). *F,* Femur; *RF,* rectus femoris; *VI,* vastus intermedius; *VL,* vastus lateralis; *VM,* vastus medialis.

ultrasound image is acquired using a probe that generates a series of short, tightly focused pulses. These pass through the body and the sound waves reflected back to the probe by successive boundaries are recorded. Each pulse produces a single line of data, and a single image may be made up of over a hundred such lines (Fig. 21.1).

With each image taking as little as 1/100th of a second to construct, it can be updated continuously, giving a real-time cinematic view of the body that allows fast-moving structures, such as the heart and active muscles, and even small children to be imaged.

SCANNERS

Scanners are typically made up of one or more hand-held probes attached via flexible cables to a central unit, which

processes and displays the image (Fig. 21.2A). The probes operate at one or more fundamental frequencies, which determine the maximum depth and resolution of the images they generate. At higher frequencies, the shorter wavelengths mean that shorter pulses can be produced, giving better resolution. At lower frequencies, the resolution is reduced but the ultrasound is absorbed less readily as it passes through the body, enabling deeper structures to be examined.

The most commonly used probes are the linear and curvilinear probes (Fig. 21.2B). Linear probes are normally designed to operate at frequencies of 7.5 MHz and above; these produce high-resolution, rectangular images to a depth of around 5 cm. Curvilinear probes generate a fan-shaped image with a wider field of view than a linear probe. They operate at lower frequencies, typically between 2 and

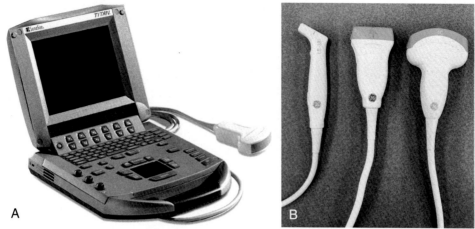

Fig. 21.2 (A) Portable ultrasound scanner (Sonosite) and (B) Hockey stick, linear and curvilinear probes (GE).

5 MHz, and can produce images to a depth of up to 15 cm but at the cost of lower resolution.

DOPPLER

The Doppler effect (Buys Ballot 1845) is used to detect and map blood flow, which is then superimposed onto the grey-scale image in real time. Using Doppler, the speed, direction and volume of flow can be assessed and displayed visually or numerically using three common formats – colour, power and spectral Doppler. Within physiotherapy this is mainly used to locate arteries and veins and identify hypervascularity associated with synovitis and tendinopathy. For these applications colour and power Doppler are usually used.

Colour Doppler

This samples the flow velocities over a wider area of the image and displays the presence of flow by adding colour to the grey scale image (Fig. 21.3A). Blue and red are typically used, although these represent flow either away or towards the ultrasound probe rather than venous and arterial flow.

Pulsed or Spectral Doppler

This detects the flow of blood through a small part of the image and displays it in the form of the spectrum of velocities detected against time (Fig. 21.3B).

Power Doppler

This variation of colour Doppler utilizes only one colour, normally orange, to display the presence of flow without directional information. This modality is more sensitive in detecting low speeds and volumes of flow.

Ultrasound Elastography

Elastography is a recent advancement in ultrasound technology that allows the stiffness of tissues to be evaluated and superimposed onto the ultrasound image. This has been successfully applied clinically in the characterization of suspicious lesions found within organs such as the liver, breast and thyroid (Ryu & Jeong 2017), and early work has suggested that it may have a role in assessing tendon pathology. There are a number of different technologies in development for this including ultrasound tissue characterization, strain and shear-wave elastography. These have yet to find widespread acceptance in clinical practice as reliability and reproducibility of findings are still problematic, but they offer the potential to characterize injury risk and enhance the ability of ultrasound to detect, monitor and quantify clinically significant changes in injured muscle and tendon structure (Drakonaki et al 2012; Washburn et al 2018).

Elastography allows information regarding the stiffness of soft tissue to be evaluated by examining the change in the ultrasound echoes caused by a strain passed simultaneously through the structures under the probe. The technology has been shown to be useful in characterizing cancers in thyroid and breast tissue (Cantisani et al 2014; Youk et al 2017). Clinical use of the technology within musculoskeletal ultrasound has yet to be established, but Demirel et al (2018) have shown that it has the potential to detect and characterize pathological changes within tendons.

Extended Field of View

This is a feature on modern scanners, which has its origins in the early static scanners of the 1970s. These types of scans were largely abandoned in the 1980s with the advent

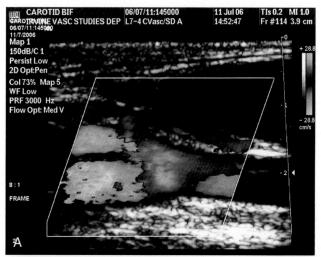

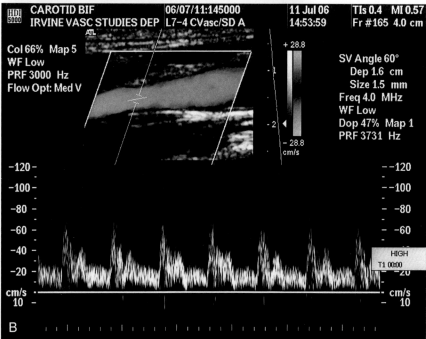

Fig. 21.3 (A) Colour Doppler image of the carotid bulb and (B) common carotid artery with spectral trace.

of high resolution real-time linear array transducers, but over recent years have made a comeback as technological improvements in computer science and motion/positions sensors occurred (Cooperberg et al 2001). Extended field of view allows a static composite image to be made of the whole length of a structure that is larger than the probe. This composite image is useful particularly when communicating anatomical relationships with other clinicians (Fig. 21.4).

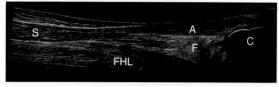

Right Achilles tendon

Fig. 21.4 Extended field of view longitudinal image of the Achilles tendon and musculotendinous junction. A, Achilles tendon; C, calcaneum; F, fat pad; S, soleus muscle belly.

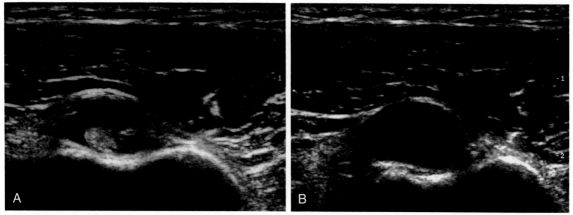

Fig. 21.5 Transverse section through the long head of biceps tendon highlighted by an effusion within the biceps sheath. Image (A) with the probe correctly aligned. In image (B) the probe is tilted slightly and the tendon appears dark due to anisotropy.

Artefacts

Artefacts are common in ultrasound and this is partly due to how the ultrasound beam propagates though tissues and the mathematical algorithms used to represent the tissues insonated by the ultrasound beam and displayed. There are numerous artefacts in ultrasound but the main ones to be considered here are anisotropy, enhancement and shadowing. Knowledge of these artefacts can help characterize tissue and reduce misdiagnosis.

Anisotropy is where the appearance of a structure seen in an image is dependent on the angle at which the ultrasound beam strikes it. This effect is particularly noticeable in tendons due to their linear architecture but is also seen when imaging nerves and muscle. When the fibres in these structures are parallel to the surface of the probe and therefore at right angles to the ultrasound beam, much of the reflected sound returns to the probe and the fibres therefore appear bright. When they are viewed at more oblique angles most of the sound is reflected away from the probe and so they appear dark, which can be misinterpreted as pathology (Fig. 21.5).

The appearance of a structure is also dependent on how much of the ultrasound beam is absorbed in the intervening tissues. Fluid filled structures such as cysts absorb significantly less of the ultrasound than fat and muscle and so the area underlying them will appear brighter. This is known as enhancement. The reverse is also true with dense material such as calcification within a tendon absorbing far more of the beam than the surrounding soft tissues. The area deep to this receives less sound and appears darker and is referred to as shadowing.

APPEARANCES: FEATURES OF AN ULTRASOUND IMAGE

Presentation

Unlike other cross-sectional imaging modalities, the orientation of an ultrasound image is not fixed and can be altered continuously to take into account the orientation of the tissues being examined.

For most applications the ultrasound image is orientated with the top of the screen representing the surface/ contact point of the probe on the body. However in musculoskeletal ultrasound there is no fixed convention regarding the direction representing proximal or distal structures which are dependent on the position and perspective of the operator. This has implications when it comes to the interpretation of stored images; however as most examinations performed in physiotherapy are evaluated in real time, this does not normally cause any difficulty.

Typical Appearance of Normal Tissue

The normal appearance of structures varies from person to person. The frequency used and the quality of the scanner also determines the amount of detail in the image. The most significant factors affecting the image, however, are the amount and nature of tissue that the sound has to pass through to reach the structure of interest.

Fig. 21.5 demonstrates some typical appearances of soft tissues:

- **Skin** appears smooth and bright (echogenic, hyperechoic, highly reflective).
- **Fat** can be bright or dark (hypoechoic, low echogenicity, low reflectivity), but subcutaneous fat is typically dark, with numerous fine bright septa running through it.

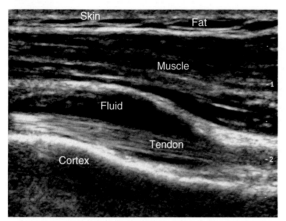

Fig. 21.6 Longitudinal section of the biceps tendon surrounded by an effusion in the tendon sheath. Note the highly reflective cortex, and the subtle reduction in brightness of the tendon from left to right as the fibres change direction (anisotropy).

- **Muscle** is also dark when viewed in cross-section. In long section, sound is reflected back by the muscle fibres and the internal structure of the muscle can be clearly visualized.
- **Fluid** whether blood, effusion or the content of cysts, is generally black (anechoic), although thicker fluids (such as pus or those containing debris) can be bright or dark. Fluid generally absorbs less sound than the surrounding soft tissue (translucence). This has the effect of making the image deep to fluid-filled structures appear relatively bright (enhancement).
- **Tendons** are typically bright, although this varies with their orientation relative to the sound waves emitted by the probe (anisotropy, Fig. 21.6).
- **Nerves** in the periphery also appear bright or dark depending on their orientation, and are distinguished from tendons dynamically, by following their course through the surrounding tissues.
- **Bone** surface appears as a particularly bright line due to the dramatic difference in acoustic impedance between bone and soft tissue. Because so much of the sound is reflected back by this boundary, very little is seen of what lies deep to the bone surface (shadowing).

Dynamic Evaluation

Unlike MRI, ultrasound can visualize structures dynamically to assess for abnormality. An obvious example of this is where the subacromial bursa may be seen to bunch as the supraspinatus tendon moves under the acromion in subacromial impingement. Other tests round the shoulder that help to demonstrate pathology would include subluxation of the long head of biceps in the bicipital groove as the

humerus externally rotates, and instability of the acromio-clavicular joint in arm elevation. This can negate the need for x-ray stress tests and reducing x-ray exposure to patients. Elsewhere, dynamic scanning can help evaluate snapping hip, iliotibial band, subluxing ulna nerve, subluxing peroneal tendons and stability of the lateral ankle ligament complex.

Image Storage

Modern ultrasounds are able to store images in multiple formats. The most common form is the still picture, but video clips can also be recorded either to scroll through an entire structure much like a magnetic resonance image (MRI) or computerized tomography (CT) sequence, or to capture movement when performing a dynamic test.

IMAGING APPLICATIONS

MUSCLE

Ultrasound is often the imaging modality of choice along with MRI for examining muscle injury (Draghi et al 2013) and in muscle research (Whittaker & Stokes 2011), as the internal structure and the interfaces between muscles are very well seen (Fig. 21.7).

Biofeedback

Ultrasound has been used in physiotherapy for many years to assess the deep muscles of the abdomen and pelvis, which are difficult to assess manually (Hides et al 1994, 1995). Muscles such as the transverse abdominis, along with the overlying internal and external oblique, can be observed simultaneously in real time (Fig. 21.8). This approach can be used for assessing almost any muscle group; for example Delft et al (2015) demonstrated the utility of transperoneal ultrasound as an alternative to digital examination for assessment of pelvic floor muscle contractility. Physiotherapists are also enabling patients to view the ultrasound themselves to observe muscle activity as visual biofeedback (Ellis et al 2018); however, evidence for the effectiveness of biofeedback in clinical practice is still lacking.

Objective Measurement

Ultrasound can be used to accurately measure the cross-sectional area of muscle (Martinson & Stokes 1991). The increase in muscle thickness during contraction can also be measured, although the correlation with effort is multifactorial and not yet fully described (Hodges et al 2003; McMeeken et al 2004). Muscle atrophy has a characteristic appearance, with the muscle appearing relatively bright. Ultrasound techniques to quantify the degree of fatty infiltration associated with muscle atrophy are still in their infancy and MRI remains the examination of choice for this (Strobel et al 2005).

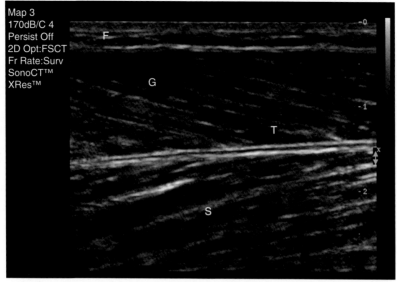

Fig. 21.7 Longitudinal section through the medial head of gastrocnemius. The thin bright layer at the top of the image is the skin; immediately below is a thin layer of relatively dark subcutaneous fat (*F*) with fine bright septations: (*G*) is the muscle belly of the medial gastrocnemius with the muscle fibres seen angling down to the bright tendon (*T*) that separates it from the underlying soleus (*S*) muscle.

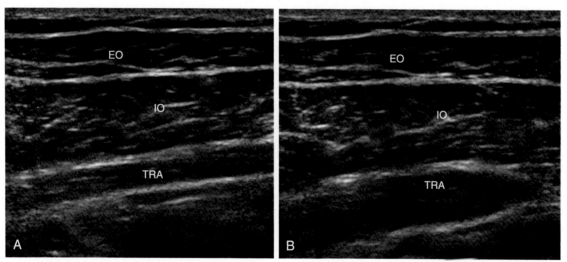

Fig. 21.8 Transverse section of the lateral abdominal wall in standing at rest (A). A significant increase in the thickness of internal oblique (*IO*) and transverse abdominus (*TRA*) is noted when the subject was asked to draw in his stomach (B). *EO,* External oblique.

Muscle Injuries

The appearance of muscle sprains and tears is highly variable; however, with experience ultrasound may have comparable efficacy to MRI in the initial assessment of injuries (Draghi et al 2013) with the advantage that it can directly assess the internal architecture. However, sensitivity is reduced for some deep muscles such as soleus (Balius et al 2014).

The appearances of low-grade tears are often very subtle, requiring experience to reliably evaluate. This is particularly true immediately after injury, as changes that can

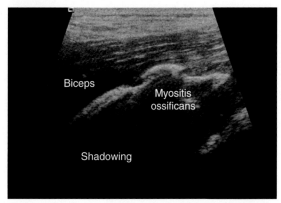

Fig. 21.9 Myositis ossificans in biceps femoris. Characteristic bright calcified outline seen within the muscle, with loss of image (shadowing) behind. (Courtesy Dr Gina Allen FRCR MF-SEM (UK), MSK radiologist, Royal Orthopaedic and University Hospitals, Birmingham.)

be detected by ultrasound may take more than a day to develop.

Larger tears are seen as a loss of continuity or a gap in the fibrous pattern, which may be highlighted by the presence of haematoma. Careful examination will also highlight muscle hernias and anatomical variations.

The appearance of a haematoma will also vary dramatically as it goes through different stages prior to being reabsorbed. Myositis ossificans is well seen with ultrasound as calcification has a bright appearance similar to bone and will typically cast a characteristic acoustic shadow artefact (Fig. 21.9).

TENDON

Most of the clinically relevant tendons in the peripheral musculoskeletal system are readily accessible to ultrasound, making it the optimal imaging method for many superficial tendons (Henderson et al 2015), with comparable and in some cases superior accuracy compared with MRI (Warden et al 2007).

The role of screening for tendon pathology is controversial, but systematic review of screening for Achilles and patella tendinopathy (McAuliffe et al 2016) showed pathological ultrasound changes were associated with a four-fold increase in risk of injury in the asymptomatic sporting population.

Normal Appearance

Normal tendon appears bright in an ultrasound image, so long as the surface of the probe is held roughly parallel with the direction of the tendon fibres. This allows incident sound to be reflected back to the probe. Once the angle changes significantly, the ultrasound no longer strikes the tendon at 90º, so much of the sound is reflected away from the probe making the tendon appear dark. This effect is known as anisotropy (Fig. 21.5).

Tendinopathy

The thickness of tendons such as the Achilles increases with tendinosis and the diameter can be compared with the unaffected side and/or normal values. The diameter and the echogenicity of the Achilles tendon return to normal as the tendon recovers (Ohberg et al 2004) and it may be that ultrasound can be used to tailor rehabilitation, although much work still needs to be done on this.

Focal tendinosis appears as dark areas within a tendon. This appearance can be mimicked by areas of normal tendon due to the anisotropy described previously, and so considerable care is required in evaluating subtle tendon injuries.

The synovial sheath that is present around some tendons is not easily identified when normal. In the presence of inflammation, it becomes oedematous and has an easily identified thickened hypoechoic (darkened) appearance. Ultrasound is very effective at identifying fluid within a tendon sheath, although it should be remembered that in some sheaths a small amount of fluid may be normal.

The ability to move joints and simultaneously visualize tendons also allows subluxation to be confirmed, typically with tendons such as biceps and the peroneii. Tethering can be identified when a tendon is seen to draw the surrounding soft tissue with it as it moves rather than gliding freely. Within the hand the flexor tendons can be seen moving through their pulleys, and with good high-frequency probes the pulleys themselves can be examined (Boutry et al 2005).

Tendon Tears

Ultrasound is often used to confirm whether a tendon has ruptured (Fig. 21.10), and the relative position of the free ends. Where tendons are superficial this is a relatively straightforward task, made easier by the ability to visualize the relative movement in real time. Partial tears can also be seen, but as with muscle tears, are more difficult to evaluate when there is not a clear gap in the fibrous pattern.

Calcific Deposits

Calcification within tendons is often observed with x-ray, but ultrasound is the optimal imaging modality as the position (Fig. 21.11) and clinical significance of deposits can be evaluated easily (Chianca et al 2018). In contrast, calcifications are poorly seen on MRI and CT lacks the soft tissue contrast to determine the type of calcification or its impact on adjacent soft tissues.

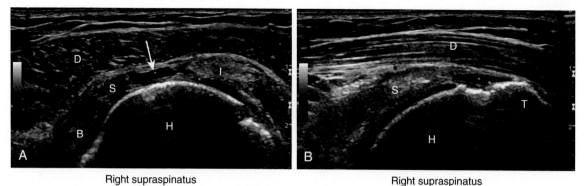

Right supraspinatus   Right supraspinatus

Fig. 21.10 (A) Short axis and (B) long axis images of the insertional zone of the right supraspinatus tendon with a small full thickness tear (*arrow*). *B*, Long head of biceps; *D*, deltoid muscle; *H*, humeral head; *I*, infraspinatus tendon; *S*, supraspinatus tendon; *T*, greater tuberosity.

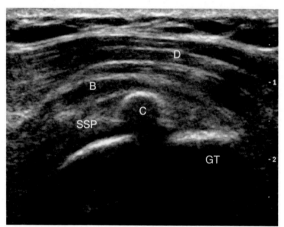

Fig. 21.11 Round calcific deposit (*C*) in the supraspinatus tendon (*SSP*) just distal to its insertion into the greater tubercle (*GT*). Note a distended subacromial bursa (*B*) deep to deltoid muscle (*D*).

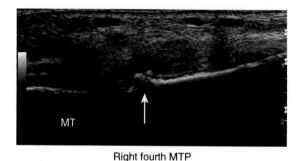

Right fourth MTP

Fig. 21.12 Stress Fracture of Fourth Metatarsal Longitudinal section taken on day 5. Metatarsal (*MT*), fracture (*arrow*).

BONES

The surfaces of bones are highly reflective and are well seen with ultrasound, making this an ideal modality to assess tomographic cortical bone–soft tissue interface. Despite this, ultrasound is not generally the modality of choice to examine bone, being better visualized by x-ray, CT and MRI.

Examining the entire surface of a bone with ultrasound can be time consuming so it would not replace the need for x-rays. Nevertheless, there is a gathering body of evidence suggesting that it could be used as a first line modality to assess bony injury (Beltrame et al 2012; Waterbrook et al 2013).

Ultrasound can be advantageous in the assessment of fractures as they often appear as a clear break in the outline of the bone and it can pick up some fractures not apparent on plain-film x-ray (Rutten et al 2006; Turk et al 2010). Where x-ray has reduced sensitivity, such as for scaphoid, rib and greater tuberosity fractures, ultrasound's very high sensitivity makes it a useful adjunct (Jain et al 2018).

Patients with persistent localized pain after trauma may undergo ultrasound examinations in order to rule out soft tissue lesions. When the images are examined, cortical irregularity, discontinuities and breaks in the cortex (Zamorani & Valle 2007) can be demonstrated which are unrelated to nutrient foramen in the bone, and correlation with x-ray and clinical examination is required. It is in these circumstances along with assessment of overuse bony injuries such as stress fractures, either insufficiency fractures or fatigue type fractures, that ultrasound demonstrates good clinical utility (Amoako et al 2017; Banal et al 2006). In the early stages of stress fracture before callous formation, soft tissue hyperaemia is demonstrable on ultrasound (Fig.21.12).

In paediatrics, where ossification of the bones is not complete, ultrasound can often complement x-rays, as the cartilaginous sections are well seen, in contrast to plain

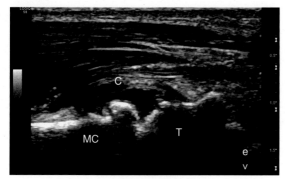

Right first CMC

Fig. 21.13 Osteoarthritis of the First Carpometacarpal Joint Long section through the palmar aspect of the right first carpometacarpal (*CMC*) joint, showing osteophyte formation at the articular margin of the first metacarpal (*MC*) and a small effusion contained by the thickened capsule (*C*). The articular margin of the trapezium (*T*) also appears irregular.

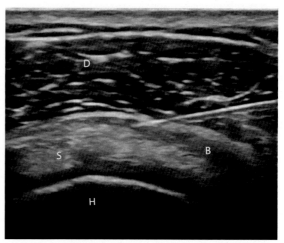

Fig. 21.14 Subacromial Injection Short axis image of the supraspinatus tendon (*S*) with a 21-gauge needle tip placed within the thickened subacromial bursa (*B*). Humeral head (*H*) and deltoid muscle (*D*).

films. Ultrasound is used to assess the depth of the acetabulum in neonates, where it has been shown to facilitate the early detection of developmental dysplasia of the hip (Laborie et al 2014).

JOINTS

The margins of peripheral joints are easily identified with ultrasound and can be examined in some detail with a high frequency probe (Fig 21.13). Although the typical appearance of different joints varies greatly, with experience synovial hypertrophy, erosions, osteophytes, ligament injuries and evidence of inflammation can be discerned. Ultrasound is particularly useful for detecting and characterizing effusions (Delaunoy et al 2003; Kane et al 2003) and for directing therapeutic injections and aspiration.

The movement of joints can also be visualized along with the surrounding soft tissue, although this can be technically challenging owing to movement of the probe in contact with the body. X-ray fluoroscopy is currently the imaging method of choice for detecting subtle carpal bone subluxation; however, with the advent of real-time three-dimensional ultrasound imaging (4D) it may be possible to evaluate movement of the carpi without the use of ionizing radiation.

Guided Injections

The accuracy of anatomically guided injections has often been questioned (Partington & Broome 1998; Simoni et al 2017; Yamakado 2002). Ultrasound guidance allows precise needle placement within a target structure (Fig. 21.14) and it has been postulated this leads to a reduced amount of drug, consequently leading to reduced complications (Roh et al 2018) and improvements in therapeutic efficacy (Aly et al 2015; Daniels et al 2018; Sibbitt et al 2009). Ultrasound guidance is the imaging modality of choice for aspiration of effusions and fluid collections (Randelli et al 2018) with superior differentiation of fluids and solids when compared to CT and fluoroscopy. Ultrasound-guided aspiration is reported to give better pain relief and higher aspiration volume than an unguided procedure (Wu et al 2016). Using ultrasound has the added benefit that structures such as blood vessels and nerves can be identified and avoided.

NERVES

The steady improvement in image quality over recent years has meant that it is now practicable to visualize nerves and nerve pathology through much of the musculoskeletal system. Visualization of the spinal cord beyond the neonatal period is extremely limited (Inklebarger et al 2018), but as the nerve roots emerge between the transverse processes in the neck, they are clearly seen. In the lower limb, the nerve roots are not well seen, until they pass into the buttock and groin as the sciatic and femoral nerves, due to their depth.

Nerve lesions (neuromas), such as schwannomas and Morton's (Fig. 21.15), as well as lacerations and compressions of peripheral nerves, such as carpal tunnel syndrome, are readily seen. Nerves are also assessed dynamically along with direct palpation, which not only enables identification of abnormal movement, as in the case of subluxing ulna nerve at the elbow, but also helps to determine if the abnormality is clinically significant.

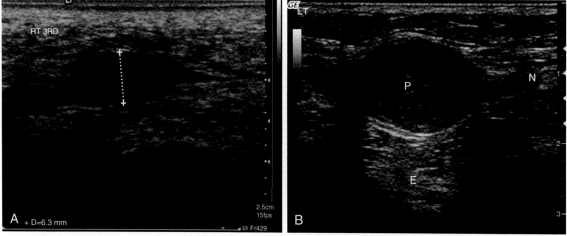

Fig. 21.15 (A) A long section through the third web space of the right foot showing a large Morton's neuroma (*between callipers*). (B) peroneal nerve tumour *(P)* just proximal to the fibular head. The lesion is in continuity with the nerve *(N)*. The region deep to the tumour *(E)* is brighter than the surrounding tissue (enhancement), suggesting that the lesion has a high fluid content.

VASCULAR

Doppler ultrasound is used in physiotherapy research to assess blood flow in the vertebral arteries (Arnold et al 2004; Mitchell et al 2004), because of concerns regarding adverse effects of cervical manipulation. The relative roles of vertebral and carotid arteries in adverse events have yet to be determined, but in the future ultrasound may have a role in premanipulation screening.

Grey-scale imaging is used to examine the structure of blood vessels, whereas Doppler is applied to evaluate the blood flow. Blood vessel walls appear as bright tubes on ultrasound, with blood appearing black (anechoic) in a grey-scale image. Arteries and veins are easily distinguished as the latter collapse with gentle probe pressure and the pulsatility of flow in arteries is unmistakable when viewed with Doppler.

Thrombus within vessels is not always visible on grey scale as it can have the same echo texture as blood; however, it can be detected in veins by dynamic testing, as the vessel will not completely collapse when compressed if there is thrombus within the lumen at that point. Within arteries, stenoses resulting from intramural thrombus cause changes in blood flow which can be detected with Doppler.

LUMPS AND BUMPS

Evaluation of palpable masses, or 'lumps and bumps' as they are commonly referred to, requires considerable experience. Ultrasound appearances may not be entirely

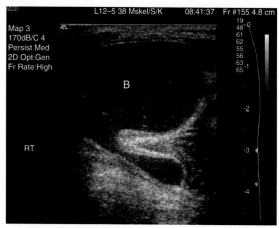

Fig. 21.16 Baker's cyst *(B)* with typical tail. Note that the cyst does not appear black (anechoic) due to the presence of blood products within it (haematoma).

specific and in ambiguous cases require clinical correlation, and often further imaging.

Ultrasound is very useful in detecting foreign bodies, especially those not well seen with x-ray, such as wood splinters. These will often appear bright, casting an acoustic shadow, and may be surrounded by a dark halo of reactive oedematous tissue. Ganglia, including Baker's cysts appear as fluid-filled sacks, and often a tail can be seen tracking towards the structure they arise from, giving them a C shape or 'speech bubble' appearance (Fig. 21.16).

Ultrasound does not suffer from the problems of MRI and CT in imaging prostheses. These generally have

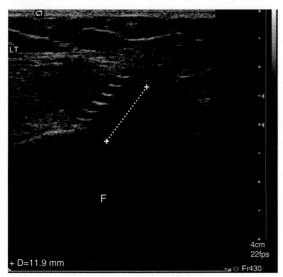

LT_

F

+ D=11.9 mm

4cm
22fps
Fr430

Fig. 21.17 Internal fixation screw protruding 12 mm through the cortex of the medial femoral condyle, not evident on check x-ray. Coronal section medial aspect of the distal femur (*F*). Screw threads (*callipers*).

sonographic qualities similar to bone, so although their internal integrity cannot be assessed, their superficial surface, effusions and collections and the overlying soft tissues can be visualized. Protruding metal work from internal fixation can be difficult to evaluate on x-ray, but is often obvious on ultrasound (Fig. 21.17).

Shoulder

Ultrasound assessment of the rotator cuff of the shoulder has consistently been shown to be comparable to MRI (Lenza et al 2013) with accuracy often reported in excess of 90%, and is easily integrated into the objective portion of a clinical assessment. Anatomical assessment of the tendons and bursa (Figs 21.10 and 21.11) is straightforward, but dynamic scanning can also demonstrate impingement (Park et al 2018) and may be particularly useful in assessing whether calcified deposits are clinically relevant. Ultrasound can also pick up causes of reduced movement such as posterior joint osteophytes and changes to the coracohumeral ligament in frozen shoulder. Performing ultrasound as part of the clinical examination rather than as a separate test makes it easier to assess the contextual relevance of both imaging findings and of the more traditional objective tests.

Elbow

Ultrasound is often used to confirm the presence of tennis elbow (enthesopathy of the common extensor origin), and

is also able to assess for compression of the posterior interosseous branch of the radial nerve, which can be responsible for similar symptoms. The distal biceps tendon is well seen, and dynamic assessment will also identify impingement with the ulna on pronation. Ultrasound will demonstrate joint abnormalities relating to the ulna nerve including subluxation which is easily assessed.

Wrist and Hand

Ultrasound greatly enhances the effectiveness of clinical assessment of the wrist and hand, with Tagliafico et al (2019) showing sonography influences both diagnosis and treatment path in around three quarters of cases where it is used. Typical examples would be radial wrist pain, where differentiating between conditions which can have similar presentations such as intersection syndrome, De Quervain's tenosynovitis and first carpometacarpal osteoarthritis can be difficult (Fig. 21.13). Ultrasound is also comparable to nerve conduction studies in the assessment of carpal tunnel syndrome (Azami et al 2014) and is able to identify causes for compression such as tenosynovitis, anatomical anomalies and space-occupying lesions such as ganglions.

Knee

MRI is the imaging modality of choice for assessing intra articular structures such as the meniscus and cruciate ligaments. Ultrasound can be used however, to evaluate tendon and collateral ligament injuries and to guide treatments.

Hip

Ultrasound of the hip joint is limited to assessment of effusion, thickening of the capsule and the overlying musculature. It is often possible to evaluate snapping tendons such as psoas major and the iliotibial band. Ultrasound is able to detect gluteus medius and minimus tendon insertion pathology and can also be used to assess muscle function.

Posteriorly, ultrasound can be used to assess the hamstrings and abductor magnus origins arising from the ischial tuberosity.

Pelvis

The abdominal wall and pelvic floor muscles can be visualized using ultrasound. This allows for direct objective evaluation of inguinal, femoral and abdominal wall hernias, along with divarifications.

Scanning through the abdominal wall, the function of the pelvic floor can be assessed indirectly by its effect on the posterior wall of the bladder. A more detailed evaluation, with direct visualization of the function and movement of the urethra, is possible by scanning through the peritoneum.

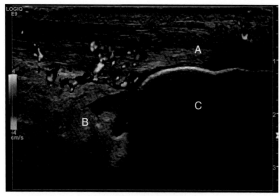

Right achilles tendon

Fig. 21.18 Tendinosis and neovascularity in the distal Achilles tendon. Colour Doppler map of blood flow superimposed on a long section image of the Achilles tendon. *A,* Achilles tendon; *B,* slightly dilated retrocalcaneal bursa; *C,* posterior aspect of the calcaneus. (A colour version of this figure is available as an insert at the end of the book)

Achilles

There is a wide differential diagnosis for posterior heel and calf pain; clinical examination is often ambiguous. Ultrasound is able to differentiate between distal and mid-section Achilles tendinosis, enthesitis, partial tears of the deep and superficial surface, and injuries to the gastrocnemius and soleus muscles (Fig. 21.18). Ultrasound can also evaluate the plantaris, the saphenous and sural nerves, the fascia cruris and can identify inflammatory changes in the superficial and retrocalcaneal bursae. Ultrasound imaging may have a role in assessment and treatment of os trigonum, but is not a sensitive test for stress fractures of the calcaneus.

Ankle and Foot

The tendons and joint lines of the foot and ankle are close to the surface and so easily and effectively assessed with ultrasound. Delzell et al (2017) found that the addition of ultrasound imaging for patients with foot and ankle problems changed the clinical diagnosis in over 60% of cases and the management in 43% of cases.

Dynamic assessment of ligaments and joint instability is particularly useful and can be performed alongside the traditional clinical tests. In the case of the anterior talofibular ligament, tears can be directly visualized while at the same time evaluating whether there is associated joint laxity.

Ultrasound is more sensitive than x-ray for detecting inflammatory and degenerative changes in the midfoot joints (Camerer et al 2017).

Assessment of metatarsalgia and Morton's neuroma (Fig. 21.15A) is technically challenging but rewarding with accuracy reported as close to 90% (Xu et al 2015). The metatarsal

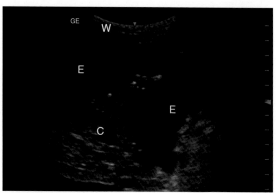

Fig. 21.19 Cross section upper left chest showing compression of the left upper lobe by a large effusion. *C,* Consolidated lung with fluid bronchograms noted; *E,* pleural effusion; *W,* chest wall. (Courtesy Simon Hayward, Specialist Physiotherapist, Blackpool Teaching Hospital NHS Foundation Trust.)

phalangeal joints can be examined at the same time for localized arthropathy or for evidence of systemic synovitis.

LUNGS

Ultrasound is increasingly being used by clinicians on patients experiencing respiratory compromise in the critical care environment (Hayward & Janssen 2018). Lung pathology can be evaluated at the bedside quickly in real time. Lung function including excursion and contraction can be assessed in addition to hypertrophy and hypotrophy of the diaphragm (Dres et al 2015). Ultrasound accurately diagnoses pleural effusions with 93% sensitivity and 98% specificity (Grimberg et al 2010) and its efficacy for assessing consolidation, pneumothorax, interstitial syndrome, pleural effusion and for monitoring was established by Volpicelli et al (2012). Meta-analysis by Winkler et al (2018) found ultrasound to have far higher sensitivity and equal specificity to chest radiograph for consolidation (Fig. 21.19), interstitial syndrome and lung contusion. This could allow clinicians to answer goal-directed questions with better accuracy. Touw et al (2018) show that it can be more effective than chest radiograph when used at the bedside in identifying post-operative pulmonary complications. The emerging technique of lung ultrasound to assess lung function and pathology more accurately in real time in any location could positively enhance a clinician's assessment and monitoring ability.

LIMITATIONS OF ULTRASOUND

Ultrasound imaging is not without its limitations both in terms of what is technically possible and in terms of the expertise needed to perform diagnostic examinations.

With the exception of specialized Doppler studies of the circle of Willis in the adult brain, ultrasound cannot be used to examine tissue lying deep to calcified bone. Air also represents a barrier to ultrasound, limiting examinations of the thorax and bowel. Other limitations include reduced image quality when examining large subjects. This can be alleviated to some extent by using lower-frequency probes, but at the cost of reduced resolution.

The accuracy of diagnostic imaging is dependent on the experience and expertise of the practitioners performing and interpreting the examinations. This is true of all imaging modalities; however ultrasound is particularly operator dependent due in part to the precision needed to acquire the optimum image and the broad range of normal and pathological appearances that are possible. Clinicians need to take into consideration the experience of the operator when interpreting ultrasound findings (Thoomes-de Graaf et al 2014). The operators themselves need to continually develop and dispassionately evaluate their practice. This is best done by continuous rigorous self audit.

SAFETY

Ultrasound is perceived as a safe form of imaging and, to date, no harmful side effects have been reported from the clinical use of real-time ultrasound in the paediatric and adult populations. Developments in ultrasound technology, however, have led to ever higher power outputs, particularly with applications such as tissue harmonic imaging and Doppler, and the possibility of tissue damage cannot be discounted. The potential risks are from heating and from mechanical effects such as cavitation (outlined in Chapter 9). These effects are likely to be negligible when using standard grey-scale imaging of musculoskeletal structures; however, it is prudent to avoid scanning over a fixed point for longer than is necessary for assessment and training purposes.

Concerns about the safety of ultrasound have been focused on in utero scanning, where ultrasound may have an effect on the rapidly developing fetus. Unnecessary scanning of the fetus should therefore be avoided (BMUS Safety Guidelines 2000; ter Haar 2012) and should be carried out only by operators with the appropriate training.

The most significant risk to the patient from the use of ultrasound comes not from the ultrasound itself but from misinterpretation of ultrasound findings, and it is essential that clinicians using ultrasound can recognize the limitations imposed by equipment, image quality and their own experience and training.

SUMMARY

Ultrasound imaging has the potential to revolutionize physiotherapy practice by allowing the clinician to directly image the structures of interest, whether the patient is on the couch or the treadmill. Muscle recruitment and its effect on other structures can be evaluated with increased accuracy. With appropriate training, focal soft-tissue lesions and pathological changes can also be evaluated and, because patients are seen regularly throughout the rehabilitation process, physiotherapists have the unique opportunity to monitor and document the healing of tendons, muscles, joints and even possibly nerve injuries. In this way, ultrasound offers physiotherapy not only a powerful adjunct to clinical assessment but also a much-needed objective tool for evaluating the effectiveness of practice, and the diverse range of treatment modalities, including those described in this text.

REFERENCES

Aly, A.-R., Rajasekaran, S., & Ashworth, N. (2015). Ultrasound-guided shoulder girdle injections are more accurate and more effective than landmark-guided injections: A systematic review and meta-analysis. *British Journal of Sports Medicine*, *49*, 1042–1049.

Amoako, A., Abid, A., Shadiack, A., & Monaco, R. (2017). Ultrasound-diagnosed tibia stress fracture: A case report. *Clinical Medicine Insights: Arthritis and Musculoskeletal Disorders*, *10*, 1–3.

Arnold, C., Bourassa, R., Langer, T., & Stoneham, G. (2004). Doppler studies evaluating the effect of a physical therapy screening protocol on vertebral artery blood flow. *Manual Therapy*, *9*, 13–21.

Azami, A., Maleki, N., Anari, H., Iranparvar Alamdari, M., Kalantarhormozi, M., & Tavosi, Z. (2014). The diagnostic value of ultrasound compared with nerve conduction velocity in carpal tunnel syndrome. *International Journal of Rheumatology Diseases*, *17*(6) 612–20.

Balius, R., Rodas, G., Pedret, C., Capdevila, L., Alomar, X., & Bong, D. A. (2014). Soleus muscle injury: Sensitivity of ultrasound patterns. *Skeletal Radiology*, *43*(6), 805–812.

Buys Ballot, C. H. D. (1845). Akustische Versuche auf der Niederländischen Eisenbahn, nebst gelegentlichen Bemerkungen zur Theorie des Hrn. *Prof. Doppler (in German) Annalen der Physik und Chemie*, *11*(11), 321–351.

Banal, F., Etchepare, F., Rouhier, B., et al. (2006). Ultrasound ability in early diagnosis of stress fracture of metatarsal bone. *Annals of the Rheumatic Diseases*, *65*, 977–978.

Beltrame, V., Stramare, R., Rebellato, N., Angelini, F., Frigo, A., & Rubaltelli, L. (2012). Sonographic evaluation of bone fractures: A reliable alternative in clinical practice? *Clinical Imaging*, *36*, 203–208.

BMUS Safety Guidelines (2000) Online. Available: http://www.bmus.org/public-info/pi-safety03.asp.

Boutry, N., Titecat, M., Demondion, X., et al. (2005). High-frequency ultrasonographic examination of the finger pulley system. *Journal of Ultrasound in Medicine*, *24*(10), 1333–1339.

Camerer, M., Ehrenstein, B., Hoffstetter, P., Fleck, M., & Hartung, W. (2017). High-resolution ultrasound of the midfoot: Sonography is more sensitive than conventional radiography in detection of osteophytes and erosions in inflammatory and non-inflammatory joint disease. *Clinical Rheumatology, 36*(9), 2145–2149.

Cantisani, V., Albano, D., Messina, C., et al. (2018). Rotator cuff calcific tendinopathy: From diagnosis to treatment. *Acta BioMedica, 89*(1-S), 186–196.

Cantisani, V., Lodise, P., Grazhdani, H., et al. (2014). Ultrasound elastography in the evaluation of thyroid pathology. Current status. *European Journal of radiology, 83*(3), 420–428.

Cooperberg, P. L., Barberie, J., Wong, T., & Fix, C. (2001). Extended field of view ultrasound. *Seminars in Ultrasound, CT and MRI, 22*(1), 65–77.

Daniels, E., Cole, D., Jacobs, B., & Phillips, S. (2018). Existing evidence on ultrasound-guided injections in sports medicine. *Orthopaedic Journal of Sports Medicine, 6*(2).

Delaunoy, I., Feipel, V., Appelboom, T., & Hauzeur, J. (2003). Sonography detection threshold for knee effusion. *Clinical Rheumatology, 22*(6), 391–392.

Delzell, P., Tritle, B., Bullen, J., Chiunda, S., & Forney, M. (2017). Clinical utility of high-frequency musculoskeletal ultrasonography in foot and ankle pathology: How ultrasound imaging influences diagnosis and management. *Journal of Foot and Ankle Surgery, 56*(4), 735–739.

Draghi, F., Zacchino, M., Canepari, M., Nucci, P., & Alessandrino, F. (2013). Muscle injuries: Ultrasound evaluation in the acute phase. *Journal of Ultrasound, 16*(4), 209–214.

Drakonaki, E. E., Allen, G. M., & Wilson, D. J. (2012). Ultrasound elastography for musculoskeletal applications. *British Journal of Radiology, 85*, 1435–1445.

Dres, M., Mayaux, J., Delemazure, J., Prodanovic, H., Similowski, T., & Demoule, A. (2015). Reliability of diaphragmatic ultrasonography to detect diaphragm dysfunction in critically ill patients *Intensive Care. Medicina Experimentalis, 3*(Suppl. 1), A452.

Ellis, R., De Jong, R., Bassett, S., Helsby, J., Stokes, M., & Cairns, M. (2018). Exploring the clinical use of ultrasound imaging: A survey of physiotherapists in New Zealand. *Musculoskeletal Science and Practice, 34*, 27–37.

Grimberg, A., Shigueoka, D. C., Atallah, A. N., Ajzen, S., & Iared, W. (2010). Diagnostic accuracy of sonography for pleural effusion: Systematic review. *Sao Paulo Medical Journal, 128*(2), 90–95.

Hayward, S., & Janssen, J. (2018). Use of thoracic ultrasound by physiotherapists: A scoping review of the literature. *Physiotherapy, 103*, 70–71.

Henderson, R., Walker, B., & Young, K. (2015). The accuracy of diagnostic ultrasound imaging for musculoskeletal soft tissue pathology of the extremities: A comprehensive review of the literature. *Chiropr Man Therap, 23*, 31.

Hides, J., Richardson, C., & Jull, G. (1995). Magnetic resonance imaging and ultrasonography of the lumbar multifidus muscle. Comparison of two different modalities. *Spine, 20*(1), 54–58.

Hides, J., Stokes, M., Saide, M., et al. (1994). Evidence of multifidus wasting ipsilateral to symptoms in patients with acute/subacute low back pain. *Spine, 19*(2), 165–177.

Hodges, P., Pengel, L., Herbert, R., & Gandevia, S. (2003). Measurement of muscle contraction with ultrasound imaging. *Muscle & Nerve, 27*(6), 682–692.

Inklebarger, J., Leddy, J., Turner, A., & Abbas, B. (2018). Transabdominal imaging of the lumbar spine with portable ultrasound. *International Journal of Medical Science and Clinical Invention, 5*(1), 3407–3412.

Jain, R., Jain, N., Sheikh, T., & Yadav, C. (2018). Early scaphoid fractures are better diagnosed with ultrasonography than X-rays: A prospective study over 114 patients. *Chinese Journal of Traumatology, 21*(4), 206–210.

Kane, D., Balint, P., & Sturrock, R. (2003). Ultrasonography is superior to clinical examination in the detection and localization of knee joint effusion in rheumatoid arthritis. *Journal of Rheumatology, 30*(5), 966–971.

Laborie, L., Markestad, T., Davidsen, H., et al. (2014). Selective ultrasound screening for developmental hip dysplasia: Effect on management and late detected cases. A prospective survey during 1991-2006. *Pediatric Radiology, 44*(4), 410–424.

Lenza, M., Buchbinder, R., Takwoingi, Y., Johnston, R. V., Hanchard, N. C., & Faloppa, F. (2013). Magnetic resonance imaging, magnetic resonance arthrography and ultrasonography for assessing rotator cuff tears in people with shoulder pain for whom surgery is being considered. *Cochrane Database of Systematic Reviews, 24*(9).

Martinson, H., & Stokes, M. (1991). Measurement of anterior tibial muscle size using real-time ultrasound imaging. *European Journal of Applied Physiology and Occupational Physiology, 63*(3–4), 250–254.

McAuliffe, S., McCreesh, K., Culloty, F., Purtill, H., & O'Sullivan, K. (2016). Can ultrasound imaging predict the development of Achilles and patellar tendinopathy? A systematic review and meta-analysis. *British Journal of Sports Medicine, 50*(24), 1516–1523.

McMeeken, J., Beath, I., Newham, D., et al. (2004). The relationship between EMG and change in thickness of transverse abdominis. *Clinical Biomechanics, 19*(4), 337–342.

Mitchell, J., Keen, D., Dyson, C., et al. (2004). Is cervical spin rotation, as used in the standard vertebrobasilar insufficiency test, associated with a measurable change in intracranial vertebral artery blood flow? *Manual Therapy, 9*(4), 220–227.

Ohberg, L., Lorentzon, R., & Alfredson, H. (2004). Eccentric training in patients with chronic Achilles tendinosis: Normalised tendon structure and decreased thickness at follow up. *British Journal of Sports Medicine, 38*(1), 8–11.

Park, J., Chai, J., Kim, D., Cha, S. (2018). Dynamic ultrasonography of the shoulder. *Ultrasonography, 37*(3), 190–199.

Partington, P. F., & Broome, G. H. (1998). Diagnostic injection around the shoulder: Hit and miss? A cadaveric study of injection accuracy. *Journal of Shoulder and Elbow Surgery, 7*(2), 147–150.

Randelli, F., Brioschi, M., Randelli, P., Ambrogi, F., Sdao, S., & Aliprandi, A. (2018). Fluoroscopy- vs ultrasound-guided aspiration techniques in the management of periprosthetic joint infection: Which is the best? *Radiologia Medica, La, 123*(1), 28–35.

Roh, Y., Hong, S., Gong, H. S. 2, & Baek, G. (2018). Ultrasound-guided versus blind corticosteroid injections for De Quervain tendinopathy: A prospective randomized trial. *Journal of Hand Surgery, 43*(8), 820–824.

Rutten, M., Jager, G., de Waal Malefijt, M., et al. (2006). Double line sign: A helpful sonographic sign to detect occult fractures of the proximal humerus. *European Radiology, 17,* 762–767.

Ryu, J., & Jeong, W. (2017). Current status of musculoskeletal application of shear wave elastography. *Ultrasonography, 36*(3), 185–197.

Sibbitt, W. L., Jr., Peisajovich, A., Michael, A. A., et al. (2009). Does sonographic needle guidance affect the clinical outcome of intraarticular injections? *Journal of Rheumatology, 36*(9), 1892–1902.

Simoni P, Grumolato M, Malaise O, et al (2017) Are blind injections of gleno-humeral joint (GHJ) really less accurate imaging-guided injections? A narrative systematic review considering multiple anatomical approaches. *Radiol Med, 122*(9), 656–675.

Strobel, K., Hodler, J., Meyer, D., et al. (2005). Fatty atrophy of supraspinatus and infraspinatus muscles: Accuracy of US. *Radiology, 237*(2), 584–589.

Tagliafico, A., Bignotti, B., Rossi, F., Rubino, M., Civani, A., & Martinoli (2019). Clinical contribution of wrist and hand sonography: Pilot study. *Journal of Ultrasound in Medicine, 38*(1), 141–148.

ter Haar, G. (2012). Guidelines and recommendations for the safe use of diagnostic ultrasound: The user's responsibilities. In G. ter Haar (Ed.), *The safe use of ultrasound in medical diagnosis* (3rd ed.). London: The British Institute of Radiology.

Thoomes-de Graaf, M., Scholten-Peeters, G., Duijn, E., et al. (2014). Inter-professional agreement of ultrasound-based diagnoses in patients with shoulder pain between physical therapists and radiologists in The Netherlands. *Manual Therapy, 19*(5), 478–483.

Touw, H. R., Parlevliet, K. L., Beerepoot, M., et al. (2018). Lung ultrasound compared with chest X-ray in diagnosing postoperative pulmonary complications following cardiothoracic surgery: A prospective observational study. *Anaesthesia, 73*(8), 946–954.

Turk, F., Kurt, A., & Saglam, S. (2010). Evaluation by ultrasound of traumatic rib fractures missed by radiography. *Emergency Radiology, 17*(6), 473–477.

van Delft, K., Thakar, R., & Sultan, A. H. (2015). Pelvic floor muscle contractility: Digital assessment vs transperineal ultrasound. *Ultrasound in Obstetrics and Gynecology, 45*(2), 217–222.

Volpicelli, G., Elbarbary, M., Blaivas, M., et al. (2012). International Liaison Committee on Lung ultrasound (ILC-LUS) for International Consensus Conference on Lung ultrasound (ICC-LUS) International evidence-based recommendations for point-of-care lung ultrasound. *Intensive Care Medicine, 38*(4), 577–591.

Warden, S., Kiss, Z., Malara, F., Ooi, A., Cook, J., & Crossley, K. (2007). Comparative accuracy of magnetic resonance imaging and ultrasonography in confirming clinically diagnosed patellar tendinopathy. *The American Journal of Sports Medicine, 35*(3), 427–436.

Washburn, N., Onishi, K., & Wang, J. H. -C. (2018). Ultrasound elastography and ultrasound tissue characterisation for tendon evaluation. *Journal of Orthopaedic Translation, 15,* 9–20.

Waterbrook, A., Adhikari, S., Stolz, U., & Adrion, C. (2013). The accuracy of point-of-care ultrasound to diagnose long bone fractures in the ED. *American Journal of Emergency Medicine, 31,* 1352–1356.

Whittaker, J., & Stokes, M. (2011). Ultrasound imaging and muscle function. *The Journal of Orthopaedic and Sports Physical Therapy, 41*(8), 572–580.

Winkler, M. H., Touw, H. R., van de Ven, P. M., Twisk, J., & Tuinman, P. (2018). Diagnostic accuracy of chest radiograph, and when concomitantly studied lung ultrasound, in critically ill patients with respiratory symptoms: A systematic review and meta-analysis. *Critical Care Medicine, 46*(7), e707–e714.

Wu, T., Dong, Y., Song, H., Fu, Y., & Li, J. (2016). Ultrasound-guided versus landmark in knee arthrocentesis: A systematic review. *Seminars in Arthritis and Rheumatism, 45*(5), 627–632.

Xu, Z., Duan, X., Yu, X., Wang, H., Dong, X., & Xiang, Z. (2015). The accuracy of ultrasonography and magnetic resonance imaging for the diagnosis of Morton's neuroma: A systematic review. *Clinical Radiology, 70*(4), 351–358.

Yamakado, K. (2002). The targeting accuracy of subacromial injection to the shoulder: An arthrographic evaluation. *Arthroscopy, 18*(8), 887–891.

Youk, J., Gweon, H., & Son, E. (2017). Shear-wave elastography in breast ultrasonography: the state of the art: the state of the art. *Ultrasonography, 36*(4), 300–309.

Zamorani, M. P., & Valle, M. (2007). Bone and joint. In S. Bianchi & C. Martinoli (Eds.), *Ultrasound of the musculoskeletal system.* Berlin/Heidelberg, Springer-Verlag.